A GUIDED APPROACH TO

INTERMEDIATE
and ADVANCED
CODING

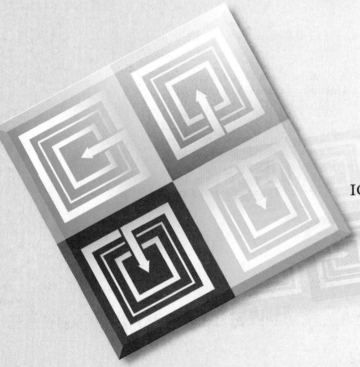

Jennifer Lamé, MPH, RHIT

ICD-10-CM/PCS AHIMA Approved Trainer
Medical Coding Program Coordinator
Southwest Wisconsin Technical College

Glenna Young, RHIA, CCS

Program Director/ Master Instructor
Health Information Technology Program
Health Occupations Department
Idaho State University

PEARSON

Boston   Columbus   Indianapolis   New York   San Francisco   Upper Saddle River   Amsterdam
Cape Town   Dubai   London   Madrid   Milan   Munich   Paris   Montréal   Toronto   Delhi
Mexico City   São Paulo   Sydney   Hong Kong   Seoul   Singapore   Taipei   Tokyo

Publisher: Julie Levin Alexander
Publisher's Assistant: Regina Bruno
Editor-in-Chief: Marlene McHugh Pratt
Executive Editor: Joan Gill
Development Editor: Alexis Breen Ferraro, iD8-TripleSSS Media Development, LLC
Associate Editor: Bronwen Glowacki
Editorial Assistant: Stephanie Kiel
Director of Marketing: David Gesell
Marketing Manager: Katrin Beacom
Senior Marketing Coordinator: Alicia Wozniak
Marketing Specialist: Michael Sirinides
Marketing Assistant: Crystal Gonzalez
Managing Production Editor: Patrick Walsh
Production Liaison: Julie Boddorf
Production Editor: Peggy Kellar/Aptara®, Inc.
Senior Media Editor: Matt Norris
Media Project Manager: Lorena Cerisano
Manufacturing Manager: Lisa McDowell
Creative Director: Andrea Nix
Art Director: Christopher Weigand
Cover and Interior Designer: Christine Cantera
Cover Image: Shutterstock/K. Oksana
Chapter Opening Design Image: pizia09/Shutterstock.com
Interior Design Image: Cihan Demirok, CIDEPIX/Shutterstock.com
Composition: Aptara®, Inc.
Printing and Binding: R.R. Donnelley/Willard
Cover Printer: Lehigh-Phoenix Color/Hagerstown
Text Font: 10/12, Plantin Std

Credits and acknowledgments for material borrowed from other sources and reproduced, with permission, in this textbook appear on the appropriate page within the text.

Every effort has been made to provide accurate and current Internet information in this book. However, the Internet and information posted on it are constantly changing, so it is inevitable that some of the Internet addresses listed in this textbook will change.

Library of Congress Cataloging-in-Publication Data

Lamé, Jennifer.
A Guided Approach to Intermediate and Advanced Coding / Jennifer Lamé, Glenna Young. — 1st ed.
    p. ; cm.
Includes bibliographical references and index.
ISBN-13: 978-0-13-292071-1
ISBN-10: 0-13-292071-9
I. Young, Glenna. II. Title.
[DNLM: 1. Clinical Coding—Problems and Exercises. W 18.2]
LC Classification not assigned
610.69076—dc23

                            2012042261

10 9 8 7 6 5 4 3

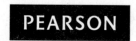

ISBN 10:   0-13-292071-9
ISBN 13: 978-0-13-292071-1

DEDICATION

This book has been a dream of mine for more than a decade and I want to thank everyone who has helped me work toward accomplishing my dream. I have a wonderful husband who has been instrumental in supporting me in my decision to write the book as well as through the countless hours of writing it. My three children have been very selfless during this time and allowed me the extra time needed to work on this text. My friends and family have been very supportive, and I could not have reached this dream without their encouragement and support.
—*Jennifer Lamé*

I would like to thank my husband and three sons for their love and support.
—*Glenna Young*

Brief Contents

Contents

Section III Advanced Coding 271

A Guided Approach to Intermediate and Advanced Coding is a hands-on coding textbook that is designed for students in intermediate or advanced coding classes who have already had a basic ICD-9 and/or ICD-10 and CPT® coding class. This text is appropriate for students enrolled in coding programs or health information management programs at career colleges, community colleges, and universities.

The United States is currently experiencing a shortage of professional medical coders, and many new graduates of coding or health information management programs struggle to find a coding job as employers seek coders with experience. This text was written to bridge the gap between beginning and intermediate/advanced level coding to help recent graduates gain employment.

THE DEVELOPMENT OF THIS TEXT

The authors of this text are both long-term educators who have struggled to find an advanced-level coding text that meets the needs of their students. None of the texts currently available provides the steps students need to get from a basic level of coding to an intermediate and advanced level, nor do these texts guide students through how to decipher medical documentation.

Both authors teach advanced medical coding courses and spend the majority of their time explaining the key elements presented in this book: how to decipher the medical documentation, what to code and what not to code from this documentation, and how to apply the coding guidelines to the medical documentation. This unique text provides examples of the various types of medical documentation students will encounter on the job, as well as what a coder needs to do with each type of medical documentation. Students are guided through the process of breaking down what is in the medical documentation and shown how to apply the skills learned in basic coding classes to the documentation they will see as practicing coders.

ORGANIZATION OF THE TEXT

This text is divided into three sections. Section I exposes the students to the role of the medical coder in healthcare, coding tools, and documentation.

Section II is a guided approach to intermediate coding. It presents a step-by-step approach to deciphering medical documentation and teaches students how to apply codes and coding guidelines to what they read in the documentation. Let's Practice exercises in this section present the reader with various medical documentation, helpful hints for deciphering the medical record, steps to follow, as well

as the final codes to assign. End-of-chapter review cases provide the student with ample opportunity to apply the intermediate coding skills they've learned on their own.

Section III contains advanced coding cases that require the students to continue practicing what they learned in Section II. In this section, students are required to apply their knowledge and skills to code the cases on their own. Note that you may see the same case presented in different chapters; this was done to represent how each facility type, service, or provider would code that individual case, and to help students understand how each provider and facility specifically handles each case.

The chapters are broken down by patient type so that students learn how the patient types correlate with documentation seen and coded in a real-world scenario. This text gives hands-on, guided practice to coding real-world records from a variety of settings (physician's office, emergency department, same-day surgery, and inpatient), and illustrates how to break down the medical records into understandable data that can be coded.

FEATURES OF THIS TEXT

Consistent pedagogical elements appear throughout the text to facilitate instruction and learning:

- **Learning Objectives**—Each chapter begins with a list of the primary skills students should have acquired after completing the chapter.

- **Key Terms**—A list of the important terms students need to know, along with their definitions, appears at the beginning of Chapters 1 through 5. The terms appear in bold on first introduction in the text, and are defined in a comprehensive glossary.

- **Introduction**—Introductory sections introduce the reader to important concepts presented in each chapter.

- **Coding Tips**—Professional coding tips appear throughout the text and provide additional information the student might use in the classroom or on the job.

- **Figures**—Anatomical line art drawings and photos are presented to illustrate key concepts.

- **Let's Practice**—Guided coding exercises appear throughout Chapters 3, 4, and 5, and present helpful hints that refer the students to coding guidelines, UHDDS guidelines, and other important coding concepts; step-by-step directions for determining the correct codes; and final code assignment.

CPT is a registered trademark of the American Medical Association.

- **Chapter Summary**—Chapter summaries provide an overview of the key topic areas presented in each chapter.
- **Chapter Review**—Chapters 1 through 5 include Multiple Choice and True/False questions to assess student mastery of content.
- **Review Cases**—Chapters 3 through 5 include multiple end-of-chapter review cases for student practice of coding various types of medical documentation. For these cases, students are expected to apply their coding skills to decipher the medical documentation and assign the correct codes on their own.
- **Advanced Cases**—Chapters 6 through 8 provide case scenarios from a variety of coding settings and specialties and help students practice advanced level coding skills.

SUPPLEMENTAL PACKAGE/ANCILLARY MATERIALS

The following robust supplementary package is available to accompany this text:

- Instructor's Resource Manual with lesson plans
- PowerPoints
- MyTest (test bank)
- MyHealthProfessionsLab: Online Workbook

ABOUT THE AUTHORS

Jennifer Lamé, MPH, RHIT, is an AHIMA-approved ICD-10-CM/PCS Trainer with over 15 years of experience in health information management (HIM) and coding. She worked as a coder and coding consultant for many years before moving into the world of teaching. She has been teaching for over 10 years and has taught primarily in HIM and coding programs. Jennifer's understanding of coding and what coders need to know in order to have a successful career is what convinced her to co-author this book. She is a long-term member of both AHIMA and IdHIMA. She has served as a reviewer of many coding, medical terminology, and health reimbursement texts. Jennifer is also an author of various supplemental materials, including instructor resources, PowerPoint lecture slides, and test bank items for coding, health reimbursement, and medical terminology products.

Glenna Young, RHIA, CCS, has over 25 years of experience in HIM and coding. Glenna has held many management positions as well as coding positions in HIM, and has been teaching in the HIM field for over 17 years. Glenna has taught coding and advanced coding for most of those 17 years and has trained many coders who are professional coders today. Glenna is a long-term member of both AHIMA and IdHIMA and has served in many IdHIMA board positions, volunteering countless hours of time to the profession. Glenna was honored with the Idaho State University Outstanding Achievement Faculty Award in 2003, the IdHIMA Distinguished Member award in 2002, and the Bingham Memorial Hospital Manager of the Year award in 1994.

ACKNOWLEDGMENTS

The authors are forever grateful to the entire team at Pearson. Our editor, Joan Gill, was instrumental in helping us move in the direction needed to create our text and accompanying supplemental package. Our development editor, Alexis Breen Ferraro, dedicated countless hours to ensure that our vision was executed in an easy-to-follow and understandable format and kept us on track for deadlines and processes. Associate Editor Bronwen Glowacki was very helpful in ensuring that we stayed on track and that our product was in the correct form and detailed. The authors also wish to thank production project manager Peggy Kellar and her team, as well as copyeditor, Lorretta Palagi—without their hard work our vision would not have been accomplished.

REVIEWERS

The publisher and authors would like to thank the reviewers for their feedback and suggestions, which helped guide the development of this text:

Michelle Edwards, CPMB, CMRS
Lead MBC Instructor
University of Antelope Valley, CA

Melissa Hibbard, BS, CEHRS, CMRS, CPC, CPhT
Program Chair, Medical Business
Miami Jacobs Career College, OH

Kristen Knox, AS, CCS, CPC, MA
Allied Health Instructor
Techskills, FL

Sheila Malahowski, CCA, MBA
Associate Professor, Health Information
 Management Coordinator
Luzerne County Community College, PA

George Peters, MS, RHIA
HIT Program Coordinator
Lehigh Carbon Community College, PA

Trasey Pfluger, RMA, CMAA, CBCS, NCICS
Program Director, Health Information Technology
Fortis College–Winter Park Campus, FL

Linda Scarborough, RN, CPC, BSM, MSHA
Healthcare Management Program Director
Lanier Technical College, GA

Devonica Vaught, MSHI, RHIA
Health Information Management Program Director
Indian River State College, FL

Learning Objectives open each chapter and provide a list of the primary skills that students should have after completing the chapter.

Learning Objectives

After reading this chapter, you should be able to:

- Spell and define the key terms presented in this chapter.
- Distinguish between an inpatient and an outpatient in the hospital setting.
- Describe coding in the emergency department.
- Describe Medicare's Ambulatory Payment Classification (APC) system.
- List and apply the steps required to properly code emergency department cases.
- Describe coding for same-day surgeries and observations.
- List and apply the steps required to properly code same-day surgery and observation cases.

Key Terms are listed and defined at the beginning of Chapters 1 through 5, appear boldface on first introduction, and are defined in the comprehensive glossary.

Key Terms

Ambulatory Payment Classification (APC) system— the outpatient prospective payment system (OPPS) used by Medicare to reimburse hospitals for outpatient services and procedures

ancillary services—outpatient services in the hospital such as lab, x-ray, and therapy services

critical access hospital (CAH)—a hospital that provides 24-hour emergency services in a rural area and that is located

An **Introduction** in each chapter alerts the reader to important concepts presented in each chapter.

INTRODUCTION

In this chapter, we explore the world of coding for the outpatient hospital coder. Hospital outpatient coders are typically responsible for coding all outpatient accounts, which can include ancillary services, such as laboratory, radiology, and physical therapy; however, the majority of outpatient hospital coding typically involves coding emergency room (ER) accounts, same-day surgery (SDS) accounts, and observation (OBSV) accounts. In all outpatient accounts the ICD-9-CM official outpatient coding guidelines are followed. Outpatient coders report ICD-9-CM codes for diagnoses and CPT® codes for procedures; they do *not* use the ICD-9-CM, Volume 3, procedure codes in an outpatient setting. (*Note:* Outpatient coders will report ICD-10-CM codes when they replace the ICD-9-CM codes on October 1, 2014.)

Coding Tips appear throughout the text and provide additional information the student might use in the classroom or on the job.

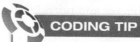

CODING TIP

Remember: Code only what was done and documented by the physician. Do not read the notes prepared by nurses, respiratory therapists, speech therapists, physical therapists, and so forth, unless you need more explanation than provided by the doctor. For example, if you are coding an encounter for a patient who is obese, you can use the dietary notes to determine the patient's body mass index; however, if the doctor did not document that the patient was obese and this is stated only in the dietary notes, it cannot be coded.

Anatomical line art and **photos** are presented to illustrate key concepts.

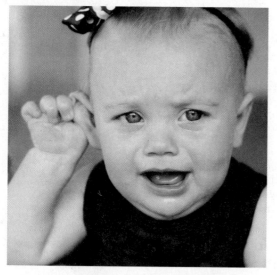

Figure 4-2 ■ This young child is pulling at the ear, a sign of otitis
Source: daynamore/Fotolia

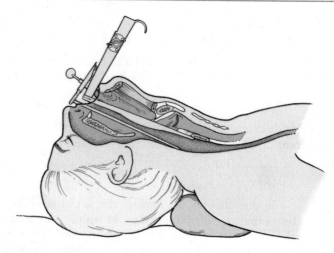

Figure 4-3 ■ Laryngoscopy.
Source: Jessica Wilson/Science Source/Photo Researchers

Let's Practice guided coding exercises appear throughout Chapters 3, 4, and 5, and present helpful hints that refer the students to coding guidelines, UHDDS guidelines, and other important coding concepts; step-by-step directions for determining the correct codes; and final code assignment with associated Outpatient Prospective Payment Classification (APC).

LET'S PRACTICE 4-3

Emergency Room

Identification: This is a 2-year-old African American male.

Chief Complaint: Ear pain

History of Present Illness: The patient is here because of left ear pain for part of the day preceded by several days of runny nose.

Allergies: None.

Current Medications: None.

Previous Illnesses: Denies any.

● **HELPFUL HINTS:** The ear pain is a sign/symptom of the otitis media and is not coded separately.

- "Codes for symptoms, signs, and ill-defined conditions from Chapter 16 are not to be used as principal diagnosis when a related definitive diagnosis has been established," per the ICD-9-CM *Official Guidelines for Coding and Reporting*, Section II, "Selection of Principal Diagnosis."

  For ICD-10 we need to note that it is the left ear.

Steps:

1. Look up otitis, media. It is not specified as another type, so select the code right by the subterm media.

Physical Examination:

HEENT: Very striking inflammation present to his left tympanic membrane. Normal exam of the right ear. Mild inflammation present to his throat. Exam of the heart and lungs is normal.

Impression:

1. Left otitis media.

Plan: Amoxicillin 500 mg tid for 10 days. Auralgan otic solution 3 drops to left ear q4h prn pain along with Tylenol and Motrin.

2. Procedure—locate E/M ER range, 99281–99285 and select the code where the key components match the documentation (■ Figure 4-2).

3. Verify codes in the Tabular Index.

4. *Optional:* using an encoder, generate APC assignment.

Codes:

ICD-9: 382.9

ICD-10: H66.92

CPT: 99282

APC: 613

Chapter summaries provide an overview of the key topic areas presented in each chapter.

SUMMARY

Hospital outpatient coding is comprised of ancillary services, emergency department services, same-day surgeries, and observations. A hospital outpatient coder is responsible for fully understanding and applying the ICD 10 CM official coding guidelines as well as understanding how to code using the CPT-4 coding manual. Coders who are coding for the emergency department, same-day surgery department, or observation encounters will assign diagnosis codes using ICD 10 CM, and procedures using the CPT-4 coding manual. Coders may also use an APC encoder to generate APC assignment. Not all of the ancillary services and supplies are reported by the hospital outpatient coder because most are captured in the chargemaster. The chargemaster typically captures the CPT codes in the 70000–99999 range. An exception is the E/M codes, which an ER hospital coder may need to code.

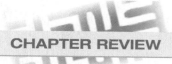

CHAPTER REVIEW

Chapter review questions in multiple-choice and true/false formats appear at the end of Chapters 1 through 5 to assess student mastery of content.

Multiple Choice

Choose the letter that best answers each question or completes each statement.

1. Which of the following is NOT a type of outpatient account?

   a. Emergency room

   b. Nursing home

   c. Observation

   d. Same-day surgery

2. Outpatient hospital claims are paid on which system?

   a. APCs

   b. DRGs

   c. RVU

   d. RBRVS

3. Hospital Facility E/M level codes are:

   a. Developed by each individual facility.

   b. CMS assigned to each facility based on APC assignment.

   c. Developed as part of the APC system.

   d. Payment based on CPT code assignment.

4. Outpatient coders utilize which procedure coding nomenclature?

   a. CPT

   b. HCPCS

   c. ICD 10 PCS

   d. Snomed

5. Demographic information for the patient is found in the health record on the:

   a. History and Physical

   b. Health Record Face Sheet

   c. Operative Report

   d. Nursing Daily Notes

True or False

Determine whether each question is true or false. In the space provided, write "T" for true or "F" for false.

_____ 1. The chargemaster houses all CPT codes in the range of 70000–99999.

_____ 2. Each facility may have its own E/M ER facility-level determination.

_____ 3. APCs were implemented in 1998.

_____ 4. Observation is a type of inpatient status.

_____ 5. The outpatient coding guidelines tell us to code a sign/symptom as well as the disease or condition with which it is associated.

_____ 6. Hard coding is coding that is completed by a hospital coder.

_____ 7. The most common types of outpatient coding for coders are ER and SDS encounters.

_____ 8. Hospital outpatient coders will need to learn ICD-10-PCS to report these codes for hospital outpatients.

_____ 9. Hospital outpatient coders follow the ICD 10 CM outpatient coding guidelines for diagnosis code assignment.

_____ 10. HCPCS codes are housed in the chargemaster.

Review Case 4-9

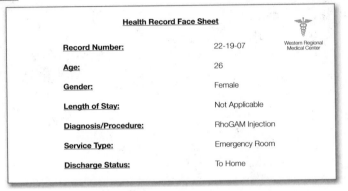

Health Record Face Sheet

Western Regional Medical Center

Record Number: 22-19-07

Age: 26

Gender: Female

Length of Stay: Not Applicable

Diagnosis/Procedure: RhoGAM Injection

Service Type: Emergency Room

Discharge Status: To Home

Multiple cases appear in the chapter review sections of Chapters 3, 4, and 5 and throughout Chapters 6, 7, and 8 that are designed to give students practice at coding various types of medical documentation. For these cases, students are expected to apply their coding skills to decipher the medical documentation and assign the correct codes on their own.

MEDICAL RECORDS

EMERGENCY TREATMENT RECORD

E.D. # 22-19-07

PATIENT NAME	PHYSICIAN
Madison Moorehead	Dr. Smith

CHIEF COMPLAINT
REQ SHOT

PHYSICIAN'S NOTES

DISABILITY
Estimated No.

DIAGNOSIS
Prenatal Rho

DISCHARGE C(
☑ Stable
☐ Admitted

P.A., F.P. RESIDE

E.D. PHYSICIAN

CONSENT FOR

CONSENT FO
and/or outpatien consent to the n and medical tre gional Medical (their professiona that no guarante tion or treatment

PATIENT OR RE

R   L

DATE: 6/14/xx

WITNESS SIGN,

WITNESS SIGN,

PHYSICIAN'S ORI

E.D. # 22-19-07

DATE	TIME	1	2	3	ORDERS
6/14/xx	10:30				Prenatal RhoGam Inject

PATIENT NAME:	Arrival Date:	Time:	Birth Date:	Record Number: 22-19-07
Moorehead, Madison, M.	6/14/xxxx	13:05	5/05/88	

Private	Means of Arrival:
	☒ Ambulatory ☐ Carry ☒ Self
☒ Pt./Family Request E.D. M.D.	☐ W/C ☐ Fam/Friend ☐ Police
	☐ Stretcher ☐ Helicopter ☐ Ambulance

CHIEF COMPLAINT:
For Rhoghen Inj   PREVIOUS ADM: ☐ YES ☒ NO

ALLERGIES: ☒ NKA ☐ CODIENE ☐ PCN   LAST TETANUS
☒ NA ☐ UNKNOWN

CURRENT MEDS. AND DOSAGE: ☐ NONE ☐ UNKNOWN
Vits   G.B. u/s done today

PAST MEDICAL HISTORY: 6 Mos. pregnant

INITIAL V.S.	WEIGHT	LMP
B.P. 110/70 T. 96° P. 76 R. 16		OD OS

IN ROOM ___6___ AT _1015_ A.M./P.M. VIA _Amb._
☐ HELD ☐ CHAIR ☐ FOEB ☐ STRETCHER ☐ SIDE RAILS UPS ☐ STANDING ☐ CALL LIGHT IN REACH

PHYSICIAN CALLED	TIME/WHERE	E = EXCHANGE/BEEPER O = OFFICE I = IN HOSPITAL H = HOME	TIME RESPONDED

TIME	ASSESSMENT AND HISTORY	TIME	MEDICATION & TREATMENTS
1000	26 y.o. ♀ presents to E.D.		Rhogam given IM
	for above Rhogam injection	11:00	lot # RHL 151
1030	Dr. contated. Lab test results from office faxed to ns.		
1130	D/C		

LAB WORK AND PROCEDURES (check work done)

		TIME	
☐ UA ☐ RANDOM ☐ C.C. ☐ CATH			MONITOR APPLIED
☐ CBC	☐ H&H _____		
☐ SMAC	☐ HOLD ADMIT		NASAL CANNULA MASK
☐ BUN	☐ CREATININE		
☐ ELECTROLYTES ☐ Na ☐ K		O₂ _____ LET TUBE	
☐ GLUCOSE	☐ AMYLASE		EKG
☐ PROTIME	☐ APTT		
☐ ABG _____		**TIME**	**X-RAYS ORDERED**
☐ CPK ☐ CARDIAC ISOENZYME		TO:	
☐ TYPE & SCREEN		RETURN	
☐ T & C _____ UNITS		TO:	
☐ BLOOD ALCOHOL ☐ LEGAL		RETURN	
☐ DRUG SCREEN URINE		TO:	
☐ THROAT CULTURE ☐ STREPSCREEN		RETURN	
☐ C&S - SOURCE _____		TO X-RAY	
☐ GM STAIN		☐ AMB ☐ W/C ☐ STRETCHER ☐ CARRY	
☐ GC - SOURCE _____		SEE	
☐ CHLAMYDIA		☐ EMS RUN SHEET	
☐ _____		☐ CODE BLUE DATA SHEET	
☐ _____		☐ I & O / NEURO	
☐ _____		☐ TRANSFER FORM	
☐ _____		☐ _____	
		☐ _____	

	ORDERED	LAB DRAWN	RETURNED

ICD-9-CM diagnosis code(s): _____

ICD-10-CM diagnosis code(s): _____

CPT code(s) with modifier, if applicable: _____

APC: _____

INTERMEDIATE and **ADVANCED** CODING

SECTION ONE

Medical Coding Overview

In this section, students are introduced to the role of the medical coder in healthcare and provided with an introduction to intermediate and advanced documentation and coding. The chapters in this section review the types of practice settings in which a professional medical coder might work, and provide a review of the various coding tools used in the profession. Students are also exposed to the different types of documentation seen in both physicians' offices and hospital settings, and the relationship between this documentation and coding is discussed.

Chapter 1: The Role of the Medical Coder in Healthcare

Chapter 2: Documentation and Coding Review

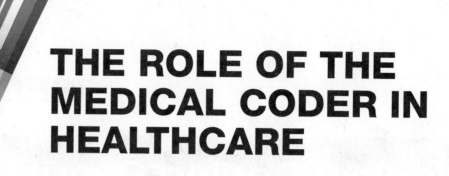

THE ROLE OF THE MEDICAL CODER IN HEALTHCARE

1

Learning Objectives

After reading this chapter, you should be able to:

- Spell and define the key terms presented in this chapter.
- Describe the role of the medical coder in healthcare.
- Discuss the healthcare record as a primary source document in the medical setting.
- Describe the classification systems in coding.
- Discuss ethical standards and the coding process.
- Describe the various settings in which the professional coder might be employed, and the code sets utilized in each setting.
- List and describe the coding tools used by professional medical coders.
- Describe the prospective payment system.
- Discuss the use of computer software in medical coding.
- List and describe the authoritative coding references used by professional medical coders.
- Discuss the importance of a corporate compliance plan.
- Understand medical coding as a profession, and list the various career pathways available to a professional coder.
- Discuss the importance of national coding certifications and membership in professional organizations.

Key Terms

AAPC—formerly the American Academy of Professional Coders; the national organization that provides education and professional certification to medical coders in the specialized areas of physician's office, hospital outpatient, interventional radiology, and cardiology

American Health Information Management Association (AHIMA)—national organization that focuses on the management of personal health information required in healthcare settings; offers resources for education, accreditation, and a variety of certification options

case-mix index—the average relative weight of all cases treated at a given healthcare facility, which reflects the intensity of the resources utilized or clinical severity of a specific group of patients in relation to other groups of patients in a classification system associated with the CMS prospective payment system(s)

Centers for Medicare and Medicaid Services (CMS)—the division of the Department of Health and Human Services that is responsible for developing healthcare policy in the United States and for administering the Medicare program and the federal portion of the Medicaid program

charge description master (CDM) or chargemaster—a comprehensive list of eligible charges for an individual provider or healthcare facility

CPT is a registered trademark of the American Medical Association.

classification system—a system that takes identified nomenclatures and arranges related entries. In coding, the nomenclature assigns code numbers to diagnoses and procedures.

clinical terminology—a set of standardized terminology used for a nomenclature

Commission on Accreditation for Health Informatics and Information Management Education (CAHIIM)—accrediting organization for educational programs in health informatics and information management

completeness—the degree to which a professional coder captures all of the diagnoses and procedures documented by the physician in the health record

compliance plan—provides the mechanism by which a facility or provider ensures that they are providing and billing for services according to the laws, regulations, and guidelines that govern billing and coding practices to prevent fraud and abuse.

decision support system—utilized for administrative and business activities in a healthcare organization or physician practice to produce information regarding the actual cost, charges, and reimbursement for hospital services provided to one or multiple patients with the same diagnosis(es) and procedure(s) performed

Department of Health and Human Services (DHHS)—cabinet-level federal agency that oversees all of the health and human services activities of the federal government and administers federal regulations

fiscal intermediary (FI)—third-party payer that has the Medicare contract for a specific state and administers the state's Medicare program, including processing the state's Medicare claims

hard coding—coding that is not done by a coder, but is instead done by a facility's chargemaster system

Health Insurance Portability and Accountability Act of 1996 (HIPAA)—federal legislation enacted to provide continuity of health coverage, control fraud and abuse in healthcare, reduce healthcare costs, and guarantee the security and privacy of health information

health record—a document created to record a patient's health and the services received during healthcare visits

Medicare Code Edits (MCE) software—software that finds and reports errors in the coding of claims data. The MCE editor will identify and indicate the nature of the error but will not correct the error

National Correct Coding Initiative (NCCI)—a series of code edits on Medicare Part B claims that identifies incorrect CPT-4® code combinations being reported; incorrect code combinations result in improper payment to a provider

nomenclature—a set of terms used in a particular discipline

patient record—the health record for a patient in a hospital setting

prospective payment system (PPS)—a reimbursement methodology that uses a predetermined payment amount rate based on the treatment for a specific illness; first utilized by Medicare but now used by many payers to reimburse for healthcare services

reliability—the degree to which the same codes are consistently assigned to the same health record by different coding professionals

resident record—the health record for a patient in a long-term care setting

resource-based relative value scale (RBRVS)—Medicare payment system that reimburses physicians treating Medicare patients. Work performed by the physician, practice expenses, overhead, equipment, supplies, and medical malpractice insurance are all taken into account. This system is utilized to ensure that fair and accurate reimbursement is provided to physicians in all services and specialties

timeliness—the amount of time it takes for the health record to be coded

validity—the degree to which the codes assigned accurately reflect the physician documentation for diagnoses and procedures in an episode of care

World Health Organization (WHO)—the United Nations' coordinating authority on international public health

INTRODUCTION

Coding professionals have a very important role in today's healthcare arena. Although coding professionals are not direct patient care providers, they do have a direct impact on patients' continuum of care, delivery and reporting of healthcare services, public health research, physician credentialing, data retrieval, electronic health records, and reimbursement. They also impact the codes applied to a facility's database, which is utilized by facility administrators for various activities, including physician recruitment, facilities management, purchasing of capital equipment, and other financial purposes.

This chapter presents the role of the medical coding professional in healthcare and discusses the scope of practice of the medical coder. The major standards for healthcare data and the organizations that develop and promulgate those standards are presented, and the coding process, practice, and ethics are discussed. Professional coding organizations and coding credentials are presented, and you will learn about the various healthcare settings and how coding application is specific and unique to each setting.

The tools utilized in professional coding are explored. Coding professionals utilize data classification systems, such as the International Classification of Diseases, Clinical Modification, Tenth Revision (ICD 10 CM) and Current Procedural Terminology (CPT), to classify, index, retain, and retrieve healthcare data.

The importance of complete, accurate, timely, and available clinical data is discussed, and a description of the major documentation content required for complete and accurate code assignment is given. Coding as a concept appears to be straightforward; however, the diversity of healthcare environments, regulatory agencies, technology, and reimbursement systems is expanding and changing the way in which professional coders ply the art of medical coding.

THE HEALTH RECORD AS A PRIMARY SOURCE DOCUMENT

The primary source document utilized in medical coding is the health record. The health record is the legal documentation of the *who, what, when, where, why*, and *how* of a patient healthcare encounter. The healthcare setting usually dictates the name of the healthcare record. When a person is admitted to an acute care hospital as an inpatient, the healthcare record is generally referred to as the patient record. A patient who resides in a long-term care facility will have a resident record. In a physician's office setting, this same healthcare record is typically referred to as a medical record, personal health record, or electronic patient record.

The patient chart is the common term for a paper-based health record. The entire healthcare system in the United States is currently mandated to exclusively utilize an electronic health record (EHR) starting in the year 2015. The EHR provides the platform for the electronic collection, storage, and analysis of private patient health information. The EHR is an interactive health record. Regardless of the healthcare setting and the name attached to the health record, the health record fills the primary role of principal repository or storage medium for patient health information. The primary purpose of patient health information is to document and support patient care services with the creation of a paper-based or electronic health record. The EHR and paper-based medical record store data and information for each individual patient encounter. The terms *data* and *information* historically may have been utilized to describe the same thing; however, these terms do not have the same definition. *Data* refers to the basic facts, processes, diagnoses/procedures, measurements, images, and symbols stored in the health record. Data is then analyzed and converted into various forms, which are utilized for a very specific purpose. Data in a usable or useful form is referred to as *information*. Data is considered to be raw facts, whereas information has meaning.

The professional coder utilizes coding classification systems to apply ICD 10 CM codes and CPT codes to physician documentation of an episode of care. Physician documentation must include applicable diagnoses and procedures The end product of coding healthcare data is a clinical database comprised of ICD 10 CM diagnosis and procedure codes, CPT procedure codes, and specific abstracted health information that can be utilized for patient continuum of care, statistical information, and medical research. A clinical database combined with a patient-specific financial database that produces a source of information is referred to as a decision support system. A decision support system in healthcare is utilized for administrative and business activities in a healthcare organization or physician practice, and is able to produce information regarding the actual cost, charges, and reimbursement for hospital services provided to one or multiple patients who have had the same diagnoses and procedures performed. A decision support system provides both clinical and financial information to a hospital or physician practice.

The coding of clinical data also provides an avenue for data and subsequently health information to be tabulated, indexed, stored, and retrieved, as required to support clinical activities such as patient care, clinical research, education, and disease prevention. Clinical data includes dates of service, physicians' name(s), consulting physicians' data, and other special data as dictated by a provider for specific patient types. Coded diagnoses and procedures describe exact health issues, treatments provided, or other services. The clinical database allows for any number of questions to be answered regarding hospital or physician services, patient outcomes, best practices, and quality of care provided. These are just a few examples of the types of information that can be derived from a coded clinical database.

Coded clinical data may also be utilized for internal administrative and external reporting purposes, such as reimbursement, gathering of vital statistics, performance improvement activities, patient safety, quality of care, medical research, and licensure or accreditation purposes.

CODING NOMENCLATURE, CLASSIFICATION SYSTEMS, AND CLINICAL VOCABULARIES

The term nomenclature is defined as a set of terms used in a particular discipline. In medical coding, the term refers to a system of names utilized in medicine for naming disease processes and procedures. Clinical terminology refers to a nomenclature system. A system that takes identified nomenclature or clinical terminology and groups related entities with procedure statistical information is referred to as a classification system. The International Classification of Diseases, Tenth Revision, Clinical Modification (ICD 10 CM) is one example of a coding classification system. Classification systems create the mechanism by which an organization is able to store and retrieve diagnoses and procedure information from databanks or the electronic health record to be utilized for clinical or administrative activities. Clinical users utilize clinical vocabularies and classifications to support medical activities such as patient care, public health, disease prevention, and clinical research. Administrative applications for clinical vocabularies and classification systems support activities such as facility or provider reimbursement, statistical reporting, licensure or accreditation, physician credentialing, or other administrative activities.

The Health Insurance Portability and Accountability Act of 1996 (HIPAA) requires the use of medical data code sets. The following code sets are required by HIPAA:

- ICD 10 CM Diseases
- ICD 10 PCS Procedures
- Current Procedural Terminology (CPT)
- Healthcare Care Common Procedure Coding System (HCPCS)
- National Drug Codes (NDC)
- Codes on Dental Procedures and Nomenclature (CDT)

Professional coders utilize coded healthcare data in a number of ways that are very specific to the coding process. The specific area of healthcare in which the professional coder is employed dictates the utilization of data. The following are two examples of further use of coded data:

- Case-mix index (CMI)—The CMI provides information regarding the types of clinically similar patients who ordinarily utilize similar resources of a facility or provider. A case-mix system will ultimately reveal the level of "severity of illness" of patient served by a facility.
- Prospective payment system (PPS)—The PPS is utilized in a variety of healthcare settings as a payment system for healthcare services provided. The payment system is based on a pre-determined rate for the treatment of specific illnesses. The PPS initiated by the federal government provides rules and

regulations for hospital inpatient (MS-DRG) and outpatient ambulatory patient classification (APC) services (MS-DRGs and APCs are discussed later in this chapter.) There are also prospective payment systems in place for inpatient rehabilitation, home health, and skilled nursing facilitates. The PPS systems were originally implemented as a payment mechanism for Medicare inpatients; however, PPS systems today are utilized for reimbursement by other third-party payers, for negotiating managed care contracts using data analysis and patient population, and for utilization management.

ETHICAL STANDARDS AND THE CODING PROCESS

Coding applications vary based on the type of medical care setting, such as a hospital, same-day surgery facility, physician practice, or skilled nursing facility. Other factors that affect the coding process may be the uses of coded information by the facility or provider, coding classification system(s), and technology utilized by the facility or provider. Reimbursement for the facility or provider is determined in large part due to coding. Common to all facility or provider coding are ethical standards of coding. One of the nation's leading professional organizations for health information management, the American Health Information Management Association (AHIMA), has created a widely adopted set of standards used by coders. AHIMA's *Standards of Ethical Coding* serve as a guide for coding professionals regarding the expectation of ethical, accurate, complete, and consistent coding practices. Common to all coding settings is the need for the coding process to adhere to quality elements of reliability, validity, completeness, and timeliness. Reliability is the degree to which the same codes are consistently assigned to the same health record by different coding professionals. Validity is the degree to which the codes assigned accurately reflect the physician documentation for diagnoses and procedures in an episode of care. Completeness is the degree to which a professional coder captures all of the diagnoses and procedures documented by the physician in the health record or episode of care. Timeliness is the amount of time it takes for the health record to be coded.

AHIMA *Standards of Ethical Coding*

AHIMA's *Standards of Ethical Coding* publication provides a set of principles and professional conduct for professional coders involved in diagnostic and or procedural coding or other data abstraction from the health record. The *Standards of Ethical Coding* are designed to assist coding professionals in decision-making processes and actions during the coding process (■ FIGURE 1-1). These ethics apply regardless of the reason for applying codes such as for reimbursement or research, and regardless of the healthcare setting. These standards apply to all coding professionals and those who manage the coding professionals regardless of AHIMA membership status. The *Standards of Ethical Coding* provide guidance to all healthcare coders in accurate, complete, and consistent coding practices. Ethical coding sets the stage for quality healthcare data.

WORK SETTINGS

The most common settings where medical coding is utilized include:

- Hospital acute care inpatient
- Ambulatory care
- Physicians' offices and clinics
- Home health care
- Long-term care
- Behavioral healthcare inpatient and outpatient
- Prisons
- Insurance companies

Hospital Acute Care Inpatient

Historically the hospital acute care inpatient setting is the most common place where professional coders are employed. In an acute care setting, a patient receives short-term treatment for severe injuries, acute episodes of illness, surgical intervention for disease processes or injuries, and other interventional treatments such as chemotherapy or radiation therapy. Acute care inpatient settings may include, but are not limited to, general medical and surgical, neonatal intensive care, coronary intensive care, general medical intensive care, and cancer treatment. The length of stay of patients in an acute inpatient setting is generally around 3 to 6 days depending on the diagnosis and procedures performed. A professional coder will be looking at documentation for acute issues and associated treatments and applying the appropriate code sets that best represent the treatment provided to the patient. A professional coder will utilize

---

Standards of Ethical Coding

Coding professionals should:

1. Apply accurate, complete, and consistent coding practices for the production of high-quality healthcare data.

2. Report all healthcare data elements (e.g. diagnosis and procedure codes, present on admission indicator, discharge status) required for external reporting purposes (e.g. reimbursement and other administrative uses, population health, quality and patient safety measurement, and research) completely and accurately, in accordance with regulatory and documentation standards and requirements and applicable official coding conventions, rules, and guidelines.

3. Assign and report only the codes and data that are clearly and consistently supported by health record documentation in accordance with applicable code set and abstraction conventions, rules, and guidelines.

4. Query provider (physician or other qualified healthcare practitioner) for clarification and additional documentation prior to code assignment when there is conflicting, incomplete, or ambiguous information in the health record regarding a significant reportable condition or procedure or other reportable data element dependent on health record documentation (e.g. present on admission indicator).

5. Refuse to change reported codes or the narratives of codes so that meanings are misrepresented.

6. Refuse to participate in or support coding or documentation practices intended to inappropriately increase payment, qualify for insurance policy coverage, or skew data by means that do not comply with federal and state statutes, regulations and official rules and guidelines.

7. Facilitate interdisciplinary collaboration in situations supporting proper coding practices.

8. Advance coding knowledge and practice through continuing education.

9. Refuse to participate in or conceal unethical coding or abstraction practices or procedures.

10. Protect the confidentiality of the health record at all times and refuse to access protected health information not required for coding-related activities (examples of coding-related activities include completion of code assignment, other health record data abstraction, coding audits, and educational purposes).

11. Demonstrate behavior that reflects integrity, shows a commitment to ethical and legal coding practices, and fosters trust in professional activities.

Figure 1-1 ■ AHIMA's *Standards of Ethical Coding.*

ICD-9-CM diagnosis and procedure code sets and the inpatient prospective payment system of Medicare Severity-Diagnosis Related Groups (MS-DRGs) in his or her daily work. The type of coding found in acute inpatient settings is generally at a higher level than in outpatient settings due to acuity of illness or injury and the higher level of risk associated with inpatient procedures. Acute care coders may work at the facility or may have the option to work from home performing remote coding for a facility.

Ambulatory Care

Ambulatory care consists of care given in a "day" setting. The type of service provided delineates the care setting and the coding applications utilized. Ambulatory surgery or same-day surgery serves a population of patients who have prescheduled their procedures. The patients are generally in the facility for 4 to 6 hours after the surgical procedure before being released to home. Ambulatory surgical coding generally consists of a limited diagnosis and a single or limited number of procedures performed during an episode of care. A professional coder in this setting utilizes the ICD-9-CM diagnosis code set and CPT code set for procedures along with the ambulatory payer classification prospective payment system of APCs.

Emergency Care

The emergency department is another ambulatory care setting where urgent or emergent care is provided to patients on a limited-stay basis. Patients seen in the emergency department will either be stabilized and admitted as inpatients to an acute care facility, or treated and sent home. A professional coder in this setting utilizes the ICD-9-CM diagnosis code set and the CPT code set for procedures. Emergency department visits are paid under the APC system if the patient was discharged home or transferred to another facility. If the patient was admitted from the ER to the facility for inpatient care, the payment will be based on the MS-DRG system.

Physicians' Offices and Clinics

Physicians' offices or clinics represent a type of outpatient care that provides patients with consultation with a physician regarding acute and chronic conditions and minor surgical procedures. Physicians' offices or clinics are identified by the type of specialty or services provided such as family medicine, gynecology and obstetrics, pediatric, internal medicine, dermatology, ophthalmology, podiatry, cardiology, gastroenterology, and infectious diseases. A professional coder utilizes the ICD-9-CM code set for diagnoses and the CPT code set for procedures. The resource-based relative value scale (RBRVS) is a payment system created by Medicare to ensure that each individual physician is provided proper reimbursement for services. RBRVS payment is based on a formula that takes into account the physician's geographic region, work done, supplies, equipment, overhead, and malpractice insurance.

Home Health Care

Home health is a type of patient care that is provided in the patient's home. Clinicians provide care for patients with long-term health issues with the goal of making it possible for the patient to remain in his or her own home rather than be treated in a residential or long-term type of institutional-based care. The professional coder will utilize the ICD-9-CM code set for diagnosis reporting and the CPT code set for procedures in the home health setting. Medicare reimburses home health agencies under the Home Health Prospective Payment System (HHPPS).

Long-Term Care

The long-term care (LTC) healthcare setting provides patients with care that may include medical and nonmedical issues. A patient may be admitted to a LTC facility due to chronic or debilitating medical problems that make it impossible for the patient to care for him- or herself in the traditional home setting. Patients admitted to a LTC facility may stay for varying lengths of time ranging from a couple of months to years. Long-term care settings provide different levels of care that vary between custodial services, which are considered to be nonskilled care that does not require a licensed nurse to provide the care, and skilled care, which does require a licensed nurse or other allied health professional such as a physical therapist to provide care. While some patients admitted to a LTC facility may only stay a short time (e.g., 1 month), the majority of patients are admitted with the intent of staying the remainder of their life. LTC patients are generally referred to as "residents" in the facility.

The professional medical coder utilizes the ICD-9-CM code set for diagnosis and procedure coding for LTC facilities. These facilities are reimbursed for services by third-party payers such as Medicare, Medicaid, private insurance, and private pay. Medicare reimbursement is based on a prospective payment system for long-term care services (LTCH PPS).

Behavioral Healthcare

Behavioral healthcare inpatient and outpatient settings both deal with the mental health issues of patients. The inpatient setting deals with acute episodes of mental illness, while the outpatient setting generally deals with the maintenance of controlled mental illness. A professional coder utilizes the ICD-9-CM code set for diagnosis in both the inpatient and outpatient settings. The ICD-9-CM procedure code set is utilized in the inpatient setting for reporting procedures, and the CPT code set is utilized to report procedures in the outpatient setting.

Prison Healthcare

The prison setting provides a unique situation in addressing healthcare for prison inmates. Healthcare in this type of setting is generally provided by healthcare providers who are employed by the prison or work on a contract basis. The prison is obligated by federal law to provide healthcare to the inmates. Healthcare funding is provided by and depends on the owner of the prison, which could be the county or state or it may be privately owned for profit. Healthcare services are not reimbursed or billed per individual. Emergency and acute healthcare are provided outside the prison setting.

Medical coding for reimbursement of healthcare services is generally not performed in the prison setting. If medical coding is performed in the prison setting, the resultant codes become part of a database that is utilized for administrative purposes only, and not for reimbursement of services provided to the patient.

Insurance Companies

Insurance companies, or third-party payers, provide reimbursement for healthcare services provided to "insured" patients. Reimbursement of services is based on the medical codes submitted for an encounter of care for an individual patient by a healthcare provider to a third-party payer. Medical coders are employed by the third-party payers to review claims. They conduct medical coding accuracy reviews and provide quality reviews on claims submitted by the healthcare provider. Professional medical coders employed in this setting utilize the ICD 10 CM/PCS diagnosis and procedure code sets and the CPT code set depending on the provider healthcare setting.

CODING TOOLS

Just as the professional medical coder can work in a variety of healthcare settings, there are also a variety of coding tools the coder can utilize. These tools include various types of technology, resources, software, and hardbound publications that assist in the coding process. We next explore the most common tools utilized by professional coders.

ICD 10 CM

The International Classification of Diseases, Tenth Edition, Clinical Modification (ICD 10 CM) is currently utilized to assign diagnosis codes in the majority of healthcare settings such as acute care, long-term care, rehabilitation, emergency department, ambulatory surgery and physician office. ICD 10 CM is updated annually with new and revised codes and or descriptions applied to discharges after October 1.

ICD 10 PCS

The International Classification of Diseases, Tenth Edition, Procedural Classification System (ICD 10 PCS) is currently utilized to assign procewdure codes in healthcare acute inpatient settings. ICD 10 PCS is updated annually with new and revised codes and or descriptions applied to discharges after October 1.

Healthcare Common Procedure Coding System (HCPCS)

The Healthcare Common Procedure Coding System (HCPCS) is divided into two principle subsystems, referred to as HCPCS Level I and II. HCPCS nomenclature are utilized primarily to report physician services and ambulatory care/surgery. We now look at the two principle HCPCS subsystem code sets and their application in medical coding.

Level I codes of the HCPCS nomenclature is comprised of Current Procedural Terminology (CPT) coding nomenclature. CPT is a numeric coding system which is copyrighted and maintained by the American Medical Association (AMA). CPT coding nomenclature consists of descriptive terms and codes which are used primarily to identify physician and other allied health professionals services and procedures utilized for claims processing and reporting in the ambulatory care or outpatient settings. The AMA updates HCPCS codes annually effective Oct 1.

Level II codes of the HCPCS nomenclature is a standardized coding system to identify and describe healthcare equipment and supplies that are not identified or represented in the Level I code set. Durable medical goods, pharmacy, and supplies are examples of services or supplies. The HCPCS nomenclatue is developed and maintained by the Centers nonphysician services such as durable medical goods, drugs, and supplies. These codes are developed and maintained by the Centers for Medicare and Medicare Services (CMS), and updated as needed. CMS issues updated information to providers quarterly in a publication titled *Quarterly Provider Update*. This publication provides medical coders with the most recent CMS coding guidelines.

Charge Description Master or Chargemaster

The charge description master (CDM) or chargemaster is a computer database utilized by most facilities to house all ancillary services and charges. A CDM lists all services eligible to be reported on a patient claim by department and by charge code. At the time of order entry, the order for the ancillary service triggers the associated HCPCS code to be posted to the patient's account with a charge; this is commonly called hard coding. It is also common to see HCPCS procedure codes aligned with a CDM item to include a text description of the procedure, revenue code, and charge. The CDM information is computerized and routed automatically to a patient bill for processing. Diagnosis codes are required to support the need for any procedure performed and charged via the CDM. Diagnosis codes are assigned by coders and matched up with the appropriate HCPCS code.

Prospective Payment MS-DRG and APC Groupers

Medicare Severity–Diagnosis Related Groups (MS-DRGs) and Ambulatory Payment Classifications (APC) represent the Medicare payment system that is based on a prospective or predetermined payment for services provided by a healthcare facility in either the acute inpatient setting (MS-DRG) or outpatient ambulatory surgical setting (APCs). Diagnosis and procedure codes assigned based on physician documentation of services provided are assigned to a specific MS-DRG or APC classification by CMS for Medicare claims. APCs and MS-DRGs are part of the PPS system, and a *grouper* is a type of computer software that assigns patients to a specific classification scheme based on the codes the coder assigns. The accuracy of diagnosis and procedure code assignment by the medical coder is imperative in both of these prospective payment systems. Incorrect assignment of codes may result in the incorrect MS-DRG or APC being assigned to a claim with a resultant increase in or loss of the reimbursement amount paid to the provider. The medical coder is charged with ensuring proper code assignment in both the inpatient and outpatient setting based on documentation in the health record. This is reflected in all healthcare claims submitted to CMS or other third-party payers to ensure that correct reimbursement is obtained. Proper code assignment results in proper MS-DRG or APC assignment and ultimately proper reimbursement for services provided and resources utilized by a provider in the care of a patient during a single encounter. Improper coding and MS-DRG or APC assignment that results in improper payments to a provider and that is willful, fraudulent, or considered to be abuse is punishable by law. The provider and/or individual medical coder may face imprisonment and/or fines based on the severity of the fraud or abuse circumstances.

Computer Software Utilized in Medical Coding

Historically, the printed coding manuals of ICD-9 and CPT were the only sources of code sets, and medical coders utilized these printed books to assign codes. The use of computer-based coding or coding software is now the norm for most medical coders in most healthcare settings. The following sections explore the major types of coding software applications currently being utilized in healthcare facilities.

Encoder Software

The primary application of encoder software is to assign diagnosis and procedure codes in the acute inpatient and outpatient healthcare settings utilizing ICD-9-CM and CPT code sets. The encoder is viewed as the most effective application to assign routine code assignments for diagnoses and procedures due to benefits such as increased productivity, accuracy of code selection, coder education during code selection, coding resources, and code edits. Coding resources and coding edits help to ensure code assignment compliance with current federal legislation and payment guidelines. An encoder will also provide appropriate MS-DRG and APC assignment for applicable Medicare or other third-party payer reimbursement. Encoder software providers include companies such as 3M and QuadraMed.

AUTHORITATIVE CODING REFERENCES

A variety of coding references come directly from government and authoritative entities and must be utilized correctly. Some of the agencies that help create the authoritative coding references are the Centers for Medicare and Medicaid Services (CMS), the American Hospital Association (AHA), and the American Medical Association (AMA).

ICD-9-CM Official Coding Guidelines

The ICD-9-CM *Official Guidelines for Coding and Reporting* have been approved and are maintained by these four organizations that make up what is referred to as the Cooperating Parties: AHA, AHIMA, CMS, and the National Center for Health Statistics (NCHS). Rules, edits, interpretations, clarifications, and authoritative coding references are also part of the official guidelines. This document is maintained and updated annually. This is the "how to" document for diagnosis and procedure coding under ICD-9-CM. Directions on how to access the official ICD-9-CM guidelines online are available in Appendix A. Please be sure to reference and utilize the guidelines when completing the coding exercises in this book.

Coding Clinic

Coding Clinic is the American Hospital Association's official, primary authoritative reference publication for official ICD-9-CM coding guidelines. The Coordination and Maintenance Committee delegates the responsibility for providing official advice to coding questions posed by the medical community to the AHA and this publication. *Coding Clinic* is published quarterly, is available in paper, and is also a part of a total reference package usually provided with encoding software. The AHA's central office website is www.ahacentraloffice.com/ahacentraloffice/shtml/Products.shtml.

CPT Assistant

The American Medical Association (AMA) is responsible for maintaining the CPT code set and thus publishes the authoritative monthly publication *CPT Assistant,* which communicates CPT guidelines, changes, and coding questions. This is another coding reference that is usually a part of the reference package offered by encoding providers. You must have a subscription to *CPT Assistant* to utilize this reference. To order, go to the AMA website at www.ama-assn.org/ama/pub/physician-resources/solutions-managing-your-practice/coding-billing-insurance/cpt.page.

National Correct Coding Initiative (NCCI) Edits

The National Correct Coding Initiative (NCCI) edits were developed by CMS to promote national correct coding methodologies and to control improper coding leading to inappropriate payment for Medicare Part B claims. The purpose of the NCCI edits is to prevent improper payment when incorrect code combinations are reported by providers for payment. NCCI edits are utilized with the APC prospective payment system and CPT codes. The website for accessing the NCCI edits is www.cms.gov/NationalCorrectCodInitEd.

HCPCS Coding Guidelines

The CMS website contains information concerning HCPCS coding guidelines and conventions. Specific payer manuals may also have guidelines and conventions regarding HCPCS coding. The website for CMS HCPCS is www.cms.gov/MedHCPCSGenInfo.

Centers for Medicare and Medicaid Services

The Centers for Medicare and Medicaid Services is the authority for the United States regarding rules and application of the ICD-9-CM coding system. The ICD-9-CM code set is the official method of communicating inpatient diagnostic and procedure data between providers and Medicare/Medicaid. CMS provides access to updates to the ICD-9-CM *Official Guidelines for Coding and Reporting*; listings of new/reviewed and deleted codes; and processes to request a new/revised code. The CMS is a federal

agency and as such, any coding changes follow the federal guidelines of being published in the *Federal Register* as drafts for public comment prior to issuing final changes.

Medicare Code Edits (MCE) Software

Medicare Code Edits (MCE) software is utilized to detect and flag potential errors in either codes assigned or the billing form prior to the claim being submitted to Medicare or other third-party payers for reimbursement on a claim. The MCE editor checks for:

- Invalid diagnosis or procedure code assignment
- External cause of morbidity codes wrongfully being utilized as principal diagnosis
- Duplication of principal diagnosis code with a duplicate submission of the same code as a secondary diagnosis
- Age conflicts as applied to newborn-, pediatric-, maternal-, and adult-specific codes
- Gender conflicts as applied to diagnosis and procedure codes that are only applicable to male or female patients
- Manifestation codes applied as principal diagnosis, nonspecific principal diagnosis code, questionable admission, unacceptable principal diagnosis, nonspecific OR procedures, noncovered procedures, open biopsy check, and bilateral procedure
- Invalid age, invalid gender, and invalid discharge status, limited coverage, and wrong procedure performed

The MCE edits are part of an electronic edit program utilized by coders and by billing personnel to ensure a claim does not contain any of the above types of problems prior to being submitted for payment to Medicare.

CORPORATE COMPLIANCE

The federal government through the Office of the Inspector General (OIG) mandates that all healthcare facilities and providers establish an official corporate compliance plan with regard to medical coding practices. A compliance plan provides the mechanism by which a facility or provider ensures that it is providing and billing for services according to the laws, regulations, and guidelines that govern billing and coding practices to prevent fraud and abuse. Healthcare providers who knowingly present a false claim for payment to the government may be prosecuted; therefore, the professional coder must understand the compliance process. The professional coder must follow the policies and procedures for compliance with specific attention to those dealing with coding to ensure the following:

- All rejected claims pertaining to diagnosis and procedure codes are reviewed.
- Proper and timely documentation of all physician and other professional services is obtained prior to coding and billing.

- A process is in place to identify coding errors.
- A process is in place for reporting potential and actual violations.

The compliance plan must also address the proper selection and sequencing of diagnoses and procedures, the correct application of the *Official Guidelines for Coding and Reporting* to the health record documentation, and a process for presubmission and postsubmission review.

MEDICAL CODING AS A PROFESSION

Health record content is comprised of physician documentation and other allied healthcare professionals' detailed descriptions of an episode of care for a patient; diagnoses; procedures; the patient's response to therapy or treatment; or a diagnostic workup of an unknown medical issue. The professional coder has a working knowledge of the health record content and understands where to look to find vital information for coding. A thorough knowledge of medical terminology, anatomy and physiology, pathobiology, and pharmacology and the ability to synthesize medical documentation are required of a professional coder.

Professional coding job descriptions are generally classified into major categories consisting of hospital inpatient coder, hospital outpatient coder, emergency department coder, physician's office coder, and ambulatory or same-day surgery coder.

Coding duties and processes vary between settings and providers; however, the main role of assigning codes to diagnoses and procedures as defined and documented by physicians for an encounter of care and in accordance with the *Official Guidelines for Coding and Reporting* does not change. A medical coder is bound to apply all diagnosis and procedure codes in an ethical manner regardless of healthcare setting. A medical coder is ethically bound to follow AHIMA's *Standards of Ethical Coding* in the constant pursuit of consistent and appropriate application of diagnosis and procedure codes. A medical coder has the duty to ensure that the assignment of diagnosis and procedure codes is not neglected and that codes are not erroneously assigned based on support documentation or lack of support documentation in the health record. A medical coder has the duty to ensure that coded data sets are valid, accurate, and complete in order to support clinical applications in the care of the patient and administrative applications for the facility or provider.

CAREER PATHWAYS

According to the *Occupational Outlook Handbook* and Bureau of Labor Statistics, the demand for health information management professionals will increase by 22% from 2012 to 2022. Strong oral and written communication skills aid the coder as a liaison between physicians, healthcare facilities, third-party payers, and other entities in the healthcare continuum. A medical coder has the opportunity to choose the type of healthcare setting and career pathway to follow.

Employment and career pathways exist in various diverse settings:

- Inpatient hospital acute care
- Emergency department
- Same-day surgery
- Acute inpatient rehabilitation
- Acute inpatient psychiatric
- Long-term care
- Physician's office private practice
- Physician's office group practice
- Free-standing (not owned by a hospital) urgent care.

Medical coders may increase their career options by furthering their education and becoming certified. It is vital that a medical coder hold the right certificates and complete formal education. Most employers prefer to hire formally educated and credentialed coders. There are many opportunities for advancing one's education and formal certification through online and traditional education methods. AHIMA and AAPC are two national organizations dedicated to ensuring coding accuracy in all healthcare settings by educating and certifying medical coders.

AHIMA and the Commission on Accreditation for Health Informatics and Information Management Education (CAHIIM) are independent accrediting organizations that establish and enforce accreditation standards for health information management (HIM) educational programs, including coding programs that may be available online or through traditional educational settings.

MEMBERSHIP AND CREDENTIALING IN PROFESSIONAL ORGANIZATIONS

There is great value in being a member of a professional organization or even multiple professional organizations (■ TABLE 1-1). A professional organization provides recognition through credentials that speak to the commitment, knowledge, and proven ability in the profession of medical coding.

AHIMA offers certification examinations for the Certified Coding Specialist (CCS) and Certified Coding Specialist–Physician Based (CCS-P). The CCS reflects a high level of coding ability in the acute care setting, and the CCS-P reflects a high level of coding ability in the outpatient setting. The Certified Coding Associate (CCA) offered by AHIMA demonstrates coding competency in any healthcare setting. CAHIIM

▇ **Table 1-1** PROFESSIONAL ORGANIZATIONS

National Organization	Total Membership	Student Membership Available?	Coding Credentials Offered	Other Credentials Offered	Contact Information
American Health Information Management Association (AHIMA)	71,000>	Yes	• Certified Coding Specialist (CCS) • Certified Coding Specialist–Physician Based (CCS-P) • Certified Coding Associate (CCA)	• Registered Health Information Administrator (RHIA) • Registered Health Information Technician (RHIT) • Certified in Healthcare Privacy and Security (CHPS) • Certified Health Data Analyst (CHDA) • Certified Documentation Improvement Practitioner (CDIP)	www.ahima.org
AAPC	140,000	Yes	• Certified Professional Coder (CPC) • Certified Professional Coder–Outpatient Hospital (CPC-H) • Certified Professional Coder–Payer (CPC-P) • Certified Interventional Radiology Cardiovascular Coder (CIRCC) • Specialty Coding Credentials	• Certified Professional Medical Auditor (CPMA) • Certified Professional Compliance Officer (CPCO) • Certified Physician Practice Manager (CPPM)	www.aapc.com
Board of Medical Specialty Coding (BMSC)	Unknown at time of publication	No	• Specialty Coding Professional (SCP) • Advanced Coding Specialist (ACS) • Specialty Coding Professional in Physician Specialties (varies) • Home Care Coding Specialist–Diagnosis (HCS-D) • Home Care Clinical Specialists–OASIS (HCS-O)	• Certified Compliance Professional–Physician (CCP-P)	www.medical specialty coding.com
Professional Association of Healthcare Coding Specialists (PAHCS)	Unknown at time of publication	No	• Specialty specific credentialing	None	www.pahcs.org/
National Cancer Registrars Association (NCRA)	5,000	No	Certified Tumor Registrar (CTR)	None	www.ncra-usa.org

and AHIMA also accredit associate degree Registered Health Information Technology programs. After successful graduation from an approved program, a person is eligible to sit for the certification examination for the Registered Health Information Technician (RHIT). RHIT graduates may be offered a variety of employment opportunities, one of which is medical coding.

AAPC offers certification in coding as reflected in the CPC (physician practice), CPC-H (outpatient hospital/facility), and CPC-P (payer) coding credentials.

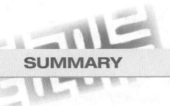

SUMMARY

The professional medical coder plays an important role in healthcare today and can work in a variety of healthcare settings. The medical coder is responsible for the accurate assignment of diagnosis and procedure codes based on physician documentation found in the health record, which provides support to clinical activities such as patient care, clinical research, education, licensing, accreditation, and medical staff credentialing.

Coders utilize ICD-9-CM and CPT-4 coding nomenclatures to assign numerical codes to diagnoses and procedures that were documented in the patient's health record. To help assign the correct codes, a variety of resources are available to coders, such as the ICD-9-CM *Official Guidelines for Coding and Reporting*, the AHA's *Coding Clinic*, and the AMA's *CPT Assistant*.

Employers recognize the value of formal education and formal certification in medical coding. It is vital that medical coders seek out formal education and certification in coding with colleges and or universities and national professional organizations. Successful completion of a coding certification exam provides the coder with formal recognition of his or her coding skills from nationally recognized professional organizations, such as AHIMA and AAPC.

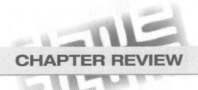

CHAPTER REVIEW

Multiple Choice

Choose the letter that best answers each question or completes each statement.

1. Which of the following is NOT an MCE edit?
   a. Incorrect fourth or fifth digit
   b. Invalid age
   c. Invalid gender
   d. All of the above are MCE edits.

2. NCCI edits were developed to help control
   a. improper coding.
   b. fraud and abuse.
   c. coding backlogs.
   d. improper data collection.

3. The Medicare Code Editor (MCE) is software that detects and flags
   a. clinically significant abnormal tests submitted to Medicare or other third-party payers for reimbursement on a claim.
   b. potential errors in either codes assigned or the billing form prior to the claim being submitted to Medicare or other third-party payer for reimbursement on a claim.
   c. any discrepancies in documentation in the electronic health record.
   d. value and volume of discharged, not final billed Medicare or third-party payer, encounters.

4. Which of the following is NOT a coding professional's role?

    a. Direct patient care

    b. Data retrieval

    c. Physician credentialing

    d. Public health research

5. NCCI edits identify

    a. incorrect code combinations being reported that result in improper payment to a provider.

    b. inappropriate charge description numbers being utilized for uniqueness and validity in provider payment.

    c. Incorrect ICD 10 CM/PCS diagnosis and procedure code assignment.

    d. nonparticipating providers who accept assignment for payment of services.

6. Medical coding for reimbursement of healthcare services is NOT generally performed in which setting?

    a. Behavioral health

    b. Home health

    c. Prison health

    d. Physicians' offices

7. Corporate Compliance Plans as mandated by the Office of Inspector General ensure all of the following except:

    a. Review of all rejected claims pertaining to diagnosis and procedure codes.

    b. Identify coding errors.

    c. Report potential and actual violations.

    d. Require all billing and coding personnel hold professional credentials.

8. Which of the following does coding data help with?

    a. Clinical research

    b. Disease prevention

    c. Education

    d. All of the above

9. A compliance plan is mandated by

    a. the American Hospital Association.

    b. the National Cancer Data Registrar Association.

    c. the Office of the Inspector General.

    d. the National Correct Coding Initiative.

10. Which of the following type of knowledge is NOT needed by a coder?

    a. Anatomy and physiology

    b. Medical terminology

    c. Pathobiology

    d. Psychology

True or False

Determine whether each question is true or false. In the space provided, write "T" for true or "F" for false.

_____ 1. ICD-10-PCS is used by every country that is part of the WHO.

_____ 2. Medicare Severity Diagnosis Related Groups (MS-DRGs) and Ambulatory Payment Classifications (APC) represent the Medicare payment system that is based on prospective payment.

_____ 3. A facility's coding policies must be aligned with the national AHIMA *Standards of Ethical Coding*.

_____ 4. Ambulatory care consists of care giving in a "day" setting (4–6 hours) with limited diagnosis and or procedure(s) performed.

_____ 5. By using an encoder, a coder will always generate the correct code assignment.

_____ 6. The NCCI edits determine and flag potential errors in age and gender conflicts in diagnosis and procedure code assignment.

_____ 7. You must have a subscription to the AMA *CPT Assistant* resource to access it.

_____ 8. CMS developed the NCCI.

_____ 9. An age conflict is not considered an MCE edit.

_____ 10. The severity of illness patient levels can be reflected in a facility's CMI.

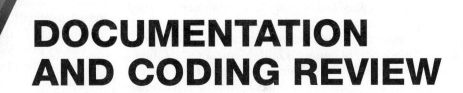

DOCUMENTATION AND CODING REVIEW

2

Learning Objectives

After reading this chapter, you should be able to:

- Spell and define the key terms presented in this chapter.
- Discuss the purpose of the healthcare record.
- Define medical necessity.
- List and describe the basic documentation found in health records and how it is used in coding.
- Describe the relationship between health record documentation and coding.

Key Terms

administrative documentation—information documented in the healthcare record regarding patient name, address, date of birth, age, next of kin, religion, physician, and insurance coverage information. Administrative information also describes why the patient is seeking services, consent for treatment, and use of private healthcare information.

chief complaint (CC)—patient-provided subjective description of the events or reason why the patient sought medical treatment

clinical documentation—information documented in the healthcare record that records the patient's current condition, course of treatment, and relevant current or past medical diagnoses or procedures along with anything "medical" such as laboratory, radiology, pathology, and cytology reports

comorbidity—condition that existed at admission and is thought to increase the length of stay by at least 1 day for approximately 75% of patients

complication—secondary condition that arises during hospitalization and is thought to increase the length of stay by at least 1 day in approximately 75% of patients

family medical history—subjective description of immediate family members' illnesses and/or diseases

medical necessity—formal process to ensure that an appropriate level of service is performed in an efficient and cost-effective manner in an appropriate setting based on the patient's physical needs and quality of life

objective documentation—the physician's assessment of the patient's current health status

past medical history—subjective description of a patient's childhood and adult illnesses and medical conditions

present illness—patient-stated subjective information regarding the current illness

principal diagnosis—condition established, after study, as the main reason for the patient's admission for inpatient treatment

principal procedure—procedure that was performed for the definitive treatment (rather than diagnosis) of the main condition or complication of the condition

progress note—a chronological record of the patient's condition during an episode of care and/or while receiving treatment from a provider

review of systems—subjective description of symptoms or illnesses pertaining to individual body systems.

social and personal history—subjective description of personal health habits and social status

standing orders—established orders that direct procedures to follow for a particular diagnosis or procedure

subjective information—information collected from the patient or other patient representative

utilization management—the process of ensuring medical necessity is met for patients receiving care in the appropriate healthcare setting

INTRODUCTION

The number one coding rule is *if it isn't documented, it didn't happen.* To code successfully, coders need to ensure that they fully understand healthcare record documentation and its components. Most introductory coding classes discuss documentation and its importance as the foundation of coding is laid. Medical coders, however, must not only know about the different types of documentation; they must also have a complete understanding of how that documentation impacts coding. To help provide this understanding, a review of documentation and its relationship to coding is provided in this chapter.

The healthcare record is the principal repository and legal business record for individual, private clinical documentation describing care and treatment for a specific patient provided by a healthcare provider or entity. This compilation of patient information and data serves the principal function of acting as a communication tool for healthcare providers in the continuum of care. Health record documentation is used to plan and manage the care provided to a patient. Evaluation of the appropriateness and timeliness of care provided and of medical necessity is another way in which clinical documentation supports and substantiates the utilization of healthcare resources.

The goal of healthcare providers is to provide the appropriate level of care in the appropriate healthcare setting according to medical necessity for each patient. This process is described as utilization management and focuses on how healthcare providers use their resources in the care of patients. Medical necessity is the expectation that a service provided will have a reasonably beneficial effect on a patient's quality of life and immediate physical needs based on the severity of patient illness or injury and the intensity of care/services needed to effectively treat the patient with the best outcome. Acute inpatient hospitalization utilizes preestablished screening criteria to ensure that the patient meets the level of acuity and intensity of services required in the acute inpatient setting. If the patient does not meet the medical necessity for inpatient care, care is provided at a lesser acuity level such as in an outpatient or physician's office setting.

The health record also substantiates reimbursement claims and provides legal protection for the patient, provider, facility, and/or allied health professionals. Finally, the health record is utilized as a data repository from which information is obtained for research, best practice, quality outcomes, education, performance improvement, administrative management, public health, and risk management. These and other functions may be classified as either a principal or secondary function of health records. A principal function is specific to the episode of care between the patient and provider. A secondary function is related to the environment where healthcare services are provided to the patient.

Regardless of where the patient receives medical care, the health record is where the source documentation relevant to the care and treatment provided to a single patient during an episode of care is stored. The medical coder's assignment of diagnostic and procedural codes is designed to communicate information about a patient's illness, services provided, treatment given, morbidity, mortality, and claim reimbursement, and coding must be performed ethically according to AHIMA's *Standards of Ethical Coding.*

Let us now look at health record documentation and medical coding through the eyes of a medical coder. This chapter reviews the most common health record documentation found in healthcare settings today, and provides examples of data collection tools along with associated documentation. You will be guided through the documentation from a "coding point of view" to ensure capture of all relevant medical diagnoses and/or procedures documented. This chapter offers a review of common questions for new coders, such as "Where do I start?" "What is this?" and "Where would I find that documented?" with regard to the health record for the most common healthcare settings.

BASIC HEALTH RECORD CONTENT

Documentation found in each basic health record, regardless of the setting in which services are provided, contains the same components and content. Basic health record content may be classified into either administrative or clinical information. Administrative documentation includes patient name, address, date of birth, age, next of kin, religion, physician, and insurance coverage information. Administrative information also describes why the patient is seeking services, consent for treatment, and use of private healthcare information. Clinical documentation records the patient's current condition, course of treatment, and relevant current or past medical diagnoses or procedures along with anything "medical" such as laboratory, radiology, pathology, and cytology reports.

Face Sheet

The face sheet, also referred to as the admission form or registration form, contains personal administrative documentation for a patient. ■ FIGURE 2-1 is an example of a face sheet you might encounter in the acute care setting; the form, however, will vary based on facility and patient type, and the face sheets you encounter within the cases in this text include basic demographic information only. Computer-based registration systems are used to generate an administrative data collection tool that generates an identification face sheet, which is generally seen at the front tab or page in a patient's health record. The healthcare face sheet contains demographic information, including basic factual information about the patient. *Demographics* is the study of statistical information surrounding human populations. The healthcare face sheet generally includes the following demographic information:

• Full name of patient

• Address of patient

Name:	Jane Doe	
Age:	76	
Gender:	Female	Western Regional Medical Center
Ethnicity:	American	
Record Number:	12-34-56	
Account Number:	123456789	
Insurance:	Medicare	
Address:	123 Adams Street	
City:	Hometown, WA Zip: 53333	
Phone Number:	(509)-555-5555	
Social Security Number:	123-12-1234	
Marital Status:	Married	
Next of Kin:	John Doe	
Relationship:	Spouse	
Account Number:	123456789-A	
Complaint:	Chest Pain	
Admit Date:	1/1/xx	
Discharge Date:	1/4/xx	
Admitting Physician:	Dr. Washington	

Figure 2-1 ■ Sample face sheet.

- Contact call number for patient
- Gender and age of patient
- Race or ethnic origin
- Marital status
- Next of kin contact information
- Social Security number

Demographic information collected in the healthcare setting is used to confirm the identity of the patient and create a statistical database from which statistical reporting and research activities can be conducted.

Financial data is also collected on the face sheet. Financial data provides information regarding the patient's employer, occupation, and insurance coverage information. Claim forms submitted by a provider to a third-party payer require financial data that is used to secure payment for substantiated healthcare encounters.

Clinical documentation in a basic form is also part of the healthcare face sheet. This clinical data includes the reason for the patient seeking care or a preliminary diagnosis as documented by the physician. This clinical documentation is vital and must be as accurate as possible because it starts the healthcare journey on which the care of the patient is based.

Obtaining the patient's consent to receive healthcare services from a provider is crucial because consent provides the legal authority for the patient to be touched by providers or allied healthcare professionals. Unlawful touching describes the legal term *battery*. Consent documents may cover other areas of healthcare to include notice of privacy practices, advance directives, patient rights information, and other administrative-type responsibilities such as damage to, or loss of, personal property.

CODING TIP

The face sheet and demographic information are considered to be "confirmatory" data that has a minimal impact on coding applications. A coder will confirm the patient's name, gender, age, and/or Social Security number to ensure accurate identification from the face sheet. The date of the episode of care confirms when services were provided. Basic clinical information or preliminary diagnosis documentation on the face sheet may be utilized as a "working diagnosis" or "admit diagnosis" but may never be utilized for the primary or principal diagnosis documentation. Some facilities have the coder write the codes assigned on the face sheet. This handwritten code information will be found only in the paper-based record and never in the electronic health record.

Medical History

The medical history is subjective information regarding an illness or medical issue from the patient's point of view (■ FIGURE 2-2). The patient is asked questions regarding current and previous medical issues and treatments or surgeries. Subjective medical history questions may include:

• Why are you seeking medical care today?

• Have you experienced these same signs and symptoms previously?

• What medications are you currently taking? (Prescription and over the counter)

• What were the circumstances or what were you doing when the problem was first experienced?

• Have you had this or similar problems previously?

• What are your current medications?

• Are you currently experiencing any other symptoms and/or signs?

Information provided by the patient to the healthcare provider should be documented in the patient's own words. The history provides background information regarding a medical condition prior to the patient seeking help from a physician. Traditional medical history elements include:

• **Chief complaint (CC)**—Patient-provided subjective description of the events or the reason why the patient sought medical treatment.

• **Present illness**—Patient-stated subjective information regarding when the present illness was first noted and what has been done in the past to help with signs and symptoms of the illness.

• **Past medical history**—Subjective description of a patient's childhood and adult illnesses and medical conditions; also includes information regarding current medications and allergies. Examples could include accidents, operations, and hospitalizations. Pregnancies, drug sensitivities, and allergies may all be documented in this section.

• **Social and personal history**—Subjective description of personal habits such as use of alcohol, tobacco, coffee, or other drugs; also occupation of patient, work status, living situation, daily routines, and marital status.

• **Family medical history**—Subjective description of illnesses and/or disease processes that have been experienced among immediate family members.

• **Review of systems**—Subjective description of symptoms or illnesses pertaining to individual body systems. The review of systems is a verbal question-and-answer exercise between the patient and provider.

Documentation found in the history is the source document for the "chief complaint" in the patient's owns words

as to the reason medical care is being sought. The history provides vital information regarding possible diagnoses or disease processes termed *comorbidities* that are already being treated or watched for in a patient. Comorbidities have the potential to exacerbate chronic or acute conditions and/or extend the time frame and resources needed to care for a patient. Comorbidity examples are diabetes mellitus, hypertension, congestive heart failure, or dependence on a ventilator due to quadriplegia.

The history also provides family history of hereditary types of disease processes or diagnoses. Family history diagnoses may include a history of coronary heart disease, colon cancer, or breast cancer. The personal medical history of a patient is also documented in the history. Personal history of cancer, exposure to potentially hazardous materials, or hip replacement are examples of personal history diagnoses. The social habits of a patient such as smoking, drinking, or drug abuse are also documented in the history. Information found in the history or history of present illness (HPI) is subjective information gathered from the patient or other patient representative.

CODING TIP

The HPI is a primary source document from which current signs, symptoms, previous medical history and correlating diagnoses, previous surgical history, allergies, personal history, family history, and diagnostic information is gathered. An HPI is taken from the patient on every encounter regardless of the setting (e.g., acute inpatient setting or physician's office). Be sure to start your "coder list" of potential diagnoses on a separate piece of paper as you read through this initial documentation.

Physical Examination

The physical examination is usually performed after the patient's medical history has been taken. The physical examination is objective documentation of a physician's assessment of a patient's current health status. The physical examination includes a main body system assessment with information gathered by observing the patient's physical condition and behavior and by palpating or touching the body of the patient. Palpating or tapping areas such as the chest and abdomen provides vital information to the physician regarding normal or abnormal sounds. The patient's breathing and heart sounds provide information about the cardiorespiratory system. Vital signs of the patient are also a part of the physical examination. Physical examination documentation includes:

• General condition: General overview of the patient's current presenting state of health to include visible signs of distress, weight, height, and skin color, and the patient's manner, communication style, and general orientation

HISTORY AND PHYSICAL EXAMINATION

JEFFREY, THOMAS
April 8, XXXX

HISTORY
This 38-year-old male was admitted through the emergency department with a history of less than 1 day of acute ureteral colic on the left side. Patient had an intravenous pyelogram in the emergency department earlier today, which shows partial to complete obstruction of the left ureter at the ureterovesical junction with a large stone, approximately 8 x 5 mm, lodged at the ureterovesical junction. Patient has no other calcifications visible. Patient denies any previous history of urinary tract stones or other genitourinary problems except for prostatitis a couple of years ago. Patient has no other significant medical problems.

PAST MEDICAL HISTORY
Otherwise negative.

ALLERGIES
None.

REVIEW OF SYSTEMS:
HEENT on the system review is essentially unremarkable. He denies headache. He has a moderate hearing deficit.
Respiratory: No upper respiratory symptoms; no cough, congestion, or hemoptysis.
Cardiac: All symptoms are denied.
Gastrointestinal: There has been no history of hematemesis or melena. He denies significant fatty food intolerance.
Genitourinary: Ureteral colic as noted in the history.
Neuromuscular: Without complaint.
Musculoskeletal: Moderate arthritis.
Endocrine: No dysuria, polyuria, or polydipsia.
Hematologic: There is no history of anemia.
Integumentary: No significant skin problem.

MEDICATIONS
None. Follows usual diet.

FAMILY HISTORY
No familial history of kidney stones or other significant hereditary disease.

PHYSICAL EXAMINATION
GENERAL: Physical exam reveals a well-nourished, well-developed male in no acute distress.
HEENT: Eyes: Pupils equal, round, react to light. Ears, nose, and throat clear.
XECK: Neck supple. No jugular venous distention or bruit.
LUNGS: Lungs clear to percussion and auscultation.
HEART: Regular rhythm, no murmur.
ABDOMEN: Abdomen soft. Slight left costovertebral angle tenderness, slight left lower quadrant tenderness. No rebound.
GENITALIA: Genitalia within normal limits. Penis: Normal male.
EXTREMITIES: No cyanosis, clubbing, or edema.
NEUROLOGIC: Neurologically oriented x3 with no gross deficits.

IMPRESSION
Left lower ureteral stone with obstruction.

RECOMMENDATION
Hydration, analgesia, observation, and if stone does not pass within 72 hours or less, will probably recommend patient for ureteroscopy and stone basketing and, if needed, ultrasonic lithotripsy. If the stone cannot be mobilized downward, push-back and extracorporeal shock wave lithotripsy might be considered.

SONYA PITT, MD

SP: hpi
D: 4/8/XXXX
T: 4/8/XXXX

Figure 2-2 ■ Sample history form/format.

Source: Health Professions Institute, Medical Transcription: Fundamentals and Practice, 3rd Ed., © 2007. Reprinted and electronically reproduced by permission of Pearson Education, Inc., Upper Saddle River, New Jersey.

- Vital signs: Blood pressure, temperature, pulse and respiration rate
- Skin: Temperature, turgor, nails, vascularity, color, edema, and lesions, as examples
- Head: Scalp, hair, and face
- Eyes: Alignment of eyes, eyelids, cornea, and irises; reaction to light and accommodation of pupils; extraocular movements and potential ophthalmoscopic examination
- Nose and sinuses: Status of airway, sinus, septum, tenderness, discharge, bleeding and capacity to smell
- Mouth: Lips, teeth, gums, tongue, and breath
- Throat: Pharynx, palate, tonsils, and uvula
- Neck: Trachea, lymph nodes, and thyroid
- Thorax: Shape, symmetry, and respiration
- Breasts: Tenderness, discharge, or masses
- Lungs: Breath sounds, friction, spoken voice, and adventitious sounds
- Heart: Trill, rhythm, pulsation, sounds, friction, murmurs, location and quality of apical impulse, carotid artery pulse, and jugular venous pressure
- Abdomen: Bowel sounds, bruits, peristalsis, scars, contour, tenderness, spasm, masses, or hernia
- Genitourinary: Discharge, lesions, penis, epididymis, hydrocele, varicocele, and scars
- Vaginal: Skene's glands, Bartholin's glands, vagina, cervix, external genitalia, uterus, and adnexa
- Rectal: Hemorrhoids, sphincter tone, masses, fissure, fistula, prostate, seminal vesicles, and feces
- Musculoskeletal: Extremities, swelling, deformities, spine, redness, tenderness, and range of motion
- Lymphatic: Axillary, inguinal nodes, consistency, location, size, mobility, and tenderness
- Blood vessels: Color, vessel walls, veins, pulses, and temperature
- Neurological: Coordination, gait, sensory, vibratory, cranial nerves, reflexes, biceps, triceps, patellar, Achilles, abdominal, cremasteric, Romberg and Babinski
- Diagnosis or diagnoses: Objective diagnosis or diagnoses as documented by the physician

Diagnostic and Therapeutic Orders

Physician orders are instructions to other healthcare professionals who perform diagnostic and therapeutic laboratory procedures, provide nursing care, provide physical therapy or respiratory therapy, administer medications, or perhaps provide nutritional services to the patient (■ Figure 2-3). Physician orders are found in all healthcare settings such as acute inpatient, physician's office, same-day surgery, long-term care, and home health. A physician order is required for all inpatient- or outpatient-based ancillary services. Examples include an order for a blood draw to check Dilantin levels from the laboratory, an x-ray on the left arm to check for a fracture, or twice-daily orders for a physical therapy protocol 12 hours post acute myocardial infarction. Only licensed physicians or clinicians are allowed to issue orders with regard to patient care. Examples of physician orders may be for medications, diagnostic tests, therapies, or other healthcare needs such as medical devices. These examples are considered routine physician orders written at the time of the patient encounter or during an acute inpatient hospitalization.

Standing orders are another type of physician order found in both acute inpatient and all outpatient healthcare settings. A standing order is established proactively by an individual physician or by a hospital medical staff. A standing order applies to a specific diagnosis, procedure, or set of protocols. Standing orders are usually established for common or routine types of care such as "preoperative standing orders" or "routine labor and delivery orders." Another example may be a standing order for a patient with an acute myocardial infarction at the local hospital to start physical therapy treatment on day 2 by sitting up at the bedside and then walking the hall. This sets a known pattern of care and speaks to delivery of "best practice" in patient care if endorsed by hospital medical staff or individual physicians.

Two other types of special orders common in acute care hospitals are the do-not-resuscitate (DNR) and restraint and seclusion orders. DNR orders are issued when the patient has verbalized and discussed with his or her physician the wish that no resuscitation attempts be made when breathing stops. DNR orders may address specifically artificial breathing or cardiopulmonary resuscitation and extend to pain control and nutrition.

Restraint and seclusion orders are given to protect the patient from harming self or others. Restraint and seclusion orders are mainly seen in acute inpatient psychiatric set-

---

CODING TIP

The physical examination is objective physician documentation regarding diagnosis or multiple diagnoses, symptoms, and/or signs of potential diagnoses the physician is currently looking at in reference to the patient and the episode of care. This is the first "solid" place to find physician information regarding the diagnosis or diagnoses and/or treatment planned for the patient during this episode of care. Look for the wording *Admit Diagnosis(es)*, and document on your "working paper" of diagnoses and procedures found during your review of the physician documentation. *Do not assume that this is the "final" diagnosis(es) and never code **only** from the history and physical examination.*

ROUTINE OB
PHYSICIAN'S STANDING ORDERS

ADMISSION ORDERS:

1. EXAM AND ADVISE PHYSICIAN.
2. NO PREP.
3. FLEETS ENEMA, IF NEEDED.
4. CLEAR LIQUIDS *UNLESS* HISTORY OF RISK FACTORS ARE PRESENT.
5. *CBC*
6. DIPSTICK UA
7. MEDS:
   A. NUBAIN 5-10 MS IV Q 3-6 HOURS PRN PAIN
   B. HOLD ROUTINE MEDS WHEN PATIENT REACHES 5 CM
   C. START IV WITH LR 1000 *CC* TRA 125 CC/HR *(CALL PHYSICIAN FIRST)*
   D. EPIDURAL/ANESTHESIA PER PATIENT REQUEST *(CALL PHYSICIAN FIRST)*

POST PARTUM ORDERS:

1. VITAL SIGNS AND UTERINE STATUS UNTIL STABLE.

2. FOLLOWING DELIVERY OF PLACENTA, ADD 20 UNITS OF PITOCIN TO 1000 *CC* IU AND RUN AT RATE PER PHYSICIAN ORDER. IF PHYSICIAN ORDERS PITOCIN 20 IN 1000 *CC* AT DELIVERY OF FETAL SHOULDERS, ANTICIPATE THIS AND PROCEED PHYSICIAN ORDERS.

3. REGULAR DIET.

4. AMBULATE AFTER 4-6 HOURS OR PRN.

5. ICE PACKS TO PERINEUM PRN.

6. AMERICAIN SPRAY OR TUCKS AT BEDSIDE FOR PRN USE.

7. SHOWER OR SITZ BATH PRN.

8. HCT 24 HOURS POST PARTUM DURING NORMAL OB HOURS.

9. REPORT ANY CONTINUED HEAVY BLEEDING.

10. MEDS:
    A. TYLENOL #3 TABLETS, 1-2 PO Q 3-4 HOURS PRN PAIN.
    B. MOM 1 OUNCE PO Q D.
    C. AMBIEN 10 MG PO AT HS PRN SLEEP.
    D. IBUPROFEN 600 MG PO Q 6 HOURS WHILE AWAKE.

Figure 2-3 ■ Sample physician order form.

tings but may also be seen in acute care, intensive care, or general medical settings. Restraint and seclusion orders are highly regulated by Medicare, state laws, and accreditation standards to ensure patient well-being and safety during the use of such orders. Physical or pharmaceutical restraints effectively prevent the patient from movement or doing harm to self or others. Seclusion room orders attempt to provide a safe, controlled environment where no outside stimulus is able to affect the behavior or thought processes of a patient. A seclusion room is also a place where a patient is unable to do harm to self or others. A seclusion room is void of any furniture and is a locked room providing constant visual nursing and one-on-one nursing observation.

The last type of physician order is the discharge order. The discharge order is utilized in the acute inpatient, same-day surgery, or emergency setting where the patient has been admitted to receive care. The discharge order provides information regarding the current medical status of the patient, where the patient is being discharged to (home, another acute care, long-term care, etc.) and follow-up plans. The physician is the only person who is able to determine if the patient is ready for discharge or needs to be transferred for further care.

The discharge order is issued by the attending physician in an acute inpatient setting and must be in writing. It states the date, time, and circumstances of the patient discharge. If a patient decides to leave an acute inpatient setting without a physician discharge order, the patient is leaving against medical advice (AMA) and presents a medical and legal risk. The proper forms must be completed with or without the patient signature advising that the patient voluntarily left inpatient care against the advice of his or her physician.

The physician orders are utilized by the coder to track patient care, identify potential diagnoses, and correlate diagnostic and/or therapeutic procedures/therapies to patient response and physician action. New or updated orders for changes in treatment or therapy are based on physician documentation and patient response. Physician orders present and/or support new diagnoses or treatments utilized during an episode of care in treating a patient.

All information found in the physician orders can be utilized in the coding process. Correlation of the physician order, physician progress note, and results of diagnostic or therapeutic treatment ordered must be evident throughout the acute inpatient health record as well as in the physician's office setting or same-day surgery setting. A coder may see that an order for the addition of an antibiotic is given in the physician orders, which then prompts for the supporting diagnosis or reason why the antibiotic is being ordered. The physician order is a great check and balance to ensure that all diagnoses, procedures, or treatments have been captured by the physician in the discharge summary and by the coder to ensure proper code assignment.

Clinical Observation Documentation

The progress note or clinical observation documentation is a chronological record of the patient's condition during an episode of care and/or while receiving treatment from a provider. Progress notes documented in the acute inpatient setting are written by physicians and other allied healthcare providers such as nurses, dietitians, and physical or occupational therapists.

The terms *clinical observation* and *progress notes* are synonymous, with the only difference being the type of healthcare facility where these terms are utilized. Clinical observations are normally associated with physicians and medical practices. Clinical observations documented in the medical practice provide a running date by date or chronological summary of the patient's status and treatment at each encounter. The observation information should provide information regarding the treatment/further care, pharmacological treatment, and the results as observed by the physician.

The progress note is generally found in acute care inpatient care. Progress notes are the physician documentation of working diagnoses, treatment plans, patient response or lack of response to a treatment plan, and the physician-adjusted treatment plan. The findings of laboratory studies, radiological studies, and/or physician-ordered therapies must have a corresponding progress note to document positive or negative patient response.

The progress note also provides a unique communication tool among healthcare providers regarding their specialized observations of the patient. In the acute care setting, the progress note is also utilized to justify continued medical necessity and treatment in the acute inpatient setting for reimbursement from third-party payers. An acute care facility may also utilize progress notes to look at coordination of services provided to the patient along with the appropriateness of services provided from a facility utilization standpoint. In the acute care setting, progress notes may be separated by discipline (i.e., physician, nursing, physical therapy, social work, or any number of licensed allied healthcare providers) or all notes may be combined in chronological order.

Progress notes may include the following types of information:

- Current health status of patient on admission, discharge, and daily during an acute inpatient stay
- Physical examination findings, including vital signs, pain assessments, and/or wound care update
- Daily record of course of patient's health status, including response or lack of response to treatment
- Documentation of patient education or family/care provider education
- Consultation requests and brief summary of consultation results
- Laboratory, radiological, other diagnostic workup results and interpretations, and plans for follow-up
- Final progress note upon discharge or death

Information found in the progress note is confirmatory of the final diagnoses and procedures. A coder can track a patient's course of treatment during an acute care episode to ensure that all procedures and potential diagnoses have been accounted for in the discharge summary. The progress note can also provide confirmatory information regarding diagnoses that have been excluded during the episode of care. The clinical observation note found in a physician's office setting provides the same type of information to a coder but is exclusive to a single episode of care for a patient.

Consultation Reports

Consultations represent the advice of another physician or physicians regarding a patient's diagnosis or therapeutic options. A primary care physician will seek the advice of another physician or specialist when it is deemed clinically necessary. An official request and/or order for a consultation must be made. The consulting physician will examine the patient and document the examination in a progress note and/or a dictated consultation report. The consultation report (■ FIGURE 2-4) usually contains the following information:

- Name of the requesting physician and reason for the consultation
- Name, credentials, and signature of consulting physician to include date and time of consultation
- Consultant's impression regarding diagnosis and/or treatment options.

CODING TIP

The consultation report is utilized as a confirmatory report regarding diagnoses or treatments in which the primary physician has requested input and advice from another physician or specialist. All information regarding diagnoses documented in the consultation reports are to be confirmed and correlated within the discharge summary in the acute care setting by the primary care physician's documentation.

Therapeutic and Diagnostic Reports: Radiology and Laboratory

In the acute care setting or physician's office setting, a patient routinely may undergo a variety of diagnostic and/or therapeutic procedures. The reasons for these types of procedures vary, including being done as part of annual general patient management. Procedures include routine laboratory analyses of blood or body fluids and radiology or other imaging examinations. Procedures are performed to determine the nature and/or extent of the patient's disease process. Definitive treatment is also provided via therapeutic procedures such as radioactive or nuclear medicine. Radiological reports may provide the exact number of ribs fractured or the exact anatomical break in the tibia and fibula. These reports provide exact and precise documentation, which supports the physician documentation and treatment of the patient. Let's look at the most common types seen in healthcare settings.

Laboratory Reports

Laboratory reports include the routine examination of sample body fluids and substances such as blood, urine, spinal fluid, and sputum collected from patients. All laboratory tests must have a corresponding physician order. No laboratory test may be performed without an order. Most routine laboratory procedures are processed by electronic equipment and a computer system, which automatically generates a test results report. Electronic copies of the results are placed in the patient health record. The report provides information regarding the name of the test performed; results of the test; date and

time in and out of the laboratory; name of the laboratory where the test was processed; and identifying information of the laboratory technologist, physician, or scientist who performed the test. Laboratory tests are to be taken under consideration and in view of the physician's documentation regarding pertinent diagnosis information.

Example: Laboratory results indicate the patient has an elevation in liver enzymes. Based on the medications and known diagnosis of the patient, the elevated liver enzymes are considered "normal for circumstances" and not addressed by the physician. The coder would not assign a code for "elevated liver enzymes" based only on the laboratory result.

Culture and sensitivity results for a "streptococcus infection" found in a sputum culture would not be coded without the physician confirming that organism to be one of the patient's conditions or diagnoses. Corresponding and correlating information should be found in the physician orders and/or progress notes with regard to organisms and treatment.

Imaging Reports

Radiology scans and images of anatomical body areas and/organs are performed on an inpatient and outpatient basis. No imaging procedure can be performed without a physician order. The interpretations of scans and images are provided by physicians whose specialty is radiology. The written reports of the radiologist's definitive findings are found in the health record.

Example: Definitive information regarding exact anatomical position of the tibia/fibula fracture and/or number and placement of ribs fractured.

Some imaging is routine and carries little to no risk of complications or adverse effects. An example is a chest x-ray. Other imaging can be very invasive with a high risk of complications or adverse effects. Examples include nuclear medicine, real-time imaging, and/or surgically guided procedures.

Radiology reports can be referenced in coding; however, a coder cannot code a diagnosis reported on a radiology report without the physician confirming that diagnosis.

CODING TIP

Diagnostic and therapeutic reports are great supportive information. A coder will utilize information that is definitive such as fracture identification to add specificity to code application. All other information is taken under advisement and in context with physician documentation and interpretation of the importance of findings.

CONSULTATION REPORT

FLINT, SHIRLEY
#989898
December 15, XXXX
Attending: Barry Topham, MD

HISTORY
The patient was admitted with a chief complaint of shortness of breath and chest pain. She is an 84-year-old female with a history of hypertension and coronary artery disease, recently discharged post admission for congestive heart failure. Her admission then was remarkable for pulmonary edema, and she responded well to diuresis.

The patient has been doing well since discharge and was taking her discharge medications until this a.m., when she woke up with shortness of breath and deep sternal chest pain that radiated toward her left arm. Associated symptoms at this time included diaphoresis, nausea, mild headache, and shortness of breath. She denied palpitations, tachycardia, or emesis.

The pain persisted and she presented to the emergency department, where she was noted to have a blood pressure of 164/112. Previous to coming into the ED, she had taken sublingual nitroglycerin without response. On EKG monitor she was noted to have a rate of 85 and rare PVCs. She was given oxygen, 40 mg of IV Lasix, and 10 mg of sublingual nifedipine, wth resolution of her chest pain and improvement in breathing. She still has mild left shoulder discomfort but is otherwise comfortable.

PAST MEDICAL HISTORY
The past medical history is well documented in past admissions and is notable for:
1. Type 2 diabetes mellitus, treated with oral agents.
2. Coronary artery disease, status post subendocardial myocardial infarction 2 years ago.
3. Episodes of atrial fibrillation on multiple occasions in the past.
4. Hypertension.
5. Anemia, unknown type.

MEDICATIONS ON ADMISSION
Glipizide 5 mg b.i.d., Lasix 40 mg b.i.d., Nitrodisc 16 mg q.d., Capoten 12.5 mg b.i.d., Procardia 10 mg t.i.d., KC1 20 mEq b.i.d., Naprosyn 375 mg b.i.d.

PHYSICAL EXAMINATION
General: A pleasant, obese female who is comfortable.
Vital signs: Current blood pressure is 118/60, respiratory rate 22, temperature 97.5, and heart rate 88.
HEENT: Extraocular muscles intact. Pupils irregular with postsurgical changes right eye. Ears, nose, and throat clear.
Neck: Supple.
Chest: Bibasilar rales with nonlabored respirations.
Cardiovascular: Carotids with mild delay and sustained upstroke. Bilateral bruits or radiated murmurs also noted. Jugular venous pressure 7 cm. The point of maximal impulse (PMI) was not palpable. Regular rate with rare ectopic beats. SI, S2 normal. Positive S4. No S3. Grade 2/6 systolic murmur heard at the lower left sternal border. Distal pulses intact and fair.
Abdomen: Soft. Positive bowel sounds. She had a pulsatile midline mass consistent with a possible abdominal aortic aneurysm that did have an overlying bruit. She had no hepatosplenomegaly or other mass.
Extremities: Extremities revealed 1+ edema to midshin, but extremities were without clubbing, cyanosis, or edema.
Rectal: Deferred.
Pelvic: Deferred.
Neurologic: Neurological examination was nonfocal.

LABORATORY
Laboratory was remarkable for a potassium of 4.0, a BUN of 94, a creatinine of 3.2, glucose of 112, hemoglobin 10, hematocrit 32, and a white count of 8.4. Platelets were normal. EKG revealed sinus rhythm at 80 with an axis of +15 and normal intervals. Left ventricular hypertrophy was identified. She had ST-segment elevation in I, II, aVL, and V4 through V6, which is unchanged, and she has a Q in lead III.

IMPRESSION
1. Chest pain with shortness of breath. Rule out congestive heart failure.
2. Possible abdominal aortic aneurysm.
3. Anemia.
4. Renal insufficiency.

PLAN
Usual rule out myocardial infarction protocol with serial EKGs and CPKs. Continue supplemental oxygen at 2 L, and obtain arterial blood gases to document PO_2. Continue Lasix. Recommend abdominal ultrasound to document the size of the aneurysm. Suggest the usual iron studies and stool guaiac to follow anemia. The worsening of the renal function could be due to congestive heart failure, and this will be followed.

MARIANNE SMITH, MD

MS:hpi
d: 12/15/XXXX
t: 12/16/XXXX

Figure 2-4 ■ Sample consultation report.

Source: Health Professions Institute, Medical Transcription: Fundamentals and Practice, 3rd Ed., © 2007. Reprinted and electronically reproduced by permission of Pearson Education, Inc., Upper Saddle River, New Jersey.

Operative Report

Documentation regarding operative sessions or procedures is vital not only to a coder as a primary source document, but also as a substantive legal and financial document for a facility or individual surgeon. The operative report or procedure note is the documentation of an operative session or surgical procedure. It is dictated by the principal surgeon, who describes the surgical procedure(s) performed on a patient (■ FIGURE 2-5). The operative report includes:

- Preoperative and postoperative diagnoses
- Procedure(s) definition and description of procedure(s) performed
- Documentation of all normal and abnormal findings
- Descriptions of all specimens removed during the operative session
- Estimated blood loss
- Description of complications or unusual events that occurred during the course of the operative session

The operative report should be dictated as close to immediately after the operative session as possible. Postoperative progress notes and/or orders also are written as required by the surgeon. The progress note is a communication tool for providers until the dictated operative report has been word processed and placed in the health record. In the physician's office setting, a procedure note provides similar information describing a low-risk type of procedure performed in the office setting.

CODING TIP

The operative report or procedure note is a primary source document for a coder. All information required to accurately assign procedure codes is contained within the operative report. The pre- and postoperative diagnoses do not have to match. A coder should always defer to the postoperative diagnoses as the definitive information at the close of the procedure. Be sure to read through the entire operative report to ensure that all procedures, complications, and techniques have been covered and taken into consideration. If a specimen was removed and sent to pathology during the operative session, do not assign codes until the definitive information from the pathologist and the official pathology report have been reviewed.

Example: Mass was taken from the breast during the operative session and sent to pathology. Pathology returned as carcinoma or pathology returned as fibrous material of the breast tissue.

Pathology Report

The pathology report is the microscopic and macroscopic evaluation of a specimen or foreign body removed from a patient during a surgical procedure (■ FIGURE 2-6). This specialized report is prepared by a physician who specializes in analyzing specimens, autopsies, and other laboratory-type services. The pathology report is the companion to the operative report when applicable. Information contained in the pathology report includes:

- Description of the tissue or foreign body examined
- Date of examination
- Microscopic and macroscopic examination of the specimen or foreign body
- Diagnosis or diagnoses for multiple specimens

CODING TIP

The pathology report is a primary source document when coding. A coder should never assign a code until the pathology report has confirmed the exact diagnoses. For example, a surgeon may document appendicitis in the operative report, and the pathology report further substantiates that diagnosis with a report of acute appendicitis.

Discharge Summary

The discharge summary is the finalized accounting of a patient's course of treatment during an acute inpatient episode of care documented by a physician (■ FIGURE 2-7). In the physician's office setting, this information is also known as the discharge abstract or clinical résumé. Regardless of the setting, the information found in the discharge summary represents an overall view of the current episode of care. The discharge summary is the main source document for coding. The principal diagnosis, secondary diagnoses, principal procedure, secondary procedures as indicated, and disposition of the patient are documented and supported in the discharge summary. Information contained in the discharge summary for acute inpatient services includes:

- Principal and secondary diagnoses, including complications and comorbidities
  - The principal diagnosis is the condition established, after study, as the main reason for the patient's admission for inpatient treatment, as per UHDDS.
  - The complication is a condition that began after the patient was admitted for inpatient care.
  - Comorbidities are defined as preexisting conditions that affect the patient's care.

OPERATIVE REPORT

MENLOVE, LYNN
575662
Date of surgery: 9/15/XXXX

PREOPERATIVE DIAGNOSIS
Cholelithiasis; recurrent biliary colic; chronic cholecystitis.

POSTOPERATIVE DIAGNOSIS
Cholelithiasis; recurrent biliary colic; chronic cholecystitis.

PROCEDURE PERFORMED
Laparoscopic cholecystectomy.

ANESTHESIA
General endotracheal anesthesia.

INDICATIONS
Presented for evaluation of recurrent, intermittent biliary colic. She needed a laparoscopic cholecystectomy in treatment for her symptoms.

PROCEDURE
After satisfactory general anesthesia was accomplished, a nasogastric tube and Foley catheter were placed for decompression of the stomach and urinary bladder. The anterior abdominal wall was sterilely prepped and draped. A curvilinear infraumbilical incision was made and the fascia grasped with two Kocher clamps. Two #1 PDS sutures were placed to assist with retraction of the fascia, and the Hasson trocar was placed in an incision in the fascia. The placement of the Hasson was preceded by digital examination of the peritoneal cavity to ensure that there were no periumbilical adhesions to the anterior abdominal wall. Pneumo-peritoneum was established, and the camera was placed through the Hasson retractor for placement of the other trocars under direct visualization. A 10-mm epigastric port was placed, and two lateral 5-mm ports were placed in the subcostal plane. Grasp-ers were placed through the lateral ports and used to retract the fundus of the gallbladder over the edge of the liver and to retract the body to facilitate dissection of the hilar structures. Before this could be accomplished, some thin, filmy adhesions between the omentum and the gallbladder were taken down bluntly with the dissector. Then attention was directed to dissection of the hilar structures.

The cystic artery and cystic duct were isolated, doubly clipped proximally and doubly clipped distally, and then divided with the parrot scissors. Dissection was commenced with cautery, and the gallbladder was removed from the hilar structures to the fun-dus. The camera was moved to the epigastric port, and the gallbladder was removed through the Hasson umbilical port. The gallbladder was inspected and indeed found to have all the clips in the appropriate place. There was an approximately 2-cm stone in the gallbladder. The Hasson retractor was replaced in the umbilical port and the camera was replaced through this. Inspection of the right upper quadrant revealed the hilar clips to be in good position. The right upper quadrant was copiously irrigated with saline and aspirated. Of note, there was no spillage of stones during the case; however, one of the graspers had disrupted the gallbladder wall early in the case, and there was some minimal spillage of clear yellow bile. All of this was irrigated and aspirated at the conclusion of the case.

The lateral ports were removed and revealed no bleeding. The epigastric port was removed and also revealed no bleeding. The Hasson retractor was withdrawn and pneumoperitoneum evacuated. The PDS sutures at the umbilical fascia were approximated to close the fascial defect, and an additional #1 PDS suture was placed to completely close this fascial defect. All skin incisions were closed with a running subcuticular 4-0 Vicryl suture. Steri-Strips were applied. The patient tolerated the procedure well and was returned to the recovery room in stable condition.

TONI DALY, MD

TD:hpi
d: 9/15/XXXX
t: 9/16/XXXX

Figure 2-5 ■ Sample operative report.

Source: Health Professions Institute, Medical Transcription: Fundamentals and Practice, 3rd Ed., © 2007. Reprinted and electronically reproduced by permission of Pearson Education, Inc., Upper Saddle River, New Jersey.

PATHOLOGY REPORT

PATIENT: Gooles, Ronald

HOS. NO: 126985

DATE OF SURGERY: 6/15/XXXX

OPERATION: HEMORRHOIDECTOMY

AGE: 34

DATE: 6/15/xxxx

DOCTOR: Dr. Salem

GROSS: Submitted are multiple, polypoid-like structures which appear grossly to be comprised of anal mucosa and submucosa. Within the submucosa are numerous, dilated, and congested blood vessels. The specimen in its entirety measures to approximately 3.0 cm. Representative portions are submitted for examination.

MICRO: The specimen reveals fragments of anal mucosa and submucosa. Within the submucosa are numerous dilated and congested blood vessels.

FINDINGS: External hemorrhoids. *Int hemorrhoids*

Robert McDonald, M.D.

Physician's Signature

Figure 2-6 ■ Sample pathology report.

DISCHARGE SUMMARY

WERNIG, INGE
#987654321
Admitted: 6/1/XXXX
Discharged: 6/10/XXXX

ADMISSION DIAGNOSES
1. Left lower leg cellulitis.
2. Left lower leg ulceration.
3. Diabetes mellitus.
4. Possible psoriasis.

DISCHARGE DIAGNOSES
1. Left lower leg cellulitis.
2. Left lower leg ulceration.
3. Diabetes mellitus.
4. Lichen simplex chronicus.

BRIEF HISTORY
This is a 48-year-old white female with obesity and diabetes who has had a smoldering left lower extremity cellulitis for the past 2-3 months. It is possibly related to her pruritus and psoriasis. She has been treated in the past with Coumadin and IV antibiotics. On the day of admission she presented to my office with worsening of the cellulitis and a new 2-cm ulceration, and was admitted for IV antibiotics and further evaluation.

EXTREMITIES
Extremities revealed bilateral edema 1 to 2+ to the knees, with erythema and diffuse excoriations with erythema from the ankle to the midshin area on the left lower extremity. She had a 2 x 2 cm superficial ulcer on the lateral aspect of the ankle.

LABORATORY
Labs on admission revealed sodium was 138. Electrolytes were normal. BUN and creatinine were normal. The creatinine was 1.4, which is probably acceptable for this obese woman. PT was slightly elevated at 15.6, PTT was normal. A subsequent chemistry panel was essentially normal. CBC revealed a white blood cell count of 6,000, hemoglobin 12, hematocrit 35, with 345,000 platelets and a normal smear.

HOSPITAL COURSE
The patient was seen in consultation by the dermatologist, who confirmed my diagnosis of cellulitis. She was placed on IV Kefzol for 48 hours with marked improvement in her cellulitis. Her skin condition was consistent with lichen simplex chronicus, and she was begun on Topicort cream b.i.d. Her Coumadin was not continued, as she had no venogram or Doppler evidence of deep venous thrombosis in the past. As well, she seems to feel that the Coumadin made her rash worse.

DISCHARGE MEDICATIONS
Glyburide 2.5 mg daily, Reflex 500 mg p.o. q.i.d., Lasix 20 mg daily, Mellaril 50 mg nightly, Topicort cream to affected are b.i.d., and normal saline and dressing changes for wound care.

NATHAN E. DAY, MD

NED:hpi
d: 6/10/XXXX
t: 6/11/XXXX

Figure 2-7 ■ Sample discharge summary.

Source: Health Professions Institute, Medical Transcription: Fundamentals and Practice, 3rd Ed., © 2007. Reprinted and electronically reproduced by permission of Pearson Education, Inc., Upper Saddle River, New Jersey.

- Principal and secondary procedures, including diagnostic and therapeutic procedures
  - The **principal procedure** is the procedure that was performed for the definitive treatment (rather than diagnosis) of the main condition or complication of the condition.
- Date, time, condition and disposition upon discharge
- Follow-up instructions, as required

CODING TIP

The discharge summary is the main source document for the coder. Physician documentation denotes the principal diagnosis, secondary diagnoses, principal procedure, and any secondary procedures for the episode of care. A coder should be guided by the physician assignment and order of diagnoses and treatments. A coder will never assign codes only from the discharge summary for an acute inpatient episode of care, physician's office visit, same-day surgery encounter, or other healthcare settings where a discharge summary or clinical discharge abstract is documented. A coder must utilize the entire complement of documentation as dictated by the setting to ensure that all appropriate diagnoses, procedures, and/or treatment codes are assigned to an episode of care.

We have looked at the basic documentation found in all areas of healthcare with an emphasis on acute care inpatient situations. Let's now look at some other common healthcare settings along with specific documentation that may cross over from the acute care inpatient setting to include specific documentation pertinent to other healthcare settings. In the following sections we look at same-day surgery, emergency department, and physician's office documentation.

Same-Day Surgery

The documentation for same-day surgery (SDS) or outpatient surgery settings closely resembles that of the acute inpatient setting. The SDS record contains the following documentation:

- History and physical examination (This can be dictated or handwritten by the physician.)
- Operative report
- Pathology report
- Physician orders and progress notes
- Discharge progress note or summary

Physician's Office

The physician's office setting utilizes the basic components seen in the acute inpatient setting with additional ambulatory-specific documentation as per setting and as the physician's specialty dictates. The physician's office utilizes basic health record documents to bill for physician services provided in the acute inpatient or SDS settings and for follow-up patient care. Documents include:

- Discharge summary
- History and physical
- Consultation reports
- Progress notes and physician orders (■ FIGURE 2-8)
- Operative report and pathology report

Physician's office–specific documentation includes:

- Medical history and physical examination
  - Medical history presents the physician's or provider's documentation regarding patient health for a specific episode of care.

ORDERS AND PROGRESS NOTES

DATE	HOUR	
3/25/xx	5-	feels 100% better, Øfurther fevers, appetite back
10:30	0-	VSS & abet
		abd erythena, induration, tenderness
		Leg rash fading
		LAB CBC WBC 10K, Next 86
		ABD Cellulitis
		much improved, on IV Levoyuin & Rocephin and oral ceflacor, awaiting culture reports.

Figure 2-8 ■ Sample physician progress notes.

- Physical examination documentation presents the physician or provider's documentation regarding the physical examination for a specific episode of care and presenting problems or maintenance of medical issues.
- The office medical history and physical differ from the inpatient history and physical with regard to addressing very specific medical history and physical findings as related to the current outpatient episode of care and presenting problem of the patient.

Example: Today, the patient presents to the physician's office with complaints of fever and pain in the ear. The physician completes the history of current illness with information specific to the fever and ear pain. Physical examination focuses on HEENT, respiratory, and cardiovascular systems. Physician diagnoses otitis media and provides a prescription for antibiotics with follow-up if conditions worsen or in 2 weeks.

- Progress note
  - This is the chronological documentation of each patient encounter, including illness, diagnoses, and treatments or procedures performed in the physician's office.
  - Each physician encounter results in a progress note to document services provided.
  - Progress notes must be legible and uniform.
  - Progress notes may be in a structured or narrative format.
  - An example of a structured progress note is the SOAP format (■ FIGURE 2-9)
    - It provides a structure for the physician to follow and utilize when making decisions.
  - A SOAP progress note is comprised of four parts:
    - S = Subjective: Patient's reason for seeking care from the physician. This section usually contains signs, symptoms, duration, level of distress, and other comments from the patient.
    - O = Objective: Physician objective findings from physical examination, review of current

---

SOAP NOTE

SUMMERS, JENNIFER
#802741
October 1, XXXX

SUBJECTIVE
Patient is here for routine gynecologic examination. She is on Ortho-Novum and is having no difficulty with the pill. She forgets to take the pill occasionally.

OBJECTIVE
Breasts reveal no masses or tenderness. Abdomen negative. Pelvic exam was entirely negative. Pap smear taken.

ASSESSMENT
Normal gynecologic examination.

PLAN
Advised to use alternative forms of contraception when she misses a pill. Given a refill of Ortho-Novum 1/35. To return in 9 months.

HIYAS FONTE, MD

HF:hpi

Figure 2-9 ■ Sample structured progress note: SOAP format.

Source: Health Professions Institute, Medical Transcription: Fundamentals and Practice, 3rd Ed., © 2007. Reprinted and electronically reproduced by permission of Pearson Education, Inc., Upper Saddle River, New Jersey.

or previous laboratory results, pathology results, radiological examinations, etc.

- A = Assessment: This is the physician's diagnosis(es) and impression regarding current episode of care.
- P = Plan: This is the physician documentation regarding the plan for the patient to include scheduled surgery, therapy, therapeutic and diagnostic procedures, referrals, patient education, and physician follow-up.

- Physician orders
  - Physician orders document instructions to other allied health professionals providing diagnostic or therapeutic treatments to the patient on an outpatient basis.

Example: Physician order for antibiotic. Physician order to laboratory to draw blood for a CBC or electrocardiogram.

- Immunization record
  - Name of immunization, date of administration, manufacturer, and lot number
  - Dosage and route of administration
  - Consent form for vaccination along with authentication of person administering
- Patient instructions
  - Communicated both verbally and in writing
  - Mirror copy of patient instructions for follow-up care as documented in the specific encounter progress note by the physician. These instructions are provided to the patient with a signature of receipt and a copy filed in the patient's health record.
- Problem list
  - Summary of all medical diagnoses and issues that are being watched or managed long term by the physician. Also includes surgical history.
- Medication list
  - Listing of all medicines the patient is currently taking along with associated diagnosis(es)
    - Specific name of medication, dosage, amounts dispensed, and dispensing instructions
    - Prescription date with refill number and/or discontinue date
  - Helps to ensure identification of potential drug interactions, drug allergies, and/or sensitivities
- Patient history questionnaire
  - Patient-completed form that describes past and current medical issues and diagnoses, including current therapy or treatments

- Questions prompt patient to provide certain information regarding presence or absence of significant conditions that may represent potential medical issues
- Updated annually
- Telephone contact
  - Documentation of instructions, prescriptions, orders, advice, medication changes, or other vital healthcare follow-up that is communicated via telephone or other medium between physician and patient
  - Documentation includes date and time of call, patient's name and reason for call, date and time of response, and response provided
  - Authentication of allied health professional speaking with patient or provider

Emergency Department

The hospital-based emergency department setting provides emergent care to patients who have a potentially life-threatening condition or traumatic injury that needs immediate diagnostic or therapeutic services provided in order to save life or limb. The emergency department (ED) is considered to be an outpatient setting. There are times when a patient is treated and stabilized in the ED and then admitted to the hospital as an inpatient for further treatment and/or observation. The health record created and maintained for emergency services contains the same basic information as inpatient documentation (■ FIGURE 2-10). Documentation found in the emergency department revolves around a very specific injury or illness per presentation of the patient. Nonpertinent medical issues and/or diagnoses may be listed but not taken into the medical decision making or the treatment provided to the patient in the emergency department. Documentation includes:

- Patient name and/or identification with time and means of arrival
  - Means of arrival refers to how the patient arrived at the ED (e.g., ambulance, walking, private vehicle, or police vehicle)
  - If transported by another person or organization, the identification of that person or organization
  - Consent to treat (may be written, verbal, or expressed)
  - Chief complaint with history of present illness
  - Physical examination (pertinent) along with treatment/procedure or medical attention provided with results or response of patient
  - Diagnostic findings
  - Condition and disposition of patient upon discharge from emergency department

EMERGENCY DEPARTMENT NOTE

BOWMAN, CYNTHIA
#012465
Date of Visit: 4/13/XXXX
Attending: Lance Owens, MD

HISTORY
The patient is a 19-year-old white female who was brought in by her mother. She has a rather long and complicated medical history. Since 16 years of age, the patient has had chronic fatigue, extreme exercise intolerance, episodes of anorexia nervosa, and recurrent syncopal attacks. She is not able to walk up a flight of stairs or walk more than one block because of fatigue and dyspnea with exertion.

EXAMINATION
The patient was noted to have a sinus bradycardia with heart rates in the 40s at times. She had an echocardiogram which showed mitral valve prolapse. She had a treadmill exercise test, at which time she was able to go into stage 3 and achieved a maximum heart rate of 185 per minute. The test was remarkable for a rather flat blood pressure response with systolic blood pressure 114 at rest and into the exercise, with no appropriate increase during the exercise test. In addition, the patient developed a prolonged PR interval of 0.34, with some blocked atrial premature contractions (APCs) during the recovery phase of the exercise. She had evidence of both sinus node dysfunction and atrioventricular (AV) nodal disease.

IMPRESSION
1. Recurrent syncopal episode of unknown etiology. Patient does not have significant postural hypotension on examination. Patient has a history of sick sinus dysfunction. It is possible that the patient has a significant bradyarrhythmia precipitating syncopal episodes.
2. Possible sinus node dysfunction.

KATHERINE HORTON, MD

KH:hpi
d&t: 4/13/XXXX

Figure 2-10 ■ Sample emergency department documentation.
Source: Health Professions Institute, Medical Transcription: Fundamentals and Practice, 3rd Ed., © 2007. Reprinted and electronically reproduced by permission of Pearson Education, Inc., Upper Saddle River, New Jersey.

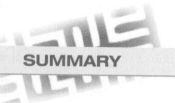

SUMMARY

This chapter focused on the various types of basic health record information found in medical practice settings. The healthcare record is the principal repository and legal record for clinical documentation relevant to care and treatment received by one specific patient during an episode of care. The principal function of the healthcare record is patient care delivery, management, and support, and it is also a communication tool among providers and patient. A secondary function of the healthcare record is billing and reimbursement, of which medical coding plays the integral part. The ability to locate, read, synthesize, and ethically assign medical codes to diagnoses and procedures found in a healthcare record is a critical function in healthcare today.

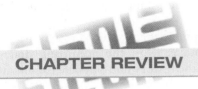

CHAPTER REVIEW

Multiple Choice

Choose the letter that best answers each question or completes each statement.

1. Which of the following is NOT a use of the health record?
   a. Data repository
   b. Legal protection
   c. Substantiates reimbursement
   d. All of the above are uses of the health record.

2. Which of the following is used for routine types of care?
   a. Diagnostic orders
   b. Progress notes
   c. Physician orders
   d. Standing orders

3. In a SOAP note, what does S stand for?
   a. Signs
   b. Subjective
   c. Suspend
   d. Symptoms

4. _____ do NOT carry out a physician order.
   a. Coders
   b. Dietitians
   c. Nurses
   d. Physical therapists

5. Which of the following reports consists of advice from another physician?
   a. Consultation
   b. Discharge summary
   c. Pathology
   d. Physician order

6. Which of the following is NOT subjective information?
   a. Patient's report of the problem's onset
   b. Patient's reason for seeking care
   c. Patient's current medications
   d. Patient's vital signs

7. Which of the following is NOT objective information?
   a. Patient's skin appearance
   b. Patient's blood pressure
   c. Patient's past medical history
   d. Patient's carotid artery pulse

8. Where would you find a liver enzyme result?
   a. Admitting diagnosis
   b. History and physical
   c. Laboratory report
   d. Nutritional consult

9. Which of the following is the main source document in coding?
   a. Consultation report
   b. Discharge summary
   c. History and physical
   d. Operative report

10. A preexisting condition that affects the patient's care is called a(n)
    a. adverse effect.
    b. comorbidity.
    c. complication.
    d. side effect.

True or False

Determine whether each question is true or false. In the space provided, write "T" for true or "F" for false.

_____ 1. An official request has to be made for a consultation.

_____ 2. A coder cannot code from information found in the progress notes.

_____ 3. A coder can use the admitting diagnosis found on a face sheet as the principal diagnosis.

_____ 4. The pathology report is a companion to the operative report when a specimen is removed.

_____ 5. A secondary diagnosis is a condition that began after the patient was admitted for inpatient care.

_____ 6. A coder must utilize a complete health record and not assign codes from only one facet of the record.

_____ 7. The review of systems is a verbal question-and-answer activity between the physician and patient.

_____ 8. Diabetes is an example of a comorbidity.

_____ 9. It is acceptable for a coder to assign the principal diagnosis from the admitting diagnosis found in the history and physical examination.

_____ 10. A progress note is generally found in the acute care inpatient record.

Intermediate Coding:
A Guided Approach

In this section, intermediate guided practice coding scenarios are presented for the physician office, outpatient hospital, and inpatient hospital settings. Each chapter in this section presents Let's Practice exercises, which guide students through the analysis of medical documentation and provide helpful hints, coding steps, and the final codes for each scenario. Each chapter ends with Review Cases, where students are expected to apply their knowledge to code various types of medical documentation on their own.

Chapter 3: Intermediate Physician Office Coding

Chapter 4: Intermediate Outpatient Hospital Coding

Chapter 5: Intermediate Inpatient Hospital Coding

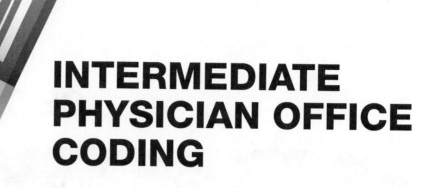

INTERMEDIATE PHYSICIAN OFFICE CODING

Learning Objectives

After reading this chapter, you should be able to:

- Spell and define the key terms presented in this chapter.
- Define the purpose of physician's office coding.
- Describe the different types and sources of physician documentation.
- Describe the guidelines used by the physician's office coder.
- Understand the difference between physician coding and facility coding.
- Differentiate among the settings physician's office coders code for.
- Apply the steps required to code physician's office cases correctly.

Key Terms

ICD-9-CM *Official Guidelines for Coding and Reporting*—official coding guidelines provided by CMS and NCHS that are to be followed when assigning ICD-9-CM codes until the October 1, 2014 implementation date of ICD-10-CM and ICD-10-PCS

inpatient—a patient who is formally admitted to a facility for treatment

outpatient—a patient who is not formally admitted to a facility

INTRODUCTION

The coding profession is a growing field and there are a variety of employment opportunities for coders. Coders can work in various settings including hospitals, physician's offices, insurance companies, law firms, public health agencies, worksite health systems, and prison systems, to name a few. This chapter discusses physician's office coding and the role and activities of a physician coder. It presents the steps a physician's office coder takes to complete the coding process for the diagnoses and procedures that a physician must report for reimbursement.

PHYSICIAN CODING

The physician's office is a unique coding setting for coding professionals. The physician's office is an outpatient setting, but the physician may see patients in both outpatient and inpatient settings. Inpatients are those who are formally admitted to a facility for treatment. **Outpatients** are those who are seen without being formally admitted to the facility. Therefore, the coding professional working in the physician's office may be assigning codes for both outpatient and inpatient services provided by the physician. The outpatient services a physician coder might code for include items a physician provides to patients in the office setting or hospital outpatient setting, whereas inpatient services a physician coder will code for are those hospital services that the physician provides to his or her patients who have been admitted to a facility as inpatients.

The purpose of coding in the physician's office setting is to obtain reimbursement for services provided and to be able to retrieve information regarding diagnoses, procedures, and other identifiers important to the individual physician. The reimbursement form utilized by physicians' offices is the CMS-1500 claim form (■ FIGURE 3-1).

Physician Documentation

Standard formats for the health records found in the physician's office were traditionally identified as source oriented, integrated, problem oriented, and other mixed formats based on individual physician preference. The electronic health record in the physician's office contains the same information as the traditional paper health record. Sources of documentation for physician services are found in many provider locations. Physician's office coders may find themselves assigning codes for patient encounters in clinics and offices, inpatient hospitals, outpatient hospitals, emergency departments, same-day surgery centers, urgent care clinics, and observation, long-term care, skilled nursing, home health, or other settings.

As discussed in Chapter 2, documentation includes administrative and clinical data. The basic documentation in the physician's office is also grouped into these categories. Administrative data includes registration information such as patient demographics, release of information forms, and financial information to include assignment of benefits. Clinical data contains the problem list; medication list; medical history; physical examination; physician orders, which are often combined with progress notes; progress notes; diagnostic reports such as radiology reports; operative reports; and/or procedure reports.

Physician's office coding currently utilized ICD 10 CM to assign diagnosis codes. Physician services and procedure services utilize CPT-4 procedure codes. Remember that ICD 10 PCS procedure code set is utilized only in the acute inpatient setting to assign procedure codes and never utilized in the physician office setting or ambulatory/outpatient setting.

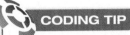
CODING TIP

Outpatient official coding guidelines state not to code any diagnosis documented as probable, suspected, questionable, rule out, working diagnosis, or other like language.

Outpatient Coding Guidelines

The physician's office coder will access administrative and clinical data for each specific patient encounter per documentation in order to properly assign diagnosis and procedure codes. The physician's office coder uses the current ICD 10 CM outpatient coding guidelines when determining the diagnostic statement(s) to be coded. (To access these guidelines, see Appendix A.)

One of the most important outpatient coding guidelines to remember as a coder is that you cannot code suspected, probable, possible, or likely diagnoses in an outpatient setting. A diagnosis that is suspected, probable, possible, or likely is only coded by inpatient facility coders.

Coding in the Physician's Office Setting

The first step in coding in the physician's office setting is to identify the appropriate setting in which you are coding, such as the physician's office, nursing home, inpatient admission, or a physician's office consultation. The second step is to determine the reason for the visit by thoroughly reading through the documentation to see what warranted the patient's visit, which would be the diagnosis(es). The third step is to determine what procedures and/or services were performed. Step 4 is to locate the correct diagnosis(es) code(s) using current year ICD 10 CM code set. Step 5 is to verify diagnosis(es) codes in the ICD 10 CM Tabular Index. Step 6 is to locate the correct procedure code using the CPT-4 coding manual. The final step is to read the procedure code description to ensure it matches your scenario, and then check to see if a modifier is also needed. In the outpatient setting, coders must adhere to the ICD 10 CM *Official Guidelines for Coding and Reporting* and *Diagnostic Coding and Reporting Guidelines for Outpatient Services,* which state that only the highest known or definitive diagnosis is assigned a code. If a definitive diagnosis has not been determined, then signs and symptoms and/or chief complaint should be utilized for coding. Do not assign codes for diagnoses documented as *probable,*

CARRIER

1500

HEALTH INSURANCE CLAIM FORM

APPROVED BY NATIONAL UNIFORM CLAIM COMMITTEE 08/05

PICA

PICA

1. MEDICARE (Medicare #) MEDICAID (Medicaid #) TRICARE CHAMPUS (Sponsor's SSN) CHAMPVA (Member ID#) GROUP HEALTH PLAN (SSN or ID) FECA BLK LUNG (SSN) OTHER (ID) 1a. INSURED'S I.D. NUMBER (For Program in Item 1)

2. PATIENT'S NAME (Last Name, First Name, Middle Initial)

3. PATIENT'S BIRTH DATE MM DD YY SEX M F

4. INSURED'S NAME (Last Name, First Name, Middle Initial)

5. PATIENT'S ADDRESS (No., Street)

6. PATIENT RELATIONSHIP TO INSURED Self Spouse Child Other

7. INSURED'S ADDRESS (No., Street)

CITY STATE

8. PATIENT STATUS Single Married Other Employed Full-Time Student Part-Time Student

CITY STATE

ZIP CODE TELEPHONE (Include Area Code) (   )

ZIP CODE TELEPHONE (Include Area Code) (   )

9. OTHER INSURED'S NAME (Last Name, First Name, Middle Initial)

10. IS PATIENT'S CONDITION RELATED TO:

11. INSURED'S POLICY GROUP OR FECA NUMBER

a. OTHER INSURED'S POLICY OR GROUP NUMBER

a. EMPLOYMENT? (Current or Previous) YES NO

a. INSURED'S DATE OF BIRTH MM DD YY SEX M F

b. OTHER INSURED'S DATE OF BIRTH MM DD YY SEX M F

b. AUTO ACCIDENT? PLACE (State) YES NO

b. EMPLOYER'S NAME OR SCHOOL NAME

c. EMPLOYER'S NAME OR SCHOOL NAME

c. OTHER ACCIDENT? YES NO

c. INSURANCE PLAN NAME OR PROGRAM NAME

d. INSURANCE PLAN NAME OR PROGRAM NAME

10d. RESERVED FOR LOCAL USE

d. IS THERE ANOTHER HEALTH BENEFIT PLAN? YES NO *If yes*, return to and complete item 9 a-d.

READ BACK OF FORM BEFORE COMPLETING & SIGNING THIS FORM.
12. PATIENT'S OR AUTHORIZED PERSON'S SIGNATURE I authorize the release of any medical or other information necessary to process this claim. I also request payment of government benefits either to myself or to the party who accepts assignment below.

SIGNED _____ DATE _____

13. INSURED'S OR AUTHORIZED PERSON'S SIGNATURE I authorize payment of medical benefits to the undersigned physician or supplier for services described below.

SIGNED _____

14. DATE OF CURRENT: MM DD YY ILLNESS (First symptom) OR INJURY (Accident) OR PREGNANCY(LMP)

15. IF PATIENT HAS HAD SAME OR SIMILAR ILLNESS. GIVE FIRST DATE MM DD YY

16. DATES PATIENT UNABLE TO WORK IN CURRENT OCCUPATION FROM MM DD YY TO MM DD YY

17. NAME OF REFERRING PROVIDER OR OTHER SOURCE 17a. 17b. NPI

18. HOSPITALIZATION DATES RELATED TO CURRENT SERVICES FROM MM DD YY TO MM DD YY

19. RESERVED FOR LOCAL USE

20. OUTSIDE LAB? YES NO $ CHARGES

21. DIAGNOSIS OR NATURE OF ILLNESS OR INJURY (Relate Items 1, 2, 3 or 4 to Item 24E by Line)
1. ___. ___ 3. ___. ___
2. ___. ___ 4. ___. ___

22. MEDICAID RESUBMISSION CODE ORIGINAL REF. NO.

23. PRIOR AUTHORIZATION NUMBER

24. A. DATE(S) OF SERVICE From MM DD YY To MM DD YY	B. PLACE OF SERVICE	C. EMG	D. PROCEDURES, SERVICES, OR SUPPLIES (Explain Unusual Circumstances) CPT/HCPCS	MODIFIER	E. DIAGNOSIS POINTER	F. $ CHARGES	G. DAYS OR UNITS	H. EPSDT Family Plan	I. ID. QUAL.	J. RENDERING PROVIDER ID. #
1									NPI	
2									NPI	
3									NPI	
4									NPI	
5									NPI	
6									NPI	

25. FEDERAL TAX I.D. NUMBER SSN EIN

26. PATIENT'S ACCOUNT NO.

27. ACCEPT ASSIGNMENT? (For govt. claims, see back) YES NO

28. TOTAL CHARGE $

29. AMOUNT PAID $

30. BALANCE DUE $

31. SIGNATURE OF PHYSICIAN OR SUPPLIER INCLUDING DEGREES OR CREDENTIALS (I certify that the statements on the reverse apply to this bill and are made a part thereof.)

SIGNED _____ DATE _____

32. SERVICE FACILITY LOCATION INFORMATION
a. NPI b.

33. BILLING PROVIDER INFO & PH # (   )
a. NPI b.

NUCC Instruction Manual available at: www.nucc.org

APPROVED OMB-0938-0999 FORM CMS-1500 (08-05)

PATIENT AND INSURED INFORMATION

PHYSICIAN OR SUPPLIER INFORMATION

Figure 3-1 ■ CMS-1500 form utilized for physician office billing.
Source: www.cms.gov

suspected, questionable, rule out, or *working diagnosis.* A chronic disease requiring ongoing treatment can be coded multiple times as long as the disease is documented and a treatment was required that affected patient care or management during each specific episode of care for the disease. Conditions that no longer exist are not assigned codes. Be sure to look for history codes if an historical condition has an impact on the current episode of care.

Physician's office coders may also code for outpatient surgery services performed by the physician and will utilize the history and physical, physician orders/progress notes, operative report, and pathology report as source documents. The postoperative diagnosis is used as the definitive diagnosis, not the preoperative diagnosis. Be sure to correlate the postoperative diagnosis with the corresponding pathology report. Read the entire operative report in order to ascertain the exact procedure that was performed, and then be guided by the procedure performed documentation on the operative report.

Inpatient setting codes for physicians are based on documentation found in the history and physical, physician orders/progress notes, operative report, and discharge summary. Physician's office coders who are coding for an inpatient service the physician provided will assign diagnosis, procedure, and evaluation and management (E/M) codes for each day of service to the patient in the hospital setting.

CODING TIP

When determining the physician's E/M, code level, it is helpful to have an E/M "cheat sheet," which can be found in a variety of resources. Most specialties will have their own specific E/M cheat sheet, and some general family practice ones are available from www.aafp.org. ■ FIGURE 3-2 shows sample E/M computer wallpaper from Brown Consulting that can be utilized to help physician coders arrive at the correct E/M level.

For additional information, visit www.aaos.org/news/bulletin/may07/managing7.asp

---

CODING TIP

A physician can choose to use either the 1995 or the 1997 E/M coding guidelines. Follow these steps to access the CMS document that includes both the 1995 and 1997 E/M coding guidelines:

1. Go to www.cms.gov.
2. Search the Outreach and Education category.
3. Go to the Medicare Learning Network (MLN) products and search for the evaluation and management services guide.

LET'S PRACTICE 3-1

Nursing Home Visit

This is an annual nursing facility history and physical and MDS/RAI evaluation for a 92-year-old female. This patient has been a resident for three years. She has CHF, COPD, and OA, all which remain stable with her current treatments.

● **HELPFUL HINT:** Go to E/M Other Nursing Facility Services.

Steps:

1. Look up failure, heart, congestive.

2. Look up disease, lung, obstructive (chronic).

3. Look up osteoarthritis.

4. Verify ICD-9 codes in the Tabular Index.

5. Determine the patient status.

6. Determine the patient service.

7. Determine the level of history, exam, and medical decision making.

8. Verify CPT codes in the Tabular Index and check for any applicable modifiers.

Codes:

ICD-9: 428.0, 496, 715.90

ICD-10: I50.9, J44.9, M19.90

CPT: 99318

Office/Clinic Coding Wallpaper 2012
Brown Consulting Associates, Inc.

New	Consult	Established	MDM (OVER) Medical Decision Making	HISTORY Minimum Requirements	EXAM Minimum Requirements	
99201	99241	99212	**Straightforward MDM**	**Problem Focused**	**Problem Focused**	New patient codes require full documentation of all three key components. For **established** patients, document two of three.
10 min	15 min	10 min	Minimal # of Dx/Tx options	1. Chief Complaints		
Self-limiting minor problem. 3 of 3 key components required for new, 99201. 2 of 3 keys required for established, 99212.			Minimal amount of data. Minimal risk for complications, morbidity or mortality	2. HPI 1 to 3 Qualifiers *HPI Qualifiers:* Location, Duration, Quality, Severity, Context, Timing, Assoc signs/smptoms, Mod. factors	1 system (1995-count systems) 1-5 elements (1997-count elements in systems)	
99202	99242		**Straightforward MDM**	**Expanded Problem Focused**	**Expanded Problem Focused**	**New** A new patient is one who has not been seen by your doctor or a same-specialty doctor in your group during the past three years. An est. pt. has been seen in past 3 years by you or other same-specialty clinician in your group. When covering for another - established.
20 min	30 min		Minimal # of Dx/Tx options	1. Chief Complaints	2-7 systems/areas (1995)	
Problems of low to moderate severity. 3 of 3 keys required.			Minimal amount of data. Min. risk comp, morbid, mortality	2. HPI X 1-3 Qualifiers 3. ROS of at least 1 system	6-11 elements (1997)	
		99213	**Low Complexity MDM**	**Expanded Problem Focused**	**Expanded Problem Focused**	
Problems of low to moderate severity. 2 of 3 key components required.	15 min		Limited # of Dx/Tx options. Limited amount of data. Low risk/comp, morbid, mortality	1. Chief Complaints 2. HPI X 1-3 Qualifiers 3. ROS of at least 1 system	2-7 systems/areas (1995) 6-11 elements (1997)	
99203	99243		**Low Complexity MDM**	**Detailed History**	**Detailed Exam**	**Wellness & illness** may both be coded on same day if illness is significant. Code the illness EM low as most of Hx/Ex would be included in the wellness. Two DX are required. Use modifier -25 on EM.
30 min	40 min		Limited # of Dx/Tx options. Limited amount of data. Low risk for complications, morbidity or mortality	1. Chief Complaints 2. HPI X 4 Qualifiers 3. ROS of at least 2 systems 4. Pertinent Med, Fam, or Soc Hx	1 sys detailed +4-6 other sys for 1995 detailed exam. Or 12 elements for 1997 GL.	
		99214	**Moderately Complex MDM**	**Detailed History**	**Detailed Exam**	
Presenting problems are of moderate to high severity. 2 of 3 key components required.	25 min		Multiple # of Dx/Tx options. Moderate amount of data. Moderate risk for complications, morbidity or mortality	1. Chief Complaints 2. HPI X 4 Qualifiers 3. ROS of at least 2 systems 4. Pertinent Med, Fam, or Soc Hx	1 sys detailed +4-6 other sys for 1995 detailed exam. Or 12 elements for 1997 GL.	
99204	99244		**Moderately Complex MDM**	**Comprehensive History**	**Comprehensive Exam**	**E/M & surgery** are frequently OK on same day. See CPT and contract payers' policies.
45 min	60 min		Multiple # of Dx/Tx options. Moderate amount of data. Moderate risk for complications, morbidity or mortality	1. Chief Complaints 2. HPI X 4 Qualifiers 3. ROS of at least 10 systems 4. Past, Med. Fam & Social Hx	8 or more systems (1995) 2 elements from each of 9 systems (1997)	
99205	99245	99215	**High Complexity MDM**	**Comprehensive History**	**Comprehensive Exam**	**A consult** is a request for opinion. It is OK to begin treatment at time of a consult. You must send report of findings and recommendations to the requestor. No consults for MCare.
60 min	80 min	40 min	Extensive # of Dx/Tx options. Extensive amount of data. Extensive risk for complications, morbidity or mortality	1. Chief Complaints 2. HPI X 4 Qualifiers 3. ROS of at least 10 systems 4. All PFSH for 99205, 99245. Two of three for 99215.	8 or more systems (1995) 2 elements from each of 9 systems (1997)	
Presenting problems are of moderate to high severity. 2 of 3 keys required for 99215.						

EXAMINATION - - Systems are numbered (1995); Elements are listed (1997)

1. Constitution
3 Vital signs (nurse doc. OK)
General appearance
2. Psychiatric
Judgment/Insight
Mood/affect Orientation X 3
Recent/remote memory
3. Skin
Inspect & palpate
4. Eyes
Conjunctivae & lids
Ex. pupils & irises
Ophthalmoscope optic disc
5. & 6. Neck & Lymph
Exam neck
Thyroid
Palpate lymph nodes (2 areas)
7. Respiratory
Auscultation of lungs
Respiratory effort
Palpation of chest
Percussion of chest

8. ENT & Mouth
External inspection ears & nose
Otoscopic ext. canals & TMs
Assess hearing, Exam oropharynx
Inspect lips, teeth and gums
Nasal mucosa, septum, turbinates
9. Cardiovascular
Auscultation of heart
Palpation of heart
Carotid arteries
Abdominal aorta
Pedal pulse
Femoral artery
Extremities for edema/varicosities
10. Gastrointestinal
Abdomen, masses/tenderness
Liver & spleen Exam for hernia
Ex. Anus/rectum
Obtain stool spec. for occult blood
11. GU - Male
Digital rectal exam of the prostate
Scrotal contents Penis

11. GU - Female & 12. (Breast)
Inspect breast Palpate breast
External genitalia Urethra
Cervix Adnexa Uterus
Bladder
13. Neurological
Test cranial nerves Sensation
Deep tendon reflexes
14. Musculoskeletal
Gait and station
Inspect/palpate digits/nails
Inspect/palpate misalignment
ROM, notation of dislocation
Assess stability, laxity etc.
Assess muscle strength/tone
Areas are: 1. Head/neck
2. Spine/Pelvis
3. RUE 4. LUE 5. RLE 6. LLE

See also 1997 Single System Exs. Download full CMS Guidelines at www.codinghelp.com

▼ REVIEW OF SYSTEMS (ROS)
Constitution, Eyes, ENT, Resp., Cardiovascular, Gastrointestinal, GU, Musculoskeletal, Neurological, Skin, Endocrine, Hematologic/Lymphatic, Allergy/Immunology & Psychiatric

EXAMPLES:
Skin: denies rashes/lesion
ENT: denies throat or ear pain
GI: has not had N/V/D
Cardio: dyspnea on exertion
99213 ROS X 1: 99214 ROS X 2:
99215, 99204 & 99205 = ROS X 10

When more than 50% of the visit is devoted to face-to-face counseling/coordination of care, you may select code based on total time. Document content and time. Clearly indicate >50% of time was counseling. **EXAMPLES:** "15/25 minutes spent counseling new DM pt on various tx plans..." OR "Entire 25 min encounter spent counseling regarding..."

Figure 3-2 ■ Brown Consulting's Office/Clinic Coding Wallpaper. Reprinted with permission.
Source: Brown Consulting

How Medical Decision Making (MDM) is Decided & Audited

A Determine total points for 1 & 2, and risk level from 3, move totals t**B** *(MDM Calculator):*

1. Number of Diagnostic/Treatment Options (scored)	2. Amount/Complexity of Data Reviewed (scored)
1 point 1 self-limiting or minor problem today *(pt. did not need to come, no particular treatment)*	1 point Order or review any number of labs
2 points 2 self-limiting/minor problems today	1 point Order or review any number of x-rays
3 points New problem(s) - no additional work-up needed (max 3 pts.)	1 point Order or review any number of diagnostic tests
4 points New problem(s) - additional work-up is planned (max 4 pts.)	1 point Reviewed any of above w/performing MD, or obtained history from another source
May have multiples of below	1 point Requested old record documented in chart today
1 pt ea Established problem stable/improved ○ ○ ○ ○	2 points Independent interp of x-ray, spec., tracing (read elsewhere)
2 pts ea Established problem worsening ○ ○ ○ ○	2 points Review & summarize old records; or history from another source; or discussed w/health care provider

Notes

3. Determine the highest level of risk for the encounter and carry that finding to **B**   *(MDM Calculator):*

	If your patient has...	If you are going to order...	If your treatment plan is like...
High Risk Level	1 or more chronic illness w/severe exacerbation *or* Acute or chronic illness which is life threatening *or* Abrupt change in neuro status	CV contrast imaging in patient w/risk factors Electrophysiological test Diagnostic endoscopy in a patient with identified risk factors Diskography (or similar)	Elective/emergent surgery w/risk factors Parenteral controlled substance *or* Drug treatment with intensive monitoring for toxicity *or* Make a "do not resuscitate" decision or a decision to de-escalate care
Moderate Risk Level	1 or more chronic problem(s) with mild exacerbation *or* 2 or more stable chronic probs. *or* An undiagnosed new problem with uncertain outcome *or* Acute illness w/systemic symptoms An acute complicated injury	Physiologic stress testing Diagnostic endoscopy in a patient who has no identified risk factors Deep needle or excisional biopsy Cardiovascular imaging procedure with contrast Obtain body cavity fluid	Elective major surgery for a patient with no identified risk factors *or* Minor surgery for a patient with identified risk factors *or* IVs with additives *or* Closed treatment of a non-displaced fracture or Prescription drug management
Low Risk Level	1 stable chronic problem *or* 1 acute uncomplicated illness *or* acute uncomplicated injury *or* 2 or more minor problems	Physiologic tests without stress Non-cardiovas. image w/contrast Superficial needle or skin biopsy Arterial puncture for labs	Over-the-counter drugs Minor surgery with no identified risk factors Physical Therapy or Occupational Therapy IVs without additives
Minimal Risk Level	1 self limiting or minor (Patient didn't need to come, no spec. Tx. plan)	Typical studies such as Labs KOH, UA, X-ray, EKG, US	Rest, gargles, Ace wraps, Dressing

B *MDM CALCULATOR* Enter 1., 2. and 3. from above. Cross out the highest and lowest. Level remaining *is* the MDM.

1. Dx/Mgt options defined as...	2. Data amount defined as...	3. Highest risk level is...	FINAL MDM
Extensive number (4 or > points)	Extensive amount (4 or > points)	High Risk	High Complexity
Multiple number (3 points)	Multiple amount (3 points)	Moderate Risk	Moderate
Limited number (2 points)	Limited amount (2 points)	Low Risk	Low Complexity
Minimal number (1 point)	Minimal or None (0-1 point)	Minimal Risk	Straightforward

C Select the E/M code based on MDM, then comply with history and/or exam requirements, or move to a lower code.

E/M Recipe Card

NEW PT - MDM	EXAM (AND)	HISTORY	New Pt	Time	Consult	Time
Straightforward MDM	1 system	CC & Brief HPI (1-3 HPI elements)	99201	10	99241	15
Straightforward MDM	2-7 (limited)	CC, HPI x1, ROS x1 system	99202	20	99242	30
Low Complexity MDM	2-7(extend)*	CC, HPI x4, ROS x2 sys., 1 Hx (PMFS)	99203	30	99243	40
Moderate MDM	8 or > sys	CC, HPI x4, ROS x10, 3 Hxs (PMFS)	99204	45	99244	60
High Complexity MDM	8 or > sys	CC, HPI x4, ROS x10, 3 Hxs (PMFS)	99205	60	99245	80

EST PT - MDM	EXAM (OR)	HISTORY	Est Pt	Time		
Straightforward MDM	1 system	CC & Brief HPI (1-3 HPI elements)	99212	10		
Low Complexity MDM	2-7 (limited)	CC, HPI x1-3, ROS x1 system	99213	15	When in doubt -	
Moderate MDM	2-7(extend)*	CC, HPI x4, ROS x2 sys., 1 Hx (PMFS)	99214	25	be conservative	
High Complexity MDM	8 or > sys	CC, HPI x4, ROS x10, 3 Hxs (PMFS)	99215	40		
"Nurse," assistant or minimal by you		Usually documented nursing, PCP is in	99211	5 minutes or more		

CODER GENERAL'S WARNING
Sometimes the MDM scores as moderate but the encounter was brief/simple. *Just because it is moderate, does not mean it is a 99214 or a 99204.*

Review CPT EMs, Apx. C, & guidelines.

*Check w/ your state administrator as Medicare payers may vary exam requirement; eg, Noridian requires 5-7 systems or areas.

Figure 3-2 ■ continued

LET'S PRACTICE 3-2

Initial Hospital Visit

This is a 23-year-old female who was brought to the emergency department because of a drug overdose. I am admitting this patient to the ICU to further monitor and treat her suicidal tendencies. The patient admitted to taking 1 bottle of Tylenol in an attempt to end her life. She has recently broken up with her boyfriend of 2 years and states that she does not wish to live without him. We will keep her on suicide watch tonight and I will reevaluate in the a.m.

● **HELPFUL HINT:** Go to the Initial Hospital Admission in the E/M section of your CPT coding manual.

Steps:

1. Go to the Table of Drugs and Chemicals.
2. Look up acetaminophen (which is the generic name for Tylenol) and locate the code for poisoning and the E-code for suicide attempt.

3. Determine the patient service level for procedure code assignment.
4. Verify ICD 10 CM codes in the Tabular Index.
5. Determine the patient status.
6. Verify codes in the procedure Tabular Index.
7. Determine the level of history, exam, and medical decision making.
8. Verify codes in the Tabular Index.

Codes:

ICD-10: T39.1X2A, F48.9

CPT: 99223

LET'S PRACTICE 3-3

Initial Hospital Consultation

I was called by Dr. Crews to see this patient. This patient is a 65-year old female with Type I diabetes mellitus. Dr. Crews is concerned about the gangrene occurring in her foot and asked for an orthopedic consult. I examined her left foot, which is obviously gangrenous and needs surgical intervention. I discussed the options, surgery, and risks with the patient and she has agreed to have this foot amputated before the gangrene spreads into her leg. We will proceed with surgery in the a.m.

● **HELPFUL HINT:** Go to the Initial Hospital Consultation in the E/M section of your CPT coding manual.

Steps:

1. Look up diabetes, Type I, with gangrene.
2. Verify ICD 10 code(s).
3. Determine the patient service level for procedure code assignment.
4. Determine the patient service.
5. Determine the level of history, exam, and medical decision making.
6. Verify codes in the procedure Tabular Index.

Codes:

ICD-10: E11.52

CPT: 99254

LET'S PRACTICE 3-4

Operative Report

The 27-year old gravida 2, para 1 presented to my office at 11 weeks' gestation. She had a normal pregnancy. Since she had a C-section with her first baby, we scheduled a C-section for today, week 39, day 5 (■ FIGURE 3-3). I performed a repeat low cervical transverse cesarean section, which went well. She delivered a healthy male weighing

8 lbs 4 oz., 21 inches long. Apgars were 8 and 9. We will follow up with her in 4 weeks.

● **HELPFUL HINT:** This is a surgery and you do not code an E/M with a surgery unless these are unrelated, so do not assign an E/M code with this visit.

LET'S PRACTICE 3-4, *continued*

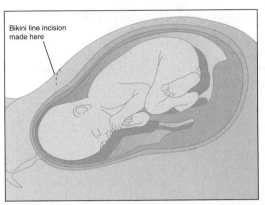
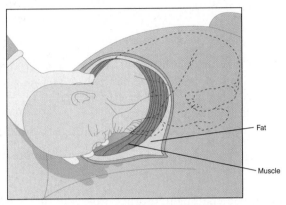

Bikini line incision made here

Fat

Muscle

A caesarean delivery may be carried out as a planned procedure (in which case it is known as an elective caesarean) or as an emergency. Usually the surgical incision is made horizontally and low down, in the position known as the "bikini line".

Figure 3-3 ■ C-section delivery.
Source: Peter Gardiner/Science Source/Photo Researchers

Steps:

1. Look up delivery, cesarean, previous cesarean section.
2. Look up Outcome of Delivery and Pregnancy, Weeks of gestation.
3. Verify ICD 10 CM codes in the Tabular Index.
4. Look up Cesarean Delivery procedure code.
5. Verify the code in the procedure Tabular Index.

Codes:

ICD-10: O34.21, Z37.0, Z3A.39

CPT: 59510

LET'S PRACTICE 3-5

Pathology Report

OPERATION: DILATATION AND CURETTAGE, HYSTEROSCOPY

#1 ENDOMETRIAL CURETTAGE

#2 ENDOCERVICAL

Gross Description: Specimen #1 indicated as endometrial curettings are multiple, irregularly shaped fragments of pink-tan tissue that together measure approximately 2.0 cm. The specimen is submitted in its entirety for examination. Specimen #2 indicated as endocervical curettings are multiple, irregularly shaped fragments of pink-tan tissue and mixed with mucus and blood and together measuring approximately 1.0 cm. The specimen is submitted in its entirety for examination.

Microscopic Description: Sections reveal multiple fragments of endometrium. There are numerous glands present with moderate tortuosity. The glands reveal secretory activity with some glands still exhibiting subnuclear vacuoles. The stroma is minimally edematous. The histology is consistent with approximately the 18th to 19th day of the menstrual cycle. Specimen #2 reveals endometrial fragments similar to those described in Specimen #1. Endocervical fragments are also present that are histologically unremarkable.

Diagnosis:

1. Specimen #1, secretory phase endometrium approximately 18th to 19th day of the menstrual cycle.
2. Specimen #2, secretory endometrial fragments consistent with approximately 18th to 19th day of the menstrual cycle.
3. Endocervical fragments, benign.

● **HELPFUL HINT:** You are coding for the pathologist, so go to the CPT pathology section (88300–88309) and find the correct specimen.

Steps:

1. Locate the pathology codes from the CPT index.
2. Read the given pathology codes and decide which code the specimen examined fits into.

Code:

CPT Pathology Code: 88305

LET'S PRACTICE 3-6

Office Visit

Chief Complaint: Congestion

History of Present Illness: This is an established 44-year-old female who presents complaining of a cold she has had for the past four days and now it has gone into her eye on the right side, which has become reddened and matted.

Past Medical History: Is otherwise healthy.

Current Medications: Zovirax.

Allergies: None known.

Review of Systems: She has no chest pain, sputum production. Sinus drainage has been clear but her cough has been productive, although she has not visualized this. She denies ear pain and no nausea or vomiting.

Physical Exam:

Vitals: BP is 120/80, temperature is 97, pulse 72, respirations 18.

HEENT: Head is normocephalic. TMs are clear. The patient has obvious conjunctivitis (■ FIGURE 3-4) with conjunctival infection on the right eye. The anterior chamber on slit-lamp exam appears clear without evidence of any substance in the anterior chamber. Oropharynx is unremarkable and neck is supple.

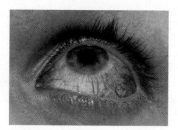

Figure 3-4 ■ Conjunctivitis or pink eye.
Source: Sergii Chepulskyi/Shutterstock

Lungs: Clear without rales, rhonchi, or rub.

Heart: Regular rate and rhythm without murmur.

Chest: The patient has upper respiratory congestion heard when she breathes in and coughs.

Diagnosis:

1. Conjunctivitis, right eye.

2. Acute bronchitis.

Plan: Amoxicillin 500 mg tid × 10 days and Garamycin drops 1–2 q 4h prn. Follow up prn.

● **HELPFUL HINT:** Go to Office Visit, Established Patient, in the E/M section of your CPT coding manual.

Steps:

1. Look up conjunctivitis.

2. Look up bronchitis, acute.

3. Verify ICD-9 codes in the Tabular Index.

4. Determine the patient status.

5. Determine the patient service.

6. Determine the level of history, exam, and medical decision making.

7. Verify codes in the Tabular Index.

Codes:

ICD-9: 372.30, 466.0

ICD-10: H10.9, J20.9

CPT: 99213

LET'S PRACTICE 3-7

Urgent Care

Identification: This is a 14-year-old Hispanic male.

Chief Complaint: Cough, fever, chills, and malaise.

History of Present Illness: The patient is a 14-year-old male who has had a cough, fever, chills and malaise for the past few days. He has had a sore throat for the past couple of days. He has had difficulty sleeping at night because of the cough. He lives at home with his mother and she is similarly sick. He has not had any wheezing per se. He has had fever and chills.

Allergies: No known allergies.

Current Medications: Aspirin this morning but none regularly.

Physical Examination: General: Shows him to be conversant without any hoarseness. He does appear slightly pale.

LET'S PRACTICE 3-7, *continued*

Vitals: O_2 saturations are 97% on room air. Temperature: 98.3. Otherwise vitals are all normal.

ENT: Without evidence of infection. Neck: Supple without any adenopathy.

Lungs: Clear without wheezes or crackles.

Heart: Regular rhythm without any murmur or rub.

Skin: Warm and dry with good capillary refill.

Impression:

1. Acute bronchitis.

Plan: The patient had symptoms fairly isolated to the bronchials. It may very well be viral but I could not tell and so I prescribed doxycycline 100 mg, 1 bid for a week and prednisone 60 mg q day for five days. For the cough itself he is to use Guiatuss AC, 2 tsp q4h prn, and was given 4 oz. He is to drink lots of fluids and rest and use Tylenol or ibuprofen as needed.

● **HELPFUL HINT:** Go to the Office Visit, New Patient, in the E/M section of your CPT coding manual.

Steps:

1. Look up bronchitis, acute.
2. Verify ICD-9 codes in the Tabular Index.
3. Determine the patient status.
4. Determine the patient service.
5. Determine the level of history, exam, and medical decision making.
6. Verify codes in the Tabular Index.

Codes:

ICD-9: 466.0

ICD-10: J20.9

CPT: 99202

LET'S PRACTICE 3-8

Office Visit

Identification: This is a 24-year-old Caucasian male.

Chief Complaint: Urticaria.

History of Present Illness: The patient is here because of urticaria since last night (■ FIGURE 3-5). This patient recently moved to town and is new to the office. Two issues might have occurred. He ate an apple last night that seemed to be imperfectly ripe. It might not have been washed. The second is he has had a cat for the past couple of days that seems to want to sleep on his bed and be near him that used to always be inside but now it goes outside and plays and rubs in the bushes, then comes back inside.

Allergies: None.

Current Medications: None.

Previous Illnesses: Denies any.

Past History: Family and past history is unremarkable.

Social History: The patient recently moved here and is a welder by trade. The patient denies smoking and drinks on occasion. He is not married.

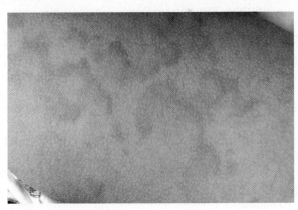

Figure 3-5 ■ Urticaria.
Source: Levent Konuk/Shutterstock

Physical Examination: Urticaria present over patchy surfaced areas of his body. The lungs are clear to auscultation. Cardiac exam is normal.

Impression:

1. Urticaria, probably food induced or cat induced.

Plan: He got rid of the cat. I told him to wash his clothes and bedding. I gave him an injection of Benadryl and

continued

LET'S PRACTICE 3-8, *continued*

epinephrine. We are going to do oral Benadryl 50 mg tid prn, and prednisone 40, 30, 20, and 10 mg daily for four days.

● **HELPFUL HINT:** Go to the Office Visit, New Patient, in your E/M section of your CPT coding manual.

Steps:

1. Look up urticaria.

2. Verify ICD-9 codes in the Tabular Index.

3. Determine the patient status.

4. Determine the patient service.

5. Determine the level of history, exam, and medical decision making.

6. Verify codes in the *Tabular Index.*

Codes:

ICD-9: 708.0

ICD-10: L50.0

CPT: 99202

LET'S PRACTICE 3-9

Emergency Care

Identification: This is a 40-year-old male.

Chief Complaint: Painful left foot.

History of Present Illness: This 40-year-old male presented to the emergency department for evaluation of a painful left foot. The patient was involved in a motor bike accident this weekend. He tells me he was riding at a low rate of speed up a trail when his motorcycle tipped over. The patient tells me he was going approximately 20 miles an hour. He tells me his left foot was caught under the bike. He twisted under the bike, although he had heavy boots on. He also sustained an abrasion to his knee, but he tells me his knee really is not hurting him. It is his mid and forefoot that is painful and quite swollen. He tells me that he was able to put weight on it initially but the next day it was increasingly painful to bear weight. He is current on his tetanus immunization and denies any other injury in this accident.

Allergies: None.

Current Medications: None.

Previous Illnesses: Denies.

Physical Examination: Reveals a well-developed, well-nourished middle-aged male. Vitals are entirely within normal limits. Exam of the extremities is limited to his lower extremity. He has an abrasion on his left lateral knee about 2.5 cm × 1.5 cm, fairly deep, but it does not appear infected. There are some other superficial abrasions on the lateral calf. His ankle is nontender. He is nontender over his proximal fibula. There is no particular swelling in the calf area. He is tender and swollen, however, over the midfoot and the distal metatarsals of his left foot. There is bruising and ecchymotic discoloration at the base of the first MTP joint. The patient has pain with motion of his toes. There is no obvious deformity, however. He does have a good dorsalis pedis pulse. An x-ray of the left foot fails to reveal any obvious fractures or bony abnormality. The abrasions on his left leg were cleaned and dressed with Neosporin ointment.

Impression:

1. Abrasion and contusion of the left knee.

2. Contusion and sprain of the left mid and forefoot.

Plan: The patient is advised to keep the foot iced and elevated. He may begin weight bearing as tolerated once he can get inside a firm lace-up boot or shoe. He really did not want any pain medication except for some Motrin. The patient tells me his work is primarily sitting work, and he thinks he can continue working without difficulty. He is cautioned that he should be rechecked if he has any further problems.

● **HELPFUL HINT:** Go to the Emergency Room Visits in the E/M section of your CPT coding manual.

Steps:

1. Look up sprain, foot.

2. Look up contusion, knee.

LET'S PRACTICE 3-9, *continued*

3. Go to the External Cause Index and look up accident, motor vehicle.

4. In the External Cause Index look up activities and status.

5. Verify ICD-9 codes in the Tabular Index.

6. Determine the patient status.

7. Determine the patient service.

8. Determine the level of history, exam, and medical decision making.

9. Verify codes in the Tabular Index.

Codes:

ICD-9: 845.11, 845.12, 924.11, E821.2, E029.9, E000.8

ICD-10: S93.622A, S93.529A, S80.02xA, V29.3xxA, Y93.89, Y99.8

CPT: 99283

LET'S PRACTICE 3-10

Radiology

History: Previous history of kidney stones with surgery on his left kidney. Now complaining of right flank pain. Will complete an intravenous KUB and renal ultrasound.

KUB: There is a cluster of small stones in the lower pole of the right kidney. There are small stones in the lower pole of the left kidney. There is a calcification in the left side of the pelvis, probably representing a phlebolith but could be a urethral calculus. No soft tissue masses seen. Gas pattern is normal.

Impression:

1. Bilateral renal calculi. Calcification in the left pelvis that could be a urethral calculus or phlebolith.

Renal Ultrasound: Both kidneys are visualized. The left kidney has a slightly irregular configuration and is not as well visualized as the right, probably related to perinephric scarring from previous surgery. The overall size and configuration of the left kidney are symmetrical compared with the right. I see no evidence of hydronephrosis, mass lesion, or other significant abnormality.

Impression:

1. Some mild irregularity of the left kidney, probably related to previous surgery, otherwise the examination is unremarkable.

● **HELPFUL HINT:** Go to the Radiology section in your CPT coding manual, because you do not report the E/M for a radiologist.

Steps:

1. Look up calculi.

2. Look up calcification, kidney.

3. Verify ICD-9 codes in the Tabular Index.

4. Look up KUB.

5. Look up ultrasound, kidney (■ FIGURE 3-6).

6. Verify codes in the Tabular Index.

Codes:

ICD-9: 592.0, 593.89

ICD-10: N20.0, N28.29

CPT: 74400, 76775

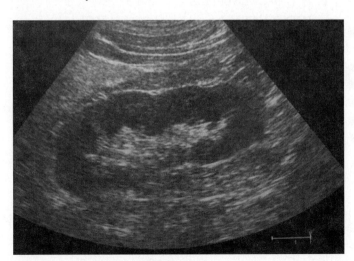

Figure 3-6 ■ Ultrasound of the kidney.
© Shipov Oleg/Shutterstock.

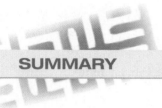

SUMMARY

As a coder you must follow the coding guidelines based on the type of provider or facility in which you are working. When coding for a physician, the coder is coding the diagnoses and services that the physician personally performed that might have occurred in a variety of settings. Some of these settings include a hospital while making inpatient rounds, a same-day surgery suite, or commonly the physician's office itself.

Regardless of the physician service being coded, the coder will follow the ICD-9-CM or ICD-10-CM official outpatient coding guidelines and assign ICD-9 or ICD-10 diagnosis codes and CPT procedure codes. The physician's office coder uses the documentation in the patient's medical record to, first, identify the setting in which the physician is providing the care; second, identify the diagnosis that warranted the care; and third, identify the service or procedure performed to treat the diagnosis.

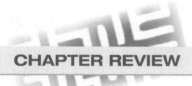

CHAPTER REVIEW

Multiple Choice

Choose the letter that best answers each question or completes each statement.

1. Which of the following code sets are currently used in physician coding?
   a. ICD-9-CM, Volumes 1 and 2
   b. ICD-9-CM, Volumes 1, 2, and 3
   c. ICD-9-CM, Volumes 1 and 2, and CPT
   d. ICD-9-CM, Volumes 1, 2, and 3, and CPT

2. Physician's office coders can code for services provided in which of the following settings?
   a. Inpatient facility
   b. Outpatient facility
   c. Physician's office
   d. All of the above

3. In a physician's office the codes are placed on which billing form?
   a. CMS-1500
   b. UB-04
   c. HIPAA-NOP
   d. UHDDS

4. In a physician's office, the patient information is divided into
   a. administrative data.
   b. clinical data.
   c. administrative and clinical data.
   d. administrative and demographic data.

5. Which of the following encounters do physician's office coders typically code for?
   a. Emergency department services
   b. Inpatient services
   c. Office visits
   d. All of the above

6. Given the following scenario, what ICD-9-CM diagnosis codes should you assign? A patient is seen by the physician for a fever and sore throat. After examination the physician determines it is strep throat.
   a. 034.0
   b. 462
   c. 780.60, 462
   d. 034.0, 780.60

7. Given the following scenario, what ICD-9-CM diagnosis codes should you assign? A patient is seen by the physician for chest pain. After examination the physician is worried about the patient having a myocardial infarction and sends the patient to the emergency department.

    a. 786.50
    b. 786.59
    c. 410.90
    d. 410.91

8. Which of the following is NOT an example of administrative data?

    a. Insurance information
    b. Mailing address
    c. Marital status
    d. Nurse's notes

9. Which of the following can be coded in a physician's office setting?

    a. Likely inguinal hernia
    b. Possibly torn medial meniscus
    c. Serous otitis media
    d. Suspected pneumonia

10. Which of the following is NOT clinical data?

    a. Gender
    b. History and physical
    c. Medication record
    d. Progress notes

True or False

Determine whether each question is true or false. In the space provided, write "T" for true or "F" for false.

_____ 1. Physician's office coders follow the same coding guidelines as inpatient facility coders.

_____ 2. In a physician's office, the coder can code probable or suspected diagnoses as they are confirmed.

_____ 3. Physician's office coders who are coding for an inpatient service their physician provided will assign diagnosis, procedure, and/or evaluation and management codes for each day of service to the patient in the hospital setting.

_____ 4. The physician's office is an outpatient setting where the physician may see patients in both the outpatient and inpatient settings.

_____ 5. In a physician's office, conditions that no longer exist are still coded by the coder.

_____ 6. ICD-9-CM procedure codes, Volume 3, or ICD-10 PCS codes are not utilized in the physician's office setting.

_____ 7. Physician's office coders will not have to start using ICD-10-CM in October 2014.

_____ 8. Chronic diseases must be documented and must require treatment or affect patient care or management in order for the physician's office coder to assign codes for these.

_____ 9. The final step in code assignment is to verify the code in the Tabular Index.

_____ 10. The Table of Drugs and Chemicals, located in Volume 2 of the ICD-9-CM coding manual, is to be used only by inpatient facility coders.

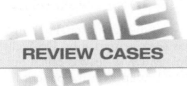

REVIEW CASES

Use these coding steps to assign the applicable codes to the review cases that follow:

1. Read the documentation contained in the medical record.

2. Determine the reason for the visit (the diagnoses).

3. Determine what treatment or service the patient received during the visit (the procedure).

4. Look up the diagnoses using your ICD-9-CM coding manual, Volumes 1 and 2. To begin preparing for the

ICD-10 conversion, you may use an electronic encoder, or refer to the ICD-10-CM draft code set, or use a website such as www.icd10data.com to either look up the ICD-10 codes or convert the ICD-9 codes to ICD-10 codes.

5. Verify ICD-9 codes in the Tabular Index.

6. Look up the procedure codes using your CPT-4 coding manual.

7. Verify CPT codes in the Tabular Index and determine if a modifier is needed.

Review Case 3-1 — Radiology
Nonenhanced CT Head Scan

History: Headache. Dizziness.

There are no abnormal areas of increased or decreased density. The subarachnoid spaces and ventricles are normal. There is no shift of midline structures. The structures at the base of the brain appear normal.

Impression:

1. Normal nonenhanced CT head scan.

ICD-10-CM diagnosis code(s): _____

_____

CPT code(s) with modifier, if applicable: _____

_____

Review Case 3-2 — Radiology
Chest X-ray

History: Preop thyroid surgery.

Chest: Two views of the chest reveal a left deviation of the trachea at the thoracic inlet to the left, suggesting the thyroid gland could be a little bit on the right. Lungs are free of infiltrates and nodules. Heart size is normal. The mediastinum has a slightly unusual configuration in that there is a double density in the area of the aortic knob. This raises the possibility of a mediastinal mass on the PA view. Nothing in the lateral view suggests a mass however. Perhaps this represents some adenopathy in the aortic window or superimposition of shadows. It is recommended that CT limited to this area be performed to exclude mass in the chest. Thoracic cage appears intact.

Impression:

1. Left tracheal deviation toward the left, suggesting the possibility of a mass in the neck. A left fullness in the region of the aortic window on the PA view raises the possibility of a mediastinal mass. The CT is the method of choice to evaluate this area.

ICD-10-CM diagnosis code(s): _____

_____

CPT code(s) with modifier, if applicable: _____

_____

Review Case 3-3 — Radiology
Acute Abdomen Series

History: Generalized Abdominal Pain.

Findings: Chest radiographic portion of the study shows clear lung fields with unremarkable heart, hila, mediastinum, and osseous structures.
Supine, erect, and lateral decubitus views of the abdomen show a normal bowel gas pattern. No organomegaly. No free air. No abnormal gas collections.

Impression:

1. Negative acute abdomen.

ICD-10-CM diagnosis code(s): _____

_____

CPT code(s) with modifier, if applicable: _____

_____

Review Case 3-4 — Radiology
Forearm X-ray

History: MVA trauma with pain in left forearm.

Left Forearm: AP and lateral views of the forearm relationships. There are no fractures. Views show normal anatomic alignment. There are no radiopaque foreign bodies.

Impression:

1. Normal forearm views.

ICD-10-CM diagnosis code(s): _____

_____

CPT code(s) with modifier, if applicable: _____

_____

Review Case 3-5 — Office Follow-Up

Subjective: This 22-month-old is brought to my office for a recheck. He was seen yesterday by Dr. Wells with fever of uncertain etiology. Dr. Wells was called out to an emergency and I will follow up with the patient for him. The patient had a workup with a blood count, CRP, and blood culture. He was treated with Motrin and Tylenol. It is significant to note that his blood count was elevated at 23,000 with 76% segs, 13.4% lymphocytes. He also had an elevated CRP, which was 7.11. Blood culture has not been read yet and will not be read until late this afternoon. Mother notes that the child has improved considerably.

The mother notes that his temperature has come down and he seems to be more playful and acting more like himself. The child does have a history of asthma and tachycardia. She tells me she is treating him with albuterol, Tylenol, ibuprofen, and Zyrtec elixir. His primary care physician is Dr. Wells. Mother also notes the child is taking fluids today quite well. She tells me he seems to be very thirsty drinking lots of fluid and he has been eating today. She notes that he has developed sort of a barky bronchial cough but that is not unusual with his history of asthma.

Objective: General exam reveals a happy, smiling 2-year-old. Temperature 97.1, heart rate 140, respiratory rate 28. I reviewed his chart from yesterday. His temperature yesterday was 105. His respiratory rate was 26. His heart rate was 200. His O_2 sat was only 93% on room air. HEENT: TMs are clear. Pharynx is minimally injected. No exudates. The neck is supple. The lungs demonstrate somewhat tubular breath sounds but I do not hear any significant wheezes, and he is moving air freely. He does have a deep bronchial cough.

Assessment:

1. Acute febrile illness, uncertain etiology.

Plan: At this point the child is improved. I would not change the treatment. I do not think he needs antibiotics. We discussed getting a chest x-ray; however, with his O_2 sats improved and his temperature down and pulse down, I really do not think that is indicated at this time. Mother is advised to follow up with Dr. Wells, primary care doctor, if she has concerns tomorrow and to check on the results of the blood culture as well.

ICD-9-CM diagnosis code(s): _____

_____

ICD-10-CM diagnosis code(s): _____

_____

CPT code(s) with modifier, if applicable: _____

_____

Review Case 3-6   **Office Visit**

Subjective: This 42-year-old new female patient presents to my office. The patient is complaining of pain in her right ear. The patient notes she has been ill now for a little over two weeks. It started with what she thought was an influenza-like illness with cough, upper respiratory congestion. She actually was seen by her primary care provider about a week and a half ago. She is unhappy with her other doctor and came to my office to seek new treatment for her symptoms. She was treated with a Z-pak, which she finished. She tells me she finished this at least 10 days ago now. She did not seem to really get a whole lot better, and her symptoms have persisted with some upper respiratory conges-

tion but her cough has resolved. She has not been running a fever; however, in the past two days she has developed pain in her right ear and pain in the right facial area above and behind her right eye. She notes that she still has greenish nasal discharge as well and thinks that she may have developed a sinus infection. The patient was treated with a Z-pak as noted about two weeks ago. She tells me at that time she was not having ear pain or facial pain. The patient notes that she is not allergic to any antibiotics.

Past Medical History: Unremarkable. She takes Effexor on a regular basis, and she has some hydrocodone, which she apparently was given for her cough several weeks ago but she is not taking this regularly.

Objective: Physical exam reveals a well-developed, well-nourished female. Temperature 97.8, respiratory rate 20, heart rate 72, blood pressure slightly elevated at 114/99, O_2 sat 97% on room air.

HEENT: Left TM is red and somewhat retracted. The right TM is dull. The pharynx shows minimal injection. No exudates. The neck is supple with no significant adenopathy. The patient is tender to percussion over her right maxillary sinus; however, her right ear is not nearly as red as her left ear. Nasal mucosa is moderately injected. The lungs were not examined. She does not have any significant cervical adenopathy.

Assessment:

1. Left otitis media and acute sinusitis.

Plan: The patient was treated with Augmentin 875 bid for 10 days. I recommend she take Sudafed 60 mg to 120 mg daily for her sinus symptoms and if she is not improving or develops new symptoms should be reevaluated.

ICD-9-CM diagnosis code(s): _____

_____

ICD-10-CM diagnosis code(s): _____

_____

CPT code(s) with modifier, if applicable: _____

_____

Review Case 3-7   **Office Visit**

Subjective: This 12-year-old established female patient is brought to the office by her mother. The child is complaining of nasal congestion, cough, and mother tells me her symptoms have gone on for a little over a week. The patient notes that her cough has actually improved. She denies any sore throat but does note the last 12 hours her right ear has started to hurt. She has not been running a fever according to her mother.

Medications: The patient does take Strattera and Lexapro. She is not on any other medications.

Allergies: No allergies to medicines.

Objective:

General: General exam reveals a well-developed, well-nourished 12-year-old.

Vitals: Temperature 97.8, respiratory rate 16, heart rate 78, normal blood pressure, O_2 sat 96% on room air.

HEENT: On exam her right TM is moderately injected. Left TM is clear. Oropharynx shows very minimal injection. She is not tender over her maxillary sinuses. Neck is supple.

Chest: The lungs are clear to auscultation.

Assessment:

1. Right otitis media and URI.

Plan: The child is treated with amoxicillin 500 tid. She is to increase fluids. I also gave her some Auralgan otic drops for symptomatic relief. Mother may give her Motrin for pain control as well. If she is not improved or has further symptoms, she should be reevaluated.

ICD-9-CM diagnosis code(s): _____

_____

ICD-10-CM diagnosis code(s): _____

_____

CPT code(s) with modifier, if applicable: _____

Review Case 3-8 Office Visit

Subjective: This 14-year-old new male patient brought to my office by his mother. He is complaining of nausea and vomiting since midnight. He also developed diarrhea about the same time. He notes that he was feeling fine yesterday. Apparently the family had a birthday party for him and everyone ate the same thing. No one else is sick. The patient, however, notes that he did spend the night at a friend's house the night before and the friend's sister was ill with vomiting and diarrhea. The patient generally is quite healthy.

Medications: He takes no medications.

Allergies: No allergies to medicines.

Review of Systems: The patient notes he has not had any black or tarry stools, although he is having watery, liquid brown stool. There was a small fleck of blood or two in the emesis he had most recently, but he has vomited almost every hour since about midnight.

History: Past, family, and social history are unremarkable.

Objective: Physical exam reveals a well-developed, well-nourished young man. He is alert and/oriented. Temperature 99, respiratory rate 20, heart rate 94, blood pressure 94/48, O_2 sat 97% on room air. The patient really is not pos-

tural, his pulse staying the same and blood pressure remaining essentially the same from supine to sitting. HEENT: On exam his TMs are clear. His pharynx is minimally injected. The neck is supple and nontender without adenopathy. The lungs are clear to auscultation. There is no CVA tenderness. The abdomen is soft. He has active bowel sounds. No peritoneal signs. He has no hepatosplenomegaly.

Assessment:

1. Acute gastroenteritis.

Plan: The patient is treated with Phenergan 25 mg IM. This did result in decrease in his nausea. We discussed giving him some IV fluids, however, at this point I do not think he is significantly volume depleted. If he goes home and stays on clear liquids for the next 24 hours and pushes fluids, he should do well. However, if he is unable to keep fluids down or develops new symptoms, he should be reevaluated. He is prescribed some Phenergan 25 mg, which he may take q4–6h prn for nausea and vomiting; total of six tablets prescribed. If he is not improved, he will be reevaluated.

ICD-9-CM diagnosis code(s): _____

_____

ICD-10-CM diagnosis code(s): _____

_____

CPT code(s) with modifier, if applicable: _____

_____

Review Case 3-9 Office Visit

Subjective: The patient is well known by me. She is a 34-year-old female who presents with several days of malaise, generalized abdominal pain, and nausea. She states that for about three days now she has had an achy feeling associated with a headache and some chills. She has had transient intermittent abdominal pain as well in multiple areas, no one area. She has had some loose bowel movements. She was nauseated somewhat and vomited once.

Objective: On examination she is noted to have normal vital signs with the exception of a low-grade fever of 100.6. She is noted to have clear lung fields bilaterally. Examination of the abdomen reveals hyperactive bowel sounds but no tenderness and there is no organomegaly. There is no costovertebral angle tenderness. HEENT: The throat is nonerythematous. Mouth shows normal mucosa with adequate saliva. The neck is supple. Extremities are unremarkable.

Assessment:

1. Viral gastroenteritis.

Plan: Fluid, clear liquid diet with increased amounts of clear liquids frequently. Tylenol or aspirin as needed for malaise or fever. Darvocet-N 100 small prescription of 10 is written to take as needed for abdominal pain. Recheck if not improving after the next three or so days.

ICD-10-CM diagnosis code(s): _____

_____

CPT code(s) with modifier, if applicable: _____

_____

Review Case 3-10 Urgent Care

Subjective: The patient is a 10-year-old brought to Urgent Care by his mother. He apparently complained of pain when he was urinating. It is not entirely clear just when this occurred but apparently he was uncomfortable enough that he called his mother from school. The mother notes that he was perfectly well this morning. She tells me that he really has not had any significant illness although he has had his appendix out and he has some mild asthma. The patient denies any nausea or vomiting. He has had no diarrhea. He denies any chills. Mother notes that he does not feel feverish. There has been no prior history of urinary symptoms and he denies any back or flank pain.

Objective: Physical exam reveals a well-developed, well-nourished 8-year-old child. He is alert and oriented. Vitals are within normal limits and he is afebrile. Exam of his abdomen reveals it is soft. He has active bowel sounds; he has no peritoneal signs. It is interesting to note that he is tender to palpation in the suprapubic area. His tenderness is exacerbated by having him contract his abdominal muscles. It turns out that he was doing sit-ups or crunches with his mother this morning. She did 30 and he apparently did 30 as well. I do not feel we need to get a urine on this child. I think this is an abdominal wall strain.

Assessment:

1. Abdominal wall tenderness.

Plan: Mother is advised to treat him with Motrin and avoid certain activities that aggravate the pain.

ICD-10-CM diagnosis code(s): _____

_____

CPT code(s) with modifier, if applicable: _____

_____

Review Case 3-11 Office Consultation

History of Present Illness: This 37-year-old Caucasian male was referred to me by Dr. Misky for evaluation of his sinuses. He has a long history of chronic pressure pain symptoms involving the left side of the face. He also has chronic cough and generalized malaise. He has been found to have a totally opacified left maxillary sinus, which has not resolved with prolonged and adequate medical treatment. He has misshapen sinuses bilaterally secondary to a congenital midface deformity

Past Medical History: Otherwise reasonable benign. Patient takes Centrax occasionally for anxiety and is currently on Ceftin as an antibiotic.

Drug Allergies: He denies any allergies

Medications: Centrax occasionally. Ceftin currently.

Family History: Noncontributory.

Social History: Noncontributory.

Review of Systems: Negative.

Physical Examination:

General: Well-developed male in no acute distress.

HEENT: Eyes are clear. Ear canals and drums are within normal limits. The nose reveals a nasal septal deviation with a spur deformity to the left that is not obstructive to the nasal airway but may very well obstruct the middle meatus. Oral cavity is clear.

Neck: Negative.

Lungs: Clear to percussion and auscultation.

Cardiovascular: Regular rate and rhythm without murmurs or gallops.

Abdomen: Benign.

Extremities: Within normal limits.

Genitorectal: Waived as clinically not necessary.

Impression: Chronic left maxillary sinusitis.

Recommendations: Schedule this patient for a Caldwell Luc procedure. The patient does not wish to proceed with nasal surgery for the septal spur.

ICD-10-CM diagnosis code(s): _____

_____

CPT code(s) with modifier, if applicable: _____

_____

Review Case 3-12 Office Visit

Chief Complaint: Abdominal adhesive disease, probable right salpingitis versus chronic interval appendicitis.

History of Present Illness: This is a 25-year-old white female with a history of right pelvic pain. She had initial flare approximately three weeks ago and I gave her five days of IV antibiotic followed by a week of po antibiotic and had near but not complete resolution of her pain. It was associated with some GI complaints, though not notable. Ultrasound was performed which showed a generously sized right ovary consistent with oophoritis or normal variant. The patient is quite large. Appendix was not visualized. She is not status postoperative laparoscopy with lysis of adhesions, appendectomy, ovarian biopsy, tubal dye perfusion. She tolerated it well but because of previous infection and likelihood of involved infection she is kept for further antibiotic therapy.

Allergies: NKDA

Medications: Proventil inhaler prn, Voltaren, 50 mg, 1 to 2 q six hours, Lortab and Vibramycin.

Past History: She has chronic hypertension and obesity. She has a history of previous cesarean section.

Family History: Significant for history of unknown malignancy in her father, specifics unknown, as well as some hypertension.

Social History: She smokes greater than one pack per day, denies significant use of alcohol or recreational drugs.

Review of Systems: Negative.

Physical Examination:

Vital Signs: Blood pressure 140/90. She is afebrile.

General: Alert and appropriate. Skin is clear.

HEENT/Neck: Unremarkable.

Lungs: Clear to auscultation with decreased pulmonary excursion secondary to habitus.

Cardiovascular: Regular rate and rhythm.

Abdomen: Soft, bowel sounds are normal. Incisions are dry.

Extremities: Unremarkable.

Genitorectal: Unremarkable.

Impression:

1. Persistent right pelvic pain.

Recommendations:

1. Proceed with a laparoscopic evaluation.

ICD-9-CM diagnosis code(s): _____

_____

ICD-10-CM diagnosis code(s): _____

_____

CPT code(s) with modifier, if applicable: _____

_____

Review Case 3-13   Urgent Care

Subjective: This 51-year-old female presents to Urgent Care. She is complaining of sore throat. Patient has been ill now for about three days with sore throat, cough, and earache. She notes her cough is productive of green sputum. She also complains of some fatigue, some backache and her chest hurts when she coughs; it is waking her at night. The patient takes no medications regularly, has no significant medical problems.

Objective: Physical exam reveals a well-developed, well-nourished female who is alert and oriented. Vitals show a temperature of 98.5, respiratory rate of 18, heart rate 90, blood pressure 113/63, her O_2 sat is 97% on room air. TMs are clear bilaterally although there is a little fluid present. They are not red or injected. Her oropharynx shows moderate injection without exudates. Neck is supple with few anterior cervical nodes. She is not tender over maxillary sinuses. Lungs are clear to auscultation.
A quick Strep test was obtained that was negative.

Assessment:

1. Acute upper respiratory infection with bronchitis and pharyngitis.

Plan: The patient was advised in symptomatic treatment, fluids, Robitussin during the day, Motrin or Tylenol. She is given some Hycodan, which she can take at bedtime for cough control. If she is not improved she should be reevaluated.

ICD-9-CM diagnosis code(s): _____

_____

ICD-10-CM diagnosis code(s): _____

_____

CPT code(s) with modifier, if applicable: _____

_____

Review Case 3-14   Office Consultation

Chief Complaint: Penile irritation

History of Present Illness: The 50-year-old male patient came in referred by Dr. Emmers. He has been experiencing a problem with his penis for six months. His general health is pretty well okay, except he did have a double bypass and hip surgery in the past. He had two heart attacks before that time. The only medications that he takes are occasional aspirin.

Drug Allergies: None.

Medications: None.

Past History: Previous bypass

Family History: Negative

Social History: Unremarkable.

Review of Systems: Skin and lymphatic normal. HEENT normal. Chest clear to auscultation, regular sinus without problems. Abdomen negative. GI negative. Back and extremities negative. Neurological negative. Hematological negative. Endocrine negative.

Physical Examination:

Vital Signs: Temperature normal. Pulse 72 and regular. Blood pressure normal. Respirations 16 and regular.

General: Well-developed male.

Ears: TMs normal, hears well in left and right.

Eyes: Pupils equal and reactive to light and accommodation.

HEENT/Neck: Head normocephalic. Neck is supple.

Neurological: Normal.

Lungs: Chest is clear to auscultation.

Cardiovascular: Regular sinus rhythm, no murmurs.

Abdomen: Soft without masses, organomegaly, tenderness, or bruits.

Extremities: Normal.

Genitorectal: Genitalia normal. Rectal exam demonstrated a normal prostate gland.

Impression:

1. Irritation of the penis underneath the foreskin, no evidence of any significant abnormality today.

Recommendations: To perform a circumcision. We will schedule this with my receptionist for next week.

ICD-10-CM diagnosis code(s): _____

_____

CPT code(s) with modifier, if applicable: _____

_____

| **Review Case 3-15** | **Pathology Report** |

Operation:
Right inguinal hernia repair.

Gross Description: Submitted from the right inguinal region are portions of purplish-tan, membranous, fibrous connective tissue that together measure approximately 4.5 cm. Representative portions are submitted for examination.

Microscopic Description: Sections reveal fibrovascular connective and adipose tissue. Portions of the tissue have a sac-like configuration with the lumen lined by mesothelial cells.

Diagnosis:

1. Hernia sac.

ICD-10-CM diagnosis code(s): _____

_____

CPT code(s) with modifier, if applicable: _____

_____

| **Review Case 3-16** | **Pathology Report** |

Operation: Laparoscopy with lysis of adhesions, left ovarian biopsy, tubal dye perfusion, and appendectomy.

Gross Description: The tortuous appendix is 11 cm in length, 5 mm in width, and blends with abundant mesoappendix. The serosal surface of the appendix is smooth; the wall is firm; the lumen contains firm brown fecal material. The specimen labeled left ovarian biopsy consists of two irregular portions of light gray or dark red hemorrhagic tissue, the larger 25 × 10 × 5 mm.

Microscopic Description: Done.

Diagnosis:

1. Appendix normal.
2. Segment, ovary, normal, left side.

Comment: The entire appendix was examined microscopically and there is no evidence of an acute or subacute appendicitis. There is also no evidence of periappendicitis such as one might expect to find in pelvic inflammatory disease.

The left ovarian biopsy reveals normal ovarian stroma containing a few primordial follicles.

ICD-10-CM diagnosis code(s): _____

_____

CPT code(s) with modifier, if applicable: _____

_____

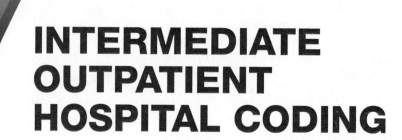

INTERMEDIATE OUTPATIENT HOSPITAL CODING

Learning Objectives

After reading this chapter, you should be able to:

- Spell and define the key terms presented in this chapter.
- Distinguish between an inpatient and an outpatient in the hospital setting.
- Describe coding in the emergency department.
- Describe Medicare's Ambulatory Payment Classification (APC) system.
- List and apply the steps required to properly code emergency department cases.
- Describe coding for same-day surgeries and observations.
- List and apply the steps required to properly code same-day surgery and observation cases.

Key Terms

Ambulatory Payment Classification (APC) system—the outpatient prospective payment system (OPPS) used by Medicare to reimburse hospitals for outpatient services and procedures

ancillary services—outpatient services in the hospital such as lab, x-ray, and therapy services

critical access hospital (CAH)—a hospital that provides 24-hour emergency services in a rural area and that is located more than 35 miles from another hospital

emergency room (ER)—the emergency room in a hospital

facility E/M—a hospital's evaluation and management (E/M) level used to capture resources utilized by the facility under the APC reimbursement system

observation (OBSV)—occurs when a patient is not formally admitted as an inpatient but whose condition warrants a hospital observation and stay to investigate further

same-day surgery (SDS)—surgery in which a patient presents for an outpatient surgery and will go home on the same day

INTRODUCTION

In this chapter, we explore the world of coding for the outpatient hospital coder. Hospital outpatient coders are typically responsible for coding all outpatient accounts, which can include ancillary services, such as laboratory, radiology, and physical therapy; however, the majority of outpatient hospital coding typically involves coding emergency room (ER) accounts, same-day surgery

(SDS) accounts, and observation (OBSV) accounts. In all outpatient accounts the ICD-9-CM official outpatient coding guidelines are followed. Outpatient coders report ICD-9-CM codes for diagnoses and CPT® codes for procedures; they do *not* use the ICD-9-CM, Volume 3, procedure codes in an outpatient setting. (*Note:* Outpatient coders will report ICD-10-CM codes when they replace the ICD-9-CM codes on October 1, 2014.)

CPT-4 codes in this chapter are from the CPT-4 2012 code set. CPT is a registered trademark of the American Medical Association.
ICD-9-CM codes in this chapter are from the ICD-9-CM 2012 code set from the Department of Health and Human Services, Centers for Disease Control and Prevention.
ICD-10-CM codes in this chapter are from the ICD-10-CM 2012 Draft code set from the Department of Health and Human Services, Centers for Disease Control and Prevention.

PATIENT TYPES IN THE HOSPITAL SETTING

As coders, we need to not only understand the different patient types but also know how to code each one of them. A hospital setting has two distinct patient types: inpatients and outpatients. Inpatients are those who are formally admitted to a hospital for treatment. Outpatients are those who are seen without being formally admitted to the hospital. The most common types of outpatients that impact coding are those seen in the ER and the SDS department. The ER is for those patients who have an emergency situation needing critical care or immediate attention, and sometimes for those who cannot get in to see their physician. SDS patients are those who are having surgery as an outpatient. SDS surgeries are performed on the same day the patient comes in for the surgery, and the SDS patient returns home on the same day of the surgery. SDS surgeries are typically routine procedures, such as hernia repairs, colonoscopies, carpal tunnel release, cataracts, and esophagogastroduodenoscopies.

CODING IN THE EMERGENCY DEPARTMENT

The emergency department or, as it is often called, the emergency room (ER) is typically a very busy place and a variety of patients are seen in the ER. Some of the patients have minor injuries and illnesses, and some have more serious emergency conditions, such as traumas, poisonings, or myocardial infarctions. As an ER coder you will be exposed to a variety of conditions and are expected to know how to code each one correctly. To start, let's discuss what is typically coded in an ER setting.

ER coders will assign a diagnosis code for any applicable diagnosis and must follow the official ICD-9-CM outpatient coding guidelines. (To access these guidelines, see Appendix A.) Any applicable diagnosis would be the primary diagnosis the patient is being seen for as well as any other complicating diagnosis that may exist, such as diabetes. ER coders do not report codes for previous conditions, such as a previous myocardial infarction, unless it relates to what the patient is being seen for in the ER. When coding a procedure in the ER setting, remember that an outpatient account gets assigned CPT procedure codes, so the ER coder will assign ICD-9 diagnoses and CPT procedures. The ER coder does not report codes that are captured via the chargemaster, which are the CPT codes that start with a 7, 8, or 9. The exception is EM codes, which are not in the chargemaster (see next section). So, ER coders will assign CPT codes in the 10000–69999 range. This is also true for HCPCS; all HCPCS codes are also kept in the chargemaster and are not reported by the coders.

ER E/M Level

If you recall your beginner course when you learned how to use E/M codes, there are E/M codes for services provided in the ER. These ER E/M codes include codes in the range of 99281–99285, 99288, and the critical care codes 99291–99292. Not every ER coder will report the ER E/M codes for an ER account—it depends on whether the ER physician is a subcontractor or an employee of the hospital. If the physician is a subcontractor, then she will typically have her own coding staff to code and bill for the services she provides. If the physician is an employee of the hospital, then the hospital coders who code for the emergency department are typically responsible for also coding the professional services, which would include those performed by the physician.

Facility E/M Level

With the implementation of Medicare's Ambulatory Payment Classifications (APC) system, Outpatient Prospective Payment System (OPPS), in 2000, hospitals were required to develop a facility E/M level in which to report a facility E/M. Hospitals that are paid based on the APC system report a facility E/M level in order to recuperate some of the monies spent on patient care in the ER, such as nursing care and respiratory and radiology services. Items such as supplies and the room are reported by using a facility E/M level. The facility E/M level is similar to the CPT ER E/M level for physicians. The APC is calculated from the CPT codes and is used to determine reimbursement in the outpatient setting.

Not every hospital is paid based on the APC system. One type of hospital that is not is a critical access hospital (CAH). A critical access hospital is one that provides 24-hour emergency services in a rural area and that is located more than 35 miles from another hospital. A CAH typically is small and does not have more than 25 inpatient beds.

When APCs were implemented on August 1, 2000, every facility was given the direction, under CMS, to devise its own E/M leveling system, so the facility E/M level may be different from facility to facility. In this book we will not report a facility E/M level because of these differences. ■FIGURE 4-1 shows an example of a facility E/M level sheet.

Coding Emergency Room Cases

The steps to coding ER visits are as follows:

1. Read through the documentation and determine the reason for the visit, that is, the primary diagnosis. Determine if any other complicating or coexisting diagnosis exists.
2. Read through the documentation and determine what service or procedure the patient received.
3. Locate the correct diagnosis codes using the ICD-9-CM coding manual, Volumes 1 and 2. To locate the correct ICD-10 code, you may utilize an electronic encoder, refer to the ICD-10-CM draft code set, or use a website such as www.icd10data.com to either look up the ICD-10 codes or convert the ICD-9 codes to ICD-10 codes.
4. Locate the correct procedure codes using your CPT-4 coding manual.
5. Check to see if a modifier is needed on the procedure code.
6. Assign the correct diagnoses and procedure codes to the patient's chart.
7. Verify codes in the Tabular Index.
8. Optional: Using an encoder, generate APC assignment.

Facility Charge Assignment		
Level	**Possible Interventions**	**Potential Symptoms/Examples That Support the Interventions**
I **CPT 99281** Type A: APC 609 Type B: APC 626 HCPCS: G0380	Initial assessment No medication or treatments Rx refill only, asymptomatic Note for work or school Wound recheck Booster or follow-up immunization, no acute injury Dressing changes (uncomplicated) Suture removal (uncomplicated) Discussion of discharge Instructions (Straightforward)	Insect bite (uncomplicated) Read Tb test

II
 	
CPT 99282
 	
Type A: APC 613
Type B: APC 627
HCPCS: G0381
	Could include interventions from previous levels,
	    plus any of:
	Tests by ED staff (urine dip, stool Hemoccult,
	    Accu-Chek or Dextrostix)
	Visual acuity (Snellen)
	Obtain clean-catch urine
	Apply Ace wrap or sling
	Prep or assist w/procedures such as minor
	    laceration repair, I&D of simple abscess, etc.
	Discussion of discharge instructions (simple)
		Localized skin rash, lesion, sunburn
		Minor viral infection
		Eye discharge–painless
		Ear pain
		Urinary frequency without fever
		Simple trauma (with no x-rays)

III
 	
CPT 99283
 	
Type A: APC 614
Type B: APC 628
HCPCS: G0382
	Could include interventions from previous levels,
	    plus any of:
	Receipt of EMS/ambulance patient
	Heparin/saline lock
	(1) Nebulizer treatment
	Preparation for lab tests described in CPT
	    (80048-87999 codes)
	Preparation for EKG
	Preparation for plain x-rays of only 1 area (hand,
	    shoulder, pelvis, etc.)
	Prescription medications administered PO
	Foley catheters; In & Out caths
	C-spine precautions
	Fluorescein stain
	Emesis/incontinence care
	Prep or assist w/procedures such as joint
	    aspiration/injection, simple fracture care, etc.
	Mental health–anxious, simple treatment
	Routine psych medical clearance
	Limited social worker intervention
	Postmortem care
	Direct admit via ED
	Discussion of discharge instructions (moderate
	    complexity)
		Minor trauma (with potential complicating factors)
		Medical conditions requiring prescription drug
		    management
		Fever that responds to antipyretics
		Headache–Hx of, no serial exam
		Head injury–without neurologic symptoms
		Eye pain
		Mild dyspnea–not requiring oxygen

Figure 4-1 ■ Sample facility E/M level sheet. Reprinted with permission of the American College of Emergency Physicians.

Facility Charge Assignment		
Level	**Possible Interventions**	**Potential Symptoms/Examples That Support the Interventions**
IV **CPT 99284** Type A: APC 615 Type B: APC 629 HCPCS: G0383	Could include interventions from previous levels, plus any of: Preparation for 2 diagnostic tests: labs, EKG, x-ray Prep for plain x-ray (multiple body areas): C-spine & foot, shoulder & pelvis Prep for special imaging study (CT, MRI, ultrasound, VQ scans) Cardiac monitoring (2) Nebulizer treatments Port-a-cath venous access Administration and monitoring of infusions or parenteral medications (IV, IM, IO, SC) NG/PEG Tube placement/replacement multiple reassessments Prep or assist w/procedures such as eye irrigation with Morgan lens, bladder irrigation with 3-way Foley, pelvic exam, etc. Sexual assault exam w/out specimen collection Psychotic patient; not suicidal Discussion of discharge instructions (complex)	Blunt/penetrating trauma–with limited diagnostic testing Headache with nausea/vomiting Dehydration requiring treatment Vomiting requiring treatment Dyspnea requiring oxygen Respiratory illness relieved with (2) nebulizer treatments Chest pain–with limited diagnostic testing Abdominal pain–with limited diagnostic testing Nonmenstrual vaginal bleeding Neurologic symptoms–with limited diagnostic testing
V **CPT 99285** Type A: APC 616 Type B: APC 630 HCPCS: G0384	Could include interventions from previous levels, plus any of: Requires frequent monitoring of multiple vital signs (i.e., O_2 sat, BP, cardiac rhythm, respiratory rate) Preparation for ≥ 3 diagnostic tests: labs, EKG, x-ray Prep for special imaging study (CT, MRI, ultrasound, VQ scan) combined with multiple tests or parenteral medication or oral or IV contrast. Administration of blood transfusion/blood products Oxygen via face mask or NRB Multiple nebulizer treatments: (3) or more (if nebulizer is continuous, each 20-minute period is considered treatment) Moderate Sedation Prep or assist with procedures such as central line insertion, gastric lavage, LP, paracentesis, etc. Cooling or heating blanket Extended social worker intervention Sexual assault exam w/specimen collection by ED staff Coordination of hospital admission/transfer or change in living situation or site Physical/chemical restraints Suicide watch Critical care less than 30 minutes	Blunt/penetrating trauma requiring multiple diagnostic tests Systemic multi-system medical emergency requiring multiple diagnostics Severe infections requiring IV/IM antibiotics Uncontrolled DM Severe burns Hypothermia New-onset altered mental status Headache (severe): CT and/or LP Chest pain–multiple diagnostic tests/treatments Respiratory illness–relieved by (3) or more nebulizer treatments Abdominal pain–multiple diagnostic tests/treatments Major musculoskeletal injury Acute peripheral vascular compromise of extremities Neurologic symptoms–multiple diagnostic tests/treatments Toxic ingestions Mental health problem–suicidal/homicidal

Figure 4-1 ■ *(Continued)*

Critical Care

Critical Care can be coded based upon either the provision of any of the listed possible interventions or by satisfying the Critical Care definition. A minimum of 30 minutes of care must be provided. Critical Care involves decision-making of high complexity to assess, manipulate, and support impairments of "one or more vital organ systems such that there is a high probability of imminent or life-threatening deterioration in the patient's condition." This includes, but is not limited to, "the treatment or prevention of further deterioration of central nervous system failure, shock-like conditions, renal, hepatic, metabolic or respiratory failure, post-operative complications or overwhelming infection." Under OPPS, the time that can be reported as Critical Care is the time spent by a physician and/or hospital staff engaged in active face-to-face critical care of a critically ill or critically injured patient. If the physician and hospital staff or multiple hospital staff members are simultaneously engaged in this active face-to-face care, the time involved can only be counted once.

Level	Facility Charge Assignment	
	Possible Interventions	**Potential Symptoms/Examples That Support the Interventions**
CPT 99291 Type A: APC 617	Could include interventions from previous levels, plus any or all of: Multiple parenteral medications requiring constant monitoring Provision of any of the following: Major trauma care/multiple surgical consultants Chest tube insertion Major burn care Treatment of active chest pain in ACS Administration of IV vasoactive meds (see guidelines) CPR Defibrillation/cardioversion Pericardiocentesis Administration of ACLS drugs in cardiac arrest Therapeutic hypothermia Bi-PAP/CPAP Endotracheal intubation Cricothyrotomy Ventilator management Arterial line placement Control of major hemorrhage Pacemaker insertion through a central line Delivery of baby	Multiple trauma; head injury with loss of consciousness Burns threatening to life or limb Coma of all etiologies (except hypoglycemic) Shock of all types: septic, cardiogenic, spinal, hypovolemic, anaphylactic Drug overdose impairing vital functions Life-threatening hyper/hypothermia Thyroid storm or Addisonian crisis Cerebral hemorrhage of any type New-onset paralysis Nonhemorrhagic strokes with vital function impairment Status epilepticus Acute myocardial infarction Cardiac arrhythmia requiring emergency treatment Aortic dissection Cardiac tamponade Aneurysm; thoracic or abdominal–leaking or ruptured Tension pneumothorax Acute respiratory failure, pulmonary edema, status asthmaticus Pulmonary embolus Embolus of fat or amniotic fluid Acute renal failure Acute hepatic failure Diabetic ketoacidosis Lactic acidosis DIC or other bleeding diatheses–hemophilia, ITP, TTP, leukemia, aplastic anemia Major envenomation by poisonous reptiles
CPT 99292	As above in additional 30-minute increments. Record the TOTAL critical care time. The first 30-74 minutes equals code 99291. If used, additional 30-minute increments (beyond the first 74 minutes) are coded 99292. Medicare does not pay for code 99292 because it is considered packaged into 99291; however, the services should be reported as appropriate.	
Critical Care with Trauma Team Activation **APC 618** **G0390**	In addition to 99291, designated trauma centers may report the Trauma Team Activation code G0390 when a trauma team was activated and all other trauma activation criteria are met.	

Copyright © 2011 American College of Emergency Physicians

Figure 4-1 ■ (Continued)

LET'S PRACTICE 4-1

Emergency Room

Chief Complaint: Left lower quadrant abdominal pain.

History of Present Illness: The patient is a 56-year-old male who presents to the emergency department with about a 30-hour history of left lower quadrant abdominal pain. The pain was severe and sudden at its onset yesterday morning. It lasted several hours and resolved completely. He had return of pain about 2:00 p.m. today and it was severe at onset, but has subsided somewhat. He has noted some frequency of urination, but denies hematuria and he denies dysuria. He has been moving his bowels normally. The pain, in recent hours, moved around to his back somewhat. He has had some slight nausea, but no vomiting. He has never had similar symptoms before. He is a generally healthy man who does not take medications on an ongoing basis. He occasionally sees Dr. Milten however, he came here because he was not available today.

Physical Examination: Objectively, the patient is alert and in no acute distress.

Abdomen: There is some mild, distinct left flank tenderness. There is no particular tenderness in the left lower quadrant, but is experiencing mild to moderate tenderness in the left midabdomen to left upper quadrant. No mass or organomegaly was noted. Bowel sounds are normal.

Genital: Normal. A urinalysis was obtained that demonstrated 3+ occult blood and one to five white blood cells, 80 to 100 red blood cells, no bacteria.

Assessment: Renal colic.

Plan: The patient was not in severe distress at the time of discharge. He was allowed to go home with Lortab elixir, one, two, or three teaspoons every four to six hours as needed for pain. A total of eight ounces were prescribed. He is unable to swallow pills. He is asked to return promptly should he worsen in any way, or vomiting develops. Also, he should see his own doctor, Dr. Milten, in one or two days if he has any persistent symptoms. I did send him home with a urine strainer and asked him to return any stone he might catch for laboratory evaluation. Further care and workup per Dr. Milten.

● **HELPFUL HINTS:** The patient came in with abdominal pain, which the physician diagnosed as renal colic. You do not code the abdominal pain because that is a sign/symptom of the renal colic and is not coded separately:

- "Codes for symptoms, signs, and ill-defined conditions from Chapter 16 are not to be used as principal diagnosis when a related definitive diagnosis has been established," per the ICD-9-CM *Official Guidelines for Coding and Reporting*, Section II, "Selection of Principal Diagnosis."

The ER E/M is assigned for the expanded problem focused history, expanded problem focused exam, and moderate medical decision making.

Steps:

1. Look up colic, kidney (which is the same as renal).

2. Procedure—locate the E/M ER range, 99281–99285 and select the code where the key components match the documentation.

3. Verify codes in the Tabular Index.

4. *Optional:* Using an encoder, generate APC assignment.

Codes:

ICD-9: 788.0

ICD-10: N23

CPT: 99283

APC: 614

LET'S PRACTICE 4-2

Emergency Room

Identification: This is a 33-year-old African American female.

Chief Complaint: Back pain.

History of Present Illness: The patient is a 33-year-old female who has been complaining of low back pain she has had for approximately two to three days. She states it feels like tight muscles that are spasming. It hurts her to get in and out of her car, to rise or sit in a chair. She has no

continued

LET'S PRACTICE 4-2, *continued*

known injury or trauma. She has had no surgeries, no back trauma in the past. She has no painful radiation of her pain. It does not go down her legs. There is no numbness, no weakness. She states she has had back pains off and on for about six weeks but did not start spasming until a couple days ago. She has had no fever. She has had no urinary frequency, urgency, burning, or other urinary symptoms.

Allergies: Codeine.

Current Medications: Premarin and Dyazide.

Previous Illnesses: Denies any.

Physical Examination:

General: Well developed, well nourished, in no acute distress. Alert and oriented and answers questions appropriately.

Vitals: Blood pressure 106/72, heart rate 85, respirations 15, temperature 97.7.

Back: Examination of the low back reveals some paravertebral tightness and pain with palpation. DTRs are 2+/4 bilaterally. Muscle strength in the lower extremities is normal.

Impression:

1. Low back spasms.

Plan: Robaxin 750 mg 2 po qid, prn for pain. Darvocet-N 100 1 to 2 po q 4–6h prn for pain. Heating pad as needed. She is to do activity as tolerated but while she is having acute spasms I told her to lie in a prone position with her legs up on a couch or a chair or some similar position that this will take the load off her back. She should get this checked in a few days if she is not improving.

● **HELPFUL HINT:** The back spasm that is documented is the cause of the back pain so the back pain is not coded.

- "Codes for symptoms, signs, and ill-defined conditions from Chapter 16 are not to be used as principal diagnosis when a related definitive diagnosis has been established," per the ICD-9-CM *Official Guidelines for Coding and Reporting*, Section II, "Selection of Principal Diagnosis."

Steps:

1. Look up spasm, muscle, back.

2. Procedure—locate E/M ER range, 99281–99285, and select the code where the key components match the documentation.

3. Verify codes in the Tabular Index.

4. *Optional:* using an encoder, generate APC assignment.

Codes:

ICD-9: 724.8

ICD-10: M62.830

CPT: 99282

APC: 613

LET'S PRACTICE 4-3

Emergency Room

Identification: This is a 2-year-old African American male.

Chief Complaint: Ear pain

History of Present Illness: The patient is here because of left ear pain for part of the day preceded by several days of runny nose.

Allergies: None.

Current Medications: None.

Previous Illnesses: Denies any.

Physical Examination:

HEENT: Very striking inflammation present to his left tympanic membrane. Normal exam of the right ear. Mild inflammation present to his throat. Exam of the heart and lungs is normal.

Impression:

1. Left otitis media.

Plan: Amoxicillin 500 mg tid for 10 days. Auralgan otic solution 3 drops to left ear q4h prn pain along with Tylenol and Motrin.

LET'S PRACTICE 4-3, *continued*

● **HELPFUL HINTS:** The ear pain is a sign/symptom of the otitis media and is not coded separately.

- "Codes for symptoms, signs, and ill-defined conditions from Chapter 16 are not to be used as principal diagnosis when a related definitive diagnosis has been established," per the ICD-9-CM *Official Guidelines for Coding and Reporting*, Section II, "Selection of Principal Diagnosis."

  For ICD-10 we need to note that it is the left ear.

Steps:

1. Look up otitis, media. It is not specified as another type, so select the code right by the subterm media.

2. Procedure—locate E/M ER range, 99281–99285 and select the code where the key components match the documentation (■ FIGURE 4-2).

3. Verify codes in the Tabular Index.

4. *Optional:* using an encoder, generate APC assignment.

Codes:

ICD-9: 382.9

ICD-10: H66.92

CPT: 99282

APC: 613

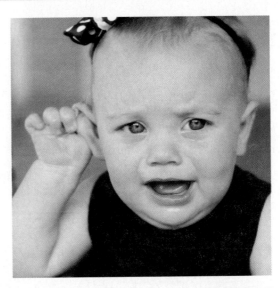

Figure 4-2 ■ This young child is pulling at the ear, a sign of otitis media.
Source: daynamore/Fotolia

LET'S PRACTICE 4-4

Emergency Room

Identification: This is a 38-year-old Caucasian female.

Chief Complaint: Sore throat.

History of Present Illness: The patient is here because of three weeks of congestion and cough with sore throat. She also had diarrhea and vomiting for a couple of days.

Allergies: None.

Current Medications: None.

Previous Illnesses: Denies any.

Physical Examination: O$_2$ saturations are 100% on room air. Temperature is 96.7. HEENT: Mild inflammation present to her throat. Fluid to the middle ear spaces bilaterally. Exam of the heart is normal. The lungs are clear. The abdomen has slightly hyperactive bowel sounds but is nontender.

Impression:

1. Pharyngitis with some sinus infection.

Plan: Z-pak and saltwater gargles.

● **HELPFUL HINTS:** The documentation does not state if these are acute or chronic, so we select the unspecified code, which is the code right beside the main term in the Alphabetic Index.

---

continued

LET'S PRACTICE 4-4, *continued*

Steps:

1. Look up pharyngitis.

2. Look up infection, sinus.

3. Procedure—locate E/M ER range, 99281–99285 and select the code where the key components match the documentation.

4. Verify the codes in the Tabular Index.

5. *Optional:* using an encoder, generate APC assignment.

Codes:

ICD-9: 462, 473.9

ICD-10: J02.9, J32.9

CPT: 99283

APC: 614

LET'S PRACTICE 4-5

Health Record Face Sheet

Western Regional
Medical Center

Record Number:	58-16-18
Age:	28
Gender:	Female
Length of Stay:	Not Applicable
Diagnosis/Procedure:	Nausea
Service Type:	Emergency Room
Discharge Status:	Home

This is the health record face sheet where you will find documentation of patient demographic information.

Coders utilize demographic information such as age, gender, service type, and discharge status.

In the clinical setting, a face sheet will also contain patient financial information.

This is the admit diagnosis.

Remember—this is not the primary diagnosis as documented by the physician on discharge.

Admit Diagnosis Code:

ICD-9: 787.02 Nausea Alone

ICD-10: R11.0 Nausea

LET'S PRACTICE 4-5, *continued*

This an Emergency Room Record - Physician Documentation.

The physician documents patient findings, physician orders for lab, radiology, and pharmacological treatment during the treatment of the patient.

The physician also documents the final discharge diagnosis and procedures, results of laboratory and or radiology tests, and discharge instructions.

Diagnosis (hand written by physician) documents the primary diagnosis as "Acute Gastroenteritis." This will be your first listed or primary diagnosis code for this episode of care.

Acute gastroenteritis codes to:

Primary diagnosis ICD-9: 558.9 Noninfectious gastroenteritis and colitis

ICD-10: K52.9 Noninfective gastroenteritis and colitis, unspecified

ALLERGIES		TETANUS STATUS	
CURRENT MEDS		LMP	
HISTORY & PHYSICAL T: P: R: BP: SaO₂: WT:		BY (INIT)	
		☐ STAT **LABS**	
		☐ ABG on _____ ℓ	
		☐ Admit Packet	
		☒ Amylase	
		☐ Cardiac Packet	
		☒ CBC ☐ DIFF.	
		☐ CBG on _____ ℓ	
		☒ Chem Profile _____	
		☐ CPK/ISO	
		☐ EKG	
		☐ Glucose	
		☐ HGD ☐ SERUM ☐ URINE	
		☐ Lytes	
		☐ PT/PTT	
		☐ Trauma Packet	
		☐ Type & Screen	
		☐ Type & Cross _____	
		☒ UA	
		☐ CSF	
		☐ Culture _____	
		☐	
		☐	
		☐	
TIME	TREATMENT ORDERS	☐	
	TIME	☐	
		X-RAYS	
		☐ Chest	
		☐ C-Spine	
		☐ Flat Plate/Upright (ABD)	
		☐ CT ☐ HEAD ☐ ABD	
	☐ STANDING ORDERS	☐	

DIAGNOSIS:

Acute Gastroenteritis

DISCHARGE TIME	DISCHARGE INSTRUCTIONS

I HAVE RECEIVED AND UNDERSTAND THE ABOVE INSTRUCTIONS.

PT/SD SIGNATURE X   *Antonia Maretti*

EMERGENCY DEPARTMENT RECORD

continued

LET'S PRACTICE 4-5, *continued*

HISTORY CHIEF COMPLAINT		MVA - RESTRAINED ☐ YES ☒ NO MORTORCYCLE - HELMET ☐ YES ☒ NO REPORTABLE INJURY ☐ YES ☒ NO	REPORTED TO: DATE TIME	

Nausea, Vertigo

TRIAGE

MENTAL STATUS _____ COLOR _____
RESPIRATIONS _____ SKIN TURGOR _____

☐ O₂ ☐ Elevate   ☐ MED. _____
☐ Splint ☐ Dressing   ☐ MED. _____
☐ Ice ☐ _____   TRIAGE NURS

PTA GCS CRAMS ☐ BLACKBOARD ☐ C-COLLAR ☐

ALLERGIES	*NKA*		
CURRENT MEDICATIONS	φ		☐ CURRENT ☐ ☐ NOT CURRENT ☐ ☐ TT ☐ Td ☐ ☐ DT ☐ DPT ☐
PMH	*12 weeks pregnant – miscarriages × 3*		

(NEURO, CARDIAC, RESPIRATORY,
GI, GU, SKIN, INCIDENT TIME)

LOT # _____

ASSESSMENT

Patient presents with nausea yesterday approximately 8 p.m,
emesis at 10 p.m. No emesis today, emesis ×1 during night.
Diarrhea during night. None today. Abdominal cramping
(intermittent). No original spotting. C/o dizziness last p.m.

VISUAL ACUITY   OD _____
OS _____
OU _____

WT

LMP

TIME	TEMP	P	R	BP	SaO₂ O₂	TIME	MEDICATION/DOSE	ROUTE	SITE	SIGNATURE
/ pm	97.5	80	20	110/60						
	OK	72	16	100/60						
	♀	72	16	110/60						
					/					
					/					

TIME	IV FLUID/AMOUNT	MEDICATION ADDED	RATE/HR	SIZE	SITE	TIME DC'D	AMT INFUSED	SIGNATURE
/30p	D5 1/2 ns - 100C		150cc					

TIME	PROBLEM/CHANGE	INTERVENTION	PATIENT RESPONSE / EVALUATION
/25p		*Lab drawn. u/A sent*	

SIGNATURE/
TITLE   X   *Mary Houser, RN*

SIGNATURE/
TITLE   X

☐ SEE ADDENDUM ED
NURSES FLOW SHEET

DISCHARGE TIME: 3:45 PM	**PATIENT BELONGINGS** BAG ON PT. NONE
DISPOSITION ☒ Discharged ☐ AMA ☐ Admit/Transfer _____ Report Given To: _____ **CONDITION ON DISCHARGE/TRANSFER** ☒ Stable ☐ Stabilized ☐ Improved ☐ Expired **DISCHARGE MODE:** ☒ Ambutatory ☐ Wheelchair ☐ Stretcher ☐ Carried Accom. by _____	Clothing _____ ☐ ☐ ☐ Wallet/Purse _____ ☐ ☐ ☐ Money _____ ☐ ☐ ☐ Jewelry _____ ☐ ☐ ☐ Glasses _____ ☐ ☐ ☐ Dentures _____ ☐ ☐ ☐ DISPOSITION: ☐ Not Disrobed ☐ Patient ☐ Family ☐ Security ☐ SEE BELONGINGS LIST

ED NURSES FLOW SHEET

Emergency Department Record – Nursing Documentation

Remember that the physician documentation is the definitive patient information.

A coder may utilize nursing documentation as a verification or clarification but MAY NOT ASSIGN codes for diagnoses or procedures that are documented only by nursing personnel.

Nursing documentation provides valuable insight to the patient and may complete the clinical picture with nursing patient care issues, concerns, and response to specific treatments.

LET'S PRACTICE 4-5, *continued*

The next record is a laboratory report. A coder MAY NOT code directly from these reports because they are not physician documentation.

However, coders typically review laboratory reports during the initial record review because the laboratory results support case-specific physician diagnoses.

There may be times when significant abnormalities such as "flags" are seen in this documentation. A "flag" attached to a laboratory value denotes a high or low value or the presence of an organism.

Look for the "L" designations for BUN, SGPT, SBGT, LDH, sodium, and cholesterol.

Be sure to look for physician documentation regarding the importance or nonimportance of high or low laboratory values.

A coder may wish to perform a "physician query" when warranted with regard to lab values and lack of documentation addressing the abnormal lab values.

Test Name	Result	Flags	Units	Low	High	Comments
LABORATORY RESULTS FOR A CHEMISTRY SCREEN						
GLUCOSE	78		mg/d	70	110	
BUN	6	L	mg/d	7	24	
CREATININE	0.6		mg/d	0.6	1.3	
BUN/ CREATININE RATIO	10.0			0.0	40.0	
URIC ACID	3.3		mg/d	2.6	5.6	
TOTAL BILIRUBIN	0.53		mg/d	0.00	1.00	
DIRECT BILIRUBIN	0.19		mg/d	0.00	0.30	
INDIRECT BILIRUBIN	0.34		mg/d	0.00	0.90	
ALK PHOSPHATASE	70		U/L	50	136	
SGPT	22	L	U/L	30	65	
SGOT	14	L	U/L	15	37	
LDH	80	L	U/L	100	190	
GTP	15		U/L	5	85	
TOTAL PROTEIN	6.7		g/dl	6.4	8.2	
ALBUMIN	4.0		g/dl	3.4	5.0	
GLOBULIN	2.7		g/dl	2.0	3.5	
A/G RATIO	1.5			1.0	2.5	
CALCIUM	9.2		mg/d	8.8	10.5	
PHOSPHORUS	3.6		mg/d	2.5	4.9	
IRON	81		ug/d	35	150	
SODIUM	137	L	mmol	140	148	
POTASSIUM	4.2		mmol	3.6	5.2	
CHLORIDE	103		mmol	100	108	
CHOLESTEROL	127	L	mg/d	130	200	
TRIGLYCERIDE	66		mg/d	30	200	
AMYLASE	48		U/L	25	115	

continued

LET'S PRACTICE 4-5, *continued*

URINALYSIS DRUG SCREEN		
☐ DRUG SCREEN	☐ RANDOM ☐ CATHETERIZED ☒ CLEAN CATCH	
ROUTINE		
COLOR	Yellow	
APPEARANCE	Hazey	
GLUCOSE	0	
BILIRUBIN	0	
KETONE	0	
SPEC GRAVITY	1.018	
BLOOD	0	
pH	9.0	
PROTEIN	30 mg/dl	
UROBILINOGEN	Normal	
NITRITE	0	
LEUKOCYTES	0	
MICROSCOPIC / HPF		
WBC	0-1	
RBC	0-1	
EPITH, CELLS	10-15	
BACTERIA	0	
MUCOUS THREADS	0	
CRYSTALS	3+ Amorpsl	
CASTS	0	
CLINITEST		
DRUG SCREEN		
AMPHETAMINE		
BARBITURATE		
BENZODIAZEPINE		
COCAINE		
MARIJUANA		
OPIATE		
TRICYCLIC ANTIDEPRESSANTS (SERUM)		
FOR CONFIRMATION OF POSITIVE SCREENS, CHECK HERE ☐		

LABORATORY REPORT SERIES

LET'S PRACTICE 4-6

Health Record Face Sheet

Documentation of patient demographic information

Demographic information utilized in coding: age, gender, service type, and discharge status

Admitting diagnosis is listed on the face sheet.

Remember – this is not the primary/principal diagnosis as documented by the physician on discharge. Remember, the final diagnosis is referred to as the principal diagnosis for inpatient coding and the primary diagnosis for outpatient coding.

Admit Diagnosis Code:

ICD-9: 784.0 Headache

ICD-10: R51 Headache

Health Record Face Sheet

Western Regional
Medical Center

Record Number:	52-98-63
Age:	44
Gender:	Male
Length of Stav:	Not Applicable
Diagnosis/Procedure:	Cephalgia
Service Type:	Emergency Room
Discharge Status:	To Home

continued

LET'S PRACTICE 4-6, continued

EMERGENCY DEPARTMENT

BRIEF HISTORY

Patient returns to ER for evaluation of headache. He was in the ER for same evaluation on Monday 2 pm.

		NOTIFIED TIME:	RELATIVE ☐ FRIEND ☐ POLICE ☐ CORONER ☐ BY WHOM		
PRESENT MEDS	PAST ILLNESSES	ALLERGIES	LAST TETANUS	WEIGHT	
Valium	*cephalgia*	*NKA*		HEIGHT	

TIME	TEMP.	PULSE	RESP.	B/P	ORDERS	TIME	MEDICATION/TREATMENT
2350	96°	92	18	132/108		0010	*75 mg Demerol 25 mg Phenegran IM*
					75 mg Demerol		*R hip*
					25 mg Phenegran		*Pt states relief*

PHYSICIAN'S CLINICAL NOTES: NURSE'S SIGNATURE

Mary Houser, RN

Dictated

Assess - Cephalgia - Possible Cluster Headache

Plan -   1) IM pain meds

2) D/C Valium

3) Vicodin ES #25

4) F/U with Neurologist as scheduled

Physician Signature:

J. Johnson, D.O.

Emergency Department Record – Nursing Documentation

Remember that the physician documentation is the definitive patient information.

A coder may utilize nursing documentation as a verification or clarification but MAY NOT ASSIGN codes for diagnoses or procedures that are documented only by nursing personnel.

Nursing documentation provides valuable insight to the patient and may complete the clinical picture with nursing patient care issues, concerns, and response to specific treatments.

This form is unique in that nursing documentation is found on the top half of the form and physician documentation may be found on the lower half of this form.

LET'S PRACTICE 4-6, *continued*

Emergency Department Record- Physician Dictated Report

Dictated by physician and then word processed by a medical transcriptionist or "clinical documentation specialist."

This report is dictated in a format known as "SOAP" format:

S = Subjective
O = Objective
A = Assessment
P = Plan

Read this entire report using the SOAP documentation to determine your E/M level and the assessment for the primary diagnosis. In this case, the cephalgia.

Subjective documentation states that the patient was given an injection of Demerol and Phenegran in the emergency room.

Injections are noninvasive procedures and are not coded by the medical coder in a hospital setting, as these services are captured in the hospital chargemaster.

Assessment documentation: Cephalgia is documented by the physician as the primary diagnosis (DX).

Cephalgia is the DX. Possible diagnosis of cluster headaches may not be coded in the outpatient setting per ICD-9-CM official outpatient coding guidelines and conventions.

DX:

ICD-9: 784.0 Headache
ICD-10: R51 Headache

Remember that outpatient coding conventions state that possible diagnoses may not be coded.

EMERGENCY DEPARTMENT VISIT

DOB: 1/15/1968

SUBJECTIVE: This 44 year old male presents to the Emergency Room complaining of persistent headache. The patient notes he has been actually having problems with headaches for over a year and a half. He has had numerous work ups with ENT specialists, family physicians, a dentist and most recently, he is scheduled to see a neurologist at the University Medical Center on 3/14/xxxx. The patient describes headaches which occur in clusters. They are quite severe, lasting six to eight hours at a time. Generally they are one-sided, either the right side or the left side of his face. He does occasionally have some nasal rhinitis with these headaches, but denies any tearing of his eyes. The patient notes he is unable to sleep and extremely miserable with these headaches. He was seen as recently as last Saturday by Dr. Hungarti in the Emergency Room, was given an injection of Demerol and Phenergan with adequate relief of the headaches for the last three days. He notes in the last 24 hours the headaches have returned, coming with increasing intensity and severity. The patient has had fairly extensive work up today, although no CT scan apparently has been done. The patient denies any recent upper respiratory infections. He has had no fever or chills. He denies any head injuries. He also denies any stiffness in his neck.

OBJECTIVE: Physical exam reveals a well developed, well nourished male. He is alert, oriented, in no acute distress. He does have some photophobia. Vitals show slightly elevated diastolic blood pressure 132/108. TMs are clear. Pharynx is clear. His neck is supple and nontender without adenopathy. There is no tenderness to palpation over his maxillary sinuses. He does have some conjunctival injection of the right eye which is the side of this current headache. However, I do not see any significant tearing nor is there obvious flushing of his skin.

ASSESSMENT: Cephalgia, possible cluster headaches by history.

PLAN: The patient is given IM pain medications. He is advised to go home to rest quietly. I suggest he not take the Valium which was prescribed last week for him. He is given Vicodin extra strength, advised to take as little of this as possible until he is evaluated by the neurologist at the University Medical Center this coming Monday.

SAME-DAY SURGERIES AND OBSERVATIONS

Coding same-day surgeries and observations is similar to coding ER encounters in that ICD diagnoses and CPT procedures are assigned. Some hospitals may also report an ICD-9 procedure code in any outpatient setting; however, that is not required for reimbursement purposes and is only used when an encoder brings up all three code sets—not because they are needed. ER encounters, OBSVs, and SDSs are paid on APCs, which are driven only by the CPT codes. Remember, in coding, we always show medical necessity by justifying the CPT procedure code with an ICD-9 diagnosis code in the outpatient setting, so the ICD-9 procedures are not needed.

As with ER coders, OBSV and SDS coders only need to report the ICD diagnosis and CPT procedure codes within the range of 10000–69999. The CPT codes that start with 7, 8, or 9 (except for E/M codes) are in the chargemaster and not reported by the coders. The diagnoses are typically simple and consists of the reason the patient is seeking medical care. Similar to ER coding, a same-day surgery coder will also assign codes for secondary diagnoses that may complicate the patient's care, conditions that were treated, or conditions that are chronic. For example, if a coder is coding an encounter for a patient with diabetes who was seen in the SDS unit for a polypectomy, the coder would read through the documentation, including the operative report and pathology, to determine the appropriate diagnosis code for the polyps and the appropriate procedure code for the polypectomy. The coder would then review the history and physical to arrive at the type of diabetes, and then assign a code for the secondary diagnosis of diabetes.

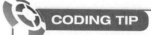

CODING TIP

Remember: Code only what was done and documented by the physician. Do not read the notes prepared by nurses, respiratory therapists, speech therapists, physical therapists, and so forth, unless you need more explanation than provided by the doctor. For example, if you are coding an encounter for a patient who is obese, you can use the dietary notes to determine the patient's body mass index; however, if the doctor did not document that the patient was obese and this is stated only in the dietary notes, it cannot be coded.

CODING TIP

You should only code for procedures performed by the physician; for example, do not code IVs, routine catheters (only if the patient had a problem and needed one), chest x-rays, or labs. Everything that is done by ancillary staff is reported in the chargemaster as a hard code and not assigned by the coder. There are some exceptions to this rule, such as when nonphysicians provide invasive care. For example, when a physical therapist completes a debridement, this would be coded by the hospital coder. Also, some hospital coders report CT scans and MRIs. Finally, when coding CPT procedures, be sure to check and see if a modifier is needed, such as RT for the right side or LT for the left, and so forth. Coders need to be fully aware of the modifiers that are applicable to the setting in which they are coding. The more a coder reviews the available coding modifiers, the easier it will be to remember the choices and uses for modifiers.

Coding Same-Day Surgery and Observation Cases

The steps to coding SDS/OBSV visits are as follows:

1. Read through the documentation and determine the reason for the visit, that is, the primary diagnosis. Determine if any other complicating or coexisting diagnosis exists.

2. Read through the documentation and determine what service or procedure the patient received.

3. Locate the correct diagnosis codes using the ICD-9-CM coding manual, Volumes 1 and 2. To begin preparing for the ICD-10 conversion, you may utilize an electronic encoder, refer to the ICD-10-CM draft code set, or use a website such as www.icd10data.com to either look up the ICD-10 codes or convert the ICD-9 codes to ICD-10 codes.

4. Locate the correct procedure code using your CPT-4 coding manual.

5. Check to see if a modifier is needed on the procedure code.

6. Remember that in outpatient hospital coding, HCPCS codes do not have to be reported by the coder because these are hard coded by the chargemaster.

7. Verify codes in the Tabular Index.

8. *Optional:* Using an encoder, generate APC assignment.

LET'S PRACTICE 4-7

Operative Report

The patient is a 63-year-old long-time smoker who smokes one pack a day and who has become increasingly hoarse during the past several months. The patient was placed on the operating table, and under general mask anesthesia an anterior commissuroscope was used to evaluate the endolaryngeal region. Excision of a nodule right true vocal cord and vocal cord stripping were performed without complications.

● **HELPFUL HINTS:** The patient is being seen for excision of a nodule on the right true vocal code. A secondary diagnosis is smoker/tobacco abuse and the procedure is the vocal cord stripping.

Steps:

1. Look up nodule, vocal code.

2. Look up abuse, tobacco.

3. Procedure—look up laryngoscopy (■ Figure 4-3), operative (this is the correct choice because the operative report says a commissuroscope was used as documented in the scenario above). Code 31540 is selected because it's worded "with excision of tumor and stripping of vocal cords."

4. Assign applicable codes.

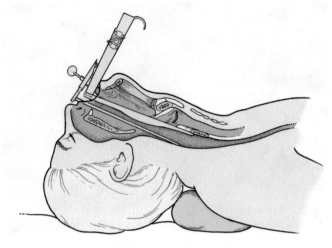

Figure 4-3 ■ Laryngoscopy.
Source: Jessica Wilson/Science Source/Photo Researchers

5. Verify codes in the Tabular Index.

6. *Optional:* Using an encoder, generate APC assignment.

Codes:

ICD-9: 478.5, 305.1

ICD-10: J38.2, F17.210

CPT: 31540

APC: 00074

LET'S PRACTICE 4-8

EGD Report

Preoperative Diagnosis: Dysphagia.

Postoperative Diagnosis: Schatzki's ring.

Operative Procedure: Esophagogastroduodenoscopy with esophageal dilation.

Description: Following informed consent the female patient was sedated with Demerol 50 mg and Versed 1 mg IV. An Olympus OES type GIF-XQI0 endoscope was introduced. A ring on the distal esophagus was best seen on retroflex exam of the cardia. There was no endoscopic esophagitis. The remainder of the stomach is unrevealing as is pylorus, duodenal bulb, and several centimeters of postbulbar duodenum. The endoscope was removed and patient was dilated with Maloney balloon dilators beginning at 46

French and advancing to 50 and 52 French. She tolerated the procedure well and there were no complications acutely.

● **HELPFUL HINTS:** The preoperative diagnosis states dysphagia; however, the postoperative diagnosis explains why the procedure was done and we code the postoperative diagnosis. The procedure was done with a scope as indicated in the second sentence of the scenario above. Balloon dilators were used to dilate the esophagus.

Steps:

1. Look up Schatzki's ring (■ Figure 4-4); it is not documented as congenital, so select acquired.

continued

LET'S PRACTICE 4-8, *continued*

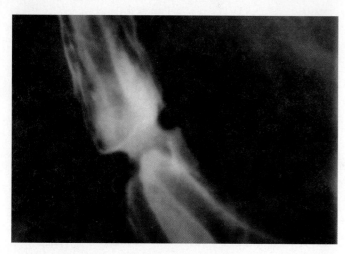

Figure 4-4 ■ X-ray image of Schatzki's ring.
Source: Bates, M.D./Custom Medical Stock Photo

2. Procedure—endoscopy, gastrointestinal, upper, dilation. Code 43249 is selected because it's worded "with balloon dilation of the esophagus."

3. Assign applicable codes.

4. Verify codes in the Tabular Index.

5. *Optional:* Using an encoder, generate APC assignment.

Codes:

ICD-9: 530.3

ICD-10: K22.2

CPT: 43249

APC: 00419

LET'S PRACTICE 4-9

Preoperative Diagnosis: Chronic left maxillary sinusitis.

Postoperative Diagnosis: Chronic left maxillary sinusitis.

Operative Procedure: Left Caldwell-Luc

Description: The patient was brought to the operating room and induced into general oral tracheal anesthesia. He was positioned, prepped, and draped in the standard fashion. 1% Xylocaine with 1:2100,000 epinephrine was infiltrated locally into the left sublabial canine fossa. 5% Cocaine on cottonoids was placed in the nostrils bilaterally. A sublabial incision was made and carried down to bone. The antrum was entered with a gouge and mallet and the enterotomy was enlarged with a Kerrison rongeur. Sinus was full of extremely thick inspissated mucus, which required a pituitary forceps to remove as it was much too thick to be suctioned. A culture was obtained. Interestingly, aside from a few very small sessile polyps along the left lateral wall, the sinus mucosa appeared reasonably healthy. A large nasal antral window was then created by egg shelling the bone over the medial wall of the sinus and creating an inferiorly based flap of nasal mucosa, which was turned into the sinus. Hemostasis was achieved with electrocoagulation. No packing was necessary. The sublabial wound was closed with interrupted 4-0 chromic.

The patient tolerated the procedure well. His throat was thoroughly suctioned and he was awakened, extu-bated, and taken to the recovery room in satisfactory condition. There were no complications.

● **HELPFUL HINTS:** In sentence 9, the physician discusses polyps that were found and then removed.

Steps:

1. Go to sinusitis, maxillary. It is not documented as acute, so select the code by the main term of maxillary.

2. Go to polyp, nose.

3. Procedure—go to Caldwell-Luc procedure, sinusotomy. Select 31032, which is the code for a Caldwell-Luc procedure with polyp removal.

4. Assign applicable codes.

5. Verify codes in the Tabular Index.

6. *Optional:* Using an encoder, generate APC assignment.

Codes:

ICD-9: 473.0, 471.8

ICD-10: J32.0, J33.8

CPT: 31032

APC: 00256

LET'S PRACTICE 4-10

Health Record Face Sheet

Western Regional
Medical Center

Record Number:	10-06-04
Age:	72
Gender:	Male
Length of Stay:	N/A
Diagnosis/Procedure:	Hernia with Repair
Service Type:	Same-Day Surgery
Discharge Status:	To Home

This is the face sheet for a same-day surgery or SDS admit.

Patient demographic information is found on the face sheet.

This is the admit diagnosis and planned procedure.

Remember—this is not the final or primary diagnosis because the primary diagnosis is determined after the actual procedure has been performed and surgical findings studied.

Admit Codes:

ICD-9: 553.1 Umbilical hernia

ICD-10: K42.9 Umbilical hernia

CPT: 49585 Repair Umbilical Hernia, 5 years and over, reducible

continued

LET'S PRACTICE 4-10, *continued*

This is the physician dictated "Discharge Summary" or the summary of care given during an episode of care.

This is the admit diagnosis. More specificity is given as to the type "umbilical" than was given on the face sheet.

This is the summary of the procedure(s) performed and the hospital course for the patient during the episode of care.

This is the final diagnosis assigned by the physician, also known as the "principal diagnosis" for inpatient coding and "primary diagnosis" for outpatient coding.

DISCHARGE SUMMARY

DATE OF ADMISSION: 05/05/XXXX

DATE OF DISCHARGE: 05/05/XXXX

ENTERING COMPLAINT:

Umbilical hernia.

PERTINENT LAB & X-RAY DATA:

There were none done.

PROCEDURES & HOSPITAL COURSE:

The patient underwent umbilical hernia repair and went home that afternoon.

DISPOSITION & REMARKS: Home and office.

CONDITION: Recovered

FINAL DIAGNOSIS:

Umbilical hernia.

OPERATION DONE: Umbilical hernia repair.

The final diagnosis generally documents the principal diagnosis for inpatient coding and the primary diagnosis for outpatient coding. The operation Done entries will document the principal procedure.

SDS or outpatient procedures utilize the ICD diagnosis code set and the CPT procedure code set.

Codes:

ICD-9: 553.1 Umbilical hernia

ICD-10: K42.9 Umbilical hernia without obstruction or gangrene

CPT: 49585 Repair Umbilical Hernia, 5 years and over, reducible

APC: 00154

This is the physician documented operation or procedure performed aka "Principle procedure".

LET'S PRACTICE 4-10, *continued*

HISTORY & PHYSICAL

DATE OF ADMISSION: 05/05/XXXX

HISTORY:

This 72-year-old man recently developed an umbilical hernia. When it first popped out it was painful. It has been painful off and on since then and whenever he is up it does bulge out. He enters now for elective repair of this small umbilical hernia because of the symptoms involved with it.

Pertinent physical findings are limited to the abdomen where he does have a small umbilical hernia. Our initial impression on this preliminary note is umbilical hernia.

This is the history and physical examination or H&P.

H&P must be dictated prior to an elective surgery or the physician must complete a handwritten H&P. If this is not done, the patient is not allowed to continue to surgery. Remember this is only for scheduled/elective surgeries.

This H&P is very minimal and really does not meet the standards of documentation required by a physician for a H&P. This type of documentation does, regretfully, happen in the real world.

Is hernia reducible? This statement by physician refers to the hernia moving inside and outside of the abdominal wall which means the hernia is reducible. Physician documentation does need to be more explicit.

continued

LET'S PRACTICE 4-10, *continued*

This is nursing pre-operative information and post-operative information for a same day surgery patient.

OUTPATIENT SURGERY

TIME	BP	TPR	NURSING REMARK:
0910	132/76	97/54/16	0910: OPS–Umbilical hernia repair. Pre op teaching done
			20 Gu NS IV started per Dr. Alvarez.
1220			RTO OPS in cart with side rails up. Awake oriente x3. States no discomfort, dress to
			umbilical in place dry intact without drainage.
1240	124/78	72/16	VS stable. Dressing without drainage. To room on floor for rest of
			recovery. Allergies: NKA or No Known Allergies

LIST ANY ALLERGIES OR OTHER SPECIAL INFORMATION:

NKA

PATIENT CONDITION ON DISCHARGE:

PHYSICIAN'S REPORT

* States blood + for Hepatitis C-can't give blood

DIAGNOSIS:

TREATMENT:

DISPOSITION:

Should this be coded? No.

The physician did not document the patient was positive for Hepatitis C. This looks to be an extension of the nursing documentation as no further physician hand written documentation is given.

The physician "dictated" this part of the report.

LET'S PRACTICE 4-10, *continued*

OPERATIVE NOTE

DATE OF PROCEDURE: 05/05/XXXX

SURGEON: Dr. Alvarez

PREOPERATIVE DIAGNOSIS: Umbilical hernia

POSTOPERATIVE DIAGNOSIS: Same

OPERATION DONE: Umbilical hernia repair.

PROCEDURE:

We prepped and draped the entire paraumbilical area. I infiltrated with 1% Xylocaine and made a 3/4 to 1" long circular incision in the upper aspects of the umbilicus. I then further infiltrated with Xylocaine and extended the incision down into the subcutaneous area and then dissected the hernia sac off the under side of the umbilicus. I then dissected the sac out circumferentially around the defect. I reduced the hernia and then inspected the defect after I freshened up the edges of the fascia. It was about 1 1/2 cm in diameter. I closed it with 3 interrupted #0 Vicryl sutures. I then closed the skin with interrupted 4–0 silk and applied a dressing to reconstitute the umbilicus. He tolerated the procedure well.

CC: Office.

This is the Operative Report as dictated by the physician.

This is the official summary of the procedure performed, pre-operative and post-operative diagnosis and step by step details for the actual procedure and or surgery performed.

Preoperative Diagnosis—Diagnosis the physician believes to be true based before procedure.

Postoperative Diagnosis—Diagnosis physician states after surgical procedure.

Official physician documentation regarding the operation performed.

This is the narrative summary of the exact procedure, steps, and findings as dictated by the physician.

Be sure to read through the entire report to ensure that nothing is dictated in the summary portion which was neglected to be noted in the Operation or Post Operative Diagnosis information.

This confirms that the hernia was reducible.

This information really should have been dictated in the "diagnosis" by the physician.

continued

LET'S PRACTICE 4-10, *continued*

This is an example of "combined" physician orders and progress notes.

Physician Orders are on the left side of the page with Physician Progress notes on the right side of the page.

PHYSICIAN'S ORDERS & PROGRESS RECORD

INSTRUCTIONS:—Note progress of case, complication, change in diagnosis, condition on discharge

Date	Orders	✓	Date	Progress
5/5/xx	① Diet as tolerated ② Tylox for pain ③ Ambulatory prn 12:30/p V.O. Home Office 1 week for follow up Rx - Vicodin		5/5/xx	**PER DICTATED REPORT** Date:_____ Diagnosis: _____ _____ Planned Procedure: _____ _____ _____ **PREOPERATIVE REVIEW OF BODY SYSTEMS** Cardiovascular_____ Pulmonary_____ Other_____ _____ Regular Medications: _____ _____ Allergies: _____ _____ Bleeding Clotting Disorders _____ Detailed H & P dictated? _____ Signature

LET'S PRACTICE 4-11

Health Record Face Sheet

Western Regional
Medical Center

Record Number: 41-08-92

Age: 4

Gender: Male

Length of Stay: Not Applicable

Diagnosis/Procedure: Tonsillitis with Tonsillectomy

Service Type: Same Day Surgery

Discharge Status: To Home

Demographic information for the patient is found on the face sheet.

Demographic information utilized in coding could be patient age, patient gender, service type, and discharge status.

Tonsillitis is the admitting diagnosis as defined in the outpatient coding guidelines.

Tonsillectomy is the procedure which is planned to be carried out.

Codes:

ICD-9: 474.02 Chronic tonsillitis and adenoiditis

ICD-10: J3503 chronic tonsillitis and adenoiditis

CPT: 42820 tonsillectomy and adenoidectomy; younger than age 12

continued

LET'S PRACTICE 4-11, *continued*

HISTORY & PHYSICAL

DATE OF ADMISSION: 7/29/XXXX

HISTORY:

This 4-year-old presents with chronic hypertrophic tonsillitis. He has had semifrequent episodes of streptococcal tonsillitis but his primary problem has been adenotonsillar hypertrophy with nocturnal airway obstruction, sleep apnea, etc. He is presently admitted for a tonsillectomy and adenoidectomy.

PAST MEDICAL HISTORY: Otherwise benign. No previous surgery. No known allergies. Takes no medications regularly.

FAMILY HISTORY: Noncontributory

REVIEW OF SYSTEMS: Negative.

PHYSICAL EXAMINATION:

Well-developed child in no acute distress.
EYES: Clear.
EARS: Canals and drums are within normal limits.
NOSE: Clear.
THROAT: Reveals 4+ tonsils which are definitely obstructive and somewhat cryptic.
NECK: Negative.
CHEST: Clear to percussion and auscultation.
HEART: Regular rate and rhythm without murmurs or gallops.
ABDOMEN: Benign.
EXTREMITIES: Within normal limits.
NEUROLOGIC: Grossly intact.

IMPRESSION:

Chronic hypertrophic adenotonsillitis.

PLAN:

T&A.

> Be sure to take note of the age, 4, of this patient.

> Impression - the pre-operative diagnosis as documented by the physician.

> Plan - What the physician has planned to treat the patient. In this case, the plan is a T&A or tonsillectomy ad adenoidectomy.
>
> Abbreviations are not to be utilized on the discharge summary and history and physical to avoid misinterpretation.

LET'S PRACTICE 4-11, *continued*

OUTPATIENT SURGERY

LAST NAME	FIRST NAME	MIDDLE NAME	AGE	BIRTH DATE	HOME PHONE	DATE	TIME AM PM
Chatterton	Coby		4	1/1/xxxx	1-555-555-1212	7/29/xxxx	

RESPONSIBLE PARTY NAME		RESP. PARTY ADDRESS	CITY STATE ZIP	EMPLOYER
LAST Parents				

INSURANCE CO. NAME	NO.	GROUP INS. WITH	POLICY NO.	CLAIM NO.	POLICY HOLDER
see file					

TIME	BP	TPR	NURSING REMARKS:
0915	92/56	97° 84/20	OPS - Tonsillectomy and adenoidectomy. Pre op teaching done.

LIST ANY ALLERGIES OR OTHER SPECIAL INFORMATION:	NURSING SIGNATURE	PATIENT CONDITION ON DISCHARGE:
None		

PHYSICIAN'S REPORT

DOCTOR:

DIAGNOSIS:

TREATMENT:

DISPOSITION:

AUTHORIZATION FOR MEDICAL and/or SURGICAL TREATMENT:

X _____

I hereby authorize Dr._____to administer   SIGNATURE OF PATIENT

such treatment as is, in his judgement, necessary.

INSTRUCTIONS
TO PATIENT:

X _____   _____   _____   X _____

PATIENT SIGNATURE   DATE   TIME   PHYSICIAN SIGNATURE

minor

> This is the nursing documentation of preoperative and postoperative patient information.

continued

LET'S PRACTICE 4-11, *continued*

This is the dictated physician documentation of the Operative Report.

OPERATIVE NOTE

DATE OF PROCEDURE: 07/29/xxxx

PREOPERATIVE DIAGNOSIS: Chronic hypertrophic adenotonsillitis.

POSTOPERATIVE DIAGNOSIS: Same

PROCEDURE PERFORMED: Tonsillectomy and adenoidectomy

DESCRIPTION:

The patient was brought to the operating room and induced into general oral tracheal anesthesia. He was positioned and draped in the Rose position. His mouth was opened with a McIvor mouth gag with a ring tongue blade attachment. A red rubber catheter was passed through the right nostril and retrieved in the oral pharynx for use as a palate retractor. The adenoids were removed with a curette. The tonsils were removed by the knife, scissors, snare technique. Hemostasis was achieved with electrocoagulation. At the close of the procedure no active bleeding was noted. The throat was thoroughly irrigated and suctioned.

The mouth gag and catheter were removed and the patient was awakened, extubated, and taken to the recovery room in satisfactory condition. There were no complications.

This documentation states the types of tools which were utilized during this adenoidectomy and tonsillectomy.

The pathology report is the definitive authority on specimens taken out during surgery. The pathologist will evaluate each specimen with a "Gross" - eye view and a "Microscopic" view.

Never code a chart without a pathology report for confirmation.

PATHOLOGY REPORT

PATIENT: Coby Chatterton

AGE: 4

MEDICAL RECORD#: 41-08-92

DATE: 7/29/xxxx

DOCTOR: Dr. Alvarez

OPERATION: TONSILLECTOMY AND ADENOIDECTOMY

GROSS: Submitted are multiple (2) grossly hyperplastic pharyngeal tonsils. They are pink-tan in color, normally lobulated, each measuring approximately 2.5 cm. in greatest dimension. Additionally present are irregularly shaped fragments of pink-tan, lobulated tissue characteristic of adenoidal tissue and together measuring approximately 2.0 cm. No gross abnormalities are noted on cut surface. Representative portions will be submitted if so requested.

This is the pathologist's (licensed physician) diagnosis regarding the specimens received for this episode of care.

This is the definitive diagnosis regarding this specimen.

FINDINGS: Multiple (2) hyperplastic pharyngeal tonsils and fragments of adenoidal tissue.

Electronically signed by:
Theodore Black, M.D.

LET'S PRACTICE 4-11, *continued*

These are the laboratory results for the urinalysis. Common items to look for on this lab will be evidence of a urinary tract infection, blood, or protein.

You will also notice drug screen items available on a UA. This lab test would only state the presence or no presence (qualitative) of the noted drugs. A different type of lab test would have to be run to identify the amount (quantity) of any drugs that are present.

URINALYSIS DRUG SCREEN	DATE DONE 7/29/xxxx
☐ **DRUG SCREEN**	CHECK ONE ☐ RANDOM ☐ CATHETERIZED ☒ CLEAN CATCH
ROUTINE	
COLOR	Yellow
APPEARANCE	Clear
GLUCOSE	∅
BILIRUBIN	1^+
KETONE	∅
SPEC GRAVITY	1.033
BLOOD	∅
pH	5.0
PROTEIN	Trace
UROBILINOGEN	Normal
NITRITE	∅
LEUKOCYTES	∅
MICROSCOPIC / HPF	
WBC	2-5
RBC	∅
EPITH. CELLS	1-3
BACTERIA	∅
MUCOUS THREADS	3^+
CRYSTALS	∅
ICTO Test	Negative
CASTS	∅
CLINITEST	
DRUG SCREEN	
AMPHETAMINE	
BARBITURATE	
BENZODIAZEPINE	
COCAINE	
MARIJUANA	
OPIATE	
TRICYCLIC ANTIDEPRESSANTS (SERUM)	
FOR CONFIRMATION OF POSITIVE SCREENS, CHECK HERE ☐	

LABORATORY REPORT SERIES

continued

LET'S PRACTICE 4-11, *continued*

COAGULATION AND SEROLOGY	TECH. R. Smith	DATE DONE 7/29/xxxx
COAGULATION		
ACT (CLOT TIME) 1-2 min.		
BLEED (SIMPLATE) TIME 2-9.5 min.		
☒ BLEED (CAPILLARY) TIME 1-3 min.	7' 10"	
☒ PROTHROMBIN TIME		
PATIENT VALUE	11.1	Sec.
NORMAL RANGE = 9.4 - 12.0		Sec.
☒ APTT		
PATIENT VALUE	24.7	Sec.
NORMAL RANGE = 23.0 - 35.5		Sec.
THROMBIN		
PATIENT VALUE		Sec.
NORMAL RANGE =		Sec.
FIBRINOGEN		
PATIENT VALUE		mg/dl
NORMAL RANGE =		mg/dl
FIBRIN DEGRADATION PRODUCTS		
PATIENT VALUE		ug/ml
NORMAL RANGE =		ug/ml
SEROLOGY		
ANA		
COLD AGGLUTININS		
MONO TEST		
RA (RHEUMATOID) TEST		
RA TITRE		
STREPTOZYME		
USR		

> This is another type of laboratory test - Coagulation and Serology.
>
> Prothrombin Time speaks to have fast the blood clots and bleeding stops. This is important when looking at surgery and potential complications.

LABORATORY REPORT SERIES

LET'S PRACTICE 4-11, *continued*

> This is an example of a "standard progress note" for a scheduled operation. This is physician documentation and should be read and considered during the coding process.

> T & A is a common abbreviation for Tonsillectomy and Adenoidectomy.

> NKA is a common abbreviation for no known allergies.

PHYSICIAN'S ORDERS & PROGRESS RECORD

INSTRUCTIONS:—NOTE PROGRESS OF CASE, COMPLICATION, CHANGE IN DIAGNOSIS, CONDITION ON DISCHARGE, INSTRUCTIONS TO PATIENT.

DATE	ORDERS	√	DATE	PROGRESS
				DATE: _07/29/xxxx_
				DIAGNOSIS: _____
				Chronic Adenotonsillitis
				PLANNED PROCEDURE: _____
				_T & A_
				INFORMED CONSENT _Yes_
				PREOPERATIVE REVIEW OF BODY SYSTEMS
				Cardiovascular_____
				Pulmonary__ _OK_
				Other_____
				Regular Medications:
				none
				Allergies: _NKA_
				Bleeding/Clotting Disorders _None_
				Detailed H&P dictated _Yes_
				Signature _Lucias Alvarez, M.D._

PHYSICIAN'S ORDERS	↑ Another brand of drugs identical in form and content may be dispensed unless checked.	PROGRESS RECORD

continued

LET'S PRACTICE 4-11, *continued*

PHYSICIAN'S ORDERS & PROGRESS RECORD

INSTRUCTIONS:—NOTE PROGRESS OF CASE, COMPLICATION, CHANGE IN DIAGNOSIS, CONDITION ON DISCHARGE, INSTRUCTIONS TO PATIENT.

STANDING ORDERS FOR:

DATE	ORDERS	√	DATE	PROGRESS
7/29/xx	**POST-OPERATIVE ORDERS:** Tonsils and Adenoids.		7/29/xx	T & A s̄ complication EBL - 20 cc
	1. Vital signs: Recovery room routine Q. 30 minutes × 6 then Q. 1 hour × 4 then Q. 4 hours × 6			
	2. Bleeding: Notify me of any bleeding.			
	3. IV's: Follow present IV with _____1000_____ CC of _____DS0. 2 NS_____ to run _____45_____ CC/hr. DC IV when tolerating fluids well.			
	4. Diet: Post T & A - Force fluids.			
	5. Position: On side or stomach until fully awake.			
	6. Humidifier at bedside.			
	7. Up with parent as tolerated when fully awake.			
	8. Tylenol Elixer (with codiene - without codiene) _____5_____ CC Q. 4 hours prn pain for hospital use.			
	9. Dispense and label for home use (8 oz. – 16 oz.) Tylenol Elixer (with codiene - without codiene).			
	10. Phenergan suppository 12.5 mg per rect q prn nausea			

PHYSICIAN'S ORDERS	Another brand of drugs identical in form and content may be dispensed unless checked.	**PROGRESS RECORD**

This is an example of "standard orders" utilized in healthcare facilities.

Note that the physician has the opportunity to add to or delete from these orders. This allows patient-specific orders to be issued with relative ease by merely adjusting standard orders.

This is the common symbol in the medical field for "without".

This progress note reads:

T&A without complication. EBL (estimated blood loss) 20 cc.

20 cc blood loss is minimal and expected during a surgical procedure. This does provide coding information regarding no complications for this patient due to blood loss.

LET'S PRACTICE 4-11, *continued*

This is the discharge order for the patient.

T.O. is the abbreviation for telephone order (from the physician)

The patient is to return to the office for re-check in 2 weeks.

p.o. is the abbreviation for "oral" route of administration for medicine.

Tol is a shortened term for "tolerated."

PHYSICIAN'S ORDERS & PROGRESS RECORD

INSTRUCTIONS:—NOTE PROGRESS OF CASE, COMPLICATION, CHANGE IN DIAGNOSIS, CONDITION ON DISCHARGE, INSTRUCTIONS TO PATIENT.

DATE	ORDERS	√	DATE	PROGRESS
07/29/xx	Discharge T. O. office ≈ 2 weeks		07/29/xx	Doing OK. Mod. uvular swelling. No. bleeding. Tol p.o. ok.

PHYSICIAN'S ORDERS

Another brand of drugs identical in form and content may be dispensed unless checked.

PROGRESS RECORD

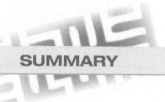

SUMMARY

Hospital outpatient coding is comprised of ancillary services, emergency department services, same-day surgeries, and observations. A hospital outpatient coder is responsible for fully understanding and applying the ICD 10 CM official coding guidelines as well as understanding how to code using the CPT-4 coding manual. Coders who are coding for the emergency department, same-day surgery department, or observation encounters will assign diagnosis codes using ICD 10 CM, and procedures using the CPT-4 coding manual. Coders may also use an APC encoder to generate APC assignment. Not all of the ancillary services and supplies are reported by the hospital outpatient coder because most are captured in the chargemaster. The chargemaster typically captures the CPT codes in the 70000–99999 range. An exception is the E/M codes, which an ER hospital coder may need to code.

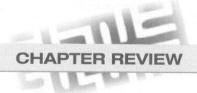

CHAPTER REVIEW

Multiple Choice

Choose the letter that best answers each question or completes each statement.

1. Which of the following is NOT a type of outpatient account?
   a. Emergency room
   b. Nursing home
   c. Observation
   d. Same-day surgery

2. Outpatient hospital claims are paid on which system?
   a. APCs
   b. DRGs
   c. RVU
   d. RBRVS

3. Hospital Facility E/M level codes are:
   a. Developed by each individual facility.
   b. CMS assigned to each facility based on APC assignment.
   c. Developed as part of the APC system.
   d. Payment based on CPT code assignment.

4. Outpatient coders utilize which procedure coding nomenclature?
   a. CPT
   b. HCPCS
   c. ICD 10 PCS
   d. Snomed

5. Demographic information for the patient is found in the health record on the:
   a. History and Physical
   b. Health Record Face Sheet
   c. Operative Report
   d. Nursing Daily Notes

6. A critical access hospital cannot be more than ____ miles from another facility.
   a. 25
   b. 35
   c. 45
   d. 55

7. Which of the following CPT codes are hard coded in the chargemaster?
   a. 70000
   b. 80000
   c. 90000
   d. All of the above

8. What is the first step in correct code assignment?
   a. Assign the correct diagnosis code.
   b. Assign the correct procedure code.
   c. Read the documentation in the medical record.
   d. Review the documentation for an applicable modifier.

9. A critical access hospital can have no more than _____ beds.
   a. 25
   b. 35
   c. 45
   d. 55

10. "SOAP" dictation format represents:
   a. Signs, Objective, Assessment, Plan
   b. Subjective, Objective, Assessment, Plan
   c. Subjective, Observed, Assessment, Plan
   d. Signs, Observed, Assessment, Plan

True or False

Determine whether each question is true or false. In the space provided, write "T" for true or "F" for false.

_____ 1. The chargemaster houses all CPT codes in the range of 70000–99999.

_____ 2. Each facility may have its own E/M ER facility-level determination.

_____ 3. APCs were implemented in 1998.

_____ 4. Observation is a type of inpatient status.

_____ 5. The outpatient coding guidelines tell us to code a sign/symptom as well as the disease or condition with which it is associated.

_____ 6. Hard coding is coding that is completed by a hospital coder.

_____ 7. The most common types of outpatient coding for coders are ER and SDS encounters.

_____ 8. Hospital outpatient coders will need to learn ICD-10-PCS to report these codes for hospital outpatients.

_____ 9. Hospital outpatient coders follow the ICD 10 CM outpatient coding guidelines for diagnosis code assignment.

_____ 10. HCPCS codes are housed in the chargemaster.

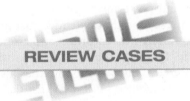

REVIEW CASES

Use these coding steps to assign the applicable codes to the review cases that follow:

1. Read through the documentation and determine the reason for the visit, that is, the primary diagnosis. Determine if any complicating or coexisting diagnosis exists.
2. Read through the documentation and determine what service or procedure the patient received.
3. Locate the correct diagnosis codes using ICD 10 CM code set.
4. Locate the correct procedure code using the CPT-4 coding manual
5. Assign the diagnoses and procedure codes to the patient's chart.
6. *Optional: Calculate* the APCs for each patient's chart.

Review Case 4-1

History of Present Illness: This is a 38-year-old lady brought to the hospital on March 22 for elective sterilization.

Drug Allergies: None.

Medications: None.

Past History: She states her health in general has been good. She was last hospitalized in 2008 for the birth of her twins.

Review of Systems: Otherwise essentially normal.

Physical Examination:

Vital Signs: Temperature 96, pulse 72, respirations 16, blood pressure 116/84.

General: 38-year-old lady in good general health, in good spirits.

HEENT/Neck: No adenopathy noted. Thyroid not palpable.

Eyes: Unremarkable.

Lungs: Clear.

Cardiovascular: Regular rhythm, no murmur noted.

Abdomen: No masses or tenderness. No organomegaly.

Extremities: Unremarkable.

Neurologic Exam: Grossly intact.

Procedure Performed:

1. Laparoscopic occlusion of tubes via a Falope ring.

ICD-9-CM diagnosis code(s): _____

_____

ICD-10-CM diagnosis code(s): _____

_____

CPT code(s) with modifier, if applicable: _____

_____

APC: _____

Review Case 4-2   Operative Report

Preoperative Diagnosis:	Left dural arteriovenous fistula; seizure disorder.
Postoperative Diagnosis:	Left dural arteriovenous fistula; seizure disorder.
Operation:	Resection of dural arteriovenous fistula.
Anesthesia:	General.

Indication for Surgery: This 10-year-old female presents with a seizure disorder that presented approximately 1 year ago. Patient underwent seizure diagnostic workup and an AV dural fistula was found. The patient has undergone previous angiography with embolization of this fistula approximately 6 months ago, but the fistula did not close completely. The patient is now presenting for definitive resection of the fistula.

Procedure: The patient was brought to the operating room and with general anesthesia given via intubation tube. The patient was placed in the supine position with Mayfield pins. The patient's head was turned to the left and the right shoulder elevated. The ear was prepped with iodine solution and properly draped in sterile fashion. Markers previously placed under MRI were clearly identified on the scalp, and an inverted-U-shaped flap clearly opened the lesion up to view. The incision was then made down to bone and dissection carried down to the periosteum using monopolar cautery. The scalp flap was reflected inferiorly and tacked into place after Raney clips were applied. Four bur holes were created, two above and two below the transverse sinus, again confirming the location of the sinus by image guidance. Once these bur holes were created, the dura was dissected free underneath the

bone and then a bit was used to cut out a craniotomy flap in this area. The flap was then set on the back table to be utilized later in the case. Once the bone flap was elevated, the dura appeared to be normal. The transverse sinus was appreciated. A C-shaped flap was made in a small fashion below the transverse sinus with the base on the transverse sinus overlying the cerebellum. This was cut through the dura, and small arterialized feeders were taken from the surface of the cerebellum to the dural AV fistula. Eventually, the entire dorsal surface of the cerebellum was freed from the tentorium and transverse sinus. Then another C-shaped flap was made above the transverse sinus with the base on the transverse sinus overlying the inferior parietal lobe. This was reflected downward and the vein of Labbé visualized anteriorly in the flap. Additional small pial and dural arterialized vessels were taken with bipolar coagulation without difficulty or significant bleeding. Eventually, at the base of the fistula, a large group of arterial vessels was seen entering a cortical vein and adjacent to the transverse sinus. This was coagulated with bipolar coagulation and divided sharply. Eventually, the entire inferior parietal area was elevated off the transverse sinus; and the small anastomotic portion of the vein of Labbé was also taken to allow for removal of the transverse sinus. Once the parietal lobe and cerebellum were lifted free of the tentorium, large Ligaclips were applied to the transverse sinus; and in slow fashion, incision was made through the anterior and posterior margins of the transverse sinus creating a resection that extended just medial to the transverse sinus along the tentorium and around to the posterior margin of the resection. No significant bleeding was encountered. This was submitted as a single specimen with Ligaclips labeled "dural AV fistula." The rest of the brain surface was normal. Furthermore, intraoperative median nerve somatosensory-evoked potentials were monitored and did not change throughout the surgery. Closure was then begun.

A piece of bovine pericardium was used to sew in the defect in the lateral dura, using a running 4-0 Nurolon stitch. The craniotomy bone flap was reattached using a small cranial plating system. The galea and muscle were closed using inverted 2-0 Vicryl sutures, followed by staples for the skin. Sterile dressings were applied.

Estimated blood loss was 400 cc. All sponge counts and needle counts were correct. I was scrubbed and present for all portions of this procedure.

ICD-9-CM diagnosis codes(s): _____

_____

ICD-10-CM diagnosis code(s): _____

_____

CPT code(s) with modifier, if applicable: _____

_____

APC: _____

Review Case 4-3

Preoperative Diagnosis: Left inguinal hernia.

Postoperative Diagnosis: Left indirect inguinal hernia.

Operative Procedure: Repair of left inguinal hernia.

A standard left groin incision was accomplished, carried down through subcutaneous tissue. The external oblique was divided in line with its fibers, the cord structures were carefully freed up and protected with a Penrose drain. The cremasteric muscle was incised and a large sac identified. This was very thin walled and had the appearance of being extremely acute. The sac was carefully freed up from the surrounding tissues, twisted and high ligation accomplished with an 0 silk followed by a 2-0 silk suture ligature. The sac was excised. The wound was then again irrigated with antibiotics after which the dermis was approximated with continuous 3-0 Vicryl and the epidermis with Steri-Strips.

ICD-9-CM diagnosis code(s): _____

_____

ICD-10-CM diagnosis code(s): _____

_____

CPT code(s) with modifier, if applicable: _____

_____

APC: _____

Review Case 4-4

Identification: This is a 36-year-old female.

Chief Complaint: Rash in both malar prominences.

History of Present Illness: The patient is a 36-year-old female who had onset yesterday of rash in both malar prominences. She has had this before. It did not respond to Zyrtec. In the past, steroids have helped it with a short course of some prednisone. There has been no shortness of breath.

Allergies: Penicillin.

Current Medication: Zyrtec.

Previous Illnesses: No diabetes, no asthma.

Social History: No tobacco. She is traveling here from Houston. Her usual physician is in Houston, and I have discussed the case with her.

Physical Examination:

General: Exam shows the patient to be alert in no acute distress. Color is good. The neck is supple.

Vitals: Vital signs are stable. Pulse ox is 96% on room air.

Heent: The pharynx is clear and moist. There is a little bit of reddened facial rash bilaterally. Tympanic membranes okay.

Chest: The lungs are clear.

Cardiac: The heart is regular rhythm.

Extremities: The extremities are without edema or tenderness.

Impression:

1. Allergic facial rash.

Plan: Do not take more Zyrtec. I have reviewed the literature. It seems that this dose should be safe, but I have discussed it with Dr. Grover, and she will see that doctor in two to three days and discuss then taking liver function tests. Also consider an ANA and other evaluations for other etiologies of the rash. She is to see a physician or go to the emergency room for any problems. A Medrol Dosepak was prescribed. The patient is stable and unchanged at discharge.

ICD-9-CM diagnosis code(s): _____

_____

ICD-10-CM diagnosis code(s): _____

_____

CPT code(s) with modifier, if applicable: _____

APC: _____

Review Case 4-5

Preoperative Diagnosis: Hemoptysis.

Postoperative Diagnosis:

1. Hemoptysis, probably secondary to pneumonia.

Operative Procedure: Fiberoptic bronchoscopy.

Description: The P20 fiberoptic bronchoscope was passed via nasal approach. The upper airway was normal. The tracheal bronchial tree was remarkable for quite prominent diffuse changes of chronic inflammation with linear striations. The segmental orifices of the left lower lobe were collapsed, probably secondary to the left hemidiaphragm paralysis. There were no other endobronchial lesions. Note that saturation by oximeter was 85% before the start of the procedure and before any sedative mediations were given.

ICD-9-CM diagnosis code(s): _____

_____

ICD-10-CM diagnosis code(s): _____

_____

CPT code(s) with modifier, if applicable: _____

_____

APC: _____

Review Case 4-6

Procedure: Utilizing local anesthetic, a 22-gauge spinal needle was inserted into the right upper uterus and about 3 cc of clear straw-colored fluid was sent to the laboratory for assessment. Amniocentesis was performed adjacent to the lower spine and left buttock region of the fetus. There were no apparent complications. The patient tolerated the procedure well. There was good fetal activity following the procedure. No evidence of Braxton Hick's contractions. Fetal cardiac activity was normal with a fetal heart rate of 147 bpm following amniocentesis. The proximal tibial ossification center (35-week marker) is present.

ICD-10-CM diagnosis code(s): _____

CPT code(s) with modifier, if applicable: _____
_____

APC: _____

Review Case 4-7

Identification: This is a 4-year-old Caucasian male.

Chief Complaint: Fever, strep throat, otitis media.

History of Present Illness: This is a 4-year-old male who was seen Tuesday in Dr. Santo's office and was diagnosed with strep throat and bilateral otitis media. He was given Keflex. He got a little bit better by Thursday, but is now sick again today. Mom thinks he also has a rash. His eyes are red. His lips are dry. His temperature was up to 102.3. Last Tylenol dose was at 12:30 p.m. today. He has been acting sick and eating less. Mom was thinking he should have been better by now.

Allergies: Amoxicillin.

Current Medications: Cephalexin and Tylenol with Codeine.

Previous Illnesses: Allergic rhinitis.

Physical Examination:

General: General exam shows a well-developed, well-nourished male. He is sleepy and ill-appearing lying on the table. His eyes are blood shot but he answers questions appropriately and is appropriate with response to my exam.

Vitals: Heart rate 137, respirations 32, temperature 100.6.

HEENT: Normocephalic, atraumatic. Eyes, the sclerae are injected bilaterally and red. There is no discharge noted. Nose has some crusted and dried rhinorrhea. Ears are erythematous bilaterally. Throat is also erythematous. The neck shows some cervical adenopathy bilaterally. I do not note any large or tender nodes.

Skin: The skin shows a very fine almost impossible to see sandpaper rash. There is no rash on the extremities or on the hands or feet. No desquamation is present.

Abdomen: The abdomen is soft and nontender. Bowel sounds are normal.

Emergency Room Course: The patient was given a dose of ibuprofen and then observed for approximately 30 minutes. I then went in and reexamined the patient. He was sitting up. He was much more alert and talkative. His eyes had cleared considerably. He was asking me if he could have Iron Man stickers and was very inquisitive and asking if there were any toys to play with. Mom states that was a big improvement. Temperature was retaken. It was still 102.3 but patient was acting remarkably better.

Impression:

1. Streptococcal pharyngitis and otitis media.

Plan: Continue the medications as he has been taking. If he is not better in the next couple of days, I would like them to call Dr. Santo's office. I did discuss briefly the possibility of other diseases with mom but I feel he lacks criteria at this point and would like him to continue his current therapy, especially in light of him having perked up and gotten so much better with a dose of ibuprofen. She is to continue the Tylenol and ibuprofen for fever. She will return with the patient sooner if he develops higher fevers or gets worse.

ICD-10-CM diagnosis code(s): _____
_____

CPT code(s) with modifier, if applicable: _____
_____

APC: _____

Health Record Face Sheet

Western Regional
Medical Center

Record Number: 16-10-02

Age: 56

Gender: Male

Length of Stay: Not Applicable

Diagnosis/Procedure: Renal Colic

Service Type: Emergency Room

Discharge Status: To Home

continued

Review Case 4-8, *continued*

ALLERGIES		TETANUS STATUS	
CURRENT MEDS		LMP	
HISTORY & PHYSICAL	T: P: R: BP: SaO₂: WT:	**BY (INIT)**	

TIME OF MD INITIAL ASSESSMENT			☐ STAT **LABS**

LABS
- ☐ ABG on _____ *l*
- ☐ Admit Packet
- ☐ Amylase
- ☐ Cardiac Packet
- ☐ CBC   ☐ DIFF.
- ☐ CBG on _____ *l*
- ☐ Chem Profile _____
- ☐ CPK/ISO
- ☐ EKG
- ☐ Glucose
- ☐ HCG   ☐ SERUM   ☐ URINE
- ☐ Lytes
- ☐ PT/PTT
- ☐ Trauma Packet
- ☐ Type & Screen
- ☐ Type & Cross _____
- ☑ UA
- ☐ CSF
- ☐ Culture _____
- ☐
- ☐

DICTATED: ☑ YES ☐ NO   ☐

TIME	TREATMENT ORDERS		☐
		TIME	☐
			X-RAYS
			☐ Chest
			☐ C-Spine
			☐ Flat Plate/Upright (ABD)
			☐ CT ☐ HEAD ☐ ABD
		☐ STANDING ORDERS	☐

DIAGNOSIS:

Renal Colic

DISCHARGE TIME	DISCHARGE INSTRUCTIONS	

Lortab Elixer (8 oz)

	Return to Work/School	
PHYSICIAN SIGNATURE	I HAVE RECEIVED AND UNDERSTAND THE ABOVE INSTRUCTIONS.	☐ SEE DISCHARGE INSTRUCTIONS SHEET
James Boyles, M.D.	PT/SD SIGNATURE X *Joseph Johnstone*	REV. BY

EMERGENCY DEPARTMENT RECORD

Review Case 4-8, *continued*

MEDICAL RECORDS

HISTORY / CHIEF COMPLAINT	MVA - RESTRAINED ☐ YES ☐ NO REPORTED TO: DATE TIME
	MOTORCYCLE - HELMET ☐ YES ☐ NO
	REPORTABLE INJURY ☐ YES ☐ NO
Lower (L) abd. pain	**TRIAGE** MENTAL STATUS _____ COLOR _____
	RESPIRATIONS _____ SKIN TURGOR _____
	☐ O₂ ☐ Elevate ☐ MED. _____
	☐ Splint ☐ Dressing ☐ MED. _____
PTA GCS CRAMS ☐ BACKBOARD ☐ C-COLLAR ☐	☐ Ice ☐ _____ TRIAGE NURSE **X**

ALLERGIES	*NKA*	**TETANUS**
CURRENT MEDICATIONS	*OTC meds without*	☐ CURRENT ☐ R
		☐ NOT CURRENT ☐ L
		☐ TT ☐ Td ☐ DEL
		☐ DT ☐ DPT ☐ TH
PMH	φ	

ASSESSMENT	(NEURO, CARDIAC, RESPIRATORY, GI, GU, SKIN, INCIDENT TIME)	**LOT #**
	Yesterday pt was eating breakfast when he had sharp pain in the (L) lower abd lasted 30 min.	
	Rested most of yesterday. Today, pain started @ 2:00 p.m. and has moved from left lower abd. to left lower back.	**VISUAL ACUITY** OD _____ OS _____ OU _____
	Urinary frequency. Some nausea. Ø vomiting.	**WT**
		LMP

TIME	TEMP	P	R	BP	SaO₂ O₂	TIME	MEDICATION/DOSE	ROUTE	SITE	SIGNATURE
5:05 pm	98	80	16	144/100	/					
					/					
					/					
					/					
					/					

TIME	IV FLUID/AMOUNT	MEDICATION ADDED	RATE/HR	SIZE	SITE	TIME Dc'd	AMT INFUSED	SIGNATURE

TIME	PROBLEM/CHANGE	INTERVENTION	PATIENT RESPONSE / EVALUATION
		UA TO Lab	

SIGNATURE/ TITLE X *Mary Houser, RN*	SIGNATURE/ TITLE X	☐ SEE ADDENDUM ED NURSES FLOW SHEET

DISCHARGE TIME: 6:00 PM	**PATIENT BELONGINGS**		BAG	ON PT.	NONE
DISPOSITION ☒ Discharged ☐ AMA	Clothing _____		☐	☐	☐
☐ Admit/Transfer _____	Wallet/Purse _____		☐	☐	☐
Report Given To: _____	Money _____		☐	☐	☐
CONDITION ON DISCHARGE/TRANSFER ☒ Stable	Jewelry _____		☐	☐	☐
☐ Stabilized ☐ Improved ☐ Expired	Glasses _____		☐	☐	☐
DISCHARGE MODE: ☒ Ambulatory	Dentures _____		☐	☐	☐
☐ Wheelchair ☐ Stretcher ☐ Carried	DISPOSITION: ☐ Not Disrobed ☐ Patient ☐ Family				
Accom. by _____	☐ Security ☐ SEE BELONGINGS LIST				

ED NURSES FLOW SHEET

continued

Review Case 4-8, *continued*

EMERGENCY DEPARTMENT VISIT

DATE OF VISIT: 8/14/xxxx

By history, the patient is a 56-year-old male who presents to the emergency department with about a 30-hour history of left lower quadrant abdominal pain. The pain was severe and sudden at its onset yesterday morning. It lasted several hours and resolved completely. He had return of pain about 2:00 p.m. today and it was severe at onset, but has subsided somewhat. He has noted some frequency of urination, but denies hematuria and he denies dysuria. He has been moving his bowels normally. The pain, in recent hours, moved around to his back somewhat. He has had some slight nausea, but no vomiting. He has never had similar symptoms before. He is a generally healthy man who does not take medications on an ongoing basis. He occasionally sees Dr. Joseph, however, he came here because he was not available today.

Objectively, the patient is alert and in no acute distress. There is some mild, distinct left flank tenderness. There is no particular tenderness in the left lower quadrant, but mild to moderate tenderness in the left mid-abdomen to left upper quadrant. No mass or organomegaly was noted. Bowel sounds are normal. Genital exam was normal. A urinalysis was obtained which demonstrated 3+ occult blood and one to five white blood cells, 80 to 100 red blood cells, no bacteria.

ASSESSMENT: Renal colic.

PLAN: The patient was not in severe distress at the time of discharge. He was allowed to go home with Lortab elixir, one, two, or three teaspoons every four to six hours as needed for pain. A total of eight ounces were prescribed. He is unable to swallow pills. He is asked to return promptly should he worsen in any way, or vomiting develops. Also, he should see his own doctor, Dr. Joseph in one or two days if he has any persistent symptoms. I did send him home with a urine strainer and asked him to return any stone he might catch for laboratory evaluation. Further care and workup per Dr. Joseph.

URINALYSIS DRUG SCREEN		
☒	□ DRUG SCREEN	□ CHECK ONE ☒ RANDOM □ CATHETERIZED □ CLEAN CATCH
ROUTINE		
COLOR	Yellow	
APPEARANCE	Sat hazy	
GLUCOSE	0	
BILIRUBIN	0	
KETONE	0	
SPEC GRAVITY	1.025	
BLOOD	3+	
pH	5.5	
PROTEIN	trace	
UROBILINOGEN	Normal	
NITRITE	0	
LEUKOCYTES	0	
MICROSCOPIC / HPF		
WBC	1-5	
RBC	80-100	
EPITH. CELLS	0-3	
BACTERIA	0	
MUCOUS THREADS	2+	
CRYSTALS	0	
CASTS	0	
CLINITEST		
DRUG SCREEN		
AMPHETAMINE		
BARBITURATE		
BENZODIAZEPINE		
COCAINE		
MARIJUANA		
OPIATE		
TRICYCLIC ANTIDEPRESSANTS (SERUM)		

LABORATORY REPORT SERIES

continued

Review Case 4-8, *continued*

ICD-9-CM diagnosis code(s): _____

ICD-10-CM diagnosis code(s): _____

CPT code(s) with modifier, if applicable: _____

APC: _____

Review Case 4-9

Health Record Face Sheet

Western Regional
Medical Center

Record Number: 22-19-07

Age: 26

Gender: Female

Length of Stay: Not Applicable

Diagnosis/Procedure: RhoGAM Injection

Service Type: Emergency Room

Discharge Status: To Home

Review Case 4-9, *continued*

	MEDICAL RECORDS

E.D. # 22-19-07	**EMERGENCY TREATMENT RECORD**	ARRIVAL DATE: 6/14/xxxx	TIME: 10:00

PATIENT NAME Madison Moorehead	PHYSICIAN Dr. Smith	AGE 26 Y	SEX F	BIRTH DATE 5/05/88

CHIEF COMPLAINT
REQ SHOT

ACTIVITY LEVEL

PHYSICIAN'S NOTES

DISABILITY
Estimated No. of Days _____   ☐ Chart Dictated   ☒ Not Dictated

DIAGNOSIS
Prenatal RhoGam

DISCHARGE CONDITION:
☒ Stable   ☐ Unchanged   ☐ Transferred   ☐ Improved   ☐ AMA
☐ Admitted   ☐ Expired   ☐ Not Seen By Physician

P.A., F.P. RESIDENT SIGNATURE

E.D. PHYSICIAN SIGNATURE
Dr. Hungarti

CONSENT FOR TREATMENT

CONSENT FOR TREATMENT: I am presenting myself for inpatient and/or outpatient care at West Valley Medical Center and I voluntarily consent to the rendering of such care including diagnostic procedures and medical treatment by authorized agents and employees of the Regional Medical Center and by its medical staff or their designees as in their professional judgment may be deemed necessary. I acknowledge that no guarantees have been made to me as to the result of examination or treatment in this hospital.

PATIENT OR REPRESENTATIVE SIGNATURE
Madison Moorehead

DATE: 6/14/xx   TIME: 11:45   IF REPRESENTATIVE, INDICATE RELATIONSHIP

WITNESS SIGNATURE: DATE
WITNESS SIGNATURE: DATE

PHYSICIAN'S ORDERS

E.D. # 22-19-07				PATIENT NAME: Madison Moorehead				
DATE	TIME	1	2	3	ORDERS			
6/14/xx	10:30				Prenatal RhoGam Injection			

	ORDERED	DRAWN	RETURNED	TO X-RAY	RETURN

continued

Review Case 4-9, *continued*

Emergency Dept. Nursing Flow Sheet
Page 1

PATIENT NAME:	Arrival Date:	Time:	Birth Date:		Record Number: 22-19-07
Moorehead, Madison, M.	6/14/xxxx	13:05	5/05/88		

Private	Means of Arrival:
	☒ Ambulatory ☐ Carry ☒ Self
☒ Pt./Family Request E.D. M.D.	☐ W/C ☐ Fam/Friend ☐ Police
	☐ Stretcher ☐ Helicopter ☐ Ambulance

CHIEF COMPLAINT:

For Rhoghen Inj   PREVIOUS ADM: ☐ YES ☒ NO

ALLERGIES: ☒ NKA ☐ CODIENE ☐ PCN   **LAST TETANUS**
_____
☒ NA ☐ UNKNOWN

CURRENT MEDS. AND DOSAGE: ☐ NONE ☐ UNKNOWN

Vits   *G.B. u/s done today*

PAST MEDICAL HISTORY: *6 Mos. pregnant*

INITIAL V.S.   WEIGHT | LMP
B.P. *110/70* T. *96°* P. *76* R. *16*   OD   OS

IN ROOM ___*6*___ AT *1015* A.M./P.M. VIA *Amb.*

☐ HELD ☐ CHAIR ☐ FOEB ☐ STRETCHER ☐ SIDE RAILS UPS ☐ STANDING ☐ CALL LIGHT IN REACH

PHYSICIAN CALLED	TIME/WHERE	E = EXCHANGE/BEEPER O = OFFICE TIME I = IN HOSPITAL H = HOME RESPONDED

LAB WORK AND PROCEDURES (check work done)

☐ UA ☐ RANDOM ☐ C.C. ☐ CATH	
☐ CBC ☐ H&H _____	
☐ SMAC ☐ HOLD ADMIT	
☐ BUN ☐ CREATININE	
☐ ELECTROLYTES ☐ Na ☐ K	
☐ GLUCOSE ☐ AMYLASE	
☐ PROTIME ☐ APTT	
☐ ABG _____ _____	
☐ CPK ☐ CARDIAC ISOENZYME	
☐ TYPE & SCREEN	
☐ T & C _____ UNITS	
☐ BLOOD ALCOHOL ☐ LEGAL	
☐ DRUG SCREEN URINE	
☐ THROAT CULTURE ☐ STREPSCREEN	
☐ C&S - SOURCE _____	
☐ GM STAIN _____	
☐ GC - SOURCE _____	
☐ CHLAMYDIA	
☐ _____	
☐ _____	
☐ _____	
☐ _____	

ORDERED	LAB DRAWN	RETURNED

TIME	
	MONITOR APPLIED
	NASAL CANNULA MASK
	O₂ _____ LET TUBE
	EKG

TIME	X-RAYS ORDERED
TO:	
RETURN	
TO:	
RETURN	
TO:	
RETURN	

TO X-RAY
☐ AMB ☐ W/C ☐ STRETCHER ☐ CARRY

SEE
☐ EMS RUN SHEET
☐ CODE BLUE DATA SHEET
☐ I & O / NEURO
☐ TRANSFER FORM
☐ _____
☐ _____

TIME	ASSESSMENT AND HISTORY	TIME	MEDICATION & TREATMENTS
1000	26 y.o. ♀ presents to E.D.		Rhogam given IM
	for above Rhogam injection	11:00	lot # RHL 151
1030	Dr. contated. Lab test results from office faxed to ns.		
1130	D/C		

PATIENT DISPOSITION/CONDITION: TIME: ___*1130*___
☐ ADMIT RM _____ REPORT TO: _____
☒ DISCHARGED ☐ TRANSFERRED _____
☒ UNCHANGED ☐ IMPROVED _____
☒ AMBULATORY ☐ W.C.   ☐ STRETCHER ☐ CARRY
☐ AFTERCARE _____

NURSING DIAGNOSIS:	DISPOSITION OF PROPERTY:	S I G N A T U R E	Nurse(s) *H. Heliop, R.N.*
Rhogam inj	☒ PATIENT ☐ FAMILY/FRIEND ☐ POLICE ☐ _____ LIST:		_____

Review Case 4-9, *continued*

ICD-9-CM diagnosis code(s): _____

ICD-10-CM diagnosis code(s): _____

CPT code(s) with modifier, if applicable: _____

APC: _____

Review Case 4-10

Health Record Face Sheet

Western Regional
Medical Center

Record Number:	03-54-42
Age:	48
Gender:	Male
Length of Stay:	N/A
Diagnosis/Procedure:	Knee Hematoma
Service Type:	Emergency Room
Discharge Status:	To Home

continued

Review Case 4-10, *continued*

		MEDICAL RECORDS		

E.D. #: 03-54-42

EMERGENCY TREATMENT RECORD

ARRIVAL DATE: 07/10/xxxx	TIME: 06:00

PATIENT: Chavez Carillo	PHYSICIAN: Dr. Vareska	AGE: 48 Y	SEX: M	BIRTH DATE: 1/30/1964

CHIEF COMPLAINT
Check R Leg

ACTIVITY LEVEL

PHYSICIAN'S NOTES

R   L

DISABILITY

Estimated No. of Days _____   ☒ Chart Dictated   ☐ Not Dictated

DIAGNOSIS:

Hematoma

DISCHARGE CONDITION:

☒ Stable   ☐ Unchanged   ☐ Transferred   ☐ Improved   ☐ AMA

☐ Admitted   ☐ Expired   ☐ Not Seen By Physician

P.A., F.P. RESIDENT SIGNATURE

E.D. PHYSICIAN SIGNATURE   *Dr. Vareska*

CONSENT FOR TREATMENT

PATIENT OR REPRESENTATIVE SIGNATURE

DATE	TIME	REPRESENTATIVE INDICATE RELATIONSHIP
WITNESS SIGNATURE		DATE
WITNESS SIGNATURE		DATE

PHYSICIAN'S ORDERS

E.D. #				PATIENT NAME				
DATE	TIME	1	2	3	ORDERS			
					ORDERED	DRAWN	RETURNED	TO X-RAY	RETURN

Review Case 4-10, *continued*

EMERGENCY ROOM REPORT

ALL EKG'S, X-RAY REPORTS AND LABORATORY TESTS NOTED IN DICTATION ARE THE INTERPRE-
TATION OF THE DICTATING PHYSICIAN UNLESS SPECIFICALLY NOTED OTHERWISE. ALL CONSULTS
WITH PHYSICIANS AS LISTED IN DICTATION ARE <u>BY</u> <u>TELEPHONE</u> UNLESS OTHERWISE SPECIFIED.

PATIENT	PHYSICIAN	DATE OF SERVICE
Chavez Carillo	*Dr. Vareska*	*7/10/xxxx*

Mr. Carillo is a very pleasant 48-year-old gentleman who presents to the emergency room for
evaluation of persistent swelling and ecchymosis in the right lower extremity below the knee.
He was evaluated on 7/7/xx by Dr. Tilley. At that time, the history revealed that 36 hours prior
to his visit on the 7th, he noticed swelling in the anterolateral aspect of the knee but not in the
knee joint proper. Subsequently this disseminated down to the ankle and to the foot. It felt tight
and was somewhat painful. He had no noted trauma other than that he has been working on
his house. He has no history of varicose veins, DVT, previous site infection. He had no systemic
symptoms such as fevers, rigors, nausea, vomiting. Dr. Tilley evaluated the patient with a right
knee film which was negative. A CBC, PT, PTT, and platelet count were all within normal limits.
Differential was normal also. He was diagnosed as having a hematoma of the right knee and
surrounding area and was instructed to elevate it. Mr. Carillo elevated it for the first 24 hours,
however he was ambulatory yesterday. He represents today because of persistent swelling.
Again he has had no fevers, rigors, no erythema, heat.

SOCIAL HISTORY: The patient lives in the city and works as a landscaper.
ALLERGIES: PENICILLIN.
LAST TETANUS: Current.
CURRENT MEDICATIONS: None.
UNDERLYING ILLNESSES: None.

PHYSICAL EXAM, Alert, pleasant gentleman in no acute distress. Blood pressure 124/78, afebrile, pulse 84, respiratory rate 16. Examination of the right lower extremity reveals ecchymosis
and swelling from just below the knee joint down to the foot. There is erythema on the posterior
aspect of the gastrocnemius muscle on the lateral aspect but this is symmetrical with the left
side. Mr. Carillo points out that he was out in the sun yesterday and got a sunburn. Dorsalis
pedis and posterior tibial pulses are intact. Capillary refill is normal. Good flexion- extension at
the knee and ankle.

DIAGNOSIS: HEMATOMA, RIGHT LOWER EXTREMITY.

ASSESSMENT/PLAN: The patient needs to faithfully elevate his leg for the next 48 hours with
a warm pack. No aspirin. He is off work and is to return for recheck on Monday. If he develops
erythema, increased swelling, or pain, he needs to be rechecked immediately.

ICD-9-CM diagnosis code(s): _____

ICD-10-CM diagnosis code(s): _____

CPT code(s) with modifier, if applicable: _____

APC: _____

Health Record Face Sheet

Western Regional
Medical Center

Record Number:	86-15-03
Age:	1
Gender:	Female
Length of Stay:	Not Applicable
Diagnosis/Procedure:	Otitis Media Tympanotomy and Tube Insertion
Service Type:	Same-Day Surgery
Discharge Status:	To Home

HISTORY & PHYSICAL

ADMISSION DATE: 2/27/xx

HISTORY: This 1-year-old child has had a long history of chronic refractory otitis media. She's been on multiple, prolonged courses of antibiotics without improvement. She has had at least one documented episode of otitis media per month for the last 8 months. She is presently admitted for bilateral tympanotomy and tube insertion.

PAST MEDICAL HISTORY: Otherwise benign. No previous surgery; no known allergies. Takes no medications regularly.

FAMILY HISTORY: Non-contributory.

REVIEW OF SYSTEMS: Negative.

EXAM: Well-developed infant in no acute distress.

EARS: The drums are somewhat thickened and retracted but there is no evidence of middle ear effusion at the present time.
NOSE & THROAT: Clear.
NECK: Negative.
CHEST: Clear.
HEART: Regular.
ABDOMEN: Benign.
EXTREMITIES: Within normal limits.

DIAGNOSIS: Chronic refractory otitis

Review Case 4-11, continued

OUTPATIENT SURGERY

PATIENT NAME LAST	FIRST NAME	MIDDLE NAME	AGE	BIRTH DATE	HOME PHONE	DATE	TIME
Kruger	Kaylee	K	1	12/14/2010	(555) 555-0202	2/27/xxxx	06:00

TIME	BP	TPR	NURSING REMARKS:
6²⁵A	96	(A)	OPSG - BDT's - pre op teaching done. Returned to OP/cart c̄
7⁴⁵A		112/24	with rails up - color good - awake - placed in mother's arms -
			no drainage noted from ears. Tol liq well - no
8¹⁵A			emesis - active & alert.
8²⁰A			Disch inst to parents by nurse. Both parents
			understand discharge inst.
8³⁵A			No drainage noted from ears - color gd -
			Disch home.

LIST ANY ALLERGIES OR OTHER SPECIAL INFORMATION: | NURSE'S SIGNATURE | PATIENT CONDITION ON DISCHARGE:

Good

PHYSICAN'S REPORT

DOCTOR:

DIAGNOSIS: Chronic refactory OM

Tubes

TREATMENT: VS per record

Diet and Act as tol

Discharege when doing well

TO office ≈ 1 week.

DISPOSITION:

AUTHORIZATION FOR MEDICAL and/or SURGICIAL TREATMENT:

X _____ Minor

I hereby authorized Dr. ___Dr. Entol___ to administer tympanotomy   SIGNATURE OF PATIENT

and tube insertion and such treatment as is, in his judgement, necessary.

INSTRUCTIONS
TO PATIENT:

X Minor	2/27/xxxx	10:00 am	X Dr. Entol
PATIENT SIGNATURE	DATE	TIME	PHYSICIAN SIGNATURE

MEDICAL RECORDS

continued

OPERATIVE NOTE

DATE OF PROCEDURE: 2/27/xxxx

PREOPERATIVE DIAGNOSIS: Chronic refractory otitis media.

POSTOPERATIVE DIAGNOSIS: Same.

PROCEDURE PERFORMED: Bilateral tympanotomy and tube insertion.

DESCRIPTION: The patient was brought to the operating room and induced into general mask anesthesia. Her ear canals were cleaned with a curet. Myringotomies were made in the anterior inferior quadrants. Shea parasol drain tubes were placed without difficulty. The middle ears were dry.

The patient tolerated the procedure well and was awakened and taken to the recovery room in satisfactory condition. There were no complications.

Review Case 4-11, *continued*

URINALYSIS DRUG SCREEN		
☐ DRUG SCREEN		CHECK ONE ☐ RANDOM ☐ CATHETERIZED ☐ CLEAN CATCH
ROUTINE		
COLOR	*Straw*	
APPEARANCE	*Slt Haze*	
SPEC. GRAVITY	*1.009*	
pH	*7.5*	
PROTEIN	∅	
GLUCOSE	∅	
KETONE	∅	
BILIRUBIN	∅	
BLOOD/ HEMOGLOBIN	∅	
MICROSCOPIC / HPF		
WBC	∅	
RBC	∅	
EPITH. CELLS	∅	
BACTERIA	∅	
MUCOUS THREADS	∅	
CRYSTALS	*2+*	
CASTS	∅	
CLINITEST		
DRUG SCREEN		
AMPHETAMINE		
BARBITURATE		
BENZODIAZEPINE		
COCAINE		
MARIJUANA		
METHADONE		
OPIATE		
TRICYCLIC ANTIDEPRESSANTS (SERUM)		

LABORATORY REPORT SERIES

continued

Review Case 4-11, *continued*

ICD-9-CM diagnosis code(s): _____

ICD-10-CM diagnosis code(s): _____

CPT code(s) with modifier, if applicable: _____

APC: _____

Review Case 4-12

Health Record Face Sheet

Western Regional
Medical Center

Record Number:	31-00-01
Age:	30
Gender:	Male
Length of Stay:	Not Applicable
Diagnosis/Procedure:	Esophageal Stricture Esophageal Dilation
Service Type:	Same-Day Surgery
Discharge Status:	To Home

Review Case 4-12, *continued*

ALLERGIES			TETANUS STATUS	
CURRENT MEDS			LMP	
HISTORY & PHYSICAL	T: P: R: BP: SaO₂: WT:		**BY (INIT)**	

TIME OF MD INITIAL ASSESSMENT				

LABS
- ☐ STAT
- ☐ ABG on _____ *l*
- ☐ Admit Packet
- ☐ Amylase
- ☐ Cardiac Packet
- ☐ CBC   ☐ DIFF.
- ☐ CBG on _____ *l*
- ☐ Chem Profile _____
- ☐ CPK/ISO
- ☐ EKG
- ☐ Glucose
- ☐ HCG   ☐ SERUM   ☐ URINE
- ☐ Lytes
- ☐ PT/PTT
- ☐ Trauma Packet
- ☐ Type & Screen
- ☐ Type & Cross _____
- ☐ UA
- ☐ CSF
- ☐ Culture _____
- ☐
- ☐
- ☐
- ☐
- ☐

DICTATED: ☐ YES ☐ NO

TIME	TREATMENT ORDERS			
		TIME		
		☐ STANDING ORDERS		

X-RAYS
- ☐ Chest
- ☐ C-Spine
- ☐ Flat Plate/Upright (ABD)
- ☐ CT   ☐ HEAD   ☐ ABD
- ☐

DIAGNOSIS:

Hiatal Hernia c̄ Esophageal Stricture and dilation

DISCHARGE TIME	DISCHARGE INSTRUCTIONS

Discharge patient when awake. Follow up Dr. Otto.

Return to Work/School

PHYSICIAN SIGNATURE X	I HAVE RECEIVED AND UNDERSTAND THE ABOVE INSTRUCTIONS. PT/SO SIGNATURE X *Michael Chien*	☐ SEE DISCHARGE INSTRUCTIONS SHEET	
Dr. Hungarti			REV. BY

EMERGENCY DEPARTMENT RECORD

continued

Review Case 4-12, *continued*

HISTORY **CHIEF COMPLAINT**	*Peanut butter caught in esophagus*	**TRIAGE**	REPORTABLE INJURY ☐ YES ☐ NO

MENTAL STATUS _____ COLOR _____
RESPIRATIONS _____ SKIN TURGOR _____

☐ O₂   ☐ Elevate   ☐ MED. _____
☐ Splint ☐ Dressing   ☐ MED. _____
☐ Ice   ☐ _____   TRIAGE NURSE **X**

PTA GCS CRAMS ☐ BACKBOARD ☐ C-COLLAR ☐

		TETANUS
	NKA	
CURRENT MEDICATIONS	*Zantac*	☐ CURRENT ☐ R ☐ NOT CURRENT ☐ L ☐ TT ☐ Td ☐ ☐ DT ☐ DPT ☐
PMH		

ASSESSMENT

(NEURO, CARDIAC, RESPIRATORY,
GI, GU, SKIN, INCIDENT TIME)

LOT # _____

Hiatal hernia - morning yesterday. Pt was eating a
peanut butter and jelly sandwich caught in upper esophagus.
Pt has a hiatal hernia and a small opening. Pt is in no
distress, cannot swallow any water.

VISUAL ACUITY OD _____ OS _____ OU _____

WT
LMP

TIME	TEMP	P	R	BP	SaO₂ O₂	TIME	MEDICATION/DOSE	ROUTE	SITE	SIGNATURE
425 pm	978	82	16	120/80	/					
		64	16	130/86	/					
				/						
				/						
				/						

TIME	IV FLUID/AMOUNT	MEDICATION ADDED	RATE/HR	SIZE	SITE	TIME Dc'd	AMT INFUSED	SIGNATURE

TIME	PROBLEM/CHANGE	INTERVENTION	PATIENT RESPONSE / EVALUATION
350	*Returned from endoscopy in stable condition. Alert, oriented, skin pink*		

SIGNATURE/ TITLE *Mary Houser, R.N.*

SIGNATURE/ TITLE X

☐ SEE ADDENDUM ED NURSES FLOW SHEET

DISCHARGE TIME:

DISPOSITION ☒ Discharged ☐ AMA
☐ Admit/Transfer _____
Report Given To: _____
CONDITION ON DISCHARGE/TRANSFER ☒ Stable
☐ Stabilized   ☐ Improved   ☐ Expired
DISCHARGE MODE: ☒ Ambulatory
☐ Wheelchair   ☐ Stretcher   ☐ Carried
Accom. by _____

PATIENT BELONGINGS	BAG	ON PT.	NONE
Clothing _____	☐	☐	☐
Wallet/Purse _____	☐	☐	☐
Money _____	☐	☐	☐
Jewelry _____	☐	☐	☐
Glasses _____	☐	☐	☐
Dentures _____	☐	☐	☐

DISPOSITION: ☐ Not Disrobed ☐ Patient ☐ Family
☐ Security ☐ SEE BELONGINGS LIST

Review Case 4-12, *continued*

DATE: 4/04/XXXX
H & P: DICTATED ☐   ATTACHED ☐
PROCEDURE REPORT: DICTATED ☐
INDICATIONS FOR PROCEDURE
Esophageal Obstruction
PRE-PROCEDURE DIAGNOSTIC STUDIES:
US - Ultrasound
PROCEDURE:
EGD c̄ with removal of obstruction
FINDINGS & TECHNIQUES:
PATIENT CONDITION:
POST DISCHARGE INSTRUCTIONS:
F/U Dr. Otto or myself 1 week
DISCHARGE DIAGNOSIS:
Esophageal Obstruction 2s to stricture

continued

Review Case 4-12, *continued*

OPERATIVE NOTE

DATE OF PROCEDURE: 4/04/xxxx

PREOPERATIVE DIAGNOSIS: Esophageal obstruction secondary to stricture.

POSTOPERATIVE DIAGNOSIS: Same.

OPERATION: Esophagogastroscopy with removal of foreign body.

ANESTHESIA: Topical plus sedation.

HISTORY: The patient is a 30-year-old Asian male who has had previous episodes of obstruction secondary to esophageal stricture. Approximately 24 hours prior to admission he again became obstructed and was unable to clear it spontaneously. He is now being admitted for EGD with removal of the obstruction.

Patient has no specific allergies to medications. Is taking Sudafed and Zantac. Has had multiple broken bones but history is otherwise negative. Heart and lungs are okay for the procedure.

PROCEDURE: The patient was brought to the endoscopy suite where he was given 100 mcg of Fentanyl and 2 mg of Versed intravenously.

The patient's oropharynx was sprayed with Cetacaine spray.

The panendoscope was passed without difficulty through the cricopharyngeus and advanced to the esophageal stricture. A large bolus of meat was within the stricture causing obstruction. Using gentle pressure, the meat was slowly extruded into the stomach. The scope was then passed into the stomach and the fundus, body and antrum of the stomach examined and found to be normal.

The scope was then removed and the procedure terminated.

FINAL DIAGNOSIS: As above.

ICD-9-CM diagnosis code(s): _____

ICD-10-CM diagnosis code(s): _____

CPT code(s) with modifier, if applicable: _____

APC: _____

Review Case 4-13

Health Record Face Sheet

Western Regional
Medical Center

Record Number:	12-88-07
Age:	78
Gender:	Female
Length of Stay:	Not Applicable
Diagnosis/Procedure:	Cataract with Extraction
Service Type:	Same-Day Surgery
Discharge Status:	To Home

HISTORY & PHYSICAL

ADMISSION DATE: 6/13/xxxx

The patient is a 78-year-old woman brought to the hospital today for elective cataract removal from her right eye and implant of intraocular lens. She has noted progressive loss of vision in her right eye to the current level of 20/50. Left eye is 20/20 best corrected, cataract having been removed in 2000 and posterior chamber implant in place.

She states her health in general has been good. She was last hospitalized in May for a hip replacement and an episode of pneumonia requiring hospitalization. She has no known allergies. She is currently taking Vasoretic for the control of blood pressure. She states blood pressure has been nicely controlled with the medication.

REVIEW OF SYSTEMS: Otherwise essentially normal.

PHYSICAL EXAM: The patient is a 78-year-old woman in good general health and spirits.

MOUTH & PHARYNX: Clear.

NECK: No adenopathy noted. Thyroid not palpable.

EYES: Best corrected vision right eye 20/50; left eye 20/20. Intraocular pressures are normal. Dilated fundus exam is clear. Exam of the anterior segment of either eye reveals cataract consistent with 20/50 vision in the right eye. In the left eye a posterior chamber implant is present. External exam and extraocular motility are normal.

CHEST: Lungs clear. Heart regular rhythm, no murmur noted.

ABDOMEN: No masses or tenderness. No organomegaly.

NEUROLOGIC EXAM: Grossly intact.

IMPRESSION:

1. Cataract removal, right eye, implant of intraocular lens.
2. Hypertension.

continued

Review Case 4-13, *continued*

OPERATIVE NOTE

DATE OF OPERATION: 6/13/xxxx

PROCEDURE: Cataract removal, right eye; implant of intraocular lens.

Before the usual prep and drape 3 1/2 cc's of 2% Xylocaine with Marcaine and Wydase were given in retrobulbar injection. 6 cc's of the same solution were injected along the superior and inferior orbital rim. After 15 minutes of super pinky intraocular pressure measured 12 with a 5 1/2 gram weight. There was excellent akinesia.

The patient was then prepped and draped in the usual manner. A self retaining lid speculum was used to separate the eyelids. A 4-0 silk suture placed under the superior rectus muscle. 140 degree limbal based conjunctival flap was made superiorly. A 120 degree limbal groove was made. The anterior chamber was entered at the 10 o'clock hour. With Amvisc in the anterior chamber, an anterior capsulotomy was performed. The limbal incision was extended with corneal scleral scissors. The lens nucleus was expressed. 10-0 nylon sutures were placed in the left hand aspect of the incision, 8-0 Vicryl in the right hand aspect. Cortical material was then irrigated and aspirated with the AMO unit. Posterior capsule was polished. Posterior chamber lens was inspected, found to be free of defects. With Amvisc in the anterior chamber, the implant was placed into the bag and centered. Residual Amvisc was irrigated and aspirated with the AMO unit. Miochol was injected. Pupil constricted round and even. Additional 10-0 nylon sutures were placed in the limbal incision. Conjunctiva was closed with a running 8-0 Vicryl. The lid speculum and silk suture were removed. The eye was patched and shielded after Maxitrol ointment was applied. Patient tolerated the procedure well. There were no complications.

PHYSICIAN'S ORDERS & PROGRESS RECORD

DATE	ORDERS	✓	DATE	PROGRESS
6/13/xx	Reg Diet shield OD Tylenol #3 $\frac{1}{1}$1 q 4h Usual meds from home		6/13/xx	ECCE c̄ RC IOL insertion s̄ complication.

Review Case 4-13, *continued*

LABORATORY REPORT						
Test Name	Result	Flags	Units	Low	High	Comments
CHEMISTRY SCREEN						
GLUCOSE	105		mg/dl	70	110	
BUN	45		mg/dl	7	24	
CREATININE	2.6		mg/dl	0.6	1.3	
BUN / CREATININE RATIO	17.3			0.0	40.0	
URIC ACID	7.6		mg/dl	2.6	5.6	
TOTAL BILIRUBIN	0.45		mg/dl	0.00	1.00	
DIRECT BILIRUBIN	0.12		mg/dl	0.00	0.30	
INDIRECT BILIRUBIN	0.33		mg/dl	0.00	0.90	
ALK PHOSPHATASE	115		U/L	50	136	
SGPT	35		U/L	30	65	
SGOT	38		U/L	15	37	
LDH	162		U/L	100	190	
GGTP	47		U/L	5	85	
TOTAL PROTEIN	7.1		g/dl	6.4	8.2	
ALBUMIN	3.7		g/dl	3.4	5.0	
GLOBULIN	3.4		g/dl	2.0	3.5	
A/G RATIO	1.1			1.0	2.5	
CALCIUM	9.0		mg/dl	8.8	10.5	
PHOSPHORUS	4.0		mg/dl	2.5	4.9	
IRON	71		ug/dl	35	150	
SODIUM	134		mmol/L	140	148	
POTASSIUM	4.0		mmol/L	3.6	5.2	
CHLORIDE	97		mmol/L	100	108	
CHOLESTEROL	208		mg/dl	130	200	
TRIGLYCERIDE	95		mg/dl	30	200	

continued

Review Case 4-13, *continued*

URINALYSIS DRUG SCREEN	
ROUTINE	
COLOR	Yellow
APPEARANCE	Clear
GLUCOSE	Ø
BILIRUBIN	Ø
KETONE	Ø
SPEC GRAVITY	1.006
BLOOD	Ø
pH	5.5
PROTEIN	30 mg/dl
UROBILINOGEN	Minimal
NITRITE	Ø
LEUKOCYTES	Trace
MICROSCOPIC / HPF	
WBC	2-5
RBC	5-10
EPITH. CELLS	1-3
BACTERIA	Ø
MUCOUS THREADS	Ø
CRYSTALS	Ø
CASTS	Ø
CLINITEST	
DRUG SCREEN	
AMPHETAMINE	
BARBITURATE	
BENZODIAZEPINE	
COCAINE	
MARIJUANA	
OPIATE	
TRICYCLIC ANTIDEPRESSANTS (SERUM)	

Review Case 4-13, *continued*

BLOOD COUNT LABORATORY RESULTS

	%	#		
WBC	7.5		RBC	3.93
			HGB	11.9
NE	60.7	4.6	HCT	35.7
LY	29.2	2.2	MCV	90.8
MO	5.1	0.4	MCH	30.2
EO	4.0	0.3	MCHC	33.2
BA	0.9	0.1	RDW	12.0

Normal WBC Pop

Normal RBC Pop   PLT   184

Normal PLT Pop   MPV   7.3

ICD-9-CM diagnosis code(s): _____

ICD-10-CM diagnosis code(s): _____

CPT code(s) with modifier, if applicable: _____

APC: _____

Review Case 4-14

Health Record Face Sheet

Western Regional
Medical Center

Record Number:	96-14-41
Age:	35
Gender:	Female
Length of Stay:	N/A
Service Type:	Same-Day Surgery
Discharge Status:	To Home
Diagnosis/Procedure:	Recurrent Carpal Tunnel
	Carpal Tunnel Decompression

continued

HISTORY & PHYSICAL

ADMISSION DATE: 9/29/xxxx

HISTORY: This is a 35-year-old female who underwent a right carpal tunnel decompression about 10 years ago and over the last several months has redeveloped signs and symptoms of carpal tunnel syndrome. She has EMG nerve conduction studies showing significant compression of her median nerve with an absent median sensory on the right. She presents for re-exploration and decompression.

PAST HISTORY: Diabetes mellitus. Hysterectomy and C-sections.

ALLERGIES: Compazine.

REGULAR MEDICATIONS: Insulin 20 NPH in the morning and 6 Regular and supplemental Insulin as needed, and Premarin.

No bleeding tendencies.

REVIEW OF SYSTEMS: In recent stable health in regard to respiratory, cardiovascular, gastrointestinal and genitourinary systems.

PHYSICAL EXAMINATION:

HEENT: Otherwise within normal limits.

NECK: Supple. No adenopathy.

CHEST: Clear anteriorly and posteriorly with equal breath sounds.

CARDIOVASCULAR: Regular sinus rhythm without murmur.

ABDOMEN: No abnormal masses.

EXTREMITIES: Pertinent findings confined to the right upper extremity. On previous exam she has a carpal tunnel incision which is somewhat more proximal than seen now. (This was done 10 years ago.) She has a Tinnel's sign at the distal edge of the incision. No thenar atrophy. A markedly positive Tinnel's sign. More proximal exam negative for thoracic outlet and no radiculopathy on neck compression.

NEUROLOGIC: Otherwise nondiagnostic.

IMPRESSION:

1. Recurrent carpal tunnel syndrome.
2. Diabetes mellitus.

PLAN: Re-exploration, carpal tunnel decompression with possible internal neurolysis.

The procedure, its risks and complications including hematoma, infection, and the guarded prognosis on relief due impart to her diabetes mellitus and also just by the nature of a recurrent carpal tunnel syndrome, has been carefully explained to the patient. Anesthetic complications have also been discussed.

Review Case 4-14, *continued*

OPERATIVE NOTE

DATE OF PROCEDURE: 9/29/xxxx

PREOPERATIVE DIAGNOSIS: Recurrent carpal tunnel syndrome.

POSTOPERATIVE DIAGNOSIS: Same.

OPERATIVE PROCEDURE: Right carpal tunnel decompression and flexor tenosynovectomy.

SURGEON: Dr. Riddle

ASSISTANT: Dr. Huvaci

INDICATIONS: This 35-year-old presents with recurrent signs and symptoms of carpal tunnel syndrome. She has had a decompression about 10 years ago. Has EMG nerve conduction findings compatible with carpal tunnel and has not responded to conservative treatment.

OPERATIVE PROCEDURE: After, satisfactory induction under general anesthesia, the entire right upper extremity was prepped and draped in the usual sterile manner. The extremity was exsanguinated and the tourniquet applied to 250 mm. of mercury.

A serpentine incision distal to the previous incision which extended into the distal forearm was outlined with methylene blue. With the use of 2 1/2 power magnification, the incision was made and carried down to the underlying transverse carpal ligament. The ligament was identified and dissection carried out with the entire release on the ulnar side of the transverse carpal ligament. There appeared to be an area of about a little over a centimeter distal to the previous incision that was involved with compression underneath what was now the transverse carpal ligament. The nerve did expand reasonably. An epineurolysis was performed as well as a tenosynovectomy of the surrounding tendons which were thickened. Dissection was carried out more proximally and no other restriction was found and distally no other compression area was identified. There were no masses in the carpal tunnel. A portion of the transverse carpal ligament was taken as a separate specimen. Hemostasis was established. 1/4% plain Marcaine was infiltrated about the skin edges. The tourniquet was released. Circulation returned promptly to the entire hand and after hemostasis was established, a small amount of dexamethasone was placed in the wound. Closure was then performed with a few 4-0 Vicryl sutures in the dermal subcutaneous layer taking care to not close the transverse carpal ligament. 5-0 Prolene suture in a horizontal mattress configuration was used on the skin.

Adaptic dry dressing was applied followed by a splint.

The patient was transported to the recovery area in satisfactory condition.

continued

Review Case 4-14, *continued*

PATHOLOGY REPORT

OPERATION: RIGHT CARPAL TUNNEL RELEASE
#1 EPINEURIUM
#2 SYNOVIUM AND TENDON
#3 VOLAR CARPAL LIGAMENT

GROSS: Specimen #1 indicated as epineurium is comprised of irregularly shaped fragments of yellow–tan tissue together measuring approximately 1.0 cm. The specimen is submitted in its entirety for examination. Specimen #2 indicated as synovium and tendon is comprised of irregularly shaped fragments of pink to yellow–tan tissue together measuring approximately 1.5 cm. The specimen is submitted in its entirety for examination. Specimen #3 indicated as volar carpal ligament is comprised of irregularly shaped fragments of pink to yellow– tan tissue together measuring approximately 1.5 cm. The specimen is submitted in its entirety for examination.

MICRO: Specimen #1 is comprised of fibrovascular connective tissue which is histologically unremarkable. The tissue is consistent with epineurium. Specimen #2 is comprised of non-inflammatory synovium and dense fibrous connective tissue consistent with tendon. The histology is unremarkable. Specimen #3 is comprised of dense fibrous connective tissue consistent with ligamentous tissue together with fibrovascular connective and adipose tissue. The histology is unremarkable.

FINDINGS: Specimen #1, fibrovascular connective tissue consistent with epineurium, removed in the course of right carpal tunnel release.
Specimen #2, non–inflammatory synovium and tissue consistent with tendon, removed in the course of right carpal tunnel release.
Specimen #3, ligamentous and associated soft tissue, removed in the course of right carpal tunnel release.

ICD-9-CM diagnosis code(s): _____

ICD-10-CM diagnosis code(s): _____

CPT code(s) with modifier, if applicable: _____

APC: _____

Review Case 4-15

Health Record Face Sheet

Western Regional
Medical Center

Record Number: 94-77-23

Age: 16

Gender: Female

Length of Stay: N/A

Service Type: Same-Day Surgery

Discharge Status: To Home

Diagnosis/Procedure: Acute Appendicitis
                                Appendectomy

continued

Review Case 4-15, *continued*

HISTORY & PHYSICAL

PATIENT: Jamara Jackson

MEDICAL RECORD NO: 94-77-23

ROOM: 516

ADMIT DATE: 12/02/xxxx

PHYSICIAN: Dr. Minut

CHIEF COMPLAINT: Abdominal pain.

HISTORY OF PRESENT ILLNESS:

This is a 16-year-old white female who began having some right-sided abdominal pain about two days ago. It is associated with some diarrhea. She had some vomiting today. No real anorexia. She ate about six hours prior to admission at Roy's Burgers. She ate a hamburger. She has an ongoing sinus infection and bladder infection that she says she has had for about a week or so.

PAST MEDICAL HISTORY:
CURRENT MEDS:	An antidepressant.
ALLERGIES:	**NO KNOWN ALLERGIES.**
SURGERIES:	She had an ovarian cyst operated on laparoscopically two years ago. She had a tonsillectomy two years ago.
MEDICAL ILLNESS:	Remarkable for depression, diagnosed, and placed on antidepressants.

PSYCHOSOCIAL HISTORY:

She is a student. Occasional rare alcohol or tobacco use. She denies any caffeine.

FAMILY HISTORY: Noncontributory.

REVIEW OF SYSTEMS:

She has had some problems with her depression and some self-mutilation off and on over the last several years.

PHYSICAL EXAM:
GENERAL:	Alert white female in mild distress secondary to abdominal pain.
HEENT:	Pupils are equal and reactive to light and accommodation. Extraocular muscles are intact. Nares are clear without any discharge. Mouth and oropharynx are pink without any exudate or lesions. Tympanic membranes are intact.
NECK:	The trachea is in midline. Thyroid is not enlarged. Carotids are equal.
CHEST:	Lungs are clear to percussion and auscultation.
HEART:	Regular rate and rhythm. No murmur.
BREASTS:	Deferred.
ABDOMEN:	Soft. There is right lower quadrant tenderness with rebound tenderness. Percussion and palpation of the left lower quadrant and right upper quadrant refer pain to the right lower quadrant.
EXTREM:	Full range of motion. All pulses present.
GU:	Pelvic examination deferred.
RECTAL:	Rectal examination deferred.
NEURO:	Grossly normal.
SKIN:	Normal color and turgor. Multiple superficial scars noted on the left forearm.

Review Case 4-15, *continued*

HISTORY & PHYSICAL CONT'D

LAB AND X-RAY:

At admission, urine HCG was negative. Urine was unremarkable. CBC showed a hemo-globin of 12.4, hematocrit 38.1, WBC 16.9. The patient had an ultrasound that showed a long appendix, the distal half of which was acutely inflamed.

IMPRESSION:

Acute appendicitis.

PLAN:

1. The plan is to take the patient to the Operating Room as soon as possible for laparoscopic appendectomy or possible open appendectomy,
2. The procedure and risks involved, benefits, and alternatives were explained to the patient and her father and they are agreeable to the surgery.

continued

OPERATIVE REPORT

PATIENT: Jamara Jackson

MEDICAL RECORD NO: 94-77-23

ROOM: 516

ADMIT DATE: 12/02/xxxx

SURGERY DATE: 12/02/xxxx

SURGEON: Dr. Minut
ASSIST: Dr. Rogerson

PREOPERATIVE DIAGNOSIS:	Acute appendicitis.
POSTOPERATIVE DIAGNOSIS:	Acute appendicitis.
OPERATIVE PROCEDURE:	Laparoscopic appendectomy.
ANESTHESIA	General endotracheal anesthesia.
ESTIMATED BLOOD LOSS:	Less than 5 cc.
IV FLUIDS:	500 cc. lactated Ringer's.

DESCRIPTION OF OPERATIVE PROCEDURE:

The patient was placed on the operating table in the supine position. General endo-tracheal anesthesia was administered. A Foley catheter and NG tube were inserted and the abdomen was prepped with Prevail and draped in the usual fashion for lapa-roscopic appendectomy. ½% Marcaine with epinephrine was used to infiltrate the skin and subcutaneous tissue and fascial planes. A total of 9 cc. was used throughout the procedure for this.

An infraumbilical incision was made first where the previous laparoscopic scar was. A Veress needle was inserted in the abdominal cavity. Saline easily flowed in, no return, positive drop test. The abdominal cavity was then insufflated to 15 mm. of mercury pressure with carbon-dioxide. Following this the Veress needle was removed and a 10 mm. trocar inserted through the infraumbilical incision. Through the port created, a laparoscope was introduced and under direct vision a 5 mm. trocar was placed in the right side of the abdomen, just above the level of the umbilicus and a 12 mm. trocar placed in the left lower quadrant.

The omentum was moved back, the cecum was exposed, and the appendix was vi-sualized. It appeared to be injected and inflamed at the tip with phlegmon present. The proximal portion of the appendix appeared unremarkable. A window was created between the appendix and its mesentery and the appendix was divided at its base by means of the EndoGIA using the bowel load. The mesentery was then divided by means of the EndoGIA using the vascular load. The appendix was removed with the Endo pouch. A culture was taken. It was sent to Pathology. A small bleeder was noted just at the end of the staple line on the mesentery. This was cauterized by means of the Bovie. The area was irrigated with warm lactated Ringer's. There was no evidence of any further bleeding. The staple lines appeared to be intact on the mesentery and on the appendiceal base. The pelvis was irrigated. The pelvis looked a little bit injected on the right side with the uterus going forward and also the right tube, though certainly not distended. The right ovary was absent. The left ovary appeared to be normal. Once ir-rigation was completed and staple lines were intact, the patient was allowed to deflate.

The fascia of the infraumbilical incision and left lower quadrant incision were approxi-mated with figure of eight #0 Vicryl sutures. The wounds were painted with Betadine solution. The subcutaneous tissue was approximated with interrupted 3-0 Dexon. The skin was closed with running 3-0 Dexon subcuticular suture. Steri-Strips, Ensure-It, and Tegaderm dressing were applied. The sponge and instrument counts were correct. The patient tolerated the procedure well and left the Operating Room in good condition.

Review Case 4-15, *continued*

TISSUE REPORT

History: ACUTE APPENDICITIS

Gross: Labeled with the patient's name and appendix, received in formalin is an 8.8 x 0.8 cm appendix with a small amount of attached mesoappendix. The serosa is tan-pink, smooth and glistening with prominent congested vessels. There is a small amount of focal fibrinous exudate along the mesoappendix. The lumen measures up to 0.5 cm and contains liquid tan purulent feces. The mucosa is tan, smooth and unremarkable. The wall measures up to 0.1 cm and is intact. There is a 0.5 x 0.5 cm fecalith identified. Representative sections are submitted in a single cassette.

MICROSCOPIC: DONE

DIAGNOSIS: ACUTE APPENDICITIS, APPENDECTOMY

ICD-9-CM diagnosis code(s): _____

ICD-10-CM diagnosis code(s): _____

CPT code(s) with modifier, if applicable: _____

APC: _____

Review Case 4-16

Health Record Face Sheet

Western Regional
Medical Center

Record Number:	02-64-12
Age:	63
Gender:	Female
Length of Stay:	N/A
Service Type:	Same-Day Surgery
Discharge Status:	To Home
Diagnosis/Procedure:	EGD with Bx

ESOPHAGOGASTRODUODENOSCOPY REPORT

DATE OF PROCEDURE: 10/2/xxxx

INDICATIONS: 63-year-old female who has a history of severe hypertriglyceridemia with pancreatitis in the past. This is presently well controlled with Atromid-S. She also has been noted to have mild hypercalcemia with a normal N-terminal parathyroid hormone assay. Recently she has been having severe headaches with nausea and vomiting. An upper GI demonstrated prominent rugal folds which were not seen on a previous upper GI series. Endoscopy with biopsy is planned.

EXAMINATION: Following informed consent, she was sedated with Demerol 50 mg and Versed 1 mg IV. An Olympus OES type GIF-XQ10 endoscope was introduced. The esophagus was unremarkable. The stomach, including retroflex exam of the fundus and cardia, is notable for prominent folds of the body of the stomach particularly along the greater curvature. Pylorus, duodenal bulb and several centimeters of post-bulbar duodenum were normal. The rugal folds were probed with a biopsy forceps and there was no induration evident. Several biopsies were taken. She tolerated the procedure well and there were no complications acutely.

FINAL IMPRESSION: Prominent rugal folds of uncertain significance. Must consider the possibility of Menetrier's disease. Doubt an infiltrating carcinoma or lymphoma.

PLAN: Home when ambulatory. Will follow up on the biopsies and communicate with her primary care physician

Review Case 4-16, *continued*

PATHOLOGY REPORT

OPERATION: ENDOSCOPY
GASTRIC TISSUE

GROSS: The specimen consists of five, pink-tan to gray-tan tissues that are up to 0.3 cm. in largest dimension. They are processed as 'received.

MICRO: Mucosal elements are well differentiated. Muscularis mucosa is at the deep edge. Glands are well differentiated. Some of the pieces show moderately severe acute gastritis with infiltration of the lamina propria and glandular elements by neutrocytes.

FINDINGS:
Moderately severe acute gastritis, gastric mucosal biopsies, esophagogastroduodenoscopy procedure.

ICD-9-CM diagnosis code(s): _____

ICD-10-CM diagnosis code(s): _____

CPT code(s) with modifier, if applicable: _____

APC: _____

Review Case 4-17

Health Record Face Sheet

Western Regional
Medical Center

Record Number:	89-01-17
Age:	15
Gender:	Female
Length of Stay:	N/A
Service Type:	Emergency Room
Discharge Status:	To Home
Diagnosis/Procedure:	Conjunctivitis

continued

EMERGENCY ROOM REPORT

CHIEF COMPLAINT: This patient is a 15-year-old white female with a chief complaint of pink eye.

HISTORY OF PRESENT ILLNESS: She awoke two days ago with both eyes stuck shut from discharge and was unable to describe the color of this discharge. That day she went to summer school and her teachers complained that her eyes looked quite red and sent her to the school nurse who sent her home with the instructions to obtain medication before she returned to school. Yesterday morning she awoke with the left eye glued shut with discharge and this morning the right eye. She complains of mild tenderness in the eyes with some itch. She has also had some sneezing. No history of hayfever or allergies. She denies any changes in vision or photophobia. She denies fever, chills, nausea, vomiting or diarrhea.

PAST MEDICAL HISTORY: Negative.

CURRENT MEDICATIONS: None.

ALLERGIES: NONE KNOWN.

PHYSICAL EXAM:

GENERAL: Alert, white, thin female in no acute distress. Vital signs: BP 116/68, temp 97, pulse 84, respirations 16.

HEENT: Head is normocephalic and atraumatic. The TMs are normal bilaterally. Eyes, PERRLA. EOMI. Sclerae are nonicteric. They are slightly injected. The limbus is spared. The discs are flat. She has no photophobia. Sinuses are nontender to palpation. The pharynx is clear.

NECK: Supple and nontender without lymphadenopathy or thyromegaly.

ASSESSMENT: ACUTE CONJUNCTIVITIS, POSSIBLY BACTERIAL.

PLAN: Sodium Sulamyd drops 1 in each eye q 3-4.hours until better. Follow up prn.

ICD-9-CM diagnosis code(s): _____

ICD-10-CM diagnosis code(s): _____

CPT code(s) with modifier, if applicable: _____

APC: _____

Review Case 4-18

<u>**Health Record Face Sheet**</u>

Western Regional
Medical Center

<u>**Record Number:**</u>	76-09-18
<u>**Age:**</u>	30
<u>**Gender:**</u>	Male
<u>**Length of Stay:**</u>	N/A
<u>**Service Type:**</u>	Consultation Emergency Room
<u>**Discharge Status:**</u>	To Home
<u>**Diagnosis/Procedure:**</u>	Fracture of Patella

continued

EMERGENCY ROOM CONSULTATION

DATE OF CONSULTATION: 4/22/xxxx

ID: 30-year-old male.

CHIEF COMPLAINT: Left knee and ankle injury.

HISTORY OF PRESENT ILLNESS: This gentleman was involved in an altercation two weeks ago, had pain in the knee, injury to his nose and left ankle, but did not seek consultation until Monday when he went into the Emergency Room where an x-ray was obtained of the knee and he was recalled in today to obtain an additional film showing a fracture of the superior lateral dome, the superior lateral patellar, nonweightbearing minimal injury. He was also told that he had an ankle fracture, but his x-rays did not accompany him. He has been weightbearing on the knee with mild limping and with only minimal complaints in the ankle. He has no other complaints so we took them again today.

PAST MEDICAL HISTORY:

MEDICAL ILLNESSES: None.

SURGERY: See previous record.

MEDICATIONS: Prescribed analgesics per

ALLERGIES: Motrin.

PHYSICAL EXAMINATION: Healthy alert male.

Vital signs: BP 132/76, pulse 64, respirations 20, temperature 96.4.

ORTHOPEDIC EXAMINATION: Reveals tenderness in the right and mid posterior rib approximately rib number eight or nine by estimation with slight swelling, no significant crepitation is noted and he is not short of breath. The left hip has full range of motion. The left knee has no effusion, extends to approximately 0, internally rotates to 60, external to 40, abduction and adduction 30 and 30. The knee is tender along the superior lateral patella, no effusion. There is no medial, lateral or AP laxity. McMurray's testing is difficult because of the discomfort in the patella. Ankle motion - he can dorsiflex 10, plantar flex 30. There is mild swelling and tenderness along the lateral malleolus, but no obvious displacement is noted clinically and he has full neurovascular pulses and sensation.

X-rays of the knee show four views with approximately 1 cm minimally displaced avulsion superior lateral patella seen on Houston view. There is also the possibility of a small intra-articular osteochondral fracture seen on lateral view, but I do not see an origin site and cannot find evidence of internal derangement. Ankle films are reviewed.

IMPRESSION:
1. Avulsion fracture left patella.
2. Rule out internal derangement, left knee.
3. Non-displaced ankle fracture, left.
4. contusion to nose

PLAN: I have recommended crutches, touch weightbearing, knee immobilization brace, and an air cast. Discussed with them the overall prognosis is good if there is no other internal derangement in the knee.

He will return to the office in approximately two weeks, notify us of increased pain, fever, chills, numbness or tingling.

RADIOLOGY REPORT

RADIOLOGY REPORT: L. Ankle

HISTORY: Rule out fracture.

LEFT ANKLE:

There is a small avulsion fracture on the tip of the lateral malleoulus. The ankle mortise is intact.

IMPRESSION:

Avulsion fracture at the tip of the lateral malleoulus.

Review Case 4-18, *continued*

ICD-9-CM diagnosis code(s): _____

ICD-10-CM diagnosis code(s): _____

CPT code(s) with modifier, if applicable: _____

APC: _____

Review Case 4-19

Health Record Face Sheet

Western Regional
Medical Center

Record Number:	52-09-77
Age:	52
Gender:	Female
Length of Stay:	N/A
Serviced Type:	Same-Day Surgery
Discharge Status:	To Home
Diagnosis/Procedure:	Colonoscopy

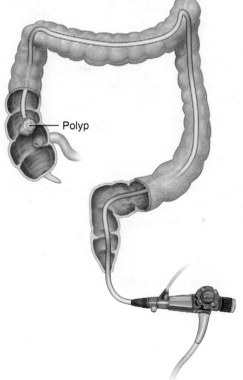

Polyp

Colonoscopy.
Source: Pearson Education/PH College

continued

COLONOSCOPY REPORT

DATE OF PROCEDURE: 12/14/xx

INDICATIONS: 52-year-old female who recently underwent perianal surgery. At the time of surgery she was found to have a rectal polyp which was removed and adenomatous. She has now undergone a prep with Fleet's Phospho-Soda and comes for total colonoscopy.

EXAMINATION: Following informed consent, she was sedated with Demerol 50 mg, Phenergan 25 mg and Versed 1 mg IV. Due to discomfort throughout the exam she was given an additional 50 mg of Demerol which resulted in some O2 desaturation requiring nasal O2. An Olympus OES type CF1T10L colonoscope was introduced and advanced to the cecum. Ileocecal valve was visualized. The scope was withdrawn with detailed circumferential inspection of the mucosa. The bowel prep was excellent. No synchronous neoplastic lesions were identified and no other abnormalities were seen. She tolerated the procedure well and there were no complications acutely.

FINAL IMPRESSION: No synchronous neoplastic lesions.

PLAN: Home when ambulatory.

H & P: DICTATED ☐   ATTACHED ☐

PROCEDURE REPORT: DICTATED ☐

INDICATIONS FOR PROCEDURE: *Rectal polyp removed reassessment*

PRE-PROCEDURE DIAGNOSTIC STUDIES: *N/A*

PROCEDURE: *Demerol Phenergan 25 Versed 1 mg IV*

FINDINGS & TECHNIQUES: *Examination for neoplasia or other lesion*

PATIENT CONDITION: *Stable*

POST DISCHARGE INSTRUCTIONS: *Home when ambulatory*

DISCHARGE DIAGNOSIS: *No synchronous neoplasia*

Physician Signature:

Michael Aguilar, M.D.

Date: *12/14/xx*

Review Case 4-19, *continued*

ICD-9-CM diagnosis code(s): _____

ICD-10-CM diagnosis code(s): _____

CPT code(s) with modifier, if applicable: _____

APC: _____

Review Case 4-20

Health Record Face Sheet

Western Regional
Medical Center

Record Number:	00-64-59
Age:	18 months
Gender:	Male
Length of Stay:	N/A
Service Type:	Emergency Room
Discharge Status:	Home
Diagnosis/Procedure:	Crush Injury Hand

continued

EMERGENCY ROOM REPORT

CHIEF COMPLAINT: Crush injury to the right hand.

ALLERGIES: NONE KNOWN

CURRENT MEDICATIONS: None.

PAST MEDICAL HISTORY: Unremarkable. Immunizations are current.

HISTORY OF PRESENT ILLNESS: This is an 18-month-old white male who got his right hand caught in a roller of a conveyer belt. His hand got crushed between the rubber belt and an aluminum roller. The roller had to be reversed in order to remove the patient's hand from the place where it was trapped. No other injuries are apparent. The roller only extended up to the level of the wrist prior to being reversed.

PHYSICAL EXAM:
GENERAL: The patient is alert, appropriate and uncomfortable appearing. He is crying, and yet is partially consolable by being held. Respirations are slow and unlabored.

RIGHT HAND: Reveals a partial thickness abrasion involving the palmar surface of the hand. No lacerations are evident. There is a moderate amount of palmar soft tissue swelling, but no soft tissue swelling dorsally. No bony deformity is evident. No sign of any trauma to the wrist. No anatomic snuffbox tenderness. The patient holds his hand in normal anatomic position. The flexor and extensor tendons appear to be intact. There is no sign of vascular compromise. No other signs of trauma.

X-ray of the left hand is read by me as normal,

ASSESSMENT: 1.   CRUSH INJURY TO THE RIGHT HAND DUE TO A WASHING MACHINE ROLLER TYPE INJURY.
2.   DEEP ABRASIONS TO THE PALMAR ASPECT OF THE RIGHT HAND, PROBABLY SECONDARY TO MECHANICAL FRICTION.

TREATMENT: 1.   A non-adherent dressing was applied to the wound followed by a double Kerlex dressing.   2.   Prescription for 4 ounces of Tylenol with Codeine elixir. While in the emergency department, he received 25 mg of Demerol and 15 mg of Vistaril IM. He appeared much more comfortable by the time of discharge.

It should also be noted that Dr. Cromali was here in the emergency department evaluating a patient in the next bed, and he was nice enough to take a look at the patient, and agreed with initial symptomatic therapy. The parents will encourage the child to keep the hand elevated and watch for signs of infection. If any signs of infection appear, they will seek immediate reevaluation. They will attempt to apply ice to the hand as much as is possible for the next couple of days.

Review Case 4-20, *continued*

CHIEF COMPLAINT:

Rt hand caught roller   PREVIOUS ADM: ☐ YES ☒ NO

ALLERGIES: ☒ NKA ☐ CODIENE ☐ PCN

LAST TETANUS
current
☐ NA ☐ UNKNOWN

CURRENT MEDS. AND DOSAGE: ☒ NONE ☐ UNKNOWN

PAST MEDICAL HISTORY:
Ø

INITIAL V.S.

B.P.   T.   H.C.   H. Crying

WEIGHT *30 lbs.*

LMP

OD   OS

IN ROOM *17* AT *12.55* A.M./P.M.   VIA *Carry*

☐ HELD ☐ CHAIR ☐ FOEB ☐ STRETCHER ☐ SIDE RAILS UPS ☐ STANDING ☐ CALL LIGHT IN REACH

PHYSICIAN CALLED	TIME/WHERE	E = EXCHANGE/BEEPER O = OFFICE I = IN HOSPITAL H = HOME	TIME RESPONDED

LAB WORK AND PROCEDURES (check work done)

☐ UA ☐ RANDOM ☐ C.C. ☐ CATH
☐ CBC ☐ H&H _____
☐ SMAC ☐ HOLD ADMIT
☐ BUN ☐ CREATININE
☐ ELECTROLYTES ☐ Na ☐ K
☐ GLUCOSE ☐ AMYLASE
☐ PROTIME ☐ APTT
☐ ABG _____
☐ CPK ☐ CARDIAC ISOENZYME
☐ TYPE OF SCREEN
☐ T&C _____ UNITS
☐ BLOOD ALCOHOL ☐ LEGAL
☐ DRUG SCREEN URINE
☐ THROAT CULTURE ☐ STREP SCREEN
☐ C&S - SOURCE _____
☐ GM STAIN _____
☐ GC - SOURCE _____
☐ CHLAMYDIA
☐ _____
☐ _____
☐ _____
☐ _____

ORDERED	LAB DRAWN	RETURNED

TIME

MONITOR APPLIED
NASAL CANNULA
MASK
O₂ _____ LET TUBE
EKG

TIME	X -RAYS ORDERED
TO: *1255*	*Rt Hand*
RETURN *1310*	
TO:	
RETURN	
TO:	
RETURN	

TO   X-RAY
☐ AMS ☐ W/C ☐ STRETCHER ☐ CARRY

SEE:
☐ EMS RUN SHEET
☐ CODE BLUE DATA SHEET
☐ I & O / NEURO
☐ TRANSFER FORM
☐ _____
☐ _____

TIME	ASSESSMENT AND HISTORY	TIME	MEDICATION & THREATMENTS
1230	18 mo old male - 15 min - 30 mintes ago caught hand conveyoir belt - under roller. Child crying. Rt palm bruised denuded across palm - radial pulse - good. Color hand - wiggling fingers -		
1245	Dr. examined	1255	Demerol 25 mg
1320	Dr. reviewed films / examined child. Child sleepy.		Vistaril 12.5/mg
1335	Mother verbalizes care	1325	Dressed c̄ heavy barelinger adaptive et gauze - in boxer type dressing
	F/U - d.c. mothers arms		

PATIENT DISPOSITION/CONDITION: TIME: *1330*
☐ ADMIT RM _____ REPORT TO: _____
☒ DISCHARGED ☐ TRANSFERRED _____
☐ UNCHANGED ☐ IMPROVED _____
☐ AMBULATORY ☐ W.C. ☐ STRETCHER ☐ CARRY

RIGHT HAND:
X-ray Report

IMPRESSION: NO BONY INJURY TO THE RIGHT HAND. NO FRACTURES OR DISLOCATIONS.

ICD-9-CM diagnosis code(s): _____

ICD-10-CM diagnosis code(s): _____

CPT code(s) with modifier, if applicable: _____

APC: _____

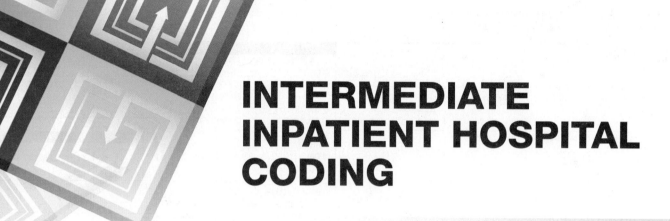

INTERMEDIATE INPATIENT HOSPITAL CODING

5

Learning Objectives

After reading this chapter, you should be able to:

- Spell and define the key terms presented in this chapter.

- Understand the inpatient coding process.

- Differentiate and apply appropriate inpatient coding nomenclature(s) in the assignment of ICD-9-CM and ICD-10-CM diagnosis and procedure codes in the hospital inpatient setting.

- List the steps to follow when coding from medical documentation.

- Accurately apply Uniform Hospital Discharge Data Set definitions to determine principal and secondary diagnoses and principal and secondary procedures.

Key Terms

chronic condition—a condition that persists for a long period of time

discharge summary—the physician's documentation of an inpatient hospital stay

history and physical (H&P)—the physician's documentation of a patient's history of illness and physical examination upon admission

operative report (OP)—the physician's documentation of a procedure that was performed

postoperative—the period of time after surgery

present on admission (POA)—indicator on inpatient claims. The POA indicates whether a diagnosis code was present or not present at the time an order for an inpatient admission occurred.

principal diagnosis—as defined by the Uniform Hospital Discharge Data Set, the condition established after study to be chiefly responsible for occasioning the admission of the patient to the hospital for care

secondary diagnosis—as defined by the Uniform Hospital Discharge Data Set, all conditions that coexist at the time of admission, or develop subsequently, which affect the treatment received and/or the length of stay in the hospital/facility

Uniform Hospital Discharge Data Set (UHDDS)—developed by the U.S. Department of Health, Education and Welfare in 1974 to ensure that all hospitals report a minimum set of data for all patient admissions and use uniform definitions when reporting that data

INTRODUCTION

Inpatient coding comprises a large portion of the coding market and is a very important process that ensures correct reimbursement in a hospital inpatient setting. As defined earlier in this text, an inpatient is a patient who has been admitted to a facility for at least one overnight stay for the purpose of receiving treatment. Note, however, that in certain instances a patient may not stay overnight; for example, the patient may expire or be transferred to another facility.

THE INPATIENT CODING PROCESS

Coders must realize the importance and impact of inpatient coding. Inpatients are typically sicker or undergoing more complex surgeries than those who are not admitted to a facility as an inpatient, which can make the patient's case more complex to code. In addition, coders must realize the difference between hospital inpatient and outpatient coding. With inpatient coding, the ICD-9-CM official coding guidelines for inpatient coding are followed when assigning diagnosis and procedure codes, whereas with outpatient coding, the ICD-9-CM official coding guidelines for outpatient coding are followed. Note that the ICD-9 coding manual is the only manual used for hospital inpatient coding; the CPT® coding manual is not used. Currently, hospital inpatient coders in the United States assign ICD-9-CM diagnosis codes and ICD-9-CM procedure codes only. As of the October 1, 2014, implementation date, they will use ICD-10-CM and ICD-10-PCS codes.

Hospital inpatient coders follow the inpatient coding guidelines, which are based on the ICD-9-CM official coding guidelines (see Appendix A), and any applicable coding policies for the facilities in which they work. Each hospital will have its own set of policies and procedures that ensure their data is coded accurately and effectively. Coding guidelines may differ from one hospital to another because one facility might want to capture information that another facility does not need to capture, for example, data about blood products being transfused, CT scans, MRIs, or other procedures or diagnoses that are not typically coded by inpatient coders.

Inpatient coders also follow another set of external policies when performing hospital inpatient coding, the **Uniform Hospital Discharge Data Set (UHDDS)** as promulgated by Medicare. The UHDDS was developed by the Department of Health, Education and Welfare in 1974 to ensure that all acute care inpatient hospitals report a minimum set of data for all patient admissions and use uniform definitions when reporting that data. Definitions for demographic information, admission date, discharge date, and disposition of the patient are included in the UHDDS. The UHDDS also includes physician identification, diagnoses, procedures, and reimbursement information for any given patient episode of care. Some of the most important data elements of the UHDDS that inpatient coders follow are those that pertain to the definition and selection of the principal diagnosis and secondary diagnosis. According to the UHDDS, an inpatient coder should report all diagnoses that affect the current hospital episode of care and require resources for clinical evaluation, therapeutic treatment, diagnostic procedures, extended length of stay, or increased nursing care and/or monitoring unless otherwise stated as per hospital policy.

Acute care hospital needs for coded data may vary depending on the type or specialty of the facility. A good example is the additional coding that may take place in research and teaching hospitals. These types of specialty hospitals often capture all pertinent medical data from an episode of care. The data is then placed in a databank or repository to be utilized in the future or as demand dictates. For example, a facility may want to capture all family history information regarding cancer or cardiovascular disease. Another example is data captured on a patient's cancer status, such as "2 years and still in remission," or data from an episode of care in the emergency department for a laceration of the thumb caused by a broken drinking glass. Be sure to always follow UHDDS and hospital/facility-specific coding guidelines. The UHDDS guidelines may be found by following the directions given in Appendix B or at the Center for Medicare and Medicaid Services website, www.cms.gov.

Now we will explore UHDDS guidelines for the selection of a principal diagnosis in hospital inpatient coding. The UHDDS definition for principal diagnosis in the acute hospital inpatient setting is "the condition established after study to be chiefly responsible for occasioning the admission of the patient to the hospital." The UHDDS definition for secondary diagnosis is "all conditions that coexist at the time of admission, or develop subsequently, which affect the treatment received and/or the length of stay (LOS)." The principal diagnosis is the first listed diagnosis and is the basis for determination of payment to acute care inpatient hospitals under the prospective payment system and MS-DRGs.

The prospective payment is also affected by two additional types of diagnosis possibilities in the inpatient setting. These two classifications of diagnoses are defined as a *complication* or *comorbidity*. The UHDDS defines a complication as "an additional diagnosis describing a condition that arises after the beginning of hospital observation and treatment that modifies the course of the patient's illness or the medical care required." The UHDDS definition for comorbidity is "pre-existing condition present at time of admission that, because of their presence, increase the patient's length of stay or resources required to treat the patient." The UHDDS also defines the principal procedure and significant procedures assigned in hospital inpatient coding. A principal procedure is defined as a "procedure that was performed for definitive treatment rather than one performed for diagnostic or exploratory purposes, or was necessary to take care of a complication. If there appear to be two procedures that are principal, then the one most related to the principal diagnosis should be selected as the principal procedure." The UHDDS defines a significant procedure as a "procedure which is surgical in nature, carries a procedural risk, carries an anesthetic risk, and/or impacts MS-DRG assignment."

The ICD 10 CM *Official Guidelines for Coding and Reporting* must also be strictly followed in code assignment in the hospital inpatient coding arena. Let's review specific guidelines that impact hospital inpatient coding. Inpatient coders are required to report a present on admission (POA) indicator on inpatient claims. The POA identifies whether a diagnosis code was present or not present at the time an order for an inpatient admission occurred. Any condition that developed during an outpatient visit is considered to be present on admission. POA indicators are only assigned to diagnosis codes that are applied and not exempt from POA reporting. The reporting options are Y = yes, N = no, E = exempt, U = unknown, and W = clinically undetermined; for those unreported or not used, this field would be left blank. The complete POA reporting guidelines are found in Appendix I of the ICD 10 CM official coding guidelines. We do not review all of the official coding guidelines in this chapter. The ICD 10 CM *Official Guidelines for Coding and Reporting* can be found on the Centers for Disease Control and Prevention official website at www.cdc.gov/nchs/data/icd10/icdguide.10.pdf.

Coding Inpatient Hospital Intermediate Cases

The steps to coding inpatient hospital intermediate visits are as follows:

1. Review the chart to ensure that all required documentation for appropriate code assignment is available in the chart. If main documentation is missing, do not code until the chart is complete. Main documentation includes the discharge summary, history and physical, operative report, pathology report, or radiology report.

2. Read through the documentation and determine the principal diagnosis (PDx) and applicable secondary diagnoses (SDx) per UHDDS guidelines.

3. Read through the documentation and determine the principal procedure (PPx) and applicable significant procedures (SPx) per UHDDS guidelines.

4. Assign correct principal diagnosis and secondary diagnoses codes using the ICD 10 CM code set.

5. Assign correct principal and significant procedure codes using the ICD 10 PCS code set.

6. Assign the correct MS-DRG.

7. Perform a final check on all assigned diagnosis and procedure codes to ensure that all applicable diagnoses and procedures have been addressed.

8. Check the assigned MS-DRG. If the MS-DRG calculated is missing complications, comorbidity, or medical severity, go back through the chart to check for any missed complications, comorbidities, or medical severity diagnoses. Assign any missing codes and recalculate the MS-DRG.

9. Assign the correct diagnoses with POA indicators and procedure codes to the patient's chart.

LET'S PRACTICE 5-1

Coding Guideline: Selection of Principal Diagnosis

Patient was admitted with right lower abdominal pain and an elevated white cell count. The physician documents acute appendicitis with an open appendectomy.

● HELPFUL HINTS:

• Lower abdominal pain is a symptom of appendicitis and is not coded.

• Elevated white cell count is also a sign and/or symptom of appendicitis and is not coded.

Steps:

1. Identify all applicable diagnoses and procedures.
   • Diagnoses found: Acute appendicitis.
   • Procedures found: Open appendectomy.

2. Assign correct ICD 10 CM diagnosis and ICD 10 PCS procedure codes following all applicable official coding guidelines.

LET'S PRACTICE 5-1, *continued*

3. Assign correct ICD-10-CM and ICD-10-PCS codes by utilizing an electronic encoder, the ICD-10-CM and ICD-10-PCS draft code sets, or a website such as www.icd10data.com to either look up the ICD-10 codes or convert the ICD-9 codes to ICD-10 codes.

   • "Codes for symptoms, signs, and ill-defined conditions from Chapter 16 are not to be used as principal diagnosis when a related definitive diagnosis has been established," per the ICD-9-CM *Official Guidelines for Coding and Reporting*, Section II, "Selection of Principal Diagnosis."

4. Verify that all diagnoses and procedures identified have been assigned a code or excluded from code assignment.

PDx: Acute appendicitis.

PPx: Open appendectomy.

5. Using the physician documentation, verify that the correct principal diagnosis, POA indicator, and principal procedure have been assigned.

6. Calculate MS-DRG assignment.

Codes:

ICD-9: PDx: 540.9-Y, PPx: 47.09

ICD-10: PDx: K35.80-Y, PPx: 0DTJ0ZZ

MS-DRG: 343

LET'S PRACTICE 5-2

Coding Guideline: Chronic Condition with Acute Exacerbation and Two Diagnoses Meeting Principal Diagnosis Criteria and Combination Codes

Patient presented to the hospital complaining of shortness of breath and a fever. The patient has COPD (■ FIGURE 5-1) and was admitted for acute exacerbation of COPD. A chest x-ray taken the day of admission shows left lower lobe infiltrates. The patient was started on IV antibiotics for pneumonia.

● HELPFUL HINTS:

• Shortness of breath and fever are both signs/symptoms of pneumonia and/or acute exacerbation of COPD. No codes assigned.

• Chronic COPD with acute exacerbation and pneumonia, per the AHA's *Coding Clinic*, First Quarter 2010, "… are two separate conditions which the patient presented with at the same time. The pneumonia is not the exacerbation of the COPD and either code may be sequenced as the principal diagnosis as per physician documentation and therapy provided" (486 and 491.21).

• Physician states the patient was admitted for acute exacerbation of COPD—this is the principal diagnosis.

• Pneumonia is listed as a secondary diagnosis.

Procedure code(s): chest x-ray and IV antibiotics treatment information not coded by an inpatient coder.

Steps:

1. Identify all applicable diagnoses and procedures.

   • Diagnoses found: COPD with acute exacerbation; pneumonia.

   • Procedures found: None.

2. Assign correct ICD-9-CM diagnosis and procedure codes following all applicable official coding guidelines:

   • Section I.B.10 – Acute and Chronic Conditions: " If the same condition is described as both acute (subacute) and chronic, and separate subentries exist in the *Alphabetic Index* at the same indentation level, code both and sequence the acute (subacute) code first."

   • Section I.B.11 – Combination Code: "Assign only the combination code when that code fully identifies the diagnostic conditions involved or when the *Alphabetic Index* so directs."

   • Section II.B – Two or more diagnoses that equally meet the definition for principal diagnosis: ". . . either condition may be sequenced first, unless the circumstances of the admission, the therapy provided, the *Tabular List*, or the *Alphabetic Index* indicates otherwise."

3. Assign correct ICD-10-CM and ICD-10-PCS codes by utilizing an electronic encoder, the ICD-10-CM and ICD-10-PCS draft code sets, or a website such as www.icd10data.com to either look up the ICD-10 codes or convert the ICD-9 codes to ICD-10 codes.

continued

LET'S PRACTICE 5-2, *continued*

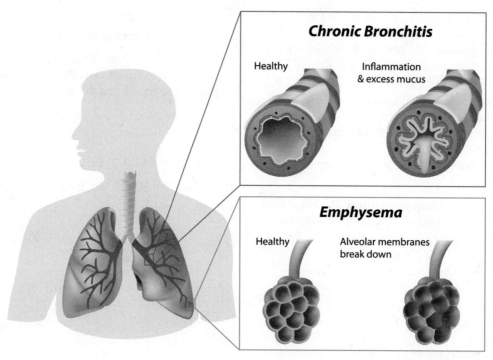

Figure 5-1 ■ Chronic obstructive pulmonary disease (COPD).

Source: Alila/Fotolia.com

4. Verify that all diagnoses and procedures identified have been assigned a code or excluded from code assignment.

PDx: Chronic COPD with acute exacerbation.

SDx: Pneumonia.

PPx and SPx: Not applicable.

5. Using the physician documentation, verify that the correct principal diagnosis, POA indicator, and principal procedure have been assigned.

6. Calculate MS-DRG assignment.

Codes:

ICD-9: PDx: 491.21-Y, SDx: 486-Y

ICD-10: PDx: J44.1-Y, SDx: J189-Y

MS-DRG: 190

LET'S PRACTICE 5-3

Coding Guideline: Other Reporting of Additional Diagnoses

Patient was admitted for dehydration and IV saline was ordered. The physician also ordered Lasix and a nebulizer treatment. Upon review of the history and physical you see that the patient has CHF and asthma.

● **HELPFUL HINTS:**

• Dehydration is the principal diagnosis because this is what occasioned the admission of the patient to the hospital.

LET'S PRACTICE 5-3, *continued*

- Treatment with IV fluids supports dehydration as the principal diagnosis. Be sure to check for the required IV rate per Medicare to support the principal diagnosis of dehydration.

- The two other coexisting diagnoses, congestive heart failure and asthma, would be coded as secondary diagnoses because both were addressed and/or treated by the physician during the episode of care.

Steps:

1. Identify all applicable diagnoses and procedures.
   - Diagnoses found: Dehydration; congestive heart failure; asthma.
   - Procedures found: Nebulizer treatment; IV; Lasix.

2. Assign correct ICD-9-CM diagnosis and procedure codes following all applicable official coding guidelines.
   - Section III – Reporting Additional Diagnoses: For reporting purposes, the definition for "other diagnoses" is interpreted as additional conditions that affect patient care in terms of requiring clinical evaluation; or therapeutic treatment; or diagnostic procedures; or extended length of hospital stay; or increased nursing care and/or monitoring.
   - UHDDS item 11-b defines other diagnoses as "all conditions that coexist at the time of admission, that develop subsequently, or that affect the treatment received and/or the length of stay. Diagnoses that relate to an earlier episode which have no bearing on the current hospital stay are to be excluded."

3. Assign correct ICD-10-CM and ICD-10-PCS codes by utilizing an electronic encoder, the ICD-10-CM and ICD-10-PCS draft code sets, or a website such as www.icd10data.com to either look up the ICD-10 codes or convert the ICD-9 codes to ICD-10 codes.

4. Verify that all diagnoses and procedures identified have been assigned a code or excluded from code assignment.
   PDx: Dehydration.
   SDx: Congestive heart failure; asthma.
   PPx: None.
   SPx: None.

5. Using the physician documentation, verify that the correct principal diagnosis, POA indicator, and principal procedure have been assigned.

6. Calculate MS-DRG assignment.

Codes:

ICD-9: PDx: 276.51-Y, SDx: 428.0-Y, SDx: 493.90-Y

ICD-10: PDx: R86.0-Y, SDx: I50.9-Y, SDx: J45.909-Y

MS-DRG: 641

LET'S PRACTICE 5-4

Coding Guideline: Principal Diagnosis Selection

A patient with hypertension (HTN) was admitted to the hospital for breast cancer of the upper-inner quadrant of the right breast. She was taken to the OR for a modified radical mastectomy. The day after surgery, she developed a urinary tract infection (UTI) and was given IV antibiotics before she was discharged home the following day.

● HELPFUL HINTS:

- The principal diagnosis code is cancer of the upper-inner quadrant of the right female breast.

- The secondary diagnosis of postoperative urinary tract infection is coded because the onset of this diagnosis occurred after admission to the facility and is a postoperative complication.

- The secondary diagnosis code of hypertension is coded as an additional diagnosis. The hypertension existed prior to the time of treatment, that is, the patient had this condition when she came to the hospital, which is referred to as a comorbidity.

- The principal procedure, "unilateral modified radical mastectomy, right, female breast," reflects the treatment and/or procedure received during the episode of care.

continued

LET'S PRACTICE 5-4, *continued*

Steps:

1. Identify all applicable diagnoses and procedures.

   • Diagnoses found: Carcinoma of the upper-inner quadrant right breast; hypertension; postoperative complication of urinary tract infection requiring additional resources and care to patient

   • Procedures found: Modified radical mastectomy, unilateral, right; IV antibiotics.

2. Assign correct ICD-9-CM diagnosis and procedure codes following all applicable official coding guidelines.

   • Section II – Selection of Principal Diagnosis: Breast carcinoma. The circumstances of the inpatient admission always govern the selection of the principal diagnosis. The principal diagnosis is defined in the UHDDS as "that condition established after study to be chiefly responsible for occasioning the admission of the patient to the hospital for care."

   • Section III – Reporting Additional Diagnoses: Hypertension is a condition that coexisted at the time of admission and meets the criteria for reporting additional diagnoses.

   • The postoperative complication of urinary tract infection meets the criteria for Section III because it extended the length of the hospital stay and/or required increased care.

3. Assign correct ICD-10-CM and ICD-10-PCS codes by utilizing an electronic encoder, the ICD-10-CM and ICD-10-PCS draft code sets, or a website such as www.icd10data.com to either look up the ICD-10 codes or convert the ICD-9 codes to ICD-10 codes.

4. Verify that all diagnoses and procedures identified have been assigned a code or excluded from code assignment.

   PDx: Carcinoma upper-inner quadrant right breast.

   SDx: Hypertension; postoperative infection urinary tract infection.

   PPx: Modified radical mastectomy, unilateral, right breast.

   SPx: Not applicable.

5. Using the physician documentation, verify that the correct principal diagnosis, POA indicator, and principal procedure have been assigned.

6. Calculate MS-DRG assignment.

Codes:

ICD-9: PDx: 174.2-Y, SDx: 998.59-N, SDx: 599.0-N, SDx: 401.9-Y, PPx: 85.43

ICD-10: PDx: C50.211-Y, SDx: T81.4xxA-N, SDx: N39.0-N, SDx: I10-Y, PPx: 0HTT0ZZ

MS-DRG: 582

CODING FROM DOCUMENTATION

Hospital inpatient coders utilize the patient health record and documentation for the applicable episode of care as the legal source documents from which to assign diagnosis and procedure codes. The inpatient coder reviews all physician documentation to identify potential applicable diagnoses.

The question "*How do I know what to code and what not to code?*" is often asked when learning to code inpatient records. In the hospital inpatient setting, a diagnosis code may be assigned for any condition that complicated the patient's care; any condition the physician mentioned as important and relevant to the specific episode of care; any condition for which a clinical evaluation was performed; and any condition or diagnosis that was addressed and treated during the episode of care or is a chronic disease and/or condition. For example, if the patient has chronic obstructive pulmonary disease (COPD) but he did not receive any respiratory therapy to treat it, you would still code it because it is a **chronic condition** (one that persists for a long period of time) that affects the patient every day

and is taken into consideration when making medical decisions about risk and any potential treatments given to or procedures performed on the patient. As a hospital inpatient coder, you will be given a complete health/medical record from which to assign codes for a single episode of care. Some of the health/medical records may be 10 pages in length, while others may be 100. The key to navigating through the health/medical record successfully is developing a routine in which you abstract out or analyze the data. Consider the following suggestions when reviewing a health/medical record:

1. First read the **discharge summary** to get an overview of what happened to the patient during the episode of care. Be sure to underline, highlight, or write on a separate piece of working paper all documented diagnoses and procedures found in the physician documentation summary of the patient's episode of care. Read and be guided by the discharge diagnosis(es) and orders as documented by the physician. Note, however, that you should *never code only from the discharge summary.*

2. Next read the history and physical (H&P) for more information about the patient's condition and historical summary of events and/or disease processes that brought the patient into the acute care setting. The H&P provides information about other conditions, past and chronic, that the patient may have, such as those listed in the medical history. Examples of documentation that may be found in the medical history include hypertension, diabetes mellitus, and fracture of tibia 10 years ago.

When looking at the H&P, remember that just because the physician records something in the medical history, it does not mean the condition is gone. For example, COPD is an ongoing condition. You only need to code the "histories of" if they are relevant, such as a history of CA, which can be related to many conditions, versus a history of pneumonia 2 years ago, which is probably not relevant to the current course of care. Also, when coding the "history of," try to focus only on the conditions and diseases being treated or those complicating care. Note, too, that oftentimes the physician will say "history of a [condition]" and coders will spend a lot of time looking for an applicable "history of" code. A patient may have many "histories of," but that does not mean that there is an ICD-9 diagnosis code that matches it. A common example of this is physician documentation of "history of asthma." Asthma is a condition that never "goes away" and as such is coded in the present tense as "asthma." The "history of" diagnosis codes are for major or complicating diagnoses, not routine diagnoses or treatments that are self-limiting and/or resolved without further impact on the patient. An example of this is "history of a motor vehicle accident (MVA) 15 years ago with a brief loss of consciousness and head laceration." Today, the patient is presenting with acute appendicitis. The MVA, head laceration, and brief loss of consciousness do not impact the current episode of care and would not be coded.

Coding Past History

A "history of" statement by a physician may include resolved conditions or diagnoses and/or a postprocedure status from previous episodes of care that have no bearing on the current stay or episode of care. Such conditions are not to be reported and are coded only if required by hospital policy per the ICD-9-CM *Official Guidelines for Coding and Reporting.*

History codes may be reported as secondary codes if the historical condition, personal, or family history has an impact on the current care or may influence treatment or medical decision making. For example, a family history of breast cancer is very appropriate to assign as a secondary diagnosis code when a patient is seeking a yearly mammogram at age 33.

Consider, however, the example of a patient who has been diagnosed with a lump in the breast and is coming in for a breast biopsy. This patient has a history of colitis that is currently well controlled with maintenance medication. If the physician were to use the term "history of colitis," that would not match the ICD-9-CM definition of "history of" because in this example, the colitis is still present and is currently being treated so it is "active," not "resolved" nor correctly considered "history of." The colitis diagnosis is not really relevant to nor does it affect the episode of care in which the breast biopsy is being performed and would not be coded for ICD-9-CM purposes; be sure, however, to check your facility's coding policy because, for example, a research/teaching medical facility may want to capture this type of "data" to be utilized in the future.

3. After reading the discharge summary and history and physical, check for other major documents such as an emergency room document, consultation, or operative report (OP). If present, read and abstract information from these reports to identify diagnoses or procedures. The operative report, if applicable, is a major document and is vital to ensuring accurate assignment of both diagnosis and procedure codes. The operative report will document preoperative diagnoses and postoperative diagnoses. The preoperative and postoperative diagnoses will not always be the same; and the postoperative diagnosis is the one that is used to guide the coder as we look at the pathology report to verify the postoperative diagnosis.

Example: A patient's preoperative diagnosis was acute abdominal pain. The postoperative diagnosis is acute appendicitis with the principal procedure of open appendectomy. The postoperative diagnosis must always be verified with a pathology report if a specimen was sent to pathology for identification.

Example: A patient's breast mass was biopsied and sent to pathology. The postoperative diagnosis stated "pending pathology." The pathology report returned as adenocarcinoma of the breast. For coding purposes, then, the coder is guided by the pathologist's diagnosis of adenocarcinoma of the breast as reflected on the pathology report. Again, always verify the postoperative diagnosis with the pathology report if a specimen was sent to pathology. Never code from the preoperative diagnosis as documented in the operative report.

Example: A physician removed a lesion from a patient's colon and sent it to pathology. The preoperative diagnosis was lesion of the colon. The postoperative diagnosis was cancer of the colon with the pathology report stating that the cancer is an adenocarcinoma. You code the adenocarcinoma because, "after study," that is what the lesion was determined to be under microscopic examination by a licensed medical physician who specializes in pathology. The pathology diagnosis as stated by the licensed pathologist is the more definitive diagnosis versus the primary care physician/surgeon's diagnosis.

4. After you have read the discharge summary, the H&P, and the emergency room, consultation, and operative reports (if applicable), the next type of documentation utilized is the physician orders and progress notes. Physician orders and progress notes are read and reviewed to confirm, correlate, and/or find documentation not found in the previous reports. Each physician order for medication, treatment, procedures, or other allied health therapies must have a correlating progress note to document the patient response or nonresponse. You may find something documented in the physician orders or progress notes that is not addressed in the major dictated reports/documents. If you find an applicable secondary diagnosis documented, such as postoperative ileus, that had not yet been documented elsewhere, you would also want to code that diagnosis.

5. Go back and reread the discharge summary and your personal coding notes to ensure that you have coded everything or addressed everything with regard to diagnoses and procedures.

CODING TIP

You may find it helpful to make notes as you are going through the health/medical record and episode-of-care documentation. A coder should make note of all signs, symptoms, diagnoses, procedures, treatments, and/or therapies found in the health/medical record documentation. Final verification of each and every item noted while reviewing the episode of care must be addressed, correlated, thrown out, or assigned a code in order to ensure that the final codes are reflective of and present an accurate picture of the episode of care being coded.

Remember that you should only code what was done and documented by the physician. Do not read the nurses' notes or notes from respiratory, speech therapy, pharmacy, or other ancillary services unless you need more explanation than what the physician provided. You will only code for significant procedures performed by the physician, not for anything that is done by ancillary staff. The UHDDS definition of a significant procedure is "one that is surgical in nature, or carries a procedural risk, carries an anesthetic risk, or requires specialized training." For example, IVs, routine catheters, chest-x-rays, and lab work do not meet the definition of a significant procedure and are not routinely coded by the inpatient coder. These types of procedures or any procedures performed by ancillary staff are reported and charged out via the facility chargemaster and are not coded by the inpatient coder.

There are some exceptions to this statement, such as skin debridement. A physical therapist may perform an excisional or nonexcisional skin debridement of an inpatient burn victim. The inpatient coder would capture and assign this procedure code. In addition, facility-specific policies and procedures vary and may mandate that the inpatient coder capture and assign codes for nonsignificant procedures. An example of this may be a facility policy requiring the coding of CT scans and MRIs even if they are in the chargemaster because they can affect the health grade status of a facility and need to be reflected in a database for statistical reporting. These types of procedure codes will not affect an MS-DRG or the facility reimbursement.

CODING TIP

Significant procedure criteria must be met for every procedure coded. Asking "Who performed the procedure?" will help to identify a significant procedure per the UHDDS.

LET'S PRACTICE 5-5

Coding Guideline: Significant Procedure

Patient was admitted for labor and delivery at 39 weeks' gestation. During the course of labor and delivery, the physician wanted to augment the woman's labor to speed it up, so IV Pitocin was ordered. The patient's labor progressed well and while she was pushing, the doctor decided to use a vacuum cup device to assist in the delivery process. A vacuum cup was applied to the baby's scalp with resultant vaginal delivery of a healthy 7 lb, 3 oz male baby. Delivery was accomplished without complication with the exception of the use of the vacuum cup to facilitate delivery. Mother and baby were transferred to postpartum care.

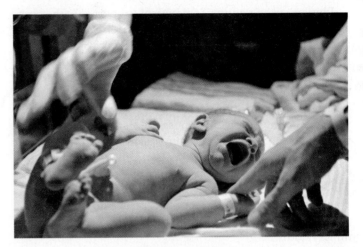

Figure 5-2 ■ Male baby delivered by vaginal delivery.
Source: Carolina K. Smith, M.D./Shutterstock.com

● HELPFUL HINTS:

- Augmentation of labor via IV Pitocin is documented to speed up labor only, not to induce labor and is not coded because it does not meet the significant procedure criteria.
- We would code for the delivery complicated by the use of a vacuum cup. Key term: Delivery, vacuum.

Steps:

1. Identify all applicable diagnoses and procedures.
   - Diagnoses found: Term pregnancy with vacuum assist vaginal delivery (■ FIGURE 5-2), single liveborn male infant.
   - Procedures found: Vacuum cup assist vaginal delivery, single liveborn infant; IV Pitocin to augment labor.

2. Assign correct ICD-9-CM diagnosis and procedure codes following all applicable official coding guidelines.

3. Assign correct ICD-10-CM and ICD-10-PCS codes by utilizing an electronic encoder, the ICD-10-CM and ICD-10-PCS draft code sets, or a website such as

www.icd10data.com to either look up the ICD-10 codes or convert the ICD-9 codes to ICD-10 codes.

4. Verify that all diagnoses and procedures identified have been assigned a code or excluded from code assignment.
   PDx: Term pregnancy with vacuum assist vaginal delivery.
   SDx: Single liveborn male infant.
   PPx: Vacuum assist delivery single liveborn infant.
   SPx: None.

5. Using the physician documentation, verify that the correct principal diagnosis, POA indicator, and principal procedure have been assigned.

6. Calculate MS-DRG assignment.

Codes:

ICD-9: PDx: 669.51-N, SDx: V27.0-E, PPx: 72.79

ICD-10: PDx: O66.5-N, SDx: Z37.0-E, PPx: 10D07Z6

MS-DRG: 775

LET'S PRACTICE 5-6

Hemoptysis with History of Tuberculosis and Acute Chest Pain

A 62-year-old female presented with shortness of breath, a feeling of tightness across the chest, and tachycardia. Patient also reported a recent bout of hemoptysis approx-imately 2 weeks ago and that she has been taking Coumadin for the past 10 years due to a deep vein thrombosis that resolved with pharmacological intervention. Patient also reported having tuberculosis as a child.

continued

LET'S PRACTICE 5-6, *continued*

Physical examination of the patient supported with chest x-ray findings of possible bleb formations in both the right and left lung required bronchoscopy to be performed. Bronchoscopy revealed two small thrombi present in the lower trachea, which were suctioned and sent to pathology. Both the right and left upper lobes were observed with no lesions detected. The right and left lower lobe and middle lobe were also free of any lesions. Diagnosis of old hemorrhage with retained thrombi and no new lung lesions present.

Cardiology consultation was performed regarding the tachycardia and chest pain the patient was experiencing. The patient was found to have AV nodal reentry tachycardia, atrial fibrillation, and atrial flutter. The patient was given IV medications, which brought the cardiac issues under control.

Impression:

1. AV nodal reentry tachycardia.

2. Atrial fibrillation.

3. Atrial flutter.

4. Hemoptysis .

5. History of tuberculosis.

6. Old thrombi present in lung.

7. Long-term Coumadin utilization.

Procedure:

1. Bronchoscopy with suction of old thrombi.

● **HELPFUL HINTS:** Our scenario indicates that the patient was admitted for hemoptysis with a history of tuberculosis. The patient also presented with cardiac arrhythmias. Be sure to follow the lead of the physician documentation in assigning the principal diagnosis in this case. Be sure to follow the findings of the bronchoscopy regarding the history of tuberculosis and the suspicion of possible new lesions.

Steps:

1. Identify all applicable diagnoses and procedures.

    • Diagnoses found: Hemoptysis; history of tuberculosis; AV nodal reentry tachycardia; atrial fibrillation; atrial flutter; history of DVT; old thrombi present in lung; long-term Coumadin utilization.

    • Procedures found: Bronchoscopy with suction of old thrombi.

2. Assign correct ICD-9-CM diagnosis and procedure codes following all applicable official coding guidelines.

3. Assign correct ICD-10-CM and ICD-10-PCS codes by utilizing an electronic encoder, the ICD-10-CM and ICD-10-PCS draft code sets, or a website such as www.icd10data.com to either look up the ICD-10 codes or convert the ICD-9 codes to ICD-10 codes.

4. Verify that all diagnoses and procedures identified have been assigned a code or excluded from code assignment.

    PDx: AV nodal reentry tachycardia.

    SDx: AV nodal reentry tachycardia; atrial fibrillation; atrial flutter; hemoptysis; history of DVT; old thrombi present in lung; long-term Coumadin utilization.

    PPx: Bronchoscopy with suction of old thrombi.

5. Using the physician documentation, verify that the correct principal diagnosis, POA indicator, and principal procedure have been assigned.

6. Calculate MS-DRG assignment.

Codes:

ICD-9: PDx: 427.89-Y, 786.30-Y, 416.2-Y, 427.32-Y, V12.01-E, 427.31-Y, V58.61-E, V12.51-E, PPx: 33.24, SPx: None

ICD-10: PDx: I49.8-Y, R04.2-Y, I27.82-Y, I48.92-Y, Z86.11-E, I48.91-Y, Z79.01-E, Z86.718-E, PPx: 0BB38ZX, SPx: None

MS-DRG: 309

LET'S PRACTICE 5-7

Dysmenorrhea and Menometrorrhagia

The patient is a 46-year-old gravida 2, para 1, AB 1, who presented with dysmenorrhea and excessive/frequent menstruation. Patient is currently using mechanical means only for birth control. The patient was admitted for a hysteroscopy and D&C on the basis of having to wear a pad almost three weeks out of the month. Patient reports that for the past few months she has had light flow and spotting occurring even for two weeks after her period is

LET'S PRACTICE 5-7, *continued*

over. She has been advised concerning options, technical aspects, and risks of this procedure.

Past History: There is no previous history of surgery, blood dyscrasias, or transfusions. The patient is on thyroid medication for hypothyroidism and has been treated with Zantac and Carafate because of an ulcer. The ulcer was diagnosed four years ago with no history recently of being bothered by ulcers. This certainly does not make her a candidate for antiprostaglandin or aspirin therapy in relation to her dysmenorrhea.

Drug Allergies: None known.

Medications: As previously mentioned.

Family History: Unremarkable except for father with Parkinson's disease.

Physical Examination:

Heent/Neck: Normal. Thyroid normal.

Lungs: Clear.

Breasts: Normal. Most recent mammogram negative.

Cardiovascular: Heart regular sinus rhythm without murmur.

Abdomen: Supple.

Extremities: Normal.

Pelvic Exam: Perineum normal. Vagina healthy. Cervix mild eversion. Pap smear normal. Uterus posterior, upper limits normal size, shape and mobile with unremarkable adnexa.

Impression:

1. Dysmenorrhea.

2. Menometrorrhagia.

Procedure: Hysteroscopy and D&C performed without complications

---

● HELPFUL HINTS:

- The patient was admitted for the treatment of dysmenorrhea and menometrorrhagia, which are both coded. Both of these diagnoses meet the criteria for principal diagnoses.
- The coder should follow the physician documentation with dysmenorrhea being listed first and thus coded as the principal diagnosis.

- The patient has a coexisting diagnosis of hypothyroidism, so we code that as well.
- The ulcer mentioned in the patient history is not a current problem nor does the physician currently treat it, so we will not code it.
- The procedures performed are a hysteroscopy and D&C, both of which are coded.

Steps:

1. Identify all applicable diagnoses and procedures.
   - Diagnoses found: Dysmenorrhea; menometrorrhagia; hypothyroidism.
   - Procedures found: Hysteroscopy; dilation and curettage

2. Assign correct ICD-9-CM diagnosis and procedure codes following all applicable official coding guidelines.

3. Assign correct ICD-10-CM and ICD-10-PCS codes by utilizing an electronic encoder, the ICD-10-CM and ICD-10-PCS draft code sets, or a website such as www.icd10data.com to either look up the ICD-10 codes or convert the ICD-9 codes to ICD-10 codes.

4. Verify that all diagnoses and procedures identified have been assigned a code or excluded from code assignment.

   PDx: Dysmenorrhea.

   SDx: Menometrorrhagia.

   PPx: Dilatation and curettage of uterus.

   SPx: Hysteroscopy.

5. Using the physician documentation, verify that the correct principal diagnosis, POA indicator, and principal procedure have been assigned.

6. Calculate MS-DRG assignment.

Codes:

ICD-9: PDx: 625.3-Y, SDx: 626.2-Y, 244.9-Y PPx: 69.09, SPx: 68.12

ICD-10: PDx: N94.6-Y, SDx: N92.0-Y, E03.9-Y, PPx: 0UDB7ZX, SPx: 0UJD8ZZ

MS-DRG: 745

LET'S PRACTICE 5-8

Discharge Summary: Asthma

Consultants: Pulmonary team.

Discharge Diagnoses:

1. Respiratory distress exacerbated by asthma (■ FIG-URE 5-3).

2. Viral upper respiratory infection.

Procedures: None.

History: This is a 12-year-old white male who came into the emergency room complaining of moderate-to-severe respiratory distress for the whole day of August 10.

The patient is a known asthmatic for the past seven years, who woke up Saturday morning with "the worst attack" he has ever had. The patient said he could barely breathe all day, until he came to the emergency room at Children's Medical Center, and received three albuterol and steroid respiratory treatments.

The patient has tried Primatene mist in the past without good control of his asthma. He said he had only had one other episode like this in the past, which was about two years ago, but it was not this severe. The patient was on Ventolin prn, for his known asthma and minor flare-ups, but he had run out, and did not have any on Saturday. Triggers for asthmatic attacks in this patient are exercise, nervousness, hot water baths, viral illnesses, and cats.

On admission, the patient had a runny nose, cough, and watery eyes that he said began about two days prior to admission. He did not complain of a temperature, nausea, or diarrhea, but did say he had one episode of emesis during the day. The patient said that sometimes he feels limited by his illness. His mother said he was not, at the present time, being followed by a regular pediatrician or anyone for his asthma, due to the family recently moving to this area.

Past Medical History: He has not had any hospitalizations or surgeries in the past. The patient was diagnosed with psoriasis that cleared up at age 5.

Family History: The father has asthma. The maternal grandfather had severe asthma, heart disease, and stomach cancer. The maternal grandmother had a brain tumor and strokes. His sister and mother have had episodes of psoriasis in the past.

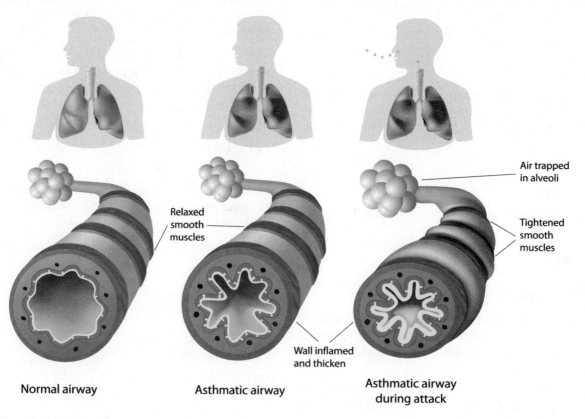

Air trapped
in alveoli

Relaxed
smooth
muscles

Tightened
smooth
muscles

Wall inflamed
and thicken

Normal airway

Asthmatic airway

Asthmatic airway
during attack

Figure 5-3 ■ Pathology of asthma.

Source: Alila/Fotolia.com

LET'S PRACTICE 5-8, *continued*

Social History: He had lived with his mother, sister, and brother-in-law, and occasionally a niece. There was positive tobacco use by the sister and brother-in-law, and the family recently moved from that living arrangement.

Review of Systems: His appetite had been low in the two days prior to admission; otherwise, as per history, above. Immunizations: This patient is up-to-date.

Allergies: The patient had no known drug allergies, but was sensitive to cats and roosters.

Physical Examination:

General: In general, he was an alert but tired male, in mild respiratory distress. He was wearing glasses. His skin did not show any rashes or lesions.

Vitals: Physical examination at the time of admission on presentation to the emergency room showed no temperature recorded. The patient had a heart rate of 130, respiratory rate of 25; his blood pressure was also not recorded. His weight was 37.5 kg on admission.

HEENT: Exam showed normocephalic, atraumatic head. Pupils equal, round, and reactive to light; extraocular motions intact; right tympanic membrane was normal; left tympanic membrane unable to visualize, due to cerumen. Nose was clear with rhinorrhea. Throat had 1–2+ tonsillar hypertrophy, without erythema. Neck showed no lymphadenopathy or masses. He was also not using his accessory muscles to breathe.

Chest: Chest showed no retractions. Lung exam showed the patient with limited respiratory effort, and end expiratory wheezing throughout.

Cardiac: Showed tachycardia; regular rhythm, without murmurs, rubs, or gallops. Abdominal exam showed positive bowel sounds in all four quadrants; soft, nontender, nondistended; no masses felt.

Genitalia: Deferred.

Extremity: Showed no cyanosis, clubbing, or edema.

Neurologically: He was grossly intact.

Laboratory Data: A chest x-ray was performed on this patient, which showed hyperinflation of his lungs; no other laboratory values were drawn on this patient.

Hospital Course: The assessment and plan from a respiratory standpoint: The patient was felt to be having an asthmatic exacerbation due to upper respiratory symptoms, probably viral. The patient had three treatments of albuterol and prednisone in the emergency room.

The patient was admitted on 2.5 liters of oxygen by nasal cannula. He was to get albuterol nebulizations, 0.5 cc in 2 cc of normal saline q 2 hours and q 1 hour prn, and to receive IV Solu-Medrol 18 mg q 6 hours. It was also felt that a pulmonary consultation would be helpful in this patient, to give a more clear picture of this patient's asthmatic status and also to help with future follow-up.

From a fluid, electrolyte, and nutrition standpoint, the patient was felt to be minimally dehydrated, and intravenous fluids were to be started of D5-1/2 normal saline plus 20 mEq/L of KCl, if the patient could not maintain 75 cc per hour minimum oral intake.

The patient showed good improvement throughout his hospital stay On his first hospital day, the patient was breathing much easier from a respiratory standpoint, and still had positive and expiratory wheezes, but was, according to him, much closer to his baseline, but not there yet.

The patient had good oral intake. The patient was able to maintain saturations of 93% to 96% on 2 liters of O_2 by nasal cannula, and it was felt at this time that we should to try to wean the patient down.

The patient's albuterol nebulizations were changed from q 2 hours and q 1 hour prn to q 4 hours and q 2 hours prn.

On the next hospital day, the patient was maintaining good oral intake. The patient said he continued to feel better. His lung exam supported this with more air movement, and less wheezing throughout his lungs. The patient was weaned down to 1 liter of oxygen by nasal cannula, with saturations in the low 90s.

The patient had PFTs done, which were reviewed by the respiratory therapist, his attending physician, and the pulmonary consult, and these PFTs showed significant chronic airway disease.

The patient received asthma teaching while he was in the hospital, to help acquaint him more with his disease.

Discharge Disposition: The patient was discharged on the next hospital day, given the fact that his lung exam showed much better air movement, and just a very rare end expiratory wheeze; the patient said he was approximately at his baseline at this point.

The patient's discharge instructions included receiving one Ace spacer to use with his AeroBid MDI 3 puffs, following his nebulizer treatments, tid. The patient was to get one home nebulizer to use with his albuterol 0.5 cc in 2 cc of Intal by nebulizer tid. The patient was also to have his IV steroids switched to po prednisone 20-mg tablets on a wean as follows: 2 tablets po bid times five days, 2 tablets po. q a.m. and 1 tablet po. q p.m. x's 5 days, then 1 tablet po bid x's 5 days, then 1 tablet p.o. q day x's 5 days.

The patient's diet was to be appropriate for age. The patient's physical activity was to be as tolerated.

continued

LET'S PRACTICE 5-8, *continued*

The patient's follow-up care was to include an appointment with me in three to six days, and an appointment at the Pulmonary Clinic with one of his consulting pulmonologists in two to four weeks.

The patient was discharged to his place of residence with his mother.

● HELPFUL HINTS:

- The patient was admitted and treated for the exacerbation of his asthma. Much of the care revolved around his breathing and treatment for asthma. Physician documentation states that triggers for the patient's asthma are exercise, nervousness, hot water baths, viral illnesses, and cats. These triggers describe both extrinsic and intrinsic triggers with the viral illnesses being the intrinsic trigger. Since there is exact documentation describing the asthmatic triggers, both intrinsic and extrinsic asthma with exacerbation should be coded.

- The mild respiratory distress is a sign/symptom of the asthma and/or URI and is not coded.

- Shortly after admission the physician felt the patient was mildly dehydrated and/ordered D5-1/2 normal saline plus 20 mL/kg. As per published treatment guidelines (*Merck Manual*), generally 50 mL/kg is given for mild dehydration and 100 mL/kg for moderate. Third-party payers such as Medicare generally require the 50 or 100 mL/kg to be prescribed as treatment in order to assign a dehydration code. Under prospective payment for Medicare, dehydration has the possibility to increase payment as it is a complication/comorbidity requiring the use of more resources.

- The URI due to viral infection is documented as the exacerbating agent for this patient's asthma. His father also has asthma, which is related and important to the current care and status of the patient's asthma, so a family history of asthma code is assigned.

- The patient did receive respiratory nebulizer treatments and oxygen therapy. These two treatments do not meet the significant procedure criteria per UHDDS, so would be coded and billed via a facility chargemaster.

Steps:

1. Identify all applicable diagnoses and procedures.
   - Diagnoses found: Asthma with acute exacerbation and triggers of exercise, cats, and upper respiratory infection (extrinsic and intrinsic); family history of asthma; mild dehydration.
   - Procedures found: Nebulizer respiratory treatments; oxygen therapy; PFTs.

2. Assign correct ICD-9-CM diagnosis and procedure codes following all applicable official coding guidelines.

3. Assign correct ICD-10-CM and ICD-10-PCS codes by utilizing an electronic encoder, the ICD-10-CM and ICD-10-PCS draft code sets, or a website such as www.icd10data.com to either look up the ICD-10 codes or convert the ICD-9 codes to ICD-10 codes.

4. Verify that all diagnoses and procedures identified have been assigned a code or excluded form code assignment.

   PDx: Asthma, intrinsic and extrinsic.

   SDx: Asthma extrinsic; upper respiratory infection, viral; family history of asthma; dehydration.

   PPx: None.

   SPx: None.

5. Using the physician documentation, verify that the correct principal diagnosis, POA indicator, and principal procedure have been assigned.

6. Calculate MS-DRG assignment.

Codes:

ICD-9: PDx: 493.12-Y, SDx: 493.02-Y, 465.9-Y, 079.99-Y, V17.5-E, 276.51-Y

ICD-10: PDx: J45.31-Y, J06.9-Y, B97.89-Y, Z82.5-E, E86.0-Y

MS-DRG: 203

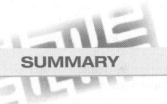

SUMMARY

With inpatient coding, physician documentation is utilized to guide code selection for diagnoses and procedures. The acute care inpatient setting typically treats patients who are sicker and require urgent or emergent care, rather than patients who are treated in the outpatient setting. The acute care inpatient setting typically involves patient lengths of stay that are between 2 and 35 days or longer depending on the severity of the diagnosis and the involvement of the treatment being provided. The longer length of stay may create large volumes of documentation, which reflect the episode of care for a patient. Therefore, inpatient coders have more documentation to read, interpret, and synthesize than is seen in the outpatient settings.

Major documentation utilized in the inpatient setting for code assignment includes the discharge summary, history and physical, emergency room report, operative report, pathology report, consultation report, progress notes, and physician orders. These major documentation sources must all be utilized to ensure the complete picture is provided regarding diagnoses, procedures, and treatments provided to a patient during a single episode of care. Inpatient coders must be familiar with and apply UHDDS and ICD-9-CM official coding guidelines when assigning diagnosis and procedure codes in the inpatient setting to ensure compliance with the assignment of principal and secondary diagnoses and principal and secondary procedures based on UHDDS and ICD-9-CM official coding guideline definitions.

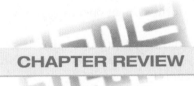

CHAPTER REVIEW

Multiple Choice

Choose the letter that best answers each question or completes each statement.

1. Which of the following code sets are used in inpatient coding?
   a. ICD-9-CM, Volumes 1 and 2
   b. ICD-9-CM, Volumes 1, 2, and 3
   c. ICD-9-CM, Volumes 1, 2, and CPT
   d. ICD-9-CM, Volumes 1, 2, and 3 and CPT

2. Which of the following is NOT typically reported in the hospital chargemaster?
   a. Debridements
   b. Labs
   c. IVs
   d. X-rays

3. What is the final step in inpatient coding?
   a. Review the documentation.
   b. Calculate the MS-DRG.
   c. Assign the E-codes.
   d. Verify the patient charges.

4. In an inpatient record, which of the following documents gives an overview of what happened to the patient?
   a. Consultation
   b. Discharge summary
   c. H&P
   d. Operative report

5. Inpatient coders only code
   a. what is in the discharge summary.
   b. what is in the history and physical.
   c. what is documented in the medical record.
   d. what is in the nurses' notes.

6. What definitions do inpatient coders use when coding?
   a. CMS
   b. ICD-9
   c. ICD-10
   d. UHDDS

7. The UHDDS was developed in
   a. 1974.
   b. 1980.
   c. 1983.
   d. 1994.

8. Which of the following is NOT the correct definition of a secondary diagnosis?
   a. Affects the treatment received.
   b. Coexists at the time of admission.
   c. Develops subsequently after admission.
   d. Relates to an earlier episode of care.

9. When coding, which of the following documents should be read first?
   a. Consultation reports
   b. Discharge summary
   c. History and physical
   d. Operative report

10. Which of the following documents is (are) used to verify what specimen was removed during an operation?
   a. Consultation reports
   b. Discharge summary
   c. Pathology report
   d. Specimen report

True or False

Determine whether each question is true or false. In the space provided, write "T" for true and "F" for false.

_____ 1. All inpatients stay at least one night in the hospital.

_____ 2. In addition to the official ICD-9-CM coding guidelines, most facilities will also have their own coding guidelines that the coder should follow.

_____ 3. A complication as defined by the UHDDS is a principal diagnosis describing a condition that arises after the beginning of hospital observation and treatment that modifies the course of the patient's illness or the medical care required.

_____ 4. According to the UHDDS, an inpatient coder should report all diagnoses that affect the current hospital stay.

_____ 5. The Uniform Hospital Discharge Data Set (UHDDS) was developed by CMS in 1974.

_____ 6. Major documentation sources found in the hospital inpatient setting include the discharge summary, operative report, history and physical, and nursing history.

_____ 7. The UHDDS definition for a significant procedure dictates that the treatment or procedure must be performed in an operating room.

_____ 8. The preoperative and postoperative diagnoses must always be the same as documented in the operative report.

_____ 9. A coder will find information regarding a patient's family history documented in the history and physical.

_____ 10. The ICD-9-CM diagnosis code set and CPT procedural code set are utilized to assign codes in the hospital inpatient setting.

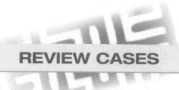

REVIEW CASES

Follow these steps to assign ICD-9-CM diagnosis and procedure codes as required to the following inpatient cases. UHDDS and ICD-9-CM official coding guidelines must be utilized in code selection and sequencing. Enter the appropriate principal diagnosis, secondary diagnosis, principal procedure, and secondary procedure codes as applicable in the space provided at the end of each review case.

1. Read the physician documents in each of the inpatient cases and assign the appropriate principal diagnosis code following the UHDDS definition for a principal diagnosis.

2. Read the physician documents in each of the inpatient cases to determine and assign codes to any secondary diagnoses as appropriate following the UHDDS definition for a secondary diagnosis and the ICD-9-CM official coding guidelines.

3. Read the physician documents in each of the inpatient cases to determine if a principal procedure code is

applicable and assign following the UHDDS definition for a principal procedure.

4. Assign applicable secondary procedure codes following the UHDDS definition for a secondary procedure and the ICD-9-CM official coding guidelines:
   - Locate and assign the correct diagnosis codes using the ICD-9-CM coding manual, Volumes 1 and 2.
   - Locate and assign the correct procedure codes using the ICD-9-CM coding manual, Volume 3.

5. Appropriately sequence and assign diagnosis, POA indicator, and procedures codes to the inpatient cases. Assign MS-DRGs (optional).

Review Case 5-1 Labor and Delivery Record

This 27-year-old gravida 2, para 1, presented to my office initially at 11 weeks' gestation seeking obstetrical services. The patient has experienced a normal and uncomplicated pregnancy to date. Patient presents today at 38 weeks' gestation for elective repeat Cesarean section. The patient underwent a Cesarean section with the delivery of her first child. A low cervical transverse Cesarean section was performed without complications. A single liveborn healthy male child weighing 8 lbs 4 oz and 21 inches long was delivered. Apgars were 8 and 9. Mom and baby progressed well and were discharged on day two. Patient will be seen in follow-up in 4 weeks or earlier if problems arise. Physician provided labor and delivery services only.

ICD-9-CM/ICD-10-CM diagnosis code(s):_____

ICD-9-CM procedure and ICD-10-PCS procedure code(s): _____

MS-DRG: _____

Review Case 5-2 Discharge Summary

DISCHARGE DIAGNOSES: 1. 28 week stillbirth vaginal delivery of nonviable male infant. 2. Oligohydramnios with premature spontaneous rupture of membranes.

History: This is a 20-year-old gravida 2, para 1, female who at approximately 28 weeks' gestation had a spontaneous rupture of membranes. Approximately one month prior to this time, the patient underwent an ultrasound which showed severe oligohydramnios.

After consultation with the perinatologist concerning the potential viability of the pregnancy, a very grim picture and prognosis were painted. The patient was advised that even though she might continue with the pregnancy for several weeks, the risk of amnionitis was inevitable and the fetus would never have lung development with the fetus being nonviable. Following this consultation and after some thought, the recommendation of the perinatologist

consultation was to induce labor. The patient was given a prostaglandin suppositories and labor was started.

Hospital Course: The prostaglandin induction suppository was explained and it was started. She did not develop fever or nausea or diarrhea. After about 6 hours, the patient delivered a nonviable stillbirth male infant weighing 15 ounces. The placenta was retained, and so the patient was taken to the operating room where a curettage was performed with removal of the placenta and a lot of retained tissue without evidence of hemorrhage. The patient was given Ancef one gram q 6 hours and followed with close observation for the first 24 hours.. By morning the patient was afebrile. Uterus was nonpalpable, lochia was mild. Hematocrit was 33%, white count 14.3. The following day the patient was discharged to home to the care of her family to be followed in my office in one week.

Disposition: Patient was discharged to home in stable condition.

Discharge Diagnosis and Procedures

1. Oligohydramnios at 28 weeks' gestation.
2. Premature spontaneous rupture of membranes.
3. Nonviable male infant.
4. Vaginal delivery, single stillborn male infant.
5. Retained placenta.
6. Curettage for removal of retained placenta.
7. Induction of labor at 28 weeks for stillbirth delivery.

ICD-9-CM/ICD-10-CM diagnosis code(s):_____

ICD-9-CM procedure and ICD-10-PCS procedure code(s): _____

MS-DRG: _____

Review Case 5-3 Discharge Summary

DISCHARGE DIAGNOSES: 1. Colon cancer resected via sigmoid colectomy previous encounter. 2. First course of chemotherapy treatment.

History: This is a 56-year-old female who was admitted to the facility today for her first treatment of chemotherapy. The patient has adenocarcinoma of the sigmoid colon, which was resected three weeks ago. She is being admitted for her first of four chemotherapy treatments.

Hospital Course: The patient received chemotherapy infusions via a peripheral vein, percutaneous approach, on day 1 of her admission. She is doing well and will go home after two more days.

Disposition: Patient was discharged to home on day 3 and will be followed with home health and will return for her next treatment in a few weeks.

Review Case 5-3, *continued*

ICD-9-CM/ICD-10-CM diagnosis code(s): _____

ICD-9-CM procedure and ICD-10-PCS procedure code(s): _____

MS-DRG: _____

Review Case 5-4

Health Record Face Sheet

Western Regional
Medical Center

Record Number: 00-01-12

Age: 38

Gender: Female

Length of Stay: 5 Days

Diagnosis/Procedure: Abdominal Wall
                            Cellulitis and
                            Hypokalemia

Service Type: INPT Medical

Discharge Status: Home

DISCHARGE SUMMARY

DISCHARGE DIAGNOSES:

1. Abdominal wall cellulitis.

2. Hypokalemia.

3. Anemia.

HOSPITAL COURSE:

The patient was admitted to the hospital with greatly inflamed lower abdominal panniculus. She has had multiple surgeries there. Her white count was 14,000, with fevers. She was placed on oral Septra, IV Roceplin and IV Levaquin, and she responded quite nicely. Over the next 2 days, her white count went from 14,000 to 6,000, the cellulitis, warmth, erythema and tenderness went down. There was still a little erythema. She was feeling much better and no longer having fevers or chills. The blood culture showed no growth. Hematocrit was 37 at admission and 33 at discharge, but this was due to dilution. Her potassium was 3.6 at discharge.

The patient was stable and sent home on Levaquin and Ceftin. Follow up with me in two weeks.

Review Case 5-4, *continued*

HISTORY & PHYSICAL

HISTORY: The patient has a long complicated medical history with multiple abdominal surgeries and multiple episodes of cellulitis. She comes in because she was a little nauseated last night and most of the day, and at about 6 o'clock today it hit with chills, her belly started getting red, tender and warm and she stated, "I've got the cellulitis again." The patient has not vomited.

PAST HISTORY:
MEDICAL/SURGICAL: Yearly episodes of cellulitis of the abdomen. Hypertension. Hypothyroidism. Chronic hypokalemia. Chronic anemia. Chronic acid reflux from the bowel and stomach. Right ear surgery with MRSA infection many years ago. Status post T&A. Cesarean section times 1. Endometriosis. Hysterectomy for endometriosis, leaving the ovaries in and doing a supracervical hysterectomy; during that surgery, they injured the bowel and the patient got a severe infection where she was opened up, had a portion of the bowel removed and left open for approximately 7 months for healing. She has had over seven surgeries for skin grafting of such, as well as a partial bowel resection. From this, the patient has had an abdominal wall with just skin and no muscle, and this causes the cellulitis problems. Appendectomy and cholecystectomy both done with the other surgeries for the bowel.

MEDICATIONS: Metformin 500 bid, for endometriosis; lisinopril; phentermine 37.5 one daily; Synthroid 0.112 two daily; daily; triamcinolone/hydrochlorothiazide 37.5/25 one daily; Prevacid 30 b.i.d.; acidophilus one daily; citalopram 20 one daily.

ALLERGIES: REGLAN and DEMEROL.

PHYSICAL EXAMINATION:

GENERAL: Alert and oriented, but appears sick.
VITAL SIGNS: Blood pressure 146/70, pulse 136, respirations 20, temperature 104.
HEENT: Unremarkable.
LUNGS: Clear.
HEART: Regular rate and rhythm.
ABDOMEN: Large, with a scar forming a large diamond in the middle without any muscle tissue, you can feel the bowel right underneath. Across the panniculus and onto the legs there is a warm erythematous rash.

ASSESSMENT: 1) Recurrent cellulitis of the legs and abdomen. 2) Anemia. 3) Hypokalemia.

PLAN: Admit. Start on Levaquin 750 mg twice daily. Place her on Rocephin 2 grams now IV, then 1 gram IV q.24h. Septra DS, two pills now then one b.i.d. Will get blood cultures, CBC, comprehensive chemistry panel, C-reactive protein, and sedimentation rate. Will treat the anemia and hypokalemia and other problems as they occur.

continued

Review Case 5-4, *continued*

PHYSICIAN'S ORDERS

Other brand of drug identical in form and content may be dispensed unless checked ☐

Orders	Medication Rationale/Diag
1. Admit	
2. Dx- Cellulitis of the Abdominal wall, Hypokalemia, Anemia	
3. Condt - fair	
4. Vitals - 40 x 24 hrs then if stable q 8h	
5. Allergies - Reglan, Demerol, Ativan	
6. Activity - as tolerated	
7. Diet - Regular	
8. IV - D₅ 1/2 NS c̄ 20 mEq KCl/l @100 cc/hr	
9. Rocephin 2 gm IV now then 1 gm IV q 24h	
10. Levaquin 750 mg IV q 24h	
11. Bactrium DS ĪĪ PO now then Ī PO BID	
12. Metformin 500 mg Ī PO BID	
13. Lisinopril - at home	
14. Synthroid 0.112 II PO QD	
15. Triamcinolone/HCl 37.5/25 + PO QD	
16. Prevacid 30mg + PO BID	
17. Citalopram 20mg + PO QD	
18. Acidophilus + PO QD (if available)	
19. Phentermine 37.5 mg+ PO QD (if available)	
20. CBC. Com. panel in AM	

PLEASE! USE BALL POINT PEN ONLY   **PHYSICIAN'S ORDER**

Review Case 5-4, *continued*

ORDERS AND PROGRESS NOTES

DATE	HOUR	
3/25/xx	5-	*feels 100% better, Øfurther fevers, appetite back*
10:30	0-	*VSS & afeb*
		abd ↓ erythema, induration, tenderness
		Leg rash fading
		LAB CBC WBC 10K, Neut 86
		ABD Cellulitis
		much improved, on IV Levaquin & Rocephin and oral Septo, awaiting culture reports.

ICD-9-CM/ICD-10-CM diagnosis code(s): _____

ICD-9-CM procedure and ICD-10-PCS procedure code(s): _____

MS-DRG: _____

Review Case 5-5

Health Record Face Sheet

Western Regional
Medical Center

Record Number:	00-02-12
Age:	36
Gender:	Female
Length of Stay:	3 Days
Diagnosis/Procedure:	Delivery at full term, vaginal, single liveborn
Service Type:	INPT Medical OB
Discharge Status:	Home

continued

HISTORY & PHYSICAL

CHIEF COMPLAINT: Frequent contractions.

HISTORY OF PRESENT ILLNESS:
This 36-year-old Gravida 4 Para 3-0-0-3 presents at 40+ weeks by an 11-week ultrasound. She states that she has been contracting off and on for a couple of days. The contractions started with more intensity at midnight and are gradually increasing. Fluid is intact. She has had no usual problems with this pregnancy. She was unsure of her last menstrual period, therefore the 11-week ultrasound was done, which established the gestational date. Her 50-gram glucose screening test was elevated; however, subsequent 3-hour test was within normal limits.

PAST OBSTETRIC HISTORY:
1st pregnancy delivered at 38 weeks with a 12-hour labor, 7-pound female vaginal delivery with epidural anesthesia, no complications 2nd pregnancy delivered at 38 weeks with a 8-hour labor, epidural anesthesia, 6-pound 11-ounce female. 3rd pregnancy delivered a 9-pound 3-ounce female without complication, induction.

PAST MEDICAL HISTORY:
No operations. No hospitalizations except for early in the pregnancy. She was actually hospitalized for a couple of days with some cellulitis and cared for by another physician.

ALLERGIES: She does have some hayfever.

FAMILY HISTORY: Unremarkable.

SOCIAL HISTORY:

She is single and uses occasional alcohol. However, none since she found out she was pregnant. She has also had some tramadol and some nonsteroidal early in the pregnancy before she realized that she was pregnant.

PHYSICAL EXAM

GENERAL: Alert and in no apparent distress.

HEENT: Clear.

NECK: Supple.

LUNGS: Clear.

ABDOMEN: Benign.

VAGINAL: She is dilated to 3 cm according to nurse.

FETUS: Fetal heart tones are okay right now, however, there was an episode shortly after placing the monitor that looked like there might be some decelerations.

LABORATORY / DIAGNOSTIC: For some reason her labs are not attached to the rest of the chart, however, I will obtain those shortly. The group B strep and so forth have been done.

ASSESSMENT: Term, multigravida in active labor.

PLAN: We will go ahead and get an epidural in and place a scalp electrode at that time. Follow her progress.

Review Case 5-5, *continued*

DELIVERY NOTE

The patient had several episodes of decelerations. We gave her some fluids that brought her blood pressure up and that seemed to help the situation. Once the heart tones were stable, we then placed an epidural. Following which, I ruptured membranes. Fluid was then clear.

A fetal scalp electrode was then placed. She did have some decelerations off and on, however, there were some periods where the activity was not very good. However, it showed good subsequent recovery and all in all the head tones were stable in between these episodes. She was not showing a lot of progress, therefore, she was started on low dose augmentation. Eventually, she got into a very quick labor pattern once she got moving. The patient was set up when she was complete and pushing.

She delivered a viable 8-pound 7-ounce male. Apgars were 9 and 9. An intact placenta with three-vessel cord was delivered by active management. Inspection revealed a very small midline tear, which was initially repaired with one 4-0 Chromic suture. However, she continued to have some bleeding in this. The small wound was then re-closed with another suture, which had much better hemostasis. The baby was taken to the newborn nursery in stable condition.

Mother is recovering in the birthing suite.

continued

Review Case 5-5, *continued*

LABOR AND DELVERY SUMMARY

FIRST STAGE

ONSET OF LABOR
- ☑ SPONTANEOUS
- ☐ AUGMENTED
- ☐ INDUCED
  - ☐ INDICATED
  - ☐ ELECTIVE
- ☐ PITOCIN IV
- ☐ CYTOTEC
- ☐ OTHER

MEMBRANE RUPTURE
- ☐ SPONTANEOUS
- ☑ ARTIFICIAL
- ☐ CLEAR
- ☐ BLOODY
- ☐ MECONIUM

MONITOR
- ☐ ELECTIVE
- ☐ INDICATED
- ☐ NONE

		FHT	UC
EXTERNAL		☐	☐
INTERNAL		☑	☐

INTRAPARTUM STATISTICS

	DATE	TIME
EDC	5-10-13	
ADMISSION	5-11-13	0512
MEMBRANES RUPTURED	5-12	0832
ONSET OF LABOR	5-12	1200
COMPLETE DILATION	5-12	1302
DELIVERY OF INFANT	5-12	1356
PLACENTA	5-12	1405
TOTAL LABOR TIME	2'5"	

VAGINAL CHECKS TO DELIVERY ___8___

DURATION	HOURS	
STAGE	HRS.	MNS.
I	1	01
II	—	54
III		2

BABY

APGAR MINUTE 1 5

HEART RATE		
ABSENT	0	0
BELOW 100	1	1
OVER 100	②	②

SEX M

RESP EFFORT		
ABSENT	0	0
WEAK CRY	1	1
STRONG CRY	②	②

WEIGHT
8 lbs 7 oz.

REFLEX STIM		
NO RESPONSE	0	0
GRIMACE	1	1
COUGH SNEEZE	②	②

VOIDED

MUSCLE TONE		
LIMP	0	0
SOME FLEXION	1	1
WELL FLEXED	②	②

CORD
- ☐ 2 VESSEL
- ☐ 3 VESSEL
- ☐ NUCHAL CORD

COLOR		
PALE BLUE	0	0
BODY PINK EXT. BLUE	①	①
ALL PINK	2	2

DELEE _____

TOTAL	9	9

RESUSCITATION
- ☑ NONE
- ☐ FREE OXYGEN
- ☐ BAG & MASK
- ☐ SUCTION
  - ☐ BULB
  - ☐ DELEE
- ☐ CORD
  - VISUALIZED
  - ☐ MECONIUM
- ☐ INTUBATION
- ☐ CARDIAC MASK

CONDITION:
- ☑ ALIVE
- ☐ STILLBORN
  - ☐ ANTEPARTUM
  - ☐ INTRAPARTUM

MULTIPLE BIRTH
- ☐ YES ☑ NO
- A B C D

SECOND STAGE

VAGINAL DELIVERY
- ☑ BIRTHING ROOM
- ☐ ROOM

VERTEX
- ☑ OA
- ☐ SPONTANEOUS
- ☐ SHOULDER DYSTOCIA
- ☐ FUNDAL PRESSURE PER _____
- ☐ OP

☐ VACUUM EXTRAC _____ MIN DEL HEAD

BREECH UMBILICUS TIME _____
- ☐ FRANK
- ☐ SINGLE FOOTLING
- ☐ DOUBLE FOOTLING
- ☐ COMPLETE
- ☐ SPONTANEOUS
- ☐ ASSIST
- ☐ TOTAL EXTRACT
- ☐ FORCEPS

EPISIOTOMY ☑ NONE   **LACERATION** ☐ NONE
- ☐ ML
- ☐ OTHER _____
- ☐ SUTURE _____
- ☑ PERINEAL
- ☐ VAGINAL
- ☐ CERVICAL
- ☐ OTHER

CESAREAN DELIVERY

PRE-OP DX _____

PROCEDURE ☐ REPEAT ☐ PRIMARY
SURGEON _____
ASSISTANT _____
ATTENDING BABY _____
CRNA _____
TYPE OF ANESTHESIA _____
CIRCULATING NURSE _____
SCRUB TECH _____
FHT (pre-scrub) _____
EBL _____

TIMES ENTER ROOM _____ SKIN INCISION _____
AMNIOTOMY _____ SKIN CLOSURE _____
EXIT ROOM _____

THIRD STAGE

PLACENTA
- ☑ SPONTANEOUS
- ☐ SIMPLE EXPRESSION
- ☐ MANUAL EXPRESSION
- ☐ CURETTAGE
- ☐ ABRUPTION _____ %
- ☐ MARGINAL
- SEPARATION _____ %
- ☐ PREVIA

ABNORMALITIES OF CORD OR PLACENTA _____

MOTHER'S MEDICATIONS/LABOR

TIME	ROUTE	MEDICATION	DOSE	PERSON

DATE	HOUR	
5/12/xx	11:50 am	S-No problems noted or unusual complaints
		O - afeb VSS
		Lungs CTA Abd soft fundus firm
		HCT 39
		A/P doing well - D/C home

Review Case 5-5, *continued*

Patient : Ashley Abbott
DOB : 3/12/76
Provider : Dr. News
Medical Record : 00-02-12

BS		Ref. Range/Females
	06:31	
SPUNHCT	39	37–47%

					Ref. Range	
WBC		7.4	mm3	4.2	-	10.0
GRAN%		66	%	45	-	75
LYMPH%		26	%	15	-	45
MONO%		5	%	2	-	10
EOS%		2.7	%	0.0	-	5.0
BASO%		0.5	%	0.0	-	3.0
RBC		4.39	mm3	4.20	-	5.00
HGB		12.4	g/dl	12.0	-	16.0
HCT		37	%	37	-	47
MCV		85	fl	81	-	101
MCH		28.3	pg	27.0	-	34.0
MCHC		33.5	g/dl	31.0	-	36.0
RDW		14.0	%	10.0	-	17.0
PLT		279	mm3	150	-	450
MPV		8.3	fl	5.5	-	10.0

T Y P E   &   S C R E E N

ABO	0
RH	POSITIVE
ANTIBODY SCREEN	NEGATIVE

RPR	NON-REACTIVE
RUBELLA	IMMUNE
HEPSAG	NON-REACTIVE

RPR, RUBELLA AND HEPATITIS TESTING DONE AT IHC LABORATORIES

Patient : Ashley Abbott
DOB : 3/12/76
Provider : Dr. News
Medical Record : 00-02-12

Age: 36
Encount

Group B Strep

KGK		Ref. Range/Females
	1	
GRPB	Negative for Group B Strep	Negative for Group B Strep

continued

Review Case 5-5, *continued*

ICD-9-CM/ICD-10-CM diagnosis code(s): _____

ICD-9-CM procedure and ICD-10-PCS procedure code(s): _____

MS-DRG: _____

Review Case 5-6

Health Record Face Sheet

Western Regional
Medical Center

Record Number:	11-13-05
Age:	Newborn
Gender:	Male
Length of Stay:	1 Day
Diagnosis/Procedure:	Newborn with Circumcision
Service Type:	Inpatient Medical
Discharge Status:	To Home

Review Case 5-6, *continued*

DISCHARGE DATE: *1/28/xx*   RECD. NO. *11-13-05*

MOTHER: AGE *21*   GRAVIDA *1*   PARA *0*

TYPE OF DELIVERY: *Vag.*

COMPLICATIONS OF DELIVERY: *Cephalohematoma*

APGARS: *9* & *9*   BIRTH WEIGHT: *8* LB *12¾* OZ   DISCHARGE WEIGHT: *8* LB *13* OZ
    1 MIN   5 MIN

GESTATIONAL AGE BY DATES: *38* WKS.   GESTATIONAL AGE BY EXAM: _____ WK

PKU Stamper: *PKU DONE*   CIRCUMCISION: [X] YES   [ ] NO

	NL	PHYSICIAN EXAMINATION ON DISCHARGE
Skin	✔	COMMENTS/IMPRESSIONS:
HEENT	✔	
Chest	✔	*normal PE*
Lungs	✔	
Heart	✔	
Abdomen	✔	
Genitalia	✔	
Anus	✔	
Back	✔	
Extremities	✔	
Hips R L	✔	
Neurological	✔	
Other		

DATE	TIME	CONDITION ON DISCHARGE/INSTRUCTIONS:	BLOOD TYPE-MATERNAL: OK	INFANT:
1/28/xx	0830	*wt 8–9 nursing fair Plan discharge today Recheck was good*		

Circumcision: [ ] gomco   [X] plasti bell   [ ] mogan
    Note

Complications/Infections: [X] NORMAL NEWBORN

continued

Review Case 5-6, *continued*

ADMISSION INFORMATION:

Physician Notified __Dr. Adol__

Delivery Time __2:25 pm__
Delivery Mode __Vag__

Weight: _____ gm °   __8__ lb __12¾__ oz   Hct: Heel _____   VENOUS _____   APGAR: 1 min...__9__... 5 min...__9__...

Length: __54½__ cm (__21¼__ in)   OFC __35½__ cm _____   Chest __36__ cm   ABD __34__ cm   Erythromycin Opth. Oint. o.u._____

Rectal Temp: __99°__   B/P __80   157__   Blood Glucose Monitor _____   Lab: Blood Glucose _____

TIME

NEWBORN ASSESSMENT:

HEART __132__/min.	HEAD	MOUTH	ANUS	CRY	COMMENTS:
☑ NORMAL	☑ NORMAL	☑ NORMAL	☐ PATENT	☑ NORMAL	0840 Male infant carried to nursery via grandmother Awake, alert & crying. Pink, weighed & measured Placed under open warer no signs of resp distress
☐ Murmur	☐ Molding	☐ Cleft lip	☐ Imperforate	☐ High pitched	
☐ Capillary refill >3 seconds	☐ Caput	☐ Cleft palate	☐	☐ Hoarse	
☐	☐ Cephalohematoma	☐ Excessive saliva		☐ Weak	
	☐ Sutures separated	☐	SPINE		
RESPIRAT. __34__/min.	☐ Anterior fontanelle large, bulging		☑ NORMAL	MUSCLE TONE	
☐ NORMAL		NECK	☐ Sacral dimple	☑ NORMAL	
☑ BS Moist	☐ Posterior fontanelle large	☑ NORMAL	☐	☐ Hypotonic	
☐ Grunting		☐ Masses		☐ Hypertonic	
☐ Nasal Flaring	☐	☐ Restricted ROM	EXTREMITIES		
☐ Retracting		☐	☑ NORMAL	ACTIVITY	
☐ Breath sounds asymmetrical	EYES		☐ Hip Click ☐ R ☐ L	☑ NORMAL	
☐	☑ NORMAL	ABDOMEN	☐ Femoral pulses weak or absent	☐ Lethargic	
	☐	☑ NORMAL		☐ Irritable	
		☐ Enlarged liver	☐ Extra digits	☐ Tremulous	
SKIN	EARS	☐ Masses	☐		
☑ NORMAL	☑ NORMAL	☐ Umbihernia		ADDITIONAL FINDINGS	
☐ Pealing		☐ Absence of bowel sounds	REFLEXES	☐ NONE	
☐ Pale	☐ Abnormal shape & position		☑ NORMAL	☐ Forceps marks	
☐ Plethoric		☐	☐ Suck weak or absent	☐ Vacuum marks	
☐ Meconium stained	☐ Canals not patent			☐ Bruising	
☐ Central cyanosis	☐	GENITALIA	☐ Palmar grasp abnormal	☐ Arm weakness	
☐ Jaundiced		☐ NORMAL BOY		☐ Laceration	
☐ Market acrocyanosis	NOSE	☐ NORMAL GIRL	☐ Plantar grasp abnormal	☐ Abrasion	
☐ Birthmarks	☑ NORMAL	☐ Hypospadius	☐ Moro absent	☐ Facial weakness	
☐ Mongolian spot(s)	☐ Nares not patent	☐ Hernia		☐ Fracture	
	☐	☐ Undesc. tes. R L	☐ Moro asymmetrical	☐ Scalp lead lesion	Nurse sig.: __H. Aguilar, RN__

R.N. ASSESSMENT COMMENTS: _____

_____

TIME: SIGNATURE:

PHYSICIAN EXAMINATION

	NL	COMMENTS/IMPRESSIONS:
Skin	✔	
HEENT	✔	
Chest	✔	*normal PE*
Lungs	✔	
Heart	✔	
Abdomen	✔	
Genitalia	✔	
Anus	✔	
Back	✔	
Extremities	✔	
Hips R L	✔	
Neurological	✔	

DATE	TIME	PROGRESS NOTES	BLOOD TYPE-MATERNAL:	INFANT:
1/27/xx	2:25 pm			

8-12 3/4 Male born to 21 yo G1P1 female mom by vag delivery with v.c assistance. Apgars 9/9 Go back in 3 weeks PE WNL HCT 56%

NEWBORN ASSESSMENT

Review Case 5-6, *continued*

STANDING ORDERS FOR NORMAL NEWBORN | PROGRESS NOTES

DELIVERY ROOM

1. Dry baby well under warmer.
2. Cover baby including most of head & keep warm.
3. Footprint & place ID bands on both arms.
4. Aqua Mephyton 1 mg IM

ADMISSION ORDERS TO NURSERY

1. Ilotycin ointment to each eye (ophthalmic ointment)
2. Weight, length and OFC
3. Bathe with soap & water, rinse well, 4–6 hours after admission or when temp is 98.6—NOT BEFORE.
4. Temperature
5. Clean cord with alcohol & watch closely for bleeding & signs of infection.
6. Keep air passages free of mucus with bulb syringe or deep suction PRN.
7. Allow mother to hold baby <u>with nurse in attendance</u>, as soon as baby is stabilized.

OBSERVE & REPORT TO DOCTOR ANY OF THE FOLLOWING:

1. Abnormal, absence of, or frequent liquid BMs
2. Absence of urination or phimosis
3. Respiratory difficulties; rapid respiration or cyanosis
4. Jaundice, especially first 24 hours
5. Elevated, low, or unstable temperatures
6. Persistent feeding problems
7. Unusual weight loss
8. Jitteriness

DAILY ROUTINE CARE

1. Daily bath with tap water or baby soap solution. Use no oil on skin.
2. Temperature each shift.
3. Feeding:
   a. NPO 2–6 hours
   b. D5W feeding x 1
   c. House formula q 4 hours
   d. Nursing babies to breast first feeding.
   e. Supplement nursing babies with D5W only unless house formula requested by mother.

DISCHARGE ORDERS

1. Discharge baby with mother.
2. Discharge instructions for Repeat PKU, PRN.

continued

Review Case 5-6, *continued*

ICD-9-CM/ICD-10-CM diagnosis code(s): _____

ICD-9-CM procedure and ICD-10-PCS procedure code(s): _____

MS-DRG: _____

Review Case 5-7

Health Record Face Sheet

Western Regional
Medical Center

Record Number:	00-03-12
Age:	58
Gender:	Female
Length of Stay:	3 Days
Diagnosis/Procedure:	Acute Labryinthitis
Service Type:	Inpatient
Discharge Status:	To Home

DISCHARGE SUMMARY

DATE OF ADMISSION: 5/4/xx

DATE OF DISCHARGE: 5/7/xx

FINAL DIAGNOSIS:

Acute labyrinthitis, probable.

ENTERING COMPLAINT: See history and physical.

COURSE IN THE HOSPITAL:

The patient's nystagmus, nausea, and vomiting improved over the next 24 hours. She still had trouble with dizziness when she got up and walked around. She was seen by neurology who felt that acute labyrinthitis was the diagnosis. Her diet was advanced. She was placed on regular doses of Meclozine. She did have some trouble with plugging and secretions. Was tried on Robitussin and then switched to Entex at the time of discharge. She improved to the point where she was able to get up and walk around, not having nausea or vomiting, able to tolerate a regular diet. Her symptoms almost entirely cleared except for some mild dizziness prior to her Meclomen dose. She is discharged home to return to the care of Dr. Williams. She will resume her home medicines. Also give her Entex LA twice a day, Meclozine 25 three times a day. She will call if problems return. She did have a sore throat and throat culture done was read as negative at time of discharge.

Pertinent laboratory studies while in the hospital include: Negative CAT scan of the head, 3.9 potassium, 114 glucose, 1.8 phosphorus, 6.2 total protein, 83 segs, 11 lymphs, and a 13 hemoglobin. EKG showed within normal limits.

HISTORY & PHYSICAL

DATE OF ADMISSION: 5/4/xx

REASON FOR ADMISSION:

Nausea, vomiting, vertigo, nystagmus.

This is a lady who is usually followed by Dr. Jones in the city, but she lives here in town. She complains of having some troubles with nausea, vomiting, some dizziness, vertigo which began acutely in the morning. States she had the flu several weeks ago and totally got over that. Had some mild upper respiratory symptoms. Had not been around anyone sick. Had some chilling through the night and came to the ER where her symptoms persisted. There she was given some phenergan IV. Improved with her vomiting but still had severe vertigo when she moved and extreme dizziness and severe nystagmus to the point that she could not open her eyes without becoming dizzy.

She is currently on Amitriptyline 25mg at bedtime. Estrogen 1.25. She took a Motrin this morning to see if it helped. She usually takes 800 twice a day for neck and back.

She is exposed to passive smoking. Drinks rarely. Lives with her 12-year-old son and a male companion.

She has had a hysterectomy in the past. Did lose the sight in her right eye. Was seen by Dr. Wright and hospitalized. Apparently Dr. Wright took care of it this time. She had a myelogram done for some reason and apparently had a reaction to it. She has also seen Dr. Williams in the past. She states her son was killed in an accident and she had trouble with her headache and nerves and a nervous breakdown then. She lost her husband several years ago. She is allergic to tranquilizers, pain pills, Dristan. The remainder of her review of systems is negative except as in history of present illness. She denies any tinnitus or headache at this time.

PHYSICAL EXAM:

VITAL SIGNS: BP is 144/100, pulse is 100, respirations are 22 and temp is 97.9.

HEENT: TM's are clear. She has no bruits, no thyromegaly, no neck vein distension.

NECK: Supple. She has nystagmus with fast component to the left.

LUNGS: Clear.

HEART: Regular rate and rhythm.

ABDOMEN: Benign. No peripheral edema. No focal weakness. She has severe vertigo when she turns in the bed.

PLAN:

To admit for IV support. Will start her on Meclozine. Continue Phenergan.

With her previous history of loss of sight wonder about a vascular problem and posterior circulation, labyrinthitis, 8th nerve problem. Will plan to treat symptomatically. Have neurology evaluate.

Apparently her CAT scan in the ER was negative and her laboratory studies disclose no critical abnormalities. She does relate that she has severe hypoglycemia.

cc: office

continued

NEUROLOGY CONSULTATION

DATE OF CONSULTATION: 5/5/xx

Attending Physician: Dr. Jones

Consulting Physician: Dr. Wise

HISTORY:

This 53-year-old white right-handed female had the very sudden onset of true vertigo yesterday with sensation of her environment spinning. This was markedly worsened with any type of movement including turning to the side while lying supine or changing position. The symptom has persisted today, but it is much improved as compared to yesterday. She was persistently nauseated, and she vomited on several occasions when this began yesterday, but this is nearly totally resolved today. She denies all visual and all neurological symptoms when associated with this when asked specifically in detail about the possibility of such occurring. She had a similar such episode lasting for several hours approximately 4 years ago. She reports that she has always been very motion sensitive and prone to "sea sickness."

The patient's past medical history is totally unremarkable, and it appears that she has enjoyed excellent health her entire life.

NEUROLOGICAL EXAMINATION:

The patient presents as a very mildly acutely ill middle-aged lady who is in no distress. I do not detect retro-orbital, intracranial, carotid artery, or subclavian artery bruits on either side.

The patient is awake, alert, oriented, and completely cooperative, and actually quite pleasant. She relates well during the interview and neurological examination, and I do not detect any evidence of deficits in higher cortical integrative functions in the process of evaluating her clinically.

The functions of the 1st through the 12th cranial nerves are all clinically intact. Both pupils are approximately 6mm, round, central, and have 4+ reactions to light and accommodation without any detectable Marcus Gunn phenomenon. The optic fundi are completely normal with sharp disc margins and normal vessel patterns, and spontaneous venous pulsations. The visual fields are clinically full to finger confrontation, and there is no extinction with minimal double simultaneous visual stimulation. The patient has intermittent very slight extremely low amplitude barely detectable counterclockwise rotatory nystagmus, which is accentuated with gaze deviation towards her right side.

Muscle, strength, muscle tone, and fine coordinated motor activity are all normal throughout bilaterally. There is no drift, pronation, or posturing of either upper extremity.

Deep tendon reflexes are all 2/4 at all sites in all 4 extremities. All deep tendon reflexes are bilaterally symmetrical, and both plantar reflexes are strongly flexor.

Finger to finger, finger to nose, rapid alternating movements, and heel to shin are all performed quite well bilaterally. After time for adjustment, the patient is basically steady while standing on a narrow base' though there is intermittent minimal swaying when her feet are together touching, and this is slightly accentuated when she closes her eyes.

Basic and higher sensory modalities are intact throughout bilaterally including for light touch, pinprick, vibratory sensation, and minimal position change. There is no sensory extinction with minimal double simultaneous tactile stimulation. The patient does take a very few steps with her gait being extremely slow and cautious and very slightly nonspecifically unsteady.

NEUROLOGY CONSULTATION—PAGE 2

IMPRESSION:

Acute labyrinthitis.

DISCUSSION:

The patient's neurological examination is entirely normal except for the rotary nystagmus and very mild truncal instability as described above. I would consider the entire clinical presentation most consistent with and suggestive of the specified diagnosis.

RECOMMENDATIONS:

At this point I would suggest that you obtain ENT consultation regarding this problem.

Thank you for asking me to see this patient at this time.

EMERGENCY ROOM REPORT

By history patient is a 58-year-old female who presents to the Emergency Department having developed severe vertigo shortly after awakening this morning. This was followed by nausea and vomiting. She has been unable to move her head without severe vertigo. She has been unable to ambulate since the symptoms began. She called an ambulance and was brought to the Emergency Department by ambulance. The patient had mild or similar symptoms about six months ago which resolved spontaneously. She denies any tinnitus or ear pain or hearing loss. She denies any numbness or tingling elsewhere in her body. She feels fully alert and well otherwise.

Objectively, the patient's vital signs are normal, except for a blood pressure of 152/86. She denies any headache. HEENT exam is not remarkable. The ears are entirely benign. Neck is supple. Carotid pulses are 2+. Facial musculature and cranial nerves 2–8 are intact. She does demonstrate gross nystagmus with a vast component to the right. The nystagmus is present in the resting condition. Cardiac exam is benign. Abdomen is soft and nontender. CBC and chem profile are not remarkable.

ASSESSMENT: Severe vertigo.

PLAN: The patient was treated with Phenergan 25 mg IV and an IV was established. Dr. Jones was contacted.

RADIOLOGY REPORT

HISTORY: Headache. Dizziness.

NONENHANCED CT HEAD SCAN:

There are no abnormal areas of increased or decreased density. The subarachnoid spaces and ventricles are normal. There is no shift of midline structures. The structures at the base of the brain appear normal.

IMPRESSION:

Normal nonenhanced CT head scan.

continued

Review Case 5-7, *continued*

☒ E.C.G.	☐ PHYSICIAN INTERP.	☐ EMER. INTERP.	☐ **RHYTHM STRIPS**

☐ MALE

☒ FEMALE   AGE _58_   HEIGHT ____   WEIGHT ____

MEDICATIONS: (LIST ALL)

_____

_____

_____

_____

CLINICAL DIAGNOSIS: (REASON FOR ECG)

_____

_____ *Dizzy* _____

_____

RHYTHM   *sinus* _____

RATE *90* _____   MEAN ORS AXIS   *T6* _____

INTERVALS: PR ___*.16*___   QRS ___*.08*___   QT ___*.38*___

DESCRIPTION:

SINCE: *no old trauma* _____

_____

ECG INTERPRETATION: _____

_____ *Probable septal QS* _____

_____

ELECTROCARDIOGRAPHIC REPORT   SIGNED

Richard Hill, M.D.
CHART COPY

Review Case 5-7, *continued*

ICD-9-CM/ICD-10-CM diagnosis code(s): _____

ICD-9-CM procedure and ICD-10-PCS procedure code(s): _____

MS-DRG: _____

Review Case 5-8

Health Record Face Sheet

Western Regional
Medical Center

Record Number: 00-04-12

Age: 29

Gender: Female

Length of Stay: 2 Days

Diagnosis/Procedure: Acute Gangrenous Suppurative
Appendicitis/Appendectomy

Service Type: Inpatient

---

continued

DISCHARGE SUMMARY

DATE OF ADMISSION: 6/1/xx
DATE OF DISCHARGE: 6/2/xx

REASON FOR ADMISSION: This is a 29-year-old female admitted with the possibility of appendicitis. She had developed abdominal pain a couple of nights before being admitted to the hospital here. She had seen both Dr. Minut and Dr. Otto with a slightly elevated white count with a slight left shift and negative pregnancy test. She had some tenderness with a slight rebound, very, very low, near the inguinal ligament in the right lower quadrant. She had ketones in the urine and was dehydrated. She said she had slept part of the night previous. She felt more comfortable with the knees flexed. She had no evidence of ulcer. Romberg sign. Rectal exam was negative. Pelvic exam completely normal. The pain was worsening, and because of the possibility of appendicitis she was admitted to the hospital, placed NPO and IV started.

ADMISSION LABORATORY: Was really unchanged. White count was 13.9 with 83 Begs, 3 bands, and 8 lymphs, and urine showed a specific gravity of 1.021 with ketones, 5-15 RBC's.

Her past medical history and review of systems was really unremarkable. Denied sore throat, cough, dysuria. Was on no medications.

Her physical exam was normal except for the findings indicated above.

We went ahead and did a barium enema on this lady with findings of an abnormal configuration of the cecum and the appendix did not fill.

Because of her continued pain that was not improving and findings on barium enema, we opted to go ahead and do an appendectomy on this lady with the findings of an acute gangrenous suppurative non-perforated appendicitis. Her postoperative course was reasonably uncomplicated except for diarrhea. We checked for Clostridium difficile which was negative. She was discharged to home the afternoon of day two, tolerating a regular diet, afebrile, vital signs stable. She was discharged on Vicodin one to two every four to six hours as needed for pain. To be followed in my office Wednesday.

SPECIAL PROCEDURES: Barium enema.

HISTORY AND PHYSICAL

This 29-year-old female was seen in consultation per request of Dr. Otto. She had developed abdominal pain Sunday night or Monday morning, she is not sure which. She had associated nausea but no vomiting. She has been evaluated by both Dr. Minut and Dr. Otto and was found to have a white count elevated slightly with slight left shift. Her pregnancy test was negative. Her abdominal findings showed rebound very low in the right lower quadrant right along the inguinal ligament. However, on my exam she really did not have much in the way of guarding or rebound when she was first seen in the emergency room on consultation. She did have ketones in her urine and was dehydrated. She said that she slept part of the night last night and felt slightly more comfortable with the knees flexed. She did not have iliopsoas sign and Romberg sign was negative. The patient's rectal exam was negative, and pelvic exam was completely negative. Because of the patient's pain worsening and the possibility of appendicitis, she was admitted to the hospital with an IV placed.

Her admission laboratory repeat HCG was negative. Urine greater than 160 mg per dcl of ketones. Specific gravity was 1.021. She had 5 to 15 RBCs. White count was 13.9 with 83 segs, 3 bands, 8 lymphs.

The patient's past medical history and review of systems were remarkable for cesarean section without appendectomy. She denied sore throat or any other recent medical problems. She has no allergies, does not smoke or drink. No current medications. She denies any significant family history and review of systems is completely negative.

PHYSICAL EXAMINATION: Head, eyes, ears, nose and throat are unremarkable. The neck is supple, trachea midline. Oral pharynx is clear. The lungs are clear. Heart: regular sinus rhythm without murmur. Abdomen: marked tenderness deep to the right, very low right lower quadrant and question of palpable lymph along the inguinal ligament. The patient is thin and easily examined. Other pertinent points of physical exam are as above.

Extremities: Normal, neuro grossly intact.

IMPRESSION: Possible appendicitis.

PLAN: Admit to the hospital, will probably obtain a barium enema. Will recheck her in two or three hours after she is hydrated.

continued

Review Case 5-8, *continued*

OPERATIVE NOTE

DATE OF PROCEDURE: 6/1/xx

PREOPERATIVE DIAGNOSIS: Acute appendicitis.
POSTOPERATIVE DIAGNOSIS: Acute nonperforated appendicitis.
PROCEDURE: Appendectomy

INDICATION FOR PROCEDURE:

The patient with right lower quadrant pain and tenderness right along the inguinal ligament with guarding and rebound after being admitted to the hospital. Dehydration with ketones in urine.

DESCRIPTION OF THE PROCEDURE:

With the patient under general anesthesia with endotracheal tube in place, having had a Betadine prep and sterile drape, a right modified incision was made just below and to the right of McBurney's point as the patient's maximum tenderness was in this location. Hemostasis was obtained with a bovie and sub Q. The fascia to the external oblique was identified and opened sharply with a knife. This was extended with the scissors. Dissection bluntly then was accomplished with muscle splitting incision through the peritoneum. There was clear fluid upon entering the abdomen. Finger was placed in the wound and the firm mass was present along the lateral pelvic wall adjacent to the inguinal ligament but adherent to the abdominal wall. Blunt dissection freed this up and it was indurated tense tissue felt to be an appendix. The cecum was mobilized through the incision but we were unable to mobilize the tip of the appendix before the appendix was clamped just above its base and 3.5 staple line was drawn on the base of the appendix. The appendix was then amputated and the mucosa was bovied. The mesentery to the appendix was taken down retrograde. This maneuver then allowed us to mobilize the appendix through a smaller incision. The appendix was finally mobilized into the operative field and found to be extremely tense, almost ready to rupture but not perforated and the appendix really was not suppurative. The patient had been given 1 gram of Cefizox prior to opening the abdomen. The mesentery of the appendix was clamped and tied off with 2-0 stick tie Vicryl. Once all of these were amputated the appendix was moved to the back table. The cecum was there placed back into the abdominal cavity and suction with guard placed on it was placed into the pelvis to suction any fluid out. Upon completion the peritoneum was closed after being grasped with clamps with 2-0 running Vicryl. Once this was accomplished the abdominal wall was irrigated and closed by me after the clips had been removed.

The external oblique fascia was closed with interrupted 2-0 Vicryl, Scarpa's fascia was closed with interrupted 4-0 Vicryl. The wound was irrigated in layers and 4-0 Vicryl was placed in the subcuticular region and steri strips used on the skin.

The patient was sent to recovery with stable normal vital signs. ESTIMATED BLOOD LOSS: Less than 25cc.

The patient extubated in OR. No tubes and drain. Family counseled postop.

Review Case 5-8, *continued*

EMERGENCY BARIUM ENEMA

HISTORY: Right lower quadrant pain.

The colon was filled in the usual fashion. There is mass effect upon the tip of the cecum. The patient is acutely tender over this area. There is also nonfilling of the appendix.

Using these three signs, I would correlate this clinically and raise the possibility of appendicitis.

IMPRESSION: Abnormal configuration of the cecum as described above. Consistent with diagnosis of appendicitis.

ICD-9-CM/ICD-10-CM diagnosis code(s): _____

ICD-9-CM procedure and ICD-10-PCS procedure code(s): _____

MS-DRG: _____

Review Case 5-9

Health Record Face Sheet

Record Number:	00-05-12	Western Regional Medical Center
Age:	57	
Gender:	Female	
Length of Stay:	22 Days	
Diagnosis/Procedure:	Myocardial Infarction	
Service Type:	Inpatient	
Discharge Status:	To Home	

continued

Review Case 5-9, *continued*

DISCHARGE SUMMARY

DATE OF ADMISSION: 3/9/xx
DATE OF DISCHARGE: 3/30/xx

HISTORY OF PRESENT ILLNESS: The patient is a 57-year-old white female admitted via ambulance from East Valley Hospital for acute inferior myocardial infarction with multiple complications.

LAB/X-RAY: Admission glucose 254, BUN 2, creatinine 1.6, uric acid 7.2, bilirubin normal, alk phos normal, SGPT 111, SGOT 253, LDH 426, GGTP 197, albumin 3.1, calcium 8.5, sodium 138, potassium 4.6, cholesterol 246, triglycerides 294. Daily SMAC profiles were obtained throughout her entire hospitalization. This was done because of her very severe disease. Her BUN and creatinine rose to a high of 37 and 0.9 on and then fell. Her potassium was maintained in a therapeutic range between 4 and 4.0 essentially throughout the hospitalization. Her liver function tests remained somewhat abnormal. They appeared to be somewhat due to the CPK rise. However, they did persist somewhat. Her SMAC on the day of discharge was 122. BUN 20, creatinine 0.8, glucose 211, bilirubin normal, alk phos 307, SGPT 28., SGOT 21, LDH 131, GGTP 323, albumin 2.8, phos 4.7, sodium 139, potassium 4.7, cholesterol 199, triglycerides 399. Urinalysis—specific gravity 1.024, pH 5.0, protein 30 mg percent, glucose 500 mg percent, ketones trace, blood trace, 2/5 white cells, 1/3 red cells, 0/1 epithelial cells, 2+ amorphous crystals.

CBC on admission. White count 14,700, hemoglobin 15.7, platelets 94,000. Serial hemoglobins etc are obtained. She did develop a progressive anemia. The last CBC was obtained yesterday. At that time white count 5,600, hemoglobin 10.3, platelets 251,000. Her PTT is maintained in a therapeutic range between 75 and 100 on IV heparin. A random glucose at 9:50 a.m. on the day of admission is 684. Magnesium is 1.6 on that date in the afternoon. Arterial blood gms on admission 7.32, pCO2 34, pO2 102, bicarb 17, saturation 96% on 100% mask O2 on admission Magnesium on 1.8 is 2.3 and is 2.0 on 1.9, is 1.6 on day 1, and is 1.6 on day 2 and is 1.8 on day 3. Very frequent potassium and electrolytes were obtained, the first couple of days of the hospitalization. Cardiac panel showed peak CK to be 1,673, drawn yesterday. Her CKs are approximately 11% MB band positive. Culture of the tip of the Swan Ganz catheter shows Staphylococcus aureus and Streptococcus agalactiae, group. These are both sensitive to Cefazolin. Blood cultures grew out Staphylococcus aureus. This is also sensitive to Cefazolin.

PA and lateral chest x-ray shows heart size at upper limits of normal. Lungs are clear. Swan Ganz catheter is present and is unchanged. Portable chest x-ray yesterday is unremarkable. Normal portable chest with Swan Ganz catheter was obtained yesterday.

SERIAL ELECTROCARDIOGRAMS: Admission ECG shows approximately 4 millimeter inferior ST elevation in 3 with somewhat less so in 2 and AVE. There is also approximately 3/4 millimeter ST depression in 1 and AVL and lead V2. First-degree AV block with a PR of about 0.40 was present. Subsequently the patient's ECGs showed resolution of the majority of the ST elevation. There did definitely remain, however, a couple of millimeters of ST elevation. The latest ECG completed yesterday shows persistent 1 to 2 millimeter ST depression in leads 1, AVL and V2 and V3, and 1-2 millimeter ST elevation in 2,3, and AVE. There are very small Q waves present in 2 and 3 which are felt not be necessarily significant.

Spirometry was obtained yesterday. Forced vital capacity 1.8, FEV 11.3, ratio of the two is 72%, FEE 2575 is 37% predicted, MVV is 51% predicted. This is diagnostic of a moderate increase in FEC which may be partly related to air trapping. Mild decrease in the FEV1/FVC ratio. Obstruction is difficult to quantitate in the presence of decreased FEC. No significant change after single bronchodilator challenge. Recommend lung volumes and DtJCO if there is a suspicion of combined restrictive and obstructive components (interpretation per Dr. Hart.

HOSPITAL COURSE: The patient initially presented with an acute MI to East Valley Hospital and Dr. Smith cared for her there until she was stable enough to transport. I was on the phone with him between 12:30 and 2:30 a.m. continuously directing and giving counsel regarding her therapy. He accompanied her here in transport, and then I first met her personally and assumed her care. She was admitted to the CCU. She treated with IV magnesium, oxygen, IV Hepariri, IV Inapsine for nausea. IV morphine sulfate for chest pain, aspirin, Zantac, dopamine for hypotension, Zol pacemaker (on standby), IV insulin bolus and IV insulin drip, IV Lopressor (15 mg total), IV Lidocaine, normal saline with 15 mEq [CCL per liter at 150 cc an hour, q. 6 hour electrolytes, and hourly Accucheks]. A Swan Ganz catheter was inserted via the right internal jugular vein without difficulty under fluoroscopic guidance at about 10 o'clock a.m. The patient was having frequent emesis productive of hemoccult positive dark brown liquid. Swan Ganz was placed because of persistent hypotension despite administration of 2 1/2 liters of normal saline and dopamine 7.5 micrograms per kilogram per minute. Blood pressure remained in the 70s where previously it had been in the 100s to 120s. Urine output was good and now poor. The Swan Ganz showed a pulmonary capillary wedge pressure of 18, right atrial pressure 18, pulmonary artery pressure 30/20, SVR 1475, pulmonary vascular resistance 125, cardiac output 3.2.

The patient's IV intake was slowed once the Swan Ganz was placed. Her Zantac was switched to a continuous drip because of her GI bleeding. Heparin was continued and titrated. She had received thrombolytics and by that afternoon, the patient's glucose on hourly finger stick checks had fallen into the 200s, and the IV insulin was slowed way down and she was switched over to subcutaneous insulin. The patient's rhythm stabilized somewhat and remained more in sinus rhythm with first-degree AV block.

Review Case 5-9, *continued*

DISCHARGE SUMMARY—PAGE 2

She was pain free by that time. Urine output was slow. It was felt that her fluid balance was very delicate secondary to a large right ventricular myocardial infarction.

At about 3:30 p.m. the patient had violent emesis and abruptly decompensated complaining of shortness of breath, but no chest pain. She became cold, diaphoretic, and her heart rate fell into the 40s with heart block. Blood pressure fell to the 70s. SAO2 fell into the mid 70s and CVP remained about 16 with a wedge of 16. She had no acute changes on her EKG except that she was in 2 or 3:1 heart block. Chest x-ray was normal. Echocardiogram was performed which showed a mobile right ventricular free wall and valves were all normal. There was no VSD or ASD. There was a small anterior pericardial effusion. At this point, Lopressor was discontinued. Her finger oximetry was monitored and her oxygen was titrated to that end point.
That evening a Nipride and Dobutamine were initiated by Dr. Gillespie who saw the patient on call for me for a few hours. She was placed on a heavy dose of Dobutamine (40 micrograms per kilogram per minute), as well as the low-dose Nipride and now low-dose Dopamine.

Overall with it she seemed to do a little bit better. The lidocaine was gradually weaned. Her F1O2 was titrated to O2 saturation of 93%. Heparin was continued and titrated to appropriate PPTs. Subcutaneous insulin was administered on a sliding scale. Later that day the rhythm remained approximately 65 with AV dissociation with junctional rhythm and some AV conduction with an atrial rate in the 130s. The Dobutamine was gradually weaned. NPH insulin was initiated. On admission multiple laboratory values were checked. She remained on gradually decreasing doses of Dobutamine (now 19 micrograms per kilogram per minute), as well as drips of Dopamine, Nipride, Lidocaine, heparin and Zantac. A Swan Ganz catheter was continuing to be used on an hourly basis. She had put on about 9 pounds of fluid. Her rhythm remained the same with junctional and MI dissociation with occasional AV conduction and an atrial rate of about 140. Overall she was slowly improving. Lasix was administered. Lidocaine was stopped. On admission, again, glucose and other laboratory values were monitored and followed. Heparin, insulin, Lasix, potassium and Zantac were all adjusted. Her weight increased another 41/2 pounds. She continued in 2:1 heart block with a ventricular rate of about 60. Her nausea was improving.

On admission the patient was given magnesium IV as well as more potassium. The Dobutamine was tapered down to 5 micrograms per kilogram per minute. She continued in 2:1 heart block with a ventricular rate of 60. She had poor appetite, but no chest pain and no nausea. On day 3 the patient was constipated. The Nipride was weaned off and the Dopamine was weaned off. Up to this point, the Swan Ganz had been used very frequently. However, it appeared that she had the new onset of infection around the catheter site. The catheter was removed and the tip was cultured. Overall the patient appeared to be doing fairly well. Antibiotics were initiated. On day 3 blood cultures were drawn and antibiotics were switched to Ancef. This was done because of a temperature spike to 103 degrees. On examination, the right internal jugular venous site where the Swan Ganz catheter had been previously placed was tender, swollen, but was in the process of gradually resolving. The patient's monitor was showing gradually improving conduction, now with sinus rhythm first-degree AV block.

On day 3 spirometry was obtained and noted. The monitor showed only sinus rhythm with first-degree AV block. Temperature maximally that day was 101.4. She seemed to be improving. She had moderate COPD. She is still somewhat febrile from her Staphylococcus sepsis from the IV line.

On day 4 the Staphylococcus aureus was identified in the blood cultures. The patient was weak, but gradually getting stronger. Her insulin was switched over to Novolin 70-30. She was increased in cardiac rehab. Heparin was continued. The patient was kept in the hospital at this point for several days to allow for strengthening and for her antibiotic treatment for her Staphylococcal line sepsis. On day 3 the patient had left heart catheterization. This showed a left ventricular end diastolic pressure of 15. Ejection fraction of the left ventricle was 75%. There was no mitral regurgitation. There was hypokinesia of the inferior wall. Coronary arteries showed total occlusion of the dominant right coronary artery with relatively faint retrograde filling. There is 50% stenosis of the midportion of the nondominant circumflex. The patient tolerated the procedure well. She was doing well at this time. She was discharged the following morning on the following medications: Aspirin enteric 5 grains daily, Lopid 600 mg b.i.d., Novolin 70–30 48 units q.a.m. and 18 units q. p.m., Velosef 250 mg q.i.d. for one week, Lasix 60 mg daily, Slow Mag one tablet b.i.d. Follow up with Dr.

Follow up with me in a week or two. SMAC and magnesium level in 3 or 4 days.

CONDITION AT DISCHARGE: Satisfactory.

DISCHARGE DIAGNO SES:
1. Large inferior wall myocardial infarction and right ventricular myocardial infarction with multiple complications.
2. Significant hypotension.
3. Significant heart block.
4. Severe hyoglycemia requiring IV insulin.
5. Hemoccult positive emesis with no overt GI bleeding.
6. Elevated liver function tests of uncertain etiology, persistent to the end of the hospitalization.
7. Anemia progressive over the hospitalization.
8. Staphylococcal aureus sepsis due to a Swan Ganz catheter.

continued

HISTORY & PHYSICAL

ADMISSION DATE: 3/9/xx

HISTORY OF PRESENT ILLNESS: The patient is a 57-year-old white female receiving primary care from Dr. Johnson who is being cared for over the past few hours by Dr. Smith who is on call for Dr. Johnson for acute MI, who is admitted now via ambulance from his office to the East Valley Hospital with acute inferior MI with multiple complications.

The patient has no prior coronary artery disease. She had first onset of chest pain yesterday at 9:30 p.m. which was fairly severe. She had an episode of syncope in the bathroom. She finally came to the emergency room about 12:30 p.m. last night with chest pain. The pain was relieved about 12:30 a.m. following nitroglycerin and morphine. At that point in time, Dr. Smith called me at home, and we visited for the next 2 hours continuously on the phone. At that time it appeared that she had stabilized enough and he accompanied her in transport here.

The patient at 12:30 was having significant heart block with bradycardia in the 30's and hypotension with blood pressure in the 60's. She was also having some ventricular ectopy and quite a bit of nausea. She was on Isuprel. She was pain free at the time, but continued to have ongoing pain off and on requiring morphine. She also continued to have nausea and had some PVC's.

With regard to her rhythm and blood pressure, the Isuprel was substituted for Dopamine beginning at 5 mcg/kg per minute, and then increased to 7.5 mcg/kg per minute. With this her blood pressure gradually rose. Her heart rate also rose into the 60's. Atropine 2 mg IV was given with no apparent benefit. She was in AV dissociation at that time. She had some ventricular ectopy about 45 minutes following the TPA (see below) and Lidocaine 50 mg intravenously was given at 1:47 a.m. Therefore her ventricular ectopy seemed to settle down quite a bit. She was discovered to be somewhat hypokalemic with a potassium of 3.5 and KCl 40 mEq intravenously was given over about 2 hours between 2 a.m. and 4 a.m. She was also found to be quite hyperglycemic with an initial blood sugar of 557. 15 units of sub Q Insulin was given at 1:25 a.m.

The patient continued to have chest pain off and on requiring morphine. Because of this and her other severe complications, TPA was administered beginning at about 1 a.m. She received a 15 mg bolus followed by 50 mg over the first 30 minutes followed by 35 mg over the next hour. About 45 minutes after the initiation of the TPA, the patient's chest pain resolved and did not return. She was given 5000 units of intravenous heparin at 12:45 a.m. She was also given 1 aspirin about that same time. Because of her hypotension she was given about a total of 1300 cc's of normal saline intravenously. Finally, at about 2:30 a.m., the patient stabilized with regard to rhythm, blood pressure, etc. with a blood pressure of about 80 and heart rate of about 60 or 70 (but still in heart block). She was having no further chest pain and no ectopy. At that point she was transferred by ambulance to here. At the present time of admission she is having no chest pain.

The patient gives history herself. Her medications at home are insulin NPH 35 units daily, Tylenol prn. She has no allergies. She takes no other medication.

She has no exertional dyspnea, orthopnea, PND, etc. She does have quite a bit of cough which she describes as a smoker's hack. She has no asthma. She was diagnosed 10 years ago as having diabetes, and has been on Insulin since that time. She smokes fairly heavily since age 21. She says that she smokes about 2 packs a day but she only completes about 1 pack worth of cigarettes a day and the other cigarettes she doesn't completely smoke. She has a history of hyperlipidemia. She says her blood pressure is usually low and runs in the 90's. Her mother had an MI at 71' and her brother had a bypass at 61. Patient's surgeries include cholecystectomy, herniorrhaphy, tonsillectomy, two D&C's, four C-sections and a tubal ligation. She has quite a bit of indigestion but no frank peptic ulcer disease or hiatal hernia. She drinks occasional coffee but no alcohol. Otherwise her general review of systems is unremarkable.

Review Case 5-9, *continued*

HISTORY & PHYSICAL—PAGE 2

PHYSICAL EXAMINATION:

BP: Ranging between 70 and 120 systolic. HEART RATE: About 60 with AV block.

SKIN: Warm and dry. The patient is sleeping. Her color is pink. Jugular venous pressure is elevated to approximately 14 cm. above the right atrium. LUNGS: Clear.

HEART: There are no murmurs, gallops or rubs.

ABDOMEN: Soft and non-tender. There is no peripheral edema. The patient is somewhat obese.

ELECTROCARDIOGRAM: Admission ECG shows incomplete right bundle branch block with junctional rate of 35 and ST elevation in 2, 3 and AVF consistent with a typical acute inferior MI. Subsequent EKG's show ST elevation still persistent in 2, 3 and AVF and also in VI. ST depression is seen more so in 1, L and V2. She has intermittent left bundle branch block. PVC's are seen. She is in sinus tachycardia vs. supraventricular tachycardia at rate 140 with 2:1 AV block.

LABORATORY DATA: The following laboratory data was obtained on admission except as noted. Sodium 140, Potassium 3.5, Glucose 557, BUN 18, Creatinine 1.2. Repeat Glucose here is 684. Repeat Potassium here is 6.3. Total Cholesterol 317, Triglycerides 1090, CK on admission to the emergency room 79. CK on admission here is 258. Hemoglobin 16.9, white count 11,700, MCV 85. Pro Time 12.4, PTT 27 (on admission). Urinalysis shows some protein. There is quite a bit of glucose with 1-2 white cells and 1-2 red cells.

CONCLUSIONS:

1. Complicated inferior MI. This is acute. It is felt that there is a right ventricular infarction complicating this. The complications are as noted below.

2. Hypotension.

3. Heart block.

Other concurrent factors are as follows:

4. Severe hyperglycemia.

5. Insulin-dependent diabetes mellitus.

6. Severe hyperlipidemia of both cholesterol and triglycerides.

7. Family history of heart disease.

8. Ongoing heavy tobacco use.

9. Significant dyspepsia.

10. Stated history of "usually low blood pressure."

PLAN: Admit for careful observation and treatment as needed.

continued

CARDIAC CATHETERIZATION LABORATORY

PROCEDURE REPORT:

PATIENT: Christine Collins

Study Date: 3/15/xx

Medical Record: 00-05-12

Referring Physician: Dr. Smith and Dr. Johnson

PROCEDURE: Left heart catheterization, selective coronary angiography, and left ventriculography.

PROCEDURE NOTE:

The patient is brought to the heart catheterization lab, and the right inguinal area is sterilely prepped and draped in the usual manner. Using the Seldinger technique, the right femoral artery is sterilely cannulated, and the 7Fr sheath introducer is positioned in the right femoral artery. Using a guidewire and fluoroscopy and high osmolar contrast, a pigtail catheter is positioned in the ascending aorta, and then in the left ventricle. Pressure measurements are made. Left ventriculography is performed in the RAO projection and is recorded on 35-mm film.

The catheter is exchanged over a guidewire for a Judkin's left coronary catheter, and left coronary cineangiography is performed in the usual manner in multiple projections. The catheter is then exchanged over a guidewire for a Judkin's right coronary catheter, and right coronary cineangiography is performed in the usual manner.

At the beginning of the case the patient arrived in the cath lab on an IV heparin drip. At the conclusion of the case heparin was discontinued and the catheters were removed. Hemostasis was obtained. The patient tolerated the procedure well with no complications.

HEMODYNAMIC DATA:

Left ventricular end diastolic pressure is normal at 15mm of mercury.

LEFT VENTRICULOGRAM:

There is no mitral regurgitation. Ejection fraction is 75%. The size of the left ventricle is normal. There is hypokinesia of the posterobasilar wall and the diaphragmatic wall. The anterior walls and apex are normal. There is definite viability of the inferior wall.

CORONARY ANGIOGRAPHY:

The LAD gives rise to two diagonal branches and a septal perforator. These are unremarkable. The circumflex gives rise to a marginal branch and a couple of posterolateral branches. The proximal to mid-circumflex has a 50% stenosis (before the takeoff of the marginal branch). Otherwise the circumflex and its branches are unremarkable.

The right coronary artery is a dominant vessel giving rise to the posterior descending artery and 2-3 right ventricular branches. The right coronary artery is totally occluded just beyond its origin. There is faint retrograde filling of the right ventricular branches via collaterals from the right coronary artery as well as some from the left coronary artery. There is moderate filling of the posterior descending artery in a retrograde manner via collaterals from the left coronary artery.

CONCLUSIONS:

1. Occluded dominant right coronary artery with limited retrograde collateral filling.

2. Moderate stenosis of the nondominant circumflex proximally.

3. Inferior hypokinesia.

Review Case 5-9, *continued*

CARDIAC PROFILE

PATIENT	:	Christine Collins	SEX	: F
ROOM #	:	306	AGE-YEARS :	57
MEDICAL RECORD :		00-05-12	PHYSICIAN :	Dr. Wright

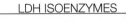

CPK ISOENZYMES   LDH ISOENZYMES

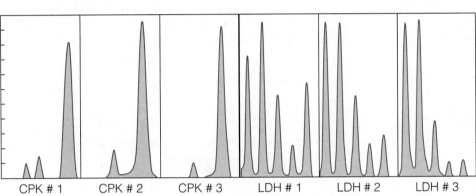

CPK # 1   CPK # 2   CPK # 3   LDH # 1   LDH # 2   LDH # 3

	CPK #1		CPK # 2		CPK # 3			LDH#1		LDH # 2		LDHt # 3	
DATE DRAWN: 3/11/xx			DATE: 3/12/xx		DATE: 3/13/xx			DATE: 3/11/xx		DATE: 3/12/xx		DATE: 3/13/xx		
TIME DRAWN: 0450			TIMEs 1650		TIME: 0600			TIME: 0450		TIME: 1650		TIME: 0600		
Frac	%	IU/L	%	IU/L	%	IU/L	Frac	%	IU/L	%	IU/L	%	IU/L
BB	4.9	12.7	0.0	0.0	0.0	0.0	LD1	23.6	42.2	32.8	139.6	38.4	191.4
MB	9.0	23.1	11.4	176.6	6.5	93.1	LD2	32.3	57.8	34.6	147.5	41.4	206.5
MM	86.1	222.2	88.6	1369.4	93.5	1344.9	LD3	18.8	33.7	17.7	75.3	13.8	68.7
							LD4	6.3	11.3	6.5	27.7	3.0	14.8
							LD5	19.0	34.0	8.4	35.9	3.5	17.6
TOTALS 258.0			1546.0		1438.0		Totals	179.0		426.0		499.0	
							LDH 1:2 RATIO 0.7			1.0		0.9	

REFERENCE RANGES (IU/L)

TOTAL CPK 21.0-232.0	BB	MB	MM 21.0-232.0
TOTAL LDH 100.0-190.0	LD1 11.0-52.0	LD2 23.0-70.0	LD3 18.0-57.0 LD4 5.0-29.0 LD5 4.0-31.0

CARDIAC PROFILE COMMENTS:

continued

Review Case 5-9, *continued*

MISC. URINES				CARDIAC PANEL		OTHER TEST REQUESTS:	
☐ 24 HR URINE (SPECIFY)		AMIKACIN, VALLEY					
		AMIKACIN, PEAK		DATE	TIME	CPK (21–215)	LDH
		DIGOXIN					(100–190)
		DILANTIN					
URINE OSMOLALITY		GENTAMYCIN, VALLEY	1	3/11/xx	0450	258	179
Na & K, RANDOM		GENTAMYCIN, PEAK	2	3/12/xx	1650	1546	426
CREATININE CLEARANCE		LIDOCAINE	3	3/13/xx	Cath LABS	1438	499
2 HR. AMYLASE		PHENOBARBITOL					
DRUG LEVELS		PROCAINAMIDE C NAPA				**MISCELLANEOUS LABORATORY**	
ACETOMINOPHEN		QUINIDINE					
SALICYLATE		TEGRETOL					
LITHIUM		THEOPHYLUNE					
		TOBRAMYCIN, VALLEY					
		TOBRAMYCIN, PEAK					

LABORATORY REPORTS

Review Case 5-9, *continued*

X	ONE CHECK FOR EACH TEST ORDERED	X	SPECIMEN
X	CULTURE		BLOOD CULT
	SMEAR (GRAM STAIN)		CSF
	AFB CULT		ABSCESS (WD)
	AFB SMEAR		THROAT
	THROAT B STEP ONLY		SPUTUM
	GC CULTURE		BRONCH OR TRACH ASP
	ANAEROBIC CULTURE		STOOL
	FUNGUS/YEAST		RECTAL SWAB
	CAMPY		URINE ☐ CATH
	INDIA INK PREP		☐ CLEAN CATCH

☐ MISC. CULTURE   SOURCE:

MICROBIOLOGY REPORT   *Swan Ganz Catheter Tip*

1-Many Coag PO2 Staph
2 Beta Hemolytic Strep Group B (Streptococcus agalactiae)

X	ONE CHECK FOR EACH TEST ORDERED	X	SPECIMEN
X	CULTURE		BLOOD CULT
	SMEAR (GRAM STAIN)		CSF
	AFB CULT		ABSCESS (WD)
	AFB SMEAR		THROAT
	THROAT B STEP ONLY		SPUTUM
	GC CULTURE		BRONCH OR TRACH ASP
	ANAEROBIC CULTURE		STOOL
	FUNGUS/YEAST		RECTAL SWAB
	CAMPY		URINE ☐ CATH
	INDIA INK PREP		☐ CLEAN CATCH

☐ MISC. CULTURE   SOURCE:

MICROBIOLOGY REPORT   *Swan Ganz Catheter Tip*

Many Coag PO2 Staph

LABORATORY REPORTS

continued

Review Case 5-9, *continued*

MICROBIOLOGY REPORT

-- Antimicrobial Susceptibility and Organism Identification Reoort --------------------------   II FINAL II

Patient Name: Christine Collins   Physician: Swan Ganz Catheter Tip   Medical Record: 00-05-12   Collected: 3/11/xx
Specimen: 4   Source: BLOOD   Room: 306   Received: 3/11/xx

Iso/Result: 01   Staphylococcus aureus
                     BOTH BOTTLES HAVE COAGULASE POSITIVE STAPH.

ANTIMICROBIC/DOSE	MIC	BLOOD	URINE	CC
AMIKACIN	<=16	S		
IM/IV 7.5 mg/Kg Q12h				
AMOX/K CLAV'ATE	<=4/2	S		
PO 1-2 tablets Q8h				
AMP/SULBACTAM	<=8/4	S		
IV I/.5-2/1 mg Q6h				
AMPICILLIN	>8	BLac		
PO 250-500 mg Q6h				
IV 1.0-2.0 mg Q4h				
CEFAZOLIN	<=2	S		
IH 0.5-1.0 gm Q8h				
IV T.0-2.0 mg Q8h				
CEPHALOTHIN	<=2	S		
PO 250-500 mg Q4h				
IV 0.5-2.0 mg 4-6h				
CHLORAMPHENICOL	<=4	S		
PO 0.5-1.0 mg Q6h				
IV 0.5^1.0 mg Q6h				
CIPROFLOXACIN	<=1	S		
PO 250-750 mg Q12h				
CLINDAMYCIN	<=0.25	S		
PO 150-300 mg Q6h				
IV 600-900 kg Q8h				
ERYTHROMYCIN	Q.5	S		
PO 250-500 kg Q6h				
GENTAMCIN	<=1	S		
IH/IV 1.0-1.7 mg/Kg Q8h				
IMIPENEM	<=1	S		
IV 0.5-1.0 mg Q6-8h				
NITROFURANTOIN	<=32			
PO 50-100 tg Q6b				
NORFLOXACIN	<=4			
PO 400 ad Q12h				
OXACILLIN	<=0.5	S5		
IV O.5-2.0 gm Q4h				
PENICILLIN	>8	BLac		
PO 250-500 mg Q6h				
TH 0.9-1.2 MILD Q6-12H				
iv i.d-3.0 NIL U				
RIFAMPIN	<=1	S		
PO 300 mg Q12h				
SULFAMETHOXAZOLE	>256			
PO 4.0'gs STAT, then				
1.0 gm 8l2h				
TETRACYCLINE	<=2	S		
PO 250-500 kg Q6h				
TLCAR/K CLAV'ATE(a)	<=1	S		
IV 2.0-3.0 gm Q4-6h				
TRIMETH/SULFA	<=2/38	S		
PO 1-2 tablets Ol2h				
IV 3.3-6.6 kg/Ko Tip Q8h				
VANCOMYC1N	<=2	S		
IV I.0 mg Q12h				

††† or S = Susceptible   R = Resistant   N/R = Not Reported   BLac = Beta Lactamase Positive
†† or NS = Moderately Susceptible   I = Intermediate   CC = Cost Code   TFG = Thymidine-dependenl Strain
† = Slightly Susceptible   MIC = mcg/mL (mg/L)   Blank = Data not available, or drug not advisable or tested
(a) Use maximum doses of drug with an aminoglycoside for P. aeruginosa in patients with granulocytopenia or serious infections.
(b) Breakpoints based on parenteral dose. For cefuroxime PO use <8=S, >4=R or urinary enteric isolates 8=S, 8-16=MS, >16=R.

†   Interpretations based on approx. adult attainable blood/urine levels, except drugs with <3 dilutions, which print
     NCCLS. Doses are guidelines; consider weight and renal/hepatic function. Urine interpretation for lower DTI only.
†† Interpretations based on NCCLS N7-A2.   Ticar/K Clav'ate for gram positives based on manufacturer's breakpoints:

Review Case 5-9, *continued*

X	ONE CHECK FOR EACH TEST ORDERED	X	SPECIMEN
	CULTURE	X	BLOOD CULT
	SMEAR (GRAM STAIN)		CSF
	AFB CULT		ABSCESS (WD)
	AFB SMEAR		THROAT
	THROAT B STEP ONLY		SPUTUM
	GC CULTURE		BRONCH OR TRACH ASP
	ANAEROBIC CULTURE		STOOL
	FUNGUS/YEAST		RECTAL SWAB
	CAMPY		URINE ☐ CATH
	INDIA INK PREP		☐ CLEAN CATCH

☐ MISC. CULTURE   SOURCE:

MICROBIOLOGY REPORT

Both bottles have coagulose positive staphylococcus
M&Cs to follow

LABORATORY REPORTS

continued

RADIOLOGY REPORTS

EXAM:

Port.Chest

HISTORY: Recent myocardial infarction.

PORTABLE CHEST:

The heart size is at the upper limits of normal. The lungs are clear. Swan-Ganz catheter is present. Compared to yesterday's film, the end of the catheter has changed positions from the right lower lobe branch to the right upper lobe branch. No other change is seen.

HISTORY: Respiratory distress.

PORTABLE CHEST:

Comparison is made with a previous portable chest earlier today for Swan-Ganz placement. The chest is a little bit different in technique. The Swan-Ganz catheter is unchanged. There seems to be a little bit more density projected over the clavicles but the chest is projected a bit more lordotic and I really can't see any definite fluid over the lung apices. Lung fields are free of infiltrates. Heart size remains normal. Pulmonary flow pattern is probably within the normal range for a portable supine film.

IMPRESSION:

HISTORY: Swan placement.

PORTABLE CHEST:

Portable AP supine view of the chest demonstrates a Swan-Ganz catheter directed out the right pulmonary outflow tract towards the right middle and lower lobe pulmonary artery. Heart size is normal. Pulmonary flow pattern is within the normal range. No pulmonary consolidation is present.

IMPRESSION:

Normal portable chest. Swan-Ganz catheter in place.

Review Case 5-9, *continued*

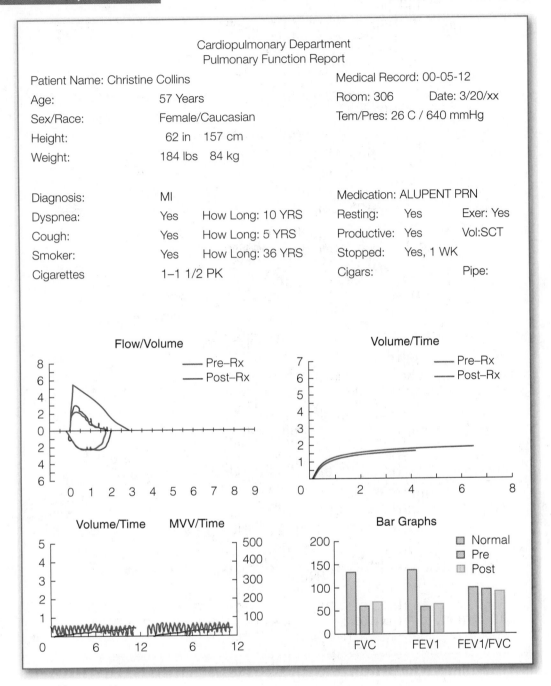

Cardiopulmonary Department
Pulmonary Function Report

Patient Name: Christine Collins   Medical Record: 00-05-12

Age: 57 Years   Room: 306   Date: 3/20/xx

Sex/Race: Female/Caucasian   Tem/Pres: 26 C / 640 mmHg

Height: 62 in   157 cm

Weight: 184 lbs   84 kg

Diagnosis: MI   Medication: ALUPENT PRN

Dyspnea: Yes   How Long: 10 YRS   Resting: Yes   Exer: Yes

Cough: Yes   How Long: 5 YRS   Productive: Yes   Vol:SCT

Smoker: Yes   How Long: 36 YRS   Stopped: Yes, 1 WK

Cigarettes   1–1 1/2 PK   Cigars: Pipe:

continued

Review Case 5-9, *continued*

Cardiopulmonary Department
Pulmonary Function Report

MI, SOB

Patient Name:	Christine Collins	Medical Record: 00-05-12	
Age:	57 Years	Room: 306	Date: 3/20/xx
Sex/Race:	Female/Caucasian	Temp/Pres: 26 C / 640 mmHg	
Height:	62 in 157 cm		
Weight:	184 lbs 84 kg		
Diagnosis:	MI	Medication: ALUPENT PRN	
Dyspnea:	Yes How Long: 10 YRS	Resting: Yes	Exer: Yes
Cough:	Yes How Long: 5 YRS	Productive: Yes	Vol:SCT
Smoker:	Yes How Long: 36 YRS	Stopped: Yes, 1 WK	
Cigarettes:	1–1 1/2 PK	Cigars:	Pipe:

		PRED	BEST	%PRED	BEST	%PRED	%CHG
			PRE–RX		POST–RX		
SPIROMETRY (BTPS)							
FVC	Liters	2.91	1.77 #	61*	2.00	69*	13
FEV1	Liters	2.16	1.28 #	59*	1.38	64*	8
FEV1/FVC	%	74	72	97	69	93	−4
FEV3	Liters		1.69		1.78		5
FEV3/FVC	%	97	95	98	89	92	−6
FEF25–75%	L/Sec	2.56	0.94 #	37*	0.90 #	35*	−4
FEF75–85%	L/Sec	0.67	0.29	43*	0.22	33*	−24
PEF	L/Sec	5.55	2.33 #	42*	3.16	57*	36
FIVC	Liters	2.91	1.93	66*	2.09	72*	8
FIF	L/Sec		2.36		2.24		−5
E Code			00000		11010		
MVV	L/Min	94	48 #	51*	52 #	55*	8
f _ _ _ _	1/Min		105		100		−5

- OUTSIDE 95% CONFIDENCE INTERVAL   * = OUTSIDE   NORMAL RANGE
CALIBRATION: PRED: 3.00   ACTUAL: EXP 2.96   INSP 3.02
IPS–0L10–01   IPS–0H10–01   N–1804-3

Review Case 5-9, *continued*

Cardiopulmonary Department
Pulmonary Function Report

MI, SOB

Patient Name:	Christine Collins		
Age:	57 Years		
Sex/Race:	Female/	Medical Record: 00-05-12	
Height:	62 in 157 cm	Room: 306	
Weight:	184 lbs 84 kg	Date: 3/20/xx	
Diagnosis:	MI	Medication: ALUPENT PRN	
Dyspnea:	Yes How Long: 10 YRS	Resting: Yes	Exer: Yes
Cough:	Yes How Long: 5 YRS	Productive: Yes	Vol:SCT
Smoker:	Yes How Long: 36 YRS	Stopped: Yes, 1 WK	
Cigarettes	1–1 1/2 PK	Cigars:	Pipe:

			PRE–RX		POST–RX		
		PRED	BEST	%PRED	BEST	%PRED	%CHG
SPIROMETRY (BTPS)							
FVC	Liters	2.91	1.77 #	61*	2.00	69*	13
FEV1	Liters	2.16	1.28 #	59*	1.38	64*	8
FEV1/FVC	%	74	72	97	69	93	−4
FEV3	Liters		1.69		1.78		5
FEV3/FVC	%	97	95	98	89	92	−6
FEF25–75%	L/Sec	2.56	0.94 #	37*	0.90 #	35*	−4
FEF75–85%	L/Sec	0.67	0.29	43*	0.22	33*	−24
PEF	L/Sec	5.55	2.33 #	42*	3.16	57*	36
FIVC	Liters	2.91	1.93	66*	2.09	72*	8
PIF	L/Sec		2.36		2.24		−5
E Code			00000		11010		
MVV	L/Min	94	48 #	51*	52 #	55*	8
f _ _ _ _	1/Min		105		100		−5

- OUTSIDE   95%   CONFIDENCE INTERVAL   * = OUTSIDE   NORMAL RANGE
CALIBRATION: PRED: 3.00   ACTUAL: EXP 2.96   INSP 3.02
IPS–0L10–01   IPS–0H10–01   N–1804–3

INTERPRETATION:

Moderate decrease in FVC which may be partly related to air trapping.

Mild deccrease in FEV1/FVC ratio; obstruction is difficult to quantitate in presence of decreased FVC.

No significant change after single bronchodilator challenge.

Recommend lung volumes, DLCO if there is suspicion of combined restrictive and obstructive components.

continued

Review Case 5-9, *continued*

ICD-9-CM/ICD-10-CM diagnosis code(s): _____

ICD-9-CM procedure and ICD-10-PCS procedure code(s): _____

MS-DRG: _____

Review Case 5-10

Health Record Face Sheet

Western Regional
Medical Center

Record Number:	00-06-12
Age:	78
Gender:	Female
Length of Stay:	5 Days
Diagnosis/Procedure:	Incontinence Marshall-Marchetti-Krantz Procedure
Service Type:	Inpatient
Discharge Status:	To Home

Review Case 5-10, *continued*

DISCHARGE SUMMARY

DATE OF ADMISSION: 8/11/xx
DATE OF DISCHARGE: 8/16/xx

Carla is well known to me and was admitted with a diagnosis of incontinence of the stress urge compound variety. We felt that if we could control the stress incontinence we may make some progress with the urge as we followed her for years and have tried to treat her and have been unsuccessful. She eventually wanted this done without any toleration of anything else. We have been over it with many discussions. She saw Dr. Wright for a 2nd opinion. He was also aware that she had severe urge incontinence but agreed that maybe some attempt to correct her stress might make the patient manageable.

Laboratory data shows a BUN of 24, albumin of 3.9, cholesterol of 340, triglyceride 227, otherwise normal. White blood count was 8,200 with a hematocrit of 39.6. Dr. Urey saw her preoperatively. She was admitted, evaluated, and taken to the operating room where a Marshall-Marchetti-Krantz procedure was carried out. Also, there was some question on this patient as to being admitted the night before, I had suggested to her she come in as an out-patient in the morning. The patient refused and said she wanted to come in the day before. We contacted her insurance company at that point in time and indicated to them that the patient was coming in the night before. They indicated to me that they would not pay for the night before. I told them to call the patient and to point out to her that they would not pay for a pre night before visit. Even with that in mind, she felt that she wanted to come into the hospital the night before. When she arrived at the hospital apparently there was some confu-sion because the people here who evaluate that were not aware of the fact that she wanted to come the night before on her own and that was not my suggestion but the patient's. At any rate, the operation went well. She tolerated the procedure well. I plan on keeping her in the hospital 5 days. That is exactly what happened. At the end of that time I removed her catheter. She voided well with residual of only 20cc.

She was discharged home on Septra. I have seen her in the office. She is doing well.

FINAL DIAGNOSIS: Incontinence.

PROCEDURE CARRIED OUT: Marshall-Marchetti-Krantz procedure.

CONSULTATIONS: Dr. Urey

continued

Review Case 5-10, *continued*

HISTORY & PHYSICAL

ADMISSION DATE:

Carla came to see me when she was 68 years old and was discovered to have a kidney just full of stones on the left side. We followed her for a long time and eventually removed the kidney. This stopped her flank pain, fever, chills, infections, etc., and she's done very well since that time. The other problem that she began having was a leakage problem. Approximately six months ago, she began to complain of urgency and cultures were negative. It was obvious it was not infection doing it and I made the diagnosis of urge incontinence. She was treated with Ditropan. She took it; it didn't really help her much, it made her dizzy, she stopped it. We tried Valium on Monday to see if that would relax her bladder. I then went to Levsinex on Friday. The frequency persisted, urine was clear. Tried Macrodantin. I cystoscoped her again. Her residual urine was 60 cc's, capacity 250. The bladder lining looked okay. There was no evidence of descensus. There was a small type vagina. Urethra was okay. There was no evidence of interstitial cystitis. I again made the diagnosis uninhibited neurogenic bladder and tried Ditropan again. I felt no DMSO was indicated. I suggested double triple voiding. We tried Ditropan Syrup instead of tablets.

She came back the following Tuesday complaining of wetting her pants, again with urge incontinence. I tried the Ditropan Syrup again. For one week we tried a little Macrodantin but this did no better. We continued the Ditropan. She did not return until one year later with nocturia 3-5 times to the bathroom. Residual urine 15 cc's, capacity 350. The leak was not so bad except with very weak cough and slight pressure. She was wearing diapers and pads and at that point in time I finally made the decision that even though her incontinence was mostly urge incontinence, I thought maybe we should try a Stamey procedure to see if it would tighten up her bladder to some extent. I knew that would not correct her urge incontinence but with some help with the stress incontinence, she may do somewhat better. She leaked when she sneezed and yet she describes an urge incontinence.

At that point in time I made a decision to do an operation. She went to Dr. Wright for second opinion. He saw her and also noted that the patient had severe urge incontinence. He agreed, however, that we had tried numerous treatments and thought maybe if we could correct her stress incontinence, it might help. She discussed this with a brother-in-law who was also a physician at that point in time. He felt it was an urge incontinence and we ought to continue to try medications. She did not return until last week again with nocturia 4-5 times. Wears diapers all the time. Has urge incontinence but also has leakage with coughing and sneezing.

She is allergic to Penicillin. She is on Septra-DS 1 po twice a day, Levsinex time capsules were tried. She got the hives secondary to the Sulfa. I gave her some Noroxin. Levsinex and Ditropan did not help her. Again, I considered the possibility of doing a Stamey elevation of her bladder. Recently refilled her Levsinex. I started talking to her about catheterizing herself prior to bedtime. I sent a nurse out to teach her intermittent catheterization to cath herself before she went to bed to see if that would help. She tried that, was unable to do so. She just totally does not want that done.

She came in on Monday nocturia voids 12:00, 4:30, 5:30, 7:30; daytime manages fairly well, but she wants something to stop her leakage. We rediscussed and I pointed out to her that I could only stop the stress incontinence not the urge incontinence. She is aware of that. She has asked for a Marshall-Marchetti procedure. She has discussed this with her family and that's what she wants.

Her medications at this point in time include: Thyroid, eye drops, Persantine. Her physician is Dr. Jackson. I tried to call him and to see her. Dr. Wright has evaluated her and feels that she would tolerate the surgery. I've called Dr. Urey. He is aware. He has agreed to write a second opinion. He again talked to me about the fact that this is urge incontinence. I do understand that but I still think that if I can tighten her bladder, I might be able to help with some of leakage and that may be enough to get us by with the use of Ditropan or Levsinex later on.

Review Case 5-10, *continued*

HISTORY & PHYSICAL—PAGE 2

This has been arranged and she's coming in tonight for surgery in the morning. This was discussed with her insurance company. They wanted her to come in as an outpatient. That was fine with me; I thought that would be okay. The patient insisted on coming in the night before and as I understand, apparently that's what she's doing just by what the insurance company has suggested to her.

PAST MEDICAL HISTORY, SOCIAL HISTORY, PSYCHIATRIC HISTORY: Otherwise unremarkable.

REVIEW OF SYSTEMS: Otherwise normal.

PHYSICAL EXAMINATION: She's an elderly female who is about 78 years old. Numerous skin changes. Aging changes.

HEAD: Normocephalic.
EARS: TM's normal; hears well in left and right.

EYES: Pupils equal, round and react to light and accommodation. Extraocular movement normal.
NOSE, MOUTH & THROAT: Normal.
NECK: Supple.
CHEST: Clear to auscultation.
COR: Regular sinus rhythm; no murmurs.
ABDOMEN: Soft without masses, organomegaly, tenderness or bruits.
BACK & EXTREMITIES: Normal.
NEUROLOGICAL: Normal.

FINAL IMPRESSION: Incontinence, probably about 60% urge incontinence, 40% stress incontinence. We're going to try a Marshall-Marchetti to see if we can help her. I recognize the dangers of doing this. This has been explained, but we're going to try it.

cc: office

continued

Review Case 5-10, *continued*

OPERATIVE NOTE

DATE OF PROCEDURE: 8/14/xx

PREOPERATIVE DIAGNOSIS: Urinary Incontinence
POSTOPERATIVE DIAGNOSIS: Urinary Incontinence

PROCEDURE CARRIED OUT: Marshall-Marchetti-Krantz Repair

PROCEDURE COMPLICATIONS: None.

ANESTHESIA: General.

PROCEDURE: Patient was placed supine on the operating table, given a general anesthetic. I then made a midline incision through the skin and subcutaneous tissues down to the rectus muscle just above the pubis. The rectus muscles were split. The space of Retzius was entered. The anterior aspect of the bladder was dissected off. The fat was cut and pushed to the side. I then placed a double row of 0 chromic sutures, figure-of-eight on each side of the urethra to the vagina. These were kept in order, changed, and then eventually attached to the pubis. They were then pulled up and tied to the pubis. When we finished, we had a good elevation of the urethra and bladder up to the pubis. Two other sutures were taken to hold the bladder up against the rectus muscle.

When this was completed, I removed two sponges that we had used. Counts were correct, and we did a closure. Closure was carried out using interrupted 2-0 PGA's to close the rectus muscles, then closing inter- rectus fascia. These were interrupted simple sutures. I then used a running 3-0 chromic suture and an 832 needle to close the subcutaneous tissue. 3-0 PGA was used subcuticularly. Steri-Strips were applied. I gave her about 30 cc's of 1% Xylocaine into the subcutaneous area at the end of the procedure.

She tolerated the procedure well and was returned to the recovery room. She did have some hypertension at the time she entered the recovery room and is getting some Apresoline at this point in time.

cc: office

Review Case 5-10, *continued*

HEMATOLOGY REPORT

HEMATOLOGY I

☒ CBC   ☐ CBC $^{WITH}_{OUT}$ DIFF
☐ RETIC   ☐ WINTROBE ESR
             ☐ WESTERGREN ESR

0 8 • 2	WBC × 10³ 4.5-11.0	
4 • 2 7	RBC × 10⁶/µ M 4.6-6.2 F 4.2-5.4	
1 2 • 9	Hgb g/dl M 13.5-18.0 F 12.0-16.0	
3 9 • 6	Hct % M 40-54 F 38-47	
0 9 3 •	MCV µ³ 80-96	
3 0 • 2	MCH pg 27-31	
3 2 • 6	MCHC % 32-36	
2 3 9 •	PLATELETS 10²/µl 150-400	

DIFFERENTIAL		RBC MORPHOLOGY	
SEGS	75	NORMAL	✗
BANDS	2	ROULEAUX	
LYMPHS	17	ANISOCYTOSIS	
		MICROCYTOSIS	
MONO	5	MACROCYTOSIS	
EOS	0	HYPOCHROMIA	
BASOS	1	POLYCHROMASIA	
		POIKILOCYTOSIS	
METAS		ELLIPTOCYTES	
MYELOS		DACRYOCYTES	
ATYP LYMPHS		CODOCYTES	
		ACANTHOCYTES	
DOHLE BODIES		ECHINOCYTES	
ABS GRANULO		BASO STIPPLING	
		NRBC/100 WBC	
ABS LYMPH.	1.4 (1.0-4.8)		

☐ SMEAR REFERRED TO PATHOLOGIST

___ mm/hr	WINTROBE SED RATE	(M 0-9) (F 0-20)
___ mm/hr	WESTERGREN SED RATE	$\left(<50\ YRS\ {M\ 0\text{-}15 \atop F\ 0\text{-}20}\right)\left(>50\ YRS\ {M\ 0\text{-}20 \atop F\ 0\text{-}30}\right)$
___ %	RETIC-CORRECTED	(0.5-1.5%)
___ %	RETIC-UNCORRECTED	(0.5-1.5%)

TEST	WBC	RBC	Hgb	Hct	MCV	MCH	MCHC
MALES	7.8±3×10³	5.4±0.8×10⁶	16± 2 gm	47± 5%	87± 7µ³	29± 2µµg	34± 2%
FEMALES	7.8±3×10³	4.8±0.8×10⁶	14± 2 gm	42± 5%	90± 9µ³	29± 2µµg	34± 2%

continued

Review Case 5-10, *continued*

ICD-9-CM/ICD-10-CM diagnosis code(s): _____

ICD-9-CM procedure and ICD-10-PCS procedure code(s): _____

MS-DRG: _____

Review Case 5-11

Health Record Face Sheet

Western Regional
Medical Center

Record Number:	00-07-12
Age:	39
Gender:	Female
Length of Stay:	2 Days
Service Type:	Inpatient
Discharge Status:	To Home
Diagnosis/Procedure:	Term Delivery Post Partum Tubal

DISCHARGE SUMMARY

PATIENT: Denise Drummond

ADMIT DATE: 10/11/xx
DISCH DATE: 10/13/xx

PHYSICIAN:

ADMITTING COMPLAINT: Ruptured membranes. Term pregnancy, sterilization desired

LABORATORY WORK: CBC showed 11,300 white count with 78 segs, 3 bands,
                      14 lymph, 4 mono, 1 eosin.

HOSPITAL COURSE: The patient didn't have much in terms of contractions after the
membranes were ruptured. Augmentation of labor was then carried out with the patient making slow but steady progress to 5 cm. and then more rapid progress was made. She delivered
spontaneously a male infant weighing 6 pounds 8 ounces. Postpartum as per the patient's
request she was taken to surgery where tubal ligation was carried out. She did require catheterization after being unable to void. Before discharge was voiding satisfactorily. She was
discharged to home, to use Motrin for pain and to return to clinic in one week for removal of
staples.

FINAL DIAGNOSIS: Normal vaginal delivery with single liveborn male infant and sterilization
postpartum.

DISCHARGE SUMMARY

continued

HISTORY AND PHYSICAL

PATIENT: Denise Drummond

ADMIT DATE: 10/11/xx

PHYSICIAN: Dr. Smith

CHIEF COMPLAINT: Ruptured membranes.

HISTORY OF PRESENT ILLNESS: The patient is a 39-year-old, almost 40-year-old gravida 8 para 6-0-1 who by menstrual history is due about the 11th of November. Ultrasound exam was carried out in July which showed a due date of about 22 November. Membranes ruptured spontaneously about midnight. The patient came to the hospital. Contractions have been irregular. The patient has progressed from about a 2 to 2.5 and maybe 50-60% effacement. Head remains very high, however. There has been good variability of fetal heart tones. There have been a couple decelerations but not severe. The pregnancy has been unremarkable. She did fail her glucose screen, however, the glucose tolerance was normal.

The patient and her husband desire no further pregnancies and request a tubal ligation following delivery. They understand the procedure should be considered permanent but that it may fail.

PAST HISTORY:
> CURRENT MEDICATIONS-She has been taking prenatal vitamins but no other medications.
> ALLERGIES-None known.
> SURGERIES-Patient in the past has had a tonsillectomy, carpal tunnel surgery on her right hand.
> MEDICAL ILLNESS-She has some hay fever.   Did have rheumatic fever at age 5.

SOCIAL HISTORY: The patient does not use tobacco or alcohol. She is a housewife.

FAMILY HISTORY: See prenatal records.

REVIEW OF SYSTEMS: Compatible with term pregnancy.

PHYSICAL EXAM:
GENERAL:
HEENT: Normal.
NECK:
CHEST: Lungs are clear.
HEART: Regular rhythm. The breasts are normal.
ABDOMEN: Gravid and appears to be close to term. Fetal heart tones are present. Vertex presentation.
EXTREMITIES: Normal. Deep tendon reflexes equal bilaterally.
GU: Pelvic exam reveals 2.5 cm. dilatation. Cervix is anterior but very high, -3 at least station and about 60% effaced. The pelvis was felt to be adequate on initial examination as it is now. Babies have ranged up to 8 pounds 5 ounces.

NEURO:

ADMISSION DIAGNOSIS:
1. Approximate 36 week gestation. Ruptured membranes. Sterilization desire. Note the patient does request an epidural anesthetic, if we are able to do this as we have planned to do the tubal ligation using the same anesthetic.

Review Case 5-11, *continued*

OPERATIVE REPORT

PATIENT: Denise Drummond

DATE: 10/12/xx

SURGEON: Dr. Smith
ASSIST: Dr. Johnson

PRE-OPERATIVE DIAGNOSIS: Sterilization desire. Recent delivery.
POSTOPERATIVE DIAGNOSIS: Same
OPERATION: Postpartum tubal ligation. Pomeroy type.
ESTIMATED BLOOD LOSS: Less than 3 cc

OPERATIVE REPORT: The patient was taken to the operating room with the epidural still in place which was used for labor. Additional medication was given until the patient was adequately numbed. Abdomen was prepped and the patient draped in the usual manner for infraumbilical incision. Bladder had been emptied previously in delivery. An infraumbilical incision was made through the thin skin. Subcutaneous tissue and anterior fascia and peritoneum. Each fallopian tube was identified in turn by its fimbriated end. Grasped in the mid portion with the Babcock clamp. A generous loop was ligated with 0-plain catgut. The ligated loop was cut away. There was good hemostasis. The peritoneum was closed with running 2-0 chrome. The fascia was closed with running 0-Vicryl. Subcutaneous tissue was approximated with interrupted 2-0 chrome and staples used in the skin. The patient tolerated the procedure well. Estimated blood loss less than 3 cc.

Review Case 5-11, *continued*

TISSUE REPORT

PATIENT: Denise Drummond
ADMIT DATE: 10/12/xx
SEX-AGE: F - 39
DOCTOR: Dr. Smith

HISTORY: None

Gross: The specimen consists of two segments of fallopian tube submitted in the same container. The right is marked with a black suture, the right is the longer, 3 cm in length. Each tube is about 5 mm in width with a smooth surface, firm wall and a pinpoint lumen. The right is marked with ink, and both are submitted in a single cassette. TM:9

MICROSCOPIC: DONE

DIAGNOSIS: **SEGMENTS, FALLOPIAN TUBES, NORMAL, RIGHT AND LEFT SIDES**

Review Case 5-11, *continued*

Health History
Summary   Date: 3/31/xx

Age : 39
Referring physician: Dr. Oles

Medical History

	Patient	Family
1. Congenital anomalies	☐	☐
2. Genetic diseases	☐	☐
3. Multiple births	☐	☒
4. Diabetes mellitus	☐	☒
5. Malignancies	☐	☒
6. Hypertension	☐	☐
7. Heart disease	☐	☒
8. Rheumatic fever	☒	
9. Pulmonary disease	☐	☐
10. GI problems	☐	
11. Renal disease	☐	☐
12. Genitourinary tract problems....	☐	
13. Abnormal uterine bleeding	☐	
14. Infertility	☐	
15. Venereal disease..................	☐	☐
16. Phlebitis, varicosities.............	☐	
17. Neurologic disorders.............	☐	☐
18. Metabol./endocrine disorders ..	☐	☐
19. Anemia/hemoglobinopathy	☐	☐
20. Blood disorders	☐	☐
21. Drug abuse........................	☐	
22. Smoking/alcohol use	☐	
23. Infectious diseases	☐	
24. Operations/accidents	☐	
25. Allergies/meds sensitivity	☒	
26. Blood transfusions...............	☐	
27. Other hospitalizations	☐	
28. _____	☐	☐
29. _____	☐	☐
30. **No known disease/problems**	☐	☐

Check and detail positive findings including date and place of treatment. Precede findings by reference number.

Maternal gmother was twin and she has twin
maternal gfather
sister/mg.father

MG.Father

age 5

Carpal Tunnel right hand/tonsillectomy
Hay fever

Preexisting Risk Guide

Indicates pregnancy/outcome at risk
31. ☐ Age < 15 or > 35
32. ☐ <8th grade education
33. ☐ Cardiac disease (class I or II)
34. ☐ Tuberculosis active
35. ☐ Chronic pulmonary disease
36. ☐ Thrombophlebitis
37. ☐ Endocrinopathy
38. ☐ Epilepsy (on medication)
39. ☐ Infertility (treated)
40. ☐ 2 abortions (spontaneous/induced)
41. ☒ 7 deliveries
42. ☐ Previous preterm or SGA infants
43. ☐ Infants > 4,000 gms
44. ☐ Isoimmunization (ABO, etc.)
45. ☐ Hemorrhage during previous preg.
46. ☐ Previous preeclampsia
47. ☐ Surgically scarred uterus
48. ☐ Preg. without familial support
49. ☐ Second pregnancy in 12 months
50. ☐ Smoking (>1 pack per day)
51. ☐ _____
52. ☐ _____
53. ☐ _____

Indicates pregnancy/outcome at high risk
54. ☑ Age > 40
55. ☐ Diabetes mellitus
56. ☐ Hypertension
57. ☐ Cardiac disease (class III or IV)
58. ☐ Chronic renal disease
59. ☐ Congenital/chromosomal anomalies
60. ☐ Hemoglobinopathies
61. ☐ Isoimmunization (Rh)
62. ☐ Alcohol or drug abuse
63. ☐ Habitual abortions
64. ☐ Incompetent cervix
65. ☐ Prior fetal or neonatal death
66. ☐ Prior neurologically damaged infant
67. ☐ Significant social problems
68. ☐ _____
69. ☐ _____
70. ☐ _____

Historical Risk Status
71. ☐ No risk factors notes
72. ☐ At risk
73. ☑ At high risk
At high risk, advanced maternal age

Menstrual History	Onset		Cycle		Length			
	13	age	28	days	5-7	days		

Pregnancy History				Grav 8	Term 6	Pret 0	Abort 1	Live 6	EDO

Month/ year	Sex	Weight at birth	Wks. gest.	Hrs. in labor	Type of delivery	Details of delivery. In and maternal or newborn complications. Use Risk Guide numbers where applicable.
	M	7'4"	40	24°	Vag	paracervical
	F	7'.	40	8°	Vag	paracervical
	F	6'4"	40	36°	Vag	paracervical
	F	7'5"	40	8°	Vag	paracervical
	M	6'10"	40	3°	Vag	paracervical
						miscarriage 5 mo
	F	8'5"	42	6°	Vag	started with Pit. epidural

Review Case 5-11, *continued*

MOTHER INTRAPARTUM

MEMBRANES RUPTURED	MONITORING			DATE	TIME	COMPLICATIONS		☐ Elevated Mat. Temp _____
TIME___*Midnight*___	☒ FSE ☐ IUPC	ONSET OF LABOR		10-23	0200	☐ ABRUPTION ☐ PREVIA ☐ PROLAPSE CORD		
	☐ EXTERNAL	COMPLETE DILATION		10-23	1540	☐ STILLBORN ☐ MULTIPLE BIRTHS X _____		
	☐ INTERMITTENT	DELIVERY TIME		10-23	1548	☐ OTHER ___*nuchal cord x 1 FHR*___		
		PLACENTA TIME		10-23	1554	FHR. ___*140's*___		

						TIME	MEDICATION DOSE	RT	SITE	NURSE SIG
2ND STAGE						1555	*Pit 20 cc*			

VAGINAL

PRESENTATION: _____*Vertex*_____

☒ SPONTANEOUS   ☐ SHOULDER DYSTOCIA   ☐ FORCEPS   ☐ ROTATION
☐ VACUUM EXTRACTION:
EPISIOTOMY: ☒ NONE ☐ ML ☐ OTHER _____
LACERATION: ☐ NONE ☐ PERINEAL: ☐ 1° ☐ 2° ☐ 3° ☐ 4°
     ☐ SULCUS ___*NA*___ ☐ CERVICAL _____
     ☐ OTHER _____
☒ URINARY CATH-TIME _____*1544*_____
ANESTHESIA: ☐ NONE ☐ LOCAL ☐ PUDENDAL ☐ PARACERVICAL ☒ EPIDURAL
ANESTH- _____
REMARKS: *Dr. Smith attended delivery*

TIME	BP	PULSE	RESP	FUNDUS	FLOW

OBSERVATIONS: _____

3RD STAGE

PLACENTA: ☒ SPONTANEOUS ☐ MANUAL ☒ INTACT ☐ FRAGMENTED ☐ CURRETAGE
ABNORMALITIES OF PLACENTA: _____
     ☒ EBL >500 cc
REMARKS: _____

TRANSFER TIME: *TO SURG 1615*

RN SIGNATURE

INFANT

APGARS	1	5
HEART RATE		
Absent 0		
Below 100 1	160	160
Above 100 2		
RESP EFFORT		
Absent 0		
Slow, Irreg 1		
Strong Cry 2	2	2
REFLEX STIM		
No Response 0		
Grimace 1	2	2
Cough Sneeze 2		
MUSCLE TONE		
Flaccid 0		
Some Flexion 1	2	2
Well Flexed 2		
COLOR		
Pale Blue 0		
Body Pink w/		
Blue Extremit. 1	0	1
All Pink 2		
TOTAL	8	9

SEX: ☒ M ☐ F
BAND# ___6761___
WEIGHT __2948__ GMS
__6__ LBS. __8__ OZ.
LENGTH_47.0_ CM_18 1/2_ IN.
☐ VOIDED ☐ STOOL

RESUSCITATION
SUCTION
☒ Prior deli. shoulders
☒ Bulb
☐ Delee _____ cc
   Color
☒ O₂ ___*slt/5 min*___
☐ Bag & Mask
☐ CORDS VISUALIZED
☐ INTUBATION
By _____
☐ ANOMALIES* _____
NURSES SIGN.: _____

INFANT INTERIM OBSERVTION				
TIME	COLOR	TEMP	RESP	ACTIVITY

OBSERVATIONS: _____

ATTENDING PHYSICIAN EXAM		
INFANT		
	NL	OTHER
HEENT		
HEART		
CHEST		
ABDOMEN		
GU		
EXTREMITIES		
REFLEXES		
Physician Sig.		

MOTHER

WAS PT MONITORED?   ☒ Yes   ☐ No
FHM PATTERN OBSERVATION:
☐ Late decels ☒ Early decels ☐ Variable decels
☐ Bradycardia ☐ Tachycardia ☐ NL/Reassuring

EVALUATION:
Good variability

CORD			TIME	MEDICATION/DOSE	RT	STE	NURSE SIG
VESSELS: ☒ 3 ☐ 2			1600	*Aqua Mephtyon 1 mg*		IM	
☒ NUCHAL CORD _X1_							
☐ OTHER _____							
☒ CORD BLOOD SENT							
☐ CORD pH _____			Transfer Time to Nursery:				
(IF INDICATED)			1625				

Review Case 5-11, *continued*

PROGRESS NOTES: DELIVERY NOTE

PATIENT: Denise Drummond

DATE: 10/12/xx

The patient had spontaneous rupture of membranes this morning. She labored, contractions didn't really become regular, however, and so finally augmentation was carried out. The patient then made slow but steady progress to about 5 cm. and dilated more rapidly. When nearly complete she was taken to delivery and there delivered spontaneously a male infant which weighed 6 pounds 8 ounces and was 18.5 inches long. Appeared to be somewhat early as the due date would indicate. The baby cried spontaneously, however and did well. There was a nuchal cord which was slipped over the shoulders during delivery. The placenta separated spontaneously and appeared to be intact. Some calcification was present. Estimated blood loss was 350 cc. Replacement none. Electronic fetal monitoring was carried out with ab-domina leads for most of the time but scalp electrode being applied in the later part of labor. The record was fairly normal with good beat to beat variation throughout. There were several instances of early decelerations and one or two late's but generally the record was reassuring.

Patient has been doing well. She is on regular diet and voiding. She has recovered well from the anesthetic as well. She is discharged to home. Prescriptions given for Motrin and she will return later in the week, for removal of staples. She will continue with prenatal vitamins. She did have to be catheterized once early this morning but has voided satisfactorily since then so will probably not have further bladder problems.

PROGRESS NOTE

continued

Review Case 5-11, *continued*

ICD-9-CM/ICD-10-CM diagnosis code(s): _____

ICD-9-CM procedure and ICD-10-PCS procedure code(s): _____

MS-DRG: _____

Review Case 5-12

Health Record Face Sheet

Western Regional
Medical Center

Record Number:	11-13-06
Age:	83
Gender:	Male
Length of Stay:	6 days
Diagnosis/Procedure:	Acute Stroke
Service Type:	INPT Medical
Discharge Status:	Home

Review Case 5-12, *continued*

HISTORY & PHYSICAL

CHIEF COMPLAINT: Cannot walk.

HISTORY OF PRESENT ILLNESS: This elderly gentleman relates a story of falling down last night and spending much of the night on the floor, not being able to stand. Previous to this, he was able to get up, move around, ride his four-wheeler and do a few chores around the farm.

PAST HISTORY:
MEDICAL/SURGICAL: History of benign prostatic hypertrophy, widespread degenerative joint disease, hypertension, diabetes mellitus, previous cholecysteclomy, and previous motor vehicle accident with partial small-bowel resection with re-obstruction requiring revision of the original anastomosis.
ALLERGIES: NONE.
MEDICATIONS: Lantus 5 units daily.

PHYSICAL EXAMINATION
GENERAL: The patient is very hard of hearing, but is otherwise alert and oriented. The patient cannot stand up and walk on his own.
VITAL SIGNS: Unremarkable with the exception of some higher blood pressure.
HEENT/NECK: No focal findings.
LUNGS: Clear.
HEART: Regular.
ABDOMEN: Soft and nontender.
EXTREMITIES: No clubbing or edema.

LABORATORY/DIAGNOSTIC: Fairly unremarkable CBC, chem-14, UA, and hemoglobin A1C; thyroid is pending. A CT scan of the head shows old strokes but no acute findings yet seen on the scan. Carotid Doppler reveals an 80-90% stenosis of the left carotid artery.

ASSESSMENT: Stroke with fall.

continued

CONSULTATION REPORT

HISTORY OF PRESENT ILLNESS: The patient is an 83-year-old gentleman who relates a history of falling down then spending a lot of time on the floor. He had quite a bit of bleeding in the lateral aspect of the left foot. Because the bleeding was extensive and because of the unexplained fall, the patient was taken to the hospital and subsequently admitted by Dr. Jackson. I have been consulted for evaluation of the 5th toe, which appears to have had a tear sustained.

PMH	Small-bowel resection. Previous admission for motor vehicle accident.
ALLERGIES:	NO KNOWN DRUG ALLERGIES.
MEDICATIONS:	Lantus 5 units daily; reviewed and up to date in the chart per Dr.

SOCIAL HISTORY: Denies alcohol, tobacco or recreational drug use past or present.

REVIEW OF SYSTEMS: Denies nausea or vomiting, fevers or chills, shortness of breath, chest pain, polydactyl polydipsia, visual changes, rapid weight gain or loss.

PHYSICAL EXAMINATION
GENERAL: Alert and oriented x3, in no acute distress. **VASCULAR:** Pedal pulses palpable 2/4 bilaterally, capillary refill time less than 2 seconds, normal pedal edema. **NEUROLOGIC:** sensations to all pedal dermatomes in a stocking glove fashion. Sharp-dull vibratory sensations are also absent in the distribution pattern. **SKIN:** Texture is dry, atrophic without pedal hair. There is a significant tear of the plantar 5th toe; full-thickness laceration/tear. The flexor tendon is identifiable. There is some oozing around the lesion. No purulent drainage. Some local erythema but no lymphangitis or popliteal lymphadenopathy. It is relatively clean. It does go down to the deep tissues, particularly down to the deep tendon. **MUSCULOSKELETAL:** Significant arthritis changes of the forefoot, particularly with hammering digits and varus 5th toes bilaterally. Slight hallux abductovalgus deformity. Muscle strength otherwise 5/5 and extension of the left 5th toe is still intact and evident.

PLAN: 1) We discussed treatment options. Realistically, because of the deep nature of this tear, the reality is that this patient may never really heal this appropriately and may have to consider amputation. This is perhaps something to consider; however, the patient would really like to consider salvage of the 5th toe. I feel it might add to stability overall. I think this is a worthwhile consideration. 2) We anesthetized the left 5th toe with 3 mL 2% lidocaine plain. The patient is relatively neuropathic but still having quite a bit of pain, so anesthesia was administered in this way. Once he was completely insensate in the 5th toe, the toe was copiously lavaged with sterile saline and Betadine bath. Once this Puisavac-type clean out was performed, any further loose debris was debrided under sterile condition with sterile instruments and sterile gloves at bedside. Once this was completed and the wound edges freshened, we reapproximated using 3-0 Prolene suture in a vertical mattress non-retention-type fashion. The wound reapproximated well. It was then dressed with a dry sterile dressing and placed in a postoperative shoe. I would like to keep the patient off this as much as possible in the shoe to try and protect any of the extension pressures in the area. Will see how well he heals. Will continue to monitor over the next week. We appreciate the consult to our clinic. The patient tolerated the procedure well and postprocedure instructions were detailed both orally and written.

PROGRESS NOTES

DATE: 6/1/xx

The patient is alert and oriented today.

I am going to start lisinopril for his blood pressure and continue the Lantus.

I will discuss the carotid Doppler findings with the family and see if we want to refer him for surgical intervention. Otherwise, I have ordered physical therapy to see if they can improve his ambulation.

DATE: 6/2/xx

The patient is improving. The nurses have had him up walking somewhat. His blood pressure is good and sugars are stable. He will probably benefit from a skilled swing bed with physical therapy for a few days starting tomorrow.

DATE: 6/3/xx

The patient was able to walk yesterday. His strength and coordination are improving, I have started Plavix. At the present time, we will probably not pursue the carotid stenosis.

RADIOLOGY

CT BRAIN

FINDINGS
Noncontrast axial CT images of the brain are obtained.

There is well-defined cerebrospinal fluid density in the left frontal lobe consistent with encephalomalacia from prior head injury or stroke,

There is no focal gyral swelling or other noncontrast CT sign of acute cerebral infarction. A subcentimeter well-defined lacune is also visible in the deep white matter of the right frontal lobe, best seen on image #20 and consistent with old infarction.

There are no parenchymal brain hyperdensities or hypodensities to suggest hemorrhagic or nonhemorrhagic cerebral contusion. There is no evidence of subdural, epidural or subarachnoid hemorrhage.

No intracranial masses are found.

There are no skull fractures.

IMPRESSION
Old left frontal lobe encephalomalacia, most likely sequelae of prior head injury or infarction. There is also a small old lacune in the deep white matter of the right frontal lobe. There is no CT evidence of acute cerebral infarction or hemorrhage, and no evidence of acute intracranial injury or skull fracture.

continued

Review Case 5-12, *continued*

RADIOLOGY

US CAROTID
Reason for Procedure:

FINDINGS
There is significant atherosclerotic plaque in the bilateral carotid arterial bulbs extending into the internal carotid arteries bilaterally in the left external carotid artery. The bilateral plaque is predominantly noncalcified.

In the proximal left internal carotid artery, the atherosclerotic plaque abnormally increases peak systolic velocity to 279 cm/sec. Tenderness left internal carotid/common carotid artery peak systolic velocity ratio is 3.5,

The plaque in the proximal right internal carotid artery abnormally increases peak systolic velocity to 125 cm/sec. The right internal carotid/common carotid artery peak systolic velocity ratio is 1.5.

Flow in the bilateral vertebral arteries is antegrade.

IMPRESSION
Significant predominantly noncalcified atherosclerotic plaque in the bilateral, carotid arterial bulbs extending into the proximal to midportions of the bilateral internal carotid arteries in the origin of left external carotid artery. The left-sided plaque produces a significant stenosis in the proximal left internal carotid artery estimated at between 80% and 99% diameter. The right-sided plaque in the proximal right internal carotid artery causes a stenosis estimated at approximately 60% diameter.

ICD-9-CM/ICD-10-CM diagnosis code(s): _____

ICD-9-CM procedure and ICD-10-PCS procedure code(s): _____

MS-DRG: _____

Review Case 5-13

Health Record Face Sheet

Western Regional
Medical Center

Record Number:	36-14-08
Age:	80
Gender:	Female
Length of Stay:	1 Day
Diagnosis/Procedure:	Acute Stress State Hypertension Flare
Service Type:	Inpatient
Discharge Status:	To Home

Review Case 5-13, *continued*

DISCHARGE SUMMARY

DATE OF ADMISSION: 5/13/xx

HISTORY: This 80-year-old was readmitted to this hospital having been discharged on 5/1/xx. At that time she was admitted with a small TIA. She had hypertension which stabilized in the hospital. She has been home. She has been doing well until today. Friends have informed us that she has been under considerable stress at home today. The patient is reluctant to acknowledge this. This afternoon she has vomiting and not doing well. Her visiting nurse reported these findings. The patient was too ill to be brought to the hospital in the car and it is my understanding that she was brought to the hospital in an ambulance. She has been restless, complains of chest pain, left shoulder pain. The shoulder pain is aggravated by any shoulder or arm motion. She has had nausea, vomiting a few times. Her blood pressure elevated this afternoon according to the visiting nurse. She was seen in the Emergency Room. Laboratory studies were done. The patient was given Captopril 25 and one half hour later the blood pressure was 200/95.

PAST HISTORY: Nephrectomy, right rotator cuff injury, Marshall-Marchetti procedure 5 years ago. The patient was in this hospital for TIA 2 years ago. The patient's medications at home are Premarin 0.625 daily, Thyroid 2 grains, thyroid 30 mg daily, Iodine drops and Pilostat for her eyes. Septra DS b.i.d. for 10 days. The patient states that she had no problems with Sulfa. She has developed a mild rash. Careful review of earlier records does indicate that at one time she did have a hive with Sulfa. Antibiotic was for urinary tract infection.

DRUG ALLERGIES: Penicillin.

PHYSICAL EXAMINATION: Blood pressure 210/110 dropping to 200/95. The patient is an adult white female complaining of nausea which receded in the Emergency Room. She has been very restless. This became less marked in the Emergency Room. She was given Captopril 25 mg at 6 p.m. EKG was normal. Head and neck are otherwise unremarkable. Lungs are clear to percussion and auscultation and without rales. Heart tones are normal. Rhythm is regular, no murmurs are heard. Motion of the left shoulder joint causes marked pain. Abdomen is soft. Liver, kidney and spleen are not palpable. Scars are present. Extremities are normal. Joints appear normal. Edema is absent.

HOSPITAL COURSE: The patient was responsive to medications and improved greatly by the next day. Labs fairly normal.

IMPRESSION:
1. Acute stressed state, hypertension flare-up.
2. Recent urinary tract infection.
3. Recent TIA.
4. Arthritis of the left shoulder.

PLAN: Will discharge home today to follow-up in office on Monday.

continued

Review Case 5-13, *continued*

Age: 80Y   Date: 5/13/xx

Test Name	Result	Flags	Units	Low	High	Comments
CHEMISTRY SCREEN						
GLUCOSE	170	H	mg/dl	70	110	
BUN	14		mg/dl	7	24	
CREATININE	0.7		mg/dl	0.6	1.3	
BUN/CREATININE RATIO	20.0			0.0	40.0	
URIC ACID	4.7		mg/dl	2.6	5.6	
TOTAL BILIRUBIN	0.56		mg/dl	0.00	1.00	
DIRECT BILIRUBIN	0.20		mg/dl	0.00	0.30	
INDIRECT BILIRUBIN	0.36		mg/dl	0.00	0.90	
ALK PHOSPHATASE	117		U/L	50	136	
SGPT	28	L	U/L	30	65	
SGOT	26		U/L	15	37	
LDH	190		U/L	100	190	
GGPT	1	L	U/L	5	85	
TOTAL PROTEIN	6.9		g/dl	6.4	8.2	
ALBUMIN	4.0		g/dl	3.4	5.0	
GLOBULIN	2.9		g/dl	2.0	3.5	
A/G RATIO	1.4			1.0	2.5	
CALCIUM	9.6		mg/dl	8.8	10.5	
PHOSPHORUS	3.8		mg/dl	2.5	4.9	
IRON	66		ug/dl	35	150	
SODIUM	137	L	mmol/L	140	148	
POTASSIUM	3.9		mmol/L	3.6	5.2	
CHLORIDE	101		mmol/L	100	108	
CHOLESTEROL	270	H	mg/dl	130	200	
TRIGLYCERIDE	142		mg/dl	30	200	

RADIOLOGY REPORT

EXAM: Lt shoulder

HISTORY: Pain.

LEFT SHOULDER:

Internal and external rotation AP views of the left shoulder show intact osseous structures and normal articular relationships. No soft tissue abnormality. No calcifications.

There is a little spurring from the margins of the glenoid typical of degenerative disease. No other abnormality.

IMPRESSION:

Minor degenerative disease.

DIAGNOSTIC IMAGING

continued

Review Case 5-13, *continued*

| TIME STAMP IN | | | **E.C.G.** | | NAME PLATE OR PRINT PATIENT'S NAME, AGE, SEX, SERVICE (M.D.) HOSPITAL NO. AND ADDRESS BELOW | | IN ☐ | **PLEASE APPLY PRESSURE YOU ARE MAKING 5 COPIES** |

DR. ORDERING TEST

OUT ☐

DATE AND TIME ORDERED
5/13/xx, 5:45   A.M.
                P.M.

TIME TO BE DONE
NOW

☐ ROU-TINE
☐ PRE-OP
☐ ASAP

☒ **E.C.G.**   ☒ **PHYSICIAN INTERP.**   ☐ **EMER. INTERP.**   ☐ **RHYTHM STRIPS**

☐ MALE   PREVIOUS   ☐ YES |
☒ FEMALE   AGE *80*   HEIGHT ___   WEIGHT ___   E.C.G.   ☐ NO |

MEDICATIONS: (LIST ALL)

Premarin, Amoxic, thyroid, iodine

_____

_____

nausea, vomiting, pain in left shoulder

CLINICAL DIAGNOSIS: (REASON FOR ECG)

_____

| | DATE DONE: 5/13/xx |

RHYTHM   *sinus*

RATE   *84*   MEAN QRS AXIS   *0°*

INTERVALS: PR   *140*   QRS   *80*   QT   *400*

DESCRIPTION: _____

_____

_____

SINCE: _____

ECG INTERPRETATION: _____

_____

Normal ECG

_____

**ELECTROCARDIOGRAPHIC
    REPORT**   SIGNED : *James Wright, M.D.*

Review Case 5-13, *continued*

ICD-9-CM/ICD-10-CM diagnosis code(s): _____

ICD-9-CM procedure and ICD-10-PCS procedure code(s): _____

MS-DRG: _____

Review Case 5-14

Health Record Face Sheet

Western Regional
Medical Center

Record Number: 25-15-05

Age: 83

Gender: Female

Length of Stay: 1 day

Diagnosis/Procedure: Peripheral Vascular Disease,
Cellulitis

Service Type: Inpatient

Discharge Status: To Skilled Nursing Facility

DISCHARGE SUMMARY

DATE OF ADMISSION: 4/11/xx

DATE OF DISCHARGE: 4/12/xx

HISTORY: This patient is an 83-year-old woman admitted because of severe edema of her lower extremities and developing leg ulcers there.

LAB/X-RAY: SMAC showed a glucose of 132, SGPT 29, albumin 3.2, cholesterol 258. The rest of the SMAC was normal. Urinalysis physiologic. Hemoglobin 13.6, hematocrit 40.7, white count was 4,800 with a normal differential. Platelets were adequate. Red blood cell morphology was essentially normal.

HOSPITAL COURSE: The patient was admitted to the hospital. She was admitted as a short stay. She was treated with Tetracycline and Lasix. It was felt that after discussion with the family that nursing home placement was the most appropriate place to care for this patient. Edema of her feet cleared rapidly with simple elevation and a dose of Lasix. She was transferred to a skilled nursing facility on Monday. She would take Synthroid 0.1 mg daily, Tetracycline 250 mg q.i.d. She would remain mostly at bedrest with the legs elevated. Heat lamp to the sacral area q.i.d. She would take Pamelor 25 mg h.s. daily as we suspected mild depression here. Follow-up would be at the nursing home.

DISCHARGE DIAGNOSIS: Severe peripheral venous insufficiency and cellulitis of the legs.

continued

HISTORY & PHYSICAL

ADMISSION DATE: 4/11/xx

This patient is an 83-year-old Caucasian female brought to the office by her daughter-in-law. Her husband died a few months ago and she has been living at home alone. They were a very reclusive couple prior to his death and would not leave the house and would not let anyone in the house except for a couple of sons and a daughter-in-law. The daughter-in-law has been going in the house three times a day getting her meals, helping her to the bathroom. This lady does not sleep in bed. She sleeps in her chairs. Her legs are swollen and her feet are down all day. She has been taking no medications up until yesterday when she was started on Tetracycline. She is awake and alert and resigned to die.

In the past she has refused hospitalization. The daughter-in-law has been having Home Health come out and trying to take care of her mother-in-law at home but simply cannot manage it any more. She has weeping infections of both the sacrum and of both feet. Cultures of these were done earlier this month and she was started yesterday on Tetracycline which all the organisms were sensitive to. She has been on no other medications.

She had a stroke 5 years ago and tires easily, and has trouble walking. She was hospitalized by Dr. Bennett in 2008 with a stroke. Had CT scan which was reported as normal, carotid angiogram showed congenital arterial abnormalities with minimal atheromatous plaquing of the right internal carotid artery. There was also a small aneurysm on the left side. She was anticoagulated at that time. Also was on a hormone shot and Thyroxin.

FAMILY HISTORY: Family history of heart disease, diabetes, skin cancers.

ALLERGIES: She is allergic to Penicillin and Aureomycin and does not tolerate Codeine.

PAST HISTORY: She has had an appendectomy, total abdominal hysterectomy, a T&A, varicose vein operations and hemorrhoidectomy.

She's had an adenomatous polyp with villous features removed from her colon in 2005. She's had skin cancers removed from her legs.

REVIEW OF SYSTEMS: At this time the patient has no complaints. She is a very reluctant patient and does not cooperate for examination. Denies any physical problems at this time. However, the daughter-in-law has obtained power of attorney.

PHYSICAL EXAMINATION: Patient is awake, alert and noncooperative.

HEAD: Normocephalic without lesions.
EYES: PERRLA, fundi normal.

Patient is grossly dirty. Has not been bathed in months. Has weeping ulcers of both feet and from her sacrum.

EARS, NOSE & THROAT: Unremarkable. She is wearing her dentures and does wear glasses. Hearing is good.
LUNGS: Clear to auscultation and percussion. No breast masses are noted.
HEART SOUNDS: Normal. Rhythm is regular.
ABDOMEN: Palpation of the abdomen reveals no masses. Bowel sounds are normal. There are no bruits.
PELVIC & RECTAL: Not attempted with this noncooperative patient. There is an area of skin breakdown over the sacrum and both feet are 4+ edematous with weeping from the dorsum of the feet.

ADMITTING DIAGNOSIS:

1. Severe edema with secondary infections of wounds of the sacrum and feet.
2. Cerebrovascular disease with previous stroke.
3. Hypothyroidism on replacement therapy.

Review Case 5-14, *continued*

PHYSICIAN'S ORDERS & PROGRESS RECORD

DATE	ORDERS	✓	DATE	PROGRESS
4/11/xx	*Sheet form admit* *Please make arrangement* *for nursing home transfer* *SMAC, CBC, U/A* *Tub bath.* *-2 gm Na+ diet* *Synthroid 0.1 mg daily* *Tetracycline 250 mg* *qid x 10 day* *-Lasix 40 mg P.O. on admission* *-(may insert Foley cath* *if necessary)* *-bed rest c̄ legs elevated* *But BRP c̄ help* *to stay off back* *heat lamp to back for* *-2 hrs qid*		4/11/xx	*83 y/o w/f unable to* *maintain herself at home* *Social Services* *Nursing facility has vacancy* *I have not been able* *to reach the family to* *have the pre-admission* *paperwork completed* *Will try again.*

continued

Review Case 5-14, *continued*

PHYSICIAN'S ORDERS & PROGRESS RECORD

INSTRUCTIONS: – NOTE PROGRESS OF CASE, COMPLICATION, CHANGE IN DIAGNOSIS, CONDITION ON DISCHARGE, INSTRUCTIONS TO PATIENT.

DATE	ORDERS	✓	DATE	PROGRESS
4/12/xx	Transfer to nursing facility		4/12/xx	Minimal edema of feet with bed rest &elevation of feet Cont this Rx alone at n.h. Add Pamelo 25 mg daily
				Social services note: necessary paperwork prepared for transfer to nursing facility. Family aware of transfer and will transport. Facility notified.

Review Case 5-14, *continued*

ICD-9-CM/ICD-10-CM diagnosis code(s): _____

ICD-9-CM procedure and ICD-10-PCS procedure code(s): _____

MS-DRG: _____

Review Case 5-15

Health Record Face Sheet

Western Regional
Medical Center

Record Number:	14-36-08
Age:	45
Gender:	Male
Length of Stay:	17 Days
Diagnosis/Procedure:	Diabetic Ketoacidosis
Service Type:	Inpatient
Discharge Status:	To Home

continued

DISCHARGE SUMMARY

DATE OF ADMISSION: 12/1/xx
DATE OF DISCHARGE: 12/18/xx

REFERRING PHYSICIAN: Dr. Baker
CONSULTING PHYSICIAN: Dr. Jones

ADMISSION DIAGNOSES:
1. Diabetic ketoacidosis.
2. Metabolic encephalopathy.

DISCHARGE DIAGNOSES:
1. Diabetic ketoacidosis.
2. Metabolic encephalopathy secondary to number one.

PERTINENT HISTORY: This 45-year-old male was transferred from urgent care for further evaluation and treatment of depressed neurological status and chemical derangements following presentation there with severe diabetic ketoacidosis on Monday. pH was as low as 7.03 and his blood sugar was 1,554.

He was treated for the diabetic ketoacidosis. The patient was also apparently agitated intermittently and required restraining. Patient received approximately 115 -mg of IV Diazepam over a 20-hour period. Because the patient's mental status had not improved with improvement of diabetes, the patient was transferred for further evaluation and treatment.

The patient has a long-standing history of insulin-dependent diabetes and has been on 60 units of Lente insulin per day. Has associated complications of diabetic neuropathy, diabetic retinopathy which has left the patient nearly blind, and nausea and vomiting and diarrhea are also felt to be related to the diabetes. There is also a history of social domestic problems contributing to the patient's lack of close medical care.

PHYSICAL EXAMINATION: On admission the blood pressure was 160/71, and pulse was 77 and regular. Afebrile. There were no spontaneous movements through most of the examination and the patient was unconscious. Other than depressed neurologic status, the examination was unremarkable.

HOSPITAL COURSE: Initial impression was that the patient had metabolic encephalopathy, probably, most likely due to the high doses of IV sedatives given. A contribution from diabetes and rapid return of blood sugar along with rapid return of blood sugar to normal as well as hypophosphatemia were felt to be possibly contributing causes. The patient was seen in consultation by Dr. Jones who felt that an unenhanced CT scan was necessary. This was done and was normal. The patient was monitored in the Intensive Care Unit. The patient's level of consciousness gradually improved as did laboratory values which improved in the fact that dehydration became progressively less and sugars became progressively under control as well as his other laboratory values. He was awake and well enough to transfer to the floor on . On the floor the patient gradually regained strength and was switched from IV Insulin to a sliding scale dosage and gradually a single morning insulin regimen was instituted. There was significant amount of trial and error and several hypoglycemic episodes were inadvertently induced. However, the patient gradually seemed to stabilize and it seemed that 20 units of Humulin T with 10 units of Humulin R was the best dosage to give him. With this particular dosage, patient was stable as blood sugars ranged from 80 to 150. The patient symptomatically felt better and stronger and also felt that he had some improvement in vision.

continued. . .

Review Case 5-15, *continued*

DISCHARGE SUMMARY—PAGE 2

One of the patient's primary problems and a significant problem before even being admitted consisted of inability of keeping meals down with significant diarrhea and vomiting with meals. It was thought that the patient had diabetic diarrhea as well as diabetic gastroparesis. The patient was started on Reglan which seemed to significantly help as did Lomotil. Stool studies did not disclose an alternative explanation for the patient's diarrhea. The patient's 24-hour stool weight was 1,096 grams. Stool specimens did not show ova or parasites, nor white blood cells. There were 2+ budding yeasts present. There were occasional muscle fibers present. There was no occult blood.

Urine studies showed the urine protein to be 1,969 mg per 24 hours. Normal is up to 150 mg per 24 hours. The creatinine clearance was 63 ml per minute. The patient's creatine at time of discharge was 1.1 with a BUN of 12 .

Other laboratory values at time of discharge: cholesterol 146, triglycerides 284, Albumin 2.4, total protein 4.7, T3 uptake was normal. Hemoglobin on was 12.7 with hematocrit of 36.5.

The patient has a referral to home health care and this was arranged.

DISCHARGE MEDICATIONS:
1. Humulin–N 100, 20 units subcutaneously every morning.
2. Humulin–R 100, 10 units subcutaneously every morning.
3. Reglan 10 mg one 20 minutes before meals three times a day at bed time for three weeks per month.
4. Viokase 1–3 with meals three times a day.
5. Zantac 150 mg twice a day.
6. Lomotil three times a day as needed for diarrhea.

DISPOSITION:
1. The patient was discharged to home. The patient's wife has a new glucose monitor which is to be used four times a day.
2. The patient is to see Dr. Baker in one week.
3. Home Health Care was arranged through Valley Home Health. They are to see the patient three times a week.
4. The patient is to follow a 2,000 to 2,400 calorie ADA diet.

DISCHARGE CONDITION: Good.

continued

Review Case 5-15, *continued*

HISTORY & PHYSICAL

DATE OF ADMISSION: 12/1/xx

CHIEF COMPLAINT:

Depressed neurologic status.

HISTORY OF PRESENT ILLNESS:

This 45-year-old white male was transferred from the urgent care to the hospital for further evaluation and treatment of depressed neurologic status and chemical derangements following a presentation with very severe diabetic ketoacidosis on Monday. History is from the patient's wife.

Approximately 2–3 days prior to his admission, the patient had been experiencing "flu like symptoms" manifested by generally feeling ill with perhaps some increase in his diarrhea and vomiting, which are chronic problems. No history, of fever, headache, injury. According to his wife, he has been taking his insulin every day although not consistently at the same time. He became progressively weaker and confused and the patient's wife took him in the morning on Monday to the urgent care. At that time, it was found that he was disoriented, combative, did not open his eyes to commands, and had incomprehensible vocalization. He did withdraw to pain. He was found to have a blood sugar of 1554. His pH was 7.03 with a PO2 of 124, PCO2 of 10. His bicarb was 2.8. The hemoglobin was 12 and the hematocrit was 33. Potassium was 6.8 and the sodium was 114. It was known from the records that his baseline creatinine was 1.5 with a BUN of 18. The patient was treated with IV fluids, IM and then IV insulin. Parameters gradually increased. It was stated that at 8 AM, his blood sugar was 1554. Approximately 20 hours later the blood sugar was 98. At the time of transfer today, the creatinine was 2.7 and the BUN was 67 at 8 AM today. The blood sugar was 201. Potassium was 3.7 and the sodium was 138. pH was 7.4 With a P02 of 66 and a PC02 of 44 on 50% mask. The hemoglobin was 13 and the hematocrit was 35.7. This was after 2 units of packed red blood cells.

The patient had been intermittently agitated and required restraining. He had been receiving several doses of IV Valium 2-5mg. He was also receiving Zantac 50mg IV every 8 hours. This was being given because of a possible history of hematemesis prior to the admission.

The patient has a 16-year history of insulin-dependent diabetes mellitus. He is currently on 60 units of Lente insulin each day. He has never taken divided doses of insulin. He takes his insulin at approximately 11:30 each day. He eats breakfast at 8 AM. His wife draws up the insulin for him because he is blind. But, she does witness him give it to himself. She does feel that he gave himself insulin on the days before this admission. She says that he eats irregularly and sleeps irregularly because of his particular lifestyle desire and perhaps some depression. He checks his own blood sugar or urine, according to his wife. She has no idea what his blood sugars usually run. She says he is private about his diabetes and doesn't keep her informed. He has had past complications of his diabetes including retinopathy with at least 1 laser therapy, left cataract removal, and supposedly there is another eye operation tentatively scheduled. He also is said to have diabetic neuropathy involving his feet. He has had no history of ulcers. He also has chronic intermittent vomiting and diarrhea which has been said to be related to his diabetes. He frequently eats a meal but then regurgitates it.

PAST MEDICAL HISTORY:

1. diabetes and its therapies and complications as listed above.
2. A nebulous history of some heart problem which he was told he had a year or two ago.

MEDICATIONS: Lente insulin 60 units each day. Occasional Lomotil. No other prescription medications. Wife says he does take large amounts of Tylenol for nonspecific pain.

ALLERGIES: None known.

SOCIAL HISTORY:

The patient is on leave for over a year from his job. He moved here 1 1/2 years ago from Alaska. He has a wife and 3 grown children. The patient smokes 1 pack of cigarettes per day and has done so since he was a teenager. His wife states that he has become progressively more depressed because of his lack of job and failing health.

Review Case 5-15, *continued*

HISTORY & PHYSICAL - PAGE 2

FAMILY HISTORY:

There is no other diabetes in the family.

REVIEW OF SYSTEMS:

Described by his wife was essentially negative. This, of course, is in exclusion of the above data.

PHYSICAL EXAMINATION:

BP is 160/71. Pulse was regular at 77 beats per minute. Respiratory rate was 16. The patient was afebrile. In general the patient appeared to be a 45-year-old man who looked his stated age. He was lying in bed with oxygen being received by mask. Arms were restrained. There were no spontaneous movements throughout most of the examination. His head was turned to the left.
HEAD & NECK: The eyes were closed. Right eye was mid range and did not react to light. Funduscopic examination could not be done. The pupil seemed dark but nonclouded. The sclera were normal bilaterally. The left eye showed pupillary changes consistent with cataract surgery. Gaze was symmetric. Nose, mouth, and ears were unremarkable. Carotids were normal.
CHEST: Chest was clear
HEART: Heart was normal.
LYMPH NODES: Negative.
ABDOMEN: Scaphoid and soft and nontender with no organomegaly, masses, or tenderness.
SKIN: Normal.
GENITAL: Unremarkable.
RECTAL: Deferred.
LOWER EXTREMITIES: Pulses were 2+. There was 2+ pedal edema.
UPPER EXTREMITIES: Normal.
NEUROLOGIC: No localizing signs. Babinski's were down bilaterally. Reflexes were 1+ to unobtainable. There appeared to be no posturing and no focal findings. Except, for the head being turned to the left. Occasionally, there were small movements of either the head or the arms.

IMPRESSION:

1. Metabolic encephalopathy related to the recent diabetic ketoacidosis and pre-renal azotemia.
2. Markedly severe diabetic ketoacidosis, somewhat resolved.
3. Some of his encephalopathy may have been related to relatively rapid decline of blood sugar from 1500 to 98 in 20 hours.
4. Renal insufficiency, gradually improving.
5. Diabetic neuropathy of the lower extremities by history.
6. Diabetic gastroparesis.
7. Pedal edema, probably secondary to the IV fluid administration.
8. Diabetic retinopathy.
9. History of depression, from the patient's wife, related to his poor health.
10. History of smoking abuse.
11. The patient's one time a day dosing of insulin seems somewhat unusual, especially at the dose of 60 units. Also, it is not known how well his control has been.

PLAN:

1. Continue rehydration.
2. Try to keep the blood sugar approximately 200–150.
3. Unenhanced CT scan of the head, rule out hemorrhage, shift, edema, or mass.
4. Try not to give sedatives.
5. Supportive care.

continued

Review Case 5-15, continued

PATIENT TRANSFER FORM
(INTER-AGENCY REFERRAL)

1. PATIENT'S LAST NAME: Barton	FIRST NAME: Bruce	MI: J	2. SEX ☒ M ☐ F	3. HEALTH INSURANCE CLAIM NUMBER: 159605-56952

4. PATIENT'S ADDRESS *(Street Number, City, State, Zip Code)*
123 Adams Ave Home Town, 55555

5. DATE OF BIRTH: 8/8/67   **RELIGION:** No Preference

7. DATE OF THIS TRANSFER: 12/18/XX

8. FACILITY NAME AND ADDRESS TRANSFERRING TO:
Valley Home Health
25 Lincoln Road
Home Town, US 55555

10. PHYSICIAN IN CHARGE AT TIME OF TRANSFER
Will this physician care for patient after admission to new facility?   ☐ YES   ☒ NO

11. DATES OF STAY AT FACILITY TRANSFERRING FROM

ADMISSION 12/1/XX   DISCHARGE 12/18/XX

14. PAYMENT SOURCE FOR CHARGES TO PATIENT

A. ☐ SELF OR FAMILY
B. ☐ PRIVATE INSURANCE
C. ☒ BLUE CROSS BLUE SHIELD
D. ☐ EMPLOYER OR UNION
E. ☐ PUBLIC AGENCY *(Give name)*
E. ☐ OTHER *(Explain)*

12-A. NAME AND ADDRESS OF FACILITY TRANSFERRING FROM
WESTERN MEDICAL CENTER
1000 HOSPITAL WAY
HOME TOWN, US, 55555

12-B. NAME AND ADDRESS OF ALL HOSPITALS AND EXTENDED CARE FACILITIES FROM WHICH PATIENT WAS DISCHARGED IN PAST 60 DAYS
none

16. DIAGNOSES AT TIME OF TRANSFER   EMPLOYMENT RELATED   A. ☐ YES   B. ☒ NO

(a) Primary   *Diabetic Ketoacidosis*

(b) Secondary

(Check if present)

Disabilities
Amputation
Paralysis
Contracture
Decub. Ulcer

Impairments
Mentality
Speech
Hearing
(Vision)
Sensation

Incontinence
Bladder
(Bowel)
Saliva

Activity Tolerance Limitations
None   Moderate   (Severe)
Patient knows diagnosis?

IMPORTANT MEDICAL INFORMATION
(State allergies if any)
   nka

DIET, DRUGS, AND OTHER THERAPY
at Time of Discharge

NPO
50U of regular insulin in 500cc of NS @ 20/hr
D5 1/2 NS c̄ 20 meq KCL @ 150cc/hr
Zantac 50 mg IV Q8H
Compazine 10 mg Q6H prn N&V IM
Valium 2mg prn agitation IV
O₂ at 50% per mask
Restrain prn   (Physician, please sign below)

Date of Last B.M. _____
Chest X-ray   date._____ result_____
C.B.C.   date._____ result_____
Serology   date._____ result_____ *sent c̄ pt.*
Urinalysis   _____ result_____

SUGGESTIONS FOR ACTIVE CARE
BED
Position in good body alignment and change position every_____hrs.
Avoid_____ position
Prone position_____ times/day as tolerated.
SIT IN CHAIR
_____ hrs. _____ times/day.

WEIGHT BEARING
Full_____Partial_____Name_____
on_____Leg
LOCOMOTION
Walk_____times/day.
EXERCISES
Range of motion_____times/day.
to_____

by patient_____nurse_____family_____
Other as outlined below_____
Stand_____Min._____times/day.
SOCIAL ACTIVITIES
Encourage group_____individual_____
within_____outside_____home.

Transport. Ambulance_____*x*_____ Car_____
Car for handicapped_____ Bus_____

Signature of Physician

Charles Baker, M.D.

Date: 12/18/xx

PATIENT TRANSFER FORM

Review Case 5-15, *continued*

ICD-9-CM/ICD-10-CM diagnosis code(s): _____

ICD-9-CM procedure and ICD-10-PCS procedure code(s): _____

MS-DRG: _____

Review Case 5-16

Health Record Face Sheet

Western Regional
Medical Center

Record Number:	14-74-52
Age:	34
Gender:	Female
Length of Stay:	4 Days
Diagnosis/Procedure:	Hemorrhoids with Excision
Service Type:	Inpatient Surgical
Discharge Status:	To Home

DISCHARGE SUMMARY

ADMISSION DATE: 4/26/xx

DISCHARGE DATE: 4/30/xx

ENTERING COMPLAINT: Severe hemorrhoids.

PERTINENT LAB & X-RAY DATA: All essentially normal.

PROCEDURES & HOSPITAL COURSE: The patient underwent a hemorrhoidectomy and had an uneventful course. At the time of discharge the operative site was healing nicely, her bowels were moving and she was up and about without problems.

DISPOSITION & REMARKS: Home and office.

CONDITION: Recovered.

FINAL DIAGNOSIS: Severe internal and external hemorrhoids.

OPERATION DONE: Hemorrhoidectomy.

continued

HISTORY & PHYSICAL

DATE OF ADMISSION: 4/26/xx

HISTORY: This 34-year-old woman has developed hemorrhoids. They came on gradually but have been especially prominent over the last year or so. They have increased dramatically in size and have become increasingly symptomatic. We treated her conservatively with sitz baths and stool softeners and so forth and she has done well for awhile but recently they have again begun bleeding and protruding and causing considerable pain. They are very marked hemorrhoids and so she has elected to have surgery and she enters now for that.

PAST HISTORY: Her health has always been good. She has had a hysterectomy with no other operations. She is on no medication now and has no allergies.

REVIEW OF SYSTEMS:

HEENT: Negative.
CARDIORESPIRATORY: She smokes but has no shortness or breath nor lung symptoms. She has never had any heart problems.
GI: Negative other than in present illness.
GU, GYN & REST: Not remarkable.

Her personal, social, and family histories are normal.

PHYSICAL EXAM:

She is a normal appearing young woman who was in no distress and had normal pulse and blood pressure.
SKIN: Negative.
HEENT: Showed no abnormalities.
NECK: Supple without masses.
LUNGS: Clear to auscultation and percussion.
HEART: Regular rhythm without murmur.
ABDOMEN: Soft and flat with no masses or tenderness.
PELVIC: Not done as she has no symptoms referable to that area.
RECTAL: Shows severe circumferential internal and external hemorrhoids.
EXTREMITIES & NEUROLOGICAL: Normal.

INITIAL IMPRESSION: Hemorrhoids

Review Case 5-16, *continued*

OPERATIVE NOTE

DATE OF PROCEDURE: 4/26/xx

SURGEON: Dr. Burkotz

PREOPERATIVE DIAGNOSIS: Severe internal and external hemorrhoids.
POSTOPERATIVE DIAGNOSIS: Same

OPERATION DONE: Hemorrhoidectomy.

PROCEDURE:

We established satisfactory general anesthesia and placed the patient up in the dorsal lithotomy position. I did insert a rigid sigmoidoscope and advanced it to 7 or 8cm but there encountered a large amount of stool. I saw nothing in the distal rectum.

We then prepped and draped the entire rectal area and I inserted a speculum and inspected the area. She had the hugest area of hemorrhoids right at about between 6 and 7 o'clock, posteriorly. This was a huge area that had a surface that was completely eroded off and was very red and inflamed. There was a small area immediately adjacent to it at 4 or 5 o'clock. The lateral edges were okay. Anteriorly at about between 11 and 12 o'clock there was another huge hemorrhoid with a smaller one just to the left of that. I initially placed a Pean clamp around the one at 7 o'clock and then placed a suture in the mucosa up in the rectum above it. I then incised under the clamp and lifted the hemorrhoid up and then tied the stitch around the base of it and amputated it. This left a bare area in which I achieved hemostasis with one 2-0 chromic cat gut stitch and then electrocautery. I then placed the Pean clamp on the hemorrhoid about 5 o'clock immediately adjacent and excised it in the same way. I did leave a small rim of mucosa in between the two. I then went anteriorly and the very large hemorrhoid there I placed a Pean clamp on and incised under the clamp and then placed a 2-0 chromic cat gut stitch through the base of the hemorrhoid up in the rectum and removed that hemorrhoid. I removed a smaller one immediately adjacent to the left of it also leaving some mucosa between. In each of the bare areas I achieved hemostasis with 3-0 plain cat gut stick ties but mostly with electrocautery. After hemostasis was secured we infiltrated the entire area with 0.25% marcaine with Epinephrine and then applied a dressing. She tolerated the procedure well.

continued

PATHOLOGY REPORT

PATIENT: Frita Falton

AGE: 34

ACC. NO: 158765209

DATE: 4/26/xx

MEDICAL RECORD: 14-74-52

DOCTOR: Dr. Burkotz

OPERATION: HEMORRHOIDECTOMY

GROSS: Submitted are multiple, polypoid-like structures which appear grossly to be comprised of anal mucosa and submucosa. Within the submucosa are numerous, dilated, and congested blood vessels. The specimen in its entirety measures to approximately 3.0 cm. Representative portions are submitted for examination.

MICRO: The specimen reveals fragments of anal mucosa and submucosa. Within the submucosa are numerous dilated and congested blood vessels.

External hemorrhoids. *and Int hemorrhoids*

Review Case 5-16, *continued*

PHYSICIAN'S ORDERS & PROGRESS RECORD

DATE	ORDERS	✓	DATE	PROGRESS
4/26/xx	Admit to surgical floor,		4/26/xx	For elective removal hemorrhoids
	CBC, SMAC, UA R/O Div			
	NPO until ambulatory and normal bowels			General Anesthesia hemorrhoids
	Clear liquids			
	now reg diet			
	prn			
	Routine po v.s. continue q 2hr up ambulate			
	with help			
	Keep supine legs 2 hours			
	IV - 0200 / keep running			
Noted 10:15	B100 - Hep lock after oral			
	diet taken			
	PCA - usual post surgical			H&P
	Compazine 10mg			OP Note Dictated

PHYSICIAN'S ORDERS	Another brand of drugs identical in form and content may be dispensed unless checked.	PROGRESS RECORD

continued

Review Case 5-16, *continued*

PHYSICIAN'S ORDERS & PROGRESS RECORD

DATE	ORDERS	✓	DATE	PROGRESS
4/27/xx	IS Cath prn inability to void		4/27/xx	
	E.S. Tylenol every 4 pn for headache			
	Keep IV at 50-75 c after diet decreased to NPO			Afebrile, alert, sterile C&S normal diet as tolerated
	Reviewed labs and elevated C&S Bact qid 30 mg			
	Colace 100 mg			
4/28/xx	DC IV and PCA		4/28/xx	doing well ok sits well and no BM yet
	Demerol 75-100 Two every 3 hours			
	Tylenol III every 3 hours for pain			
	Mon home sits after BM			
4/29/xx	Mom 30c		4/29/xx	
	Home office, follow up - colace Tylenol 3			home BM is able

PHYSICIAN'S ORDERS	**PROGRESS RECORD**

Review Case 5-16, *continued*

ICD-9-CM/ICD-10-CM diagnosis code(s): _____

ICD-9-CM procedure and ICD-10-PCS procedure code(s): _____

MS-DRG: _____

Review Case 5-17

Health Record Face Sheet

Western Regional
Medical Center

Record Number:	23-14-72
Age:	27
Gender:	Male
Length of Stay:	4 Days
Service Type:	Inpatient
Discharge Status:	To Home
Diagnosis/Procedure:	Chemical Burns to Knee

DISCHARGE SUMMARY

PATIENT: Bryson Brighton

ADMIT DATE: 5/11/xx
DISCH DATE: 5/14/xx

PHYSICIAN: Dr. Rauls

ADMITTING DIAGNOSIS: Bilateral chemical burns to the knees.

HOSPITAL COURSE:
Mr. Brighton is a young man who was admitted for bilateral chemical burns of the knee. He under went escharotomy with good results; however, due to the lack of any granulation tissue under the eschar, extensive debridement was required with dressing changes on a daily basis for approximately three days prior to re-excision and cleaning of the wounds and will re-evaluate for a split thickness skin graft. Postoperatively he remained entirely stable. Wounds were clean and dry. The dressings were changed on the third postoperative day. Overnight he remained stable. On the fourth day during dressing changes we rechecked his wound and it showed a slight improvement. We will go ahead and discharge him today with follow-up appointment post hospital day #1 in the Emergency Room, and will discuss graft at this time.

DISCHARGE DIAGNOSIS: Deep third-degree burns of the knees.

continued

Review Case 5-17, *continued*

HISTORY AND PHYSICAL

PATIENT: Bryson Brighton

ROOM #: 414

ADMIT DATE: 5/11/xx

PHYSICIAN: Dr. Lucas

CHIEF COMPLAINT:

HISTORY OF PRESENT ILLNESS:

This young man sustained burns to both knees, chemical in nature, from floor stripper. Attempts at trying to soften the eschar and debride this as an outpatient have been completely unsuccessful. He is now being admitted for further dressing changes and escharotomy with possible grafting.

PAST HISTORY:

CURRENT MEDS:	Hytrin, Xanax, and Fastin.
ALLERGIES:	No known allergies.
SURGERIES:	
MEDICAL ILLNESS:	In good health. No major medical problems.

SOCIAL HISTORY:

He is a one pack per day smoker and he occasionally uses alcohol.

FAMILY HISTORY:

No history of cancer, heart disease, asthma, kidney disease, diabetes or seizures.

REVIEW OF SYSTEMS:

PHYSICAL EXAM:
GENERAL:

HEENT:	Normocephalic, atraumatic. Pupils were equal, round and reactive. Extraocular movements are intact.
NECK:	Supple.
CHEST:	Lungs are clear.
HEART:	Regular rate and rhythm.
ABDOMEN:	Soft, flat, and nontender.
EXTREM:	Entirely normal with the exception of bilateral knees showing a 10 x 12 cm. oval area of full thickness eschar without evidence of surrounding cellulitis. Pulses are 2+ and symmetrical. Deep tendon reflexes are normal.
GU:	Unremarkable
NEURO:	Unremarkable

ADMISSION DIAGNOSIS:

1. Young man with full thickness of burns to the knees.

PLAN:

1. The patient will be admitted to the hospital for dressing changes and hydration.
2. Possible split thickness skin graft, depending on results of escharotomy.

OPERATIVE REPORT

PATIENT: Bryson Brighton

ROOM #: 414

DATE: 5/11/xx

SURGEON: Dr. Lucas

ASSIST: Dr. Rauls

PREOPERATIVE DIAGNOSIS: Third-degree burns of the bilateral knees.
PROCEDURE: Escharotomy with debridement
POSTOPERATIVE DIAGNOSIS:

DETAILS OF PROCEDURE:

The patient was taken to the Operating Room and prepped and draped in typical sterile fashion. Extensively thick eschars in both knees. Attempted to tangentially excise these with a Week blade which was unsuccessful due to the extensive thickness and mummification of the eschar. Subsequently a combination of #15 and #10 scalpel blades were used to completely excise the eschars down to clean subcutaneous tissue. Both sides, however, involved the anterior layer of the prepatellar bursa and this required excision. Patient tolerated the procedure very well and was taken to the Recovery Room in stable and satisfactory condition with the wounds dressed with 4 x 4's and Kerlix sponge. Will keep on Xeroforms, normal saline, and dressing changes and try to stimulate a good granulation bed to allow adequate grafting.

continued

ICD-9-CM/ICD-10-CM diagnosis code(s): _____

ICD-9-CM procedure and ICD-10-PCS procedure code(s): _____

MS-DRG: _____

Review Case 5-18

Health Record Face Sheet

Western Regional
Medical Center

Record Number:	42-16-08
Age:	24
Gender:	Female
Length of Stay:	2 Days
Service Type:	Inpatient
Discharge Status:	To Home
Diagnosis/Procedure:	Salmonella Enteritis

DISCHARGE SUMMARY

DATE OF ADMISSION: 1/22/xx
DATE OF DISCHARGE: 1/23/xx

DISCHARGE DIAGNOSIS:
1. Severe nausea and vomiting, and inability to keep medications down.
2. Reactive arthritis apparently secondary to Salmonella enteritis.
3. Possible gastropathy due to non-steroidal anti-inflammatory drugs.

HOSPITAL COURSE: The patient was admitted through the emergency room with nausea and vomiting, and reported inability to keep her medications down. She had been taking Codeine which was felt to possibly be contributing to her nausea.

Admission lab revealed a white count of 7,800, HCT of 33.7, MCV of 84. The differential revealed 77 segs, 1 band, 12 lymphs, 9 monos, and 1 eosinophil. Rheumatoid factor was negative. Urine HCG was negative. She remained afebrile, and the morning following admission felt markedly improved. She was able to tolerate lunch without difficulty. She required Demerol for service joint pain, but on the morning following admission was placed on Feldene 20 mg. daily. She will be discharged to home for further outpatient follow-up by her rheumatologist, Dr. Wranth in one week.

Discharge medications include Tagamet 400 mg. p.o. b.i.d., Reglan 10 mg. one-half hour before meals t.i.d. and Feldene 20 mg. each morning.

Review Case 5-18, *continued*

ADMISSION HISTORY & PHYSICAL

CHIEF COMPLAINT: 24-year-old female with severe joint pain, nausea and vomiting, unable to take medications.

HISTORY OF PRESENT ILLNESS: One month ago the patient was eating at a local restaurant. A short time later developed nausea, vomiting and diarrhea. The diarrhea became bloody. She was evaluated at the urgent care and apparently grew Salmonella on culture. She was treated with Lomotil and anti-emetics. The diarrhea lasted about 2 weeks and then resolved. A week and a half after the onset of her illness she also developed arthritis in her left knee. There was a history of a tendon repair 3 years earlier. Arthrocentesis at the urgent care raised the question of cocci being present on gram stain and the knee was explored by Dr. Brown. Although there were many white cells in the joint fluid, the cultures were negative. Since that time she has also developed pain in her right knee, both elbows and her right shoulder. She has tried a number of nonsteroidal anti-inflammatory agents including Naprosyn, Ibuprofen and most recently coated Aspirin in conjunction with Tylenol with Codeine. Unfortunately, she has continued to have a lot of nausea and vomiting, and has not been able to keep her medications down very well. She has had no further diarrhea. Some days she does relatively well but other days she is unable to do anything because of the joint pain. There has been no fever or rash. A week ago her right shoulder was injected with corticosteroids by Dr. Brown.

PAST MEDICAL HISTORY: Is otherwise unremarkable except as noted above.

REVIEW OF SYSTEMS: Is also non-contributory.

PHYSICAL EXAM: She is afebrile and vital signs are unremarkable.

HEENT: Unrevealing. Sclera anicteric.
NECK: Supple without masses.
CHEST: Clear.
CARDIAC EXAM: Reveals no murmurs, gallops or rubs.
ABDOMEN: Soft, non-tender and without palpable hepatosplenomegaly or other masses.
EXTREMITIES: She does have healing incision over the left patella. Both knees and elbows are warm to touch but not erythematous. There is also a suggestion of joint effusion. She has decreased range of motion particularly of the elbows. There is also decreased range of motion of the right shoulder. Other joints do not appear to be affected.

IMPRESSION:

1. Apparent reactive arthritis following a salmonella enteritis. Her nausea and vomiting may be due in part to Codeine and to the nonsteroidal anti-inflammatory drugs.

PLAN:

She will be admitted for hydration and treated empirically with Tagament, Reglan and will be placed on Feldene, since this has not been tried to this point.

continued

EMERGENCY DEPARTMENT VISIT

SUBJECTIVE: The patient is a 24-year-old Caucasian female who was previously seen in the Urgent Care. Her chief complaint is multiple joint pains that she has had on and off for several weeks. She indicates that she had a salmonella intestinal infection approximately five weeks ago which apparently then, according to her, developed into a septic knee joint following a star ligamentous reconstructive procedure. Her knee became infected three weeks ago. At that time, Dr. Brown took her to surgery for arthrotomy and irrigation but from the medical records all of the cultures that were obtained of the left knee fluid grew no bacteria. She states that the pain has been persistent and has spread to all different joints. She indicates that she has lost approximately 30 pounds over the last two months. She complains of stiffness, joint pain which is severe. She indicates that she is late with this period and is concerned about possibly being pregnant. She is taking Tylenol #3 and enteric coated aspirin. Both of these medications do not seem to help her with her pain. She has a history of asthma. She does not have any past medical history of rheumatoid arthritis, systemic lupus, or other arthritic conditions. Presently her temperature is 98.5, pulse 92, respirations 20, blood pressure 120/62. Presently her arthritis complaints involve mainly her large joints. She has complaints of pain and swelling in both of her knees and she had the right knee injected with steroid medication at Dr. Brown's office approximately a week and a half ago. She complains of pain and stiffness in both of her elbows and wrists and occasionally in her shoulders. For the most part, the arthritis has not bothered her small joints such as feet and hands.

OBJECTIVE: On physical examination at this time her ENT examination is not remarkable. Her neck is supple. Carotids are full. There is no jugular venous neck distention. Her heart has a regular rate and rhythm and lungs are clear to auscultation in all fields. She has no chest tenderness nor is there any thoracic tenderness to palpation or percussion. Lumbar spine she has some slight pain in the lower lumbar spine but there is not tenderness to palpation or percussion. The abdomen remains soft, flat, and not tender. She has mild swelling of primarily elbows and knees and these joints are also warm to touch compared to the rest of her skin and body surfaces. There is, however, no evidence of erythema anywhere on skin or her joint surfaces. The pain and warmth is also present over her wrists. She does not have any ankle or foot symptoms nor hip or shoulder tonight. So primarily she is knees and elbows.

LABORATORY AND X-RAY: Lab work done tonight included a CBC, sed rate, rheumatoid arthritis factor, ANA, serum pregnancy test and a Lyme Disease antibody. The CBC shows essentially normochromic, normocytic anemia with a hemoglobin of 10.7. There is no elevated white count. Sed rate is significantly elevated to 55, RA is negative. Lyme disease and ANA are pending. HCG is also negative.

The patient is extremely concerned with her inability to keep down foods and fluids and even drinking water today was impossible for her and she states she has not been able to keep down foods or liquids for approximately a four to five day period. She is feeling quite frustrated with the physician's inability to make a diagnosis and give her answers which do not seem satisfactory to her as far as the cause of her multiple joints aches and pain. I discussed her case with Dr. Wise who is on call for the rotating internist, Dr. Marven. We will admit her to the hospital for further evaluation for IV fluid and perhaps better pain control. We started an IV of D5 and half normal saline. We gave her a shot of Mepergan 2 cc intramuscularly. Dr. Wise will follow up with her in the morning.

IMPRESSION: Acute arthritis uncertain etiology.

Review Case 5-18, *continued*

LABORATORY DATA

TEST NAME		RESULT	UNITS	REFERENCE RANGE
TEST OR TEST COMPONENTS OUTSIDE THE ESTABLISHED REFERENCE RANGE				
LYME DISEASE, ELISA	*(01)	1.54		.00– .90
LYME DISEASE, IGM, IFA		TITER LESS THAN 20		LT 20

(01)   LYME DISEASE ANTIBODY, ELISA (INDEX VALUE)
     LESS THAN   0.90 – NEGATIVE
                   0.90–1.25 – EQUIVOCAL
     GREATER THAN   1.25 – POSITIVE

LYME DISEASE ANTIBODY IS NOW PERFORMED WITH A MORE

SENSITIVE ELISA TECHNIQUE THAT DETECTS BOTH IGG
AND IGM ANTIBODIES. IF THE SPECIMEN IS POSITIVE
BY THE ELISA METHOD IT WILL AUTOMATICALLY BE TESTED

FOR IGM ANTIBODY. IN EARLY DISEASE, REACTIVITY IN
THE ELISA TEST MAY BE DUE ENTIRELY TO IGM ANTIBODY.
IN LATER STAGES OF DISEASE, WHEN CARDITIS, NEURITIS

OR ARTHRITIS MAY BE PRESENT, HIGH LEVELS OF IGG ANTI-
BODY ARE USUALLY PRESENT. IGM ANTIBODY MAY OR MAY

NOT BE DETECTABLE AND ITS PRESENCE IS NOT REQUIRED TO
MAKE A DIAGNOSIS OF LYME DISEASE.

continued

Review Case 5-18, *continued*

ICD-9-CM/ICD-10-CM diagnosis code(s): _____

ICD-9-CM procedure and ICD-10-PCS procedure code(s): _____

MS-DRG: _____

Review Case 5-19, *continued*

Health Record Face Sheet

Record Number:	72-06-58	Western Regional Medical Center
Age:	50	
Gender:	Female	
Length of Stay:	2 Days	
Service Type:	Inpatient	
Discharge Status:	To Home	
Diagnosis/Procedure:	MI Cardiac Catheterization	

HISTORY AND PHYSICAL

DATE OF ADMISSION: 7/14/xx

DATE OF DISCHARGE: 7/15/xx

CHIEF COMPLAINT: Recent small myocardial infarction.

HISTORY OF PRESENT ILLNESS: This 50-year-old female patient was transferred from Valley Medical Center for further evaluation, specifically diagnostic cardiac catheterization, after a small myocardial infarction on July 12 and hospitalization until July 14 at Valley Medical Center. This was the patient's first myocardial infarction. Temporary cardiac arrest secondary to ventricular fibrillation was part of the picture.
PAST MEDICAL HISTORY: Hiatal hernia treated with Tagamet.

MEDICATIONS: None at the time taken chronically.

ALLERGIES: To Tetanus vaccine.

REVIEW OF SYSTEMS: Unremarkable.

PHYSICAL EXAMINATION: Blood pressure 112/86, pulse 68 and regular. In general the patient appeared to a 50-year-old female in no distress. HEENT was normal. Chest was clear. Heart normal. Abdomen normal. Breasts normal. Extremities normal.

ASSESSMENT: As above.

PLAN: Diagnostic catheterization.

Review Case 5-19, *continued*

CARDIAC CATHETERIZATION LABORATORY

PROCEDURE REPORT:

PATIENT: Holly Hall

Study Date: 7/14/xx

Medical Record: 72-06-58

Referring Physician: Dr. Carr

REASON FOR STUDY: 50-year-old female who has had a myocardial infarction treated with thrombolytics yesterday.

PROCEDURE: Diagnostic left heart catheterization with selective coronary angiography and left ventriculography.

PROCEDURE STATEMENTS: Following infiltration with 1% Lidocaine topical anesthesia the right femoral artery was catheterized using a Seldinger percutaneous technique and a vascular sheath was inserted. Selective coronary angiography was performed using a JL4 and JR4 catheters. A 7 French pigtail catheter was used for the left ventriculogram. The right coronary artery could not be selectively catheterized using a JR4 and a modified Amplatz was used in its place successfully. Catheters were advanced and withdrawn over flexible guidewire using fluoroscopy and high osmolor contrast. The rhythm was sinus throughout the procedure. The patient tolerated the procedure well. Following the procedure the catheters and sheath were removed and hemostasis was obtained and a pressure dressing and sand bag were applied and the patient was returned to the floor in good condition. There were no complications.

HEMODYNAMIC DATA: The aortic root pressure was measured prior to introduction of contrast. It was then remeasured prior to the left ventriculogram. Aortic root pressure was 128/80 with a mean of 92. Left ventricular pressure was 135/0 with an LVEDP of 14.

CORONARY ANGIOGRAPHY:

LEFT MAIN: The left main coronary artery was normal and bifurcated into a circumflex and anterior descending branch.

LEFT ANTERIOR DESCENDING BRANCH: This vessel was normal throughout as well as the septal and diagonal branches. The LAD extended to the cardiac apex.

LEFT POSTERIOR CIRCUMFLEX: This vessel was completely occluded after a small marginal vessel.

RIGHT CORONARY ARTERY: The right coronary artery had 2 unusual branches. The RCA was dominant. The artery was normal throughout. There was a large right ventricular branch which had its origin at the site of origin or the ostium of the RCA. There was a large atrial branch which was an extension of the distal right coronary artery. There did appear to be a small amount of collateral flow towards the occluded circumflex artery.

LEFT VENTRICULOGRAM: Overall ejection fraction was 66%. There was a small akinetic diaphragmatic area. Valvular function appeared normal.

IMPRESSIONS:

1. Recent small diaphragmatic myocardial infarction secondary to complete occlusion of the circumflex artery shortly after its origin with no reperfusion.
2. Overall normal left ventricular ejection fraction of 66%.
3. Normal left heart valvular function.
4. Normal left anterior descending artery.
5. Normal but unusual right coronary artery with an unusual right ventricular branch and an unusual atrial branch.
6. Small amount of collateralization from the right coronary artery to the circumflex.

continued

Review Case 5-19, *continued*

ICD-9-CM/ICD-10-CM diagnosis code(s): _____

ICD-9-CM procedure and ICD-10-PCS procedure code(s): _____

MS-DRG: _____

Review Case 5-20

Health Record Face Sheet

Western Regional
Medical Center

Record Number:	53-24-11
Age:	68
Gender:	Male
Length of Stay:	6 Days
Service Type:	Inpatient
Discharge Status:	To Home
Diagnosis/Procedure:	Abscess Perineum BPH

Review Case 5-20, *continued*

DISCHARGE SUMMARY

ADMITTED: 4/20/xx

DISCHARGED: 4/25/xx

The patient is a 68-year-old male admitted with acute urinary retention and a draining wound of the perineum. He has had a total proctocolectomy in January by Dr. Blake. He is morbidly obese weighing 330 pounds. He has pulmonary insufficiency related to a Pickwickian's syndrome requiring home oxygenation. He also has hypertension.

On admission his glucose was 264. He had elevation of his SGPT, SGOT, GGTP, all rather mild. Calcium was 10.8. CBC was unremarkable, Prothrombin time and PTT were normal. Blood gases on room air showed a PO2 of 43, PCO2 of 54, PH 7.35. Prostatic specific antigen was 5.7, T4 was normal at 6.5. Intravenous pyelogram Showed a bilateral hydronephrosis secondary to obstructive changes at the bladder level. The chest x-ray showed linear atelectasis. An EKG showed anterior ST-T changes, non-specific. Fistulogram and CT scan showed no evidence of the extension of the fistula into the abdominal cavity.

HOSPITAL COURSE: Initially the patient underwent an incision and drainage of the perineal abscess. Irrigation catheter was left in the abscess cavity and the cavity was irrigated on a daily basis throughout the hospitalization. On 4/21/xx, the patient underwent cystoscopy which showed a large obstructive prostate gland. This was done under local anesthesia.

We felt that he was a significant risk for anesthesia, thus had him seen in consultation by Dr. Myers. On 4/22/xx, the patient underwent cystoscopy and attempt at transurethral resection, but despite adequate relaxation, we could not reach the bladder adequately with the cystoscope to do a transurethral resection. We were fearful that if we encountered a great deal of bleeding it may be impossible to stop. In accordance, he was returned to the operating room on 4/23/xx, and underwent a suprapubic prostatectomy. The procedure was rather difficult but went well. The removed prostate gland weighed 56 grams and showed benign hyperplasia with multiple foci of infarction, no evidence of tumor. Postoperatively he did quite well. His urinary catheter was removed on the third postoperative day and he voided satisfactorily and was discharged home without a catheter.

DISCHARGE MEDICATIONS: 500 mg twice a day.

FINAL DIAGNOSIS:

1. Benign prostatic hyperplasia with secondary bilateral hydronephrosis.
2. Pulmonary insufficiency, oxygen dependent.
3. Hypertension.
4. Perineal abscess.

continued

HISTORY AND PHYSICAL

DATE OF ADMISSION: 4/20/xx

CHIEF COMPLAINT: Draining abscess from the perineum and acute urinary retention.

HISTORY: This 68-year-old white male, referred by Dr. Carter on an acute basis, having been in the hospital since Monday with acute urinary retention requiring Foley catheterization and draining wound of the perineum with purulent material that has been cultured. It was drained for further delineation of the perineal abscess and for consideration of problems with acute urinary retention. The patient's history is significant for total procto-colectomy in January by Dr. Blake with placement of an ileostomy that continues to function without problems. He had responsive ulcerative colitis, treated with maximum conservative therapy. His postoperative course was complicated by development of a perineal hematoma which drained spontaneously. Following this, he has had no problems until recent development of pressure and pain in the perineal and particularly pain in his low back in the sacral region. In addition, he was thought by Dr. Carter to have prostatitis and had been started on Cipro 400 IV along with Flagyl 500 four times a day. The patient spontaneously drained an area in his perineum where the normal rectum would be located. On evaluation here was found to have an opening that would barely admit the tip of the index finger which was probed with a Q-tip to approximately five inches. At the time of admission he had a CT scan which did not show any pelvic masses. The study was difficult, however, in an over 300-pound individual. I requested that Dr. Myers see the patient since he had previously been involved in the patient's problems with his prostate. History is significant for some difficulty with voiding in the recent past. Family reports seeing a staple in the drainage that was purulent in nature from the perineum. The patient also has had two basal cell epitheliomas completely excised from the right nostril and corner of the right eye. He is currently on Vasotec 5 mg daily for hypertension. Has not had any since Saturday.

PAST MEDICAL HISTORY/REVIEW OF SYSTEMS: Allergies to Azulfidine, Sulfa, asparagus and apparently some toothpaste. He has not been on steroids for several years. He also has a right inguinal hernia. he had history of prostatism on occasional basis with nocturia times one or two and there was some urinary hesitancy at that time.

PHYSICAL EXAMINATION: The patient is in some distress secondary to being uncomfortable due to the Foley catheter in place. His Foley catheter seemed to be draining sufficiently. The perineal wound, as indicated above, appears dry.

HEENT unremarkable. Neck is supple. Trachea midline. Thyroid is normal. Lungs are clear. Heart had a regular sinus rhythm, without murmur, gallop or rub. Abdomen is very protuberant. He has a right-sided ileostomy and a right inguinal hernia. Bowel sounds were normal. I could not discern any abdominal tenderness. Extremities are large because of the patient being overweight. He has incisions on both hips from previous bilateral hip prosthesis. Extremities appear viable.

LAB/X-RAY: Admission laboratory shows a white count of 8.8 with a hemoglobin of 13.5, hematocrit of 40.6. The patient has been Pickwickian and he has had blood cell count up into the 50s and has required phlebotomy and his own home O2. PH was 7.35, CO2 54, pO2 43, O2 saturation is 77.6. His glucose was slightly elevated at 264, however, this was nonfasting and communication with his family physician indicates that he has not had any problems with diabetes. BUN and creatinine are normal at 9 and 1.0, respectively. His SGPT was 6.7, OT 38, GPT 135, total protein was low at 5.8, as was albumin at 2.7. Sodium was 137, potassium normal at 4.8. His protime was 10.9, PTT was 31.3.

IMPRESSION:
1. Perineal abscess, status post total procto-colectomy in January, spontaneously drained, with narrow 1 cm opening. This will require placement of drain and additional exploration in the OR.
2. Acute urinary retention likely secondary to prostatic disease. Dr. Myers to consult.
3. Hypertension, treated, currently likely elevated, not on hypertensive medicine since Saturday. Will reinstitute therapy.
4. History of pulmonary disease requiring home O2 with Pickwickian syndrome with previous problems with markedly elevated red blood cell level. Currently stable.

PLAN: To the OR tomorrow for further incision and drainage of perineal abscess.

Review Case 5-20, *continued*

CONSULTATION NOTE

DATE OF CONSULTATION: 4/21

REQUESTING PHYSICIAN: Dr. Griffon

HISTORY OF PRESENT ILLNESS: This 68-year-old morbidly obese white male was admitted for drainage of a perineal abscess and found to have lower tract obstruction warranting TURP. Patient is chronically disabled from dyspnea limiting him to 50–100 feet walk on level ground. This is probably related to his morbid obesity as he has never been treated for chronic obstructive pulmonary disease or heart disease to his knowledge. He has been on continuous home oxygen at 2 liters per minute for the last year for chronic hypoxemia associated with polycythemia. He has not required phlebotomy for polycythemia since he began oxygen therapy. He has a chronic cough productive of about a tablespoon of usually clear sputum per day. He has not had paroxysmal nocturnal dyspnea or orthopnea. He has chronic pedal edema which waxes and wanes. He is a chronic loud snorer but has only mild daytime hypersomnolence. Wife is not present this evening but patient knows of no observed apneas on her part.

PAST MEDICAL HISTORY: Patient thinks he's been on hypertension therapy for about 20 years. He had a colectomy in January for ulcerative colitis. He has had both hips replaced and had a left inguinal herniorrhaphy. He has had basal cell epithelial cancers removed.

OUTPATIENT MEDICATIONS: Vasotec for hypertension.

SOCIAL HISTORY: Patient quit smoking 20 years ago after about 30 years of 1 1/2 packs per day. He was employed in farm work and some warehouse work.

FAMILY HISTORY: Patient's sister and mother died of cancer. He has four other brothers and sisters who have had hip replacement surgery. Father died age 37 of pneumonia.

REVIEW OF SYSTEMS: Negative for kidney disease, peptic ulcer disease, known heart disease, deep venous thrombosis, thyroid disease, hepatitis or liver disease. There is no prior history of pneumonia, hemoptysis and he has never been on medications for breathing difficulties.

PHYSICAL EXAM:

TEMP: 99 degrees. VITAL SIGNS: Stable.
HEENT: Unremarkable.
NECK: Without adenopathy.

continued

OPERATIVE REPORT

DATE OF OPERATION: 4/21/xx

PROCEDURE: With the patient under IV sedation in the left lateral decubitus position, because of his size, the patient had his right-buttock taped to allow adequate exposure of the perineum. After sterile Betadine prep, the area was draped and a mixture of Xylocaine 1% with 1:200,000 and Marcaine 1/2% without Epinephrine mixed 50/50 was injected to block the opening in the perineum. Once this was accomplished, digitalization was accomplished and we were allowed then to put in a proctoscope and the wound was opened to approximately 3 cm. With a head-light we were able to get good visualization of the entire pocket which extended a good five inches. There was no evidence of any clear fluid leaking from any structure nor was there any evidence of visualization from potential bowel. The operative report indicated that the perineum had been closed and the levators had been closed postop. Appears that the head of the very top of the abscess cavity was some bright red bleeding from two areas. These were coagu-lated and controlled. The area was irrigated. There did not appear to be any further abscess cavity. There did not appear to be any abnormal tissue other than the type surrounding a nor-mal abscess. There was no evidence of any tumor and there did not appear to be any further staples or stitches present. A Jackson Pratt drain with most of the tip cut off was placed, since it was soft it was secured in place to allow for irrigations in the postop period. Two packs were placed, one soaked in Betadine, the other Vaseline pack. The Vaseline pack was placed at the top of the wound where the bleeding had been present. The wound was dressed and the patient was returned to recovery with stable normal vital signs.

OPERATIVE NOTE

DATE OF PROCEDURE: 4/21/xx

PREOPERATIVE DIAGNOSIS: Chronic urinary retention and bilateral hydronephrosis.

POSTOPERATIVE DIAGNOSIS: Same.

PROCEDURE: Cystoscopy.

OPERATIVE FINDINGS: The patient has documented chronic urinary retention and bilateral hydronephrosis and is brought to the operating room with intention of doing a cystoscopy and transurethral resection under spinal anesthesia. The patient is a very large patient. He uses oxygen rather continuously. Blood gases show a CO_2 retention level of 54 and a PO_2 level of 46. There was some concern from anesthesia about the safety of an anesthetic and we finally decided to do a cystoscopy under local to see if there is significant prostatism and if we are sure he will need an anesthetic. If so, he will be seen in consultation for his lung problem before subjecting him to an anesthetic.

At local cystoscopy the urethra is very long. It has a rather high bladder neck and I am unable to get the scope entirely into the bladder. Prostatic urethra, however, is long. The prostatic lobes are markedly enlarged and they are significantly obstructive. The rest of the urethra is unremarkable. From the cystoscopy it is obvious that transurethral resection of the prostate gland would be beneficial in helping him void more satisfactorily. Because he has no rectum from a total colon resection in the past, we are unable to know for sure how large the prostate gland is or whether there is any evidence of malignancy.

The procedure was done under 4% Xylocaine anesthetic. The patient will be seen in con-sultation by Dr. Myers and will be returned hopefully tomorrow for a definitive transurethral resection.

Review Case 5-20, *continued*

OPERATIVE REPORT

DATE OF PROCEDURE: 4/22/xx

PREOPERATIVE DIAGNOSIS: Benign prostatic hyperplasia with secondary bilateral hydronephrosis.

POSTOPERATIVE DIAGNOSIS: Same.

PROCEDURE: Cystoscopy and attempted transurethral resection of the prostate gland.

OPERATIVE FINDINGS: This patient is a very large man, 330 pounds. He was cystoscoped the previous day. It was our feeling at that time that with adequate relaxation, transurethral resection of the prostate gland would be possible.

Cystoscopy at this time, however, was initially complicated by a persistent erection. This was relieved by withdrawing blood from the tunica albuginea and injecting a mg of Epinephrine 1000 cc of saline into the penis to relax the erection. Once this was done, we could, with a great deal of pressure, just barely reach the verumontanum with the resectoscope. Because of this, we sent to the other hospital and got the newer resectoscope which is slightly longer and with this we could just barely reach the bladder neck and the bladder itself could never be adequately examined. Prostatic lobes were rather markedly enlarged, did take several bites out of the prostatic tissue beginning the resection, but it became obvious that this would be extremely difficult if we encountered any significant bleeding and we would be unable to control it. We spent approximately an hour and a half attempting this procedure and finally realized that it just was not going to be technically possible and the procedure was terminated. The catheter was replaced. Bleeding was well controlled at this time. The procedure was done under spinal anesthesia.

Arrangements had been made to return the patient to the operating room on the next operative day for prostatectomy realizing that with his large weight, this will also be a difficult procedure.

continued

OPERATIVE REPORT

DATE OF PROCEDURE: 4/23/xx

PREOPERATIVE DIAGNOSIS: Benign prostatic hyperplasia.

POSTOPERATIVE DIAGNOSIS: Same.

PROCEDURE: Suprapubic prostatectomy.

OPERATIVE FINDINGS: The patient is markedly obese, making the procedure extremely difficult. The interior of the bladder was never well seen. The prostate gland, after it was shelled out, was of significant size, perhaps around 50–60 grams, appears to be grossly benign.

OPERATIVE PROCEDURE: Under suitable spinal anesthesia, the patient was placed supine on the operative table, prepped with Betadine and draped for a midline lower abdominal incision. Incision was made from the umbilicus to the symphysis pubis, deepened through a very deep layer of subcutaneous tissues. The fascia layers are finally encountered. These are incised, the rectus muscles are separated, and the bladder is located because it has been distended with normal saline prior to the procedure. Anterior bladder wall is opened through a stab wound which is bluntly enlarged. By this time, the incision is very, very deep. The normal bladder retractor would not suffice in this case. We did manage to get our hand in the prostatic fossa. The prostatic fossa was fractured anteriorly with the dissecting finger, and the prostate gland bluntly shelled from its surgical capsule and removed. Fortunately there was not much bleeding following its removal, because we were unable to see the interior of the bladder well, and certainly could not see the bladder neck for any stitch placements. We were unable to see either ureteral orifice because of the depths of the incision. A #24 French 30 cc. catheter was placed in the bladder with 40 cc. within the balloon. The bladder was closed using interrupted 0-Chromic around a #28 French Malecot catheter which was brought out through the incision. Wound was closed using #1 Vicryl for approximation of the linea alba. Multiple layers of 3–0 Vicryl for subcutaneous approximation and skin clips for skin approximation. Irrigation showed the hemostasis is adequate.

ESTIMATED BLOOD LOSS: 100 cc.

OPERATING TIME: 2 hours, which is approximately twice the normal length for this procedure.

The patient tolerated the procedure well, and left the operating room in good condition.

PATHOLOGY REPORT

SUPRAPUBIC PROSTATECTOMY
PROSTATE

GROSS: Submitted as a suprapubic prostatectomy specimen. Specimen is a lobulated pink-tan structure weighing 56 gm and measuring 5.5 x 5.0 x 3.5 cm. It is grossly characteristic of prostate. On cut surface it is multinodular. Small areas of reddish-purple nodularity are seen also on cut surface ranging in size from 1.0 to 0.5 cm. Representative portions of these sites and adjacent parenchyma are submitted for examination.

MICROSCOPIC: Multiple sections reveal prostatic tissue demonstrating adenofibromatous hyperplasia. Scattered lymphocytes and plasma cells are seen throughout some surrounding acinar structures. The areas of reddish-purple discoloration are consistent with infarction. These areas are characterized by necrosis and hemorrhage.

DIAGNOSIS:

Adenofibromatous hyperplasia of the prostate, chronic prostatitis, mild, multiple foci of infarction.

continued

Review Case 5-20, *continued*

ICD-9-CM/ICD-10-CM diagnosis code(s): _____

ICD-9-CM procedure and ICD-10-PCS procedure code(s): _____

MS-DRG: _____

Review Case 5-21

Health Record Face Sheet

Western Regional
Medical Center

Record Number:	17-39-43
Age:	64
Gender:	Female
Length of Stay:	4 days
Service Type:	Inpatient
Discharge Status:	To Home
Diagnosis/Procedure:	Bilateral L3-4 Stenosis L4 Laminar Hypertrophy
	Bilateral partial L3 laminectomy Bilateral L4-5 decompression

Review Case 5-21, *continued*

HISTORY & PHYSICAL

DATE OF ADMISSION: 3/13/xx

She has persistent right lower extremity numbness and weakness and also on physical exam today has inability to perform left heel walk, therefore, early left lower extremity weakness. She has been previously fully evaluated in the hospital with lumbar myelogram and CT scan after myelogram and has elected operative intervention and accepts banked blood.

PHYSICAL EXAM: Chest was clear to percussion and auscultation. Heart without murmur or cardiomegaly. Abdomen obese, soft, with active bowel sounds without palpable liver, spleen masses or tenderness.

IMPRESSION:
1. Bilateral moderate L3-4 lateral recess stenosis, L4-5, severe posterior facet and L4 laminar hypertrophy and regrowth with right greater than left lateral recess stenosis, with severe side to side pinching of the thecal sac, right more severely than left; widely patent canal at L5-S1 with gas in the right floor consistent with right L5-S1 disc herniation anterior to the S1 root, right L5-S1 posterior facet capsule or scar at posterior; lateral aspect of the right S1 root, scar and/or facet capsule behind the left S1 root without definite left root entrapment.
2. 14 plus years status postoperative L4, and L5 laminectomies, bilateral L4-5 diskectomy, right L5-S1 exploration without diskectomy on the right, with now new right L5-S1 floor of canal gas since CT lumbar scan from Valley Medical Center on 3/1/xx, consistent with new right L5-S1 disc herniation not present in past years.

PLAN:
1. Bilateral partial L3 laminectomy, bilateral L4 and L4-5 re-decompression with possible diskectomy, bilateral or just right L5-S1 re-exploration and probable right L5-S1 diskectomy as per operative findings.
2. She accepts banked blood.
3. We again discussed broad categories of risks. She noted wound infection with hysterectomy but not with cholecystectomy. I will plan prophylactic antibiotics as is my standard for low back operations.

continued

OPERATIVE NOTE

DATE OF PROCEDURE: 3/14/xx

PROCEDURE PERFORMED: Bilateral partial L3 laminectomy, bilateral L4 and L5 re-laminectomies, bilateral L3-4 decompression without diskectomy, bilateral L4-5 and L5-S1 re-decompressions without diskectomy, with microscope × 5 hours and 47 minutes.

SURGEON: Dr. Redi
ASSISTANT: Dr. Nichols

PREOPERATIVE DIAGNOSIS: 14+ years status post operative L4 and L5 laminectomies bilateral L4-5 diskectomy, right L5-S1 exploration without diskectomy on the right with now gas in the right floor of the canal consistent with right L5-S1 disk herniation. Bilateral moderate L3-4 lateral recess stenosis, L4-5 severe posterior facet and L4 laminar hypertrophy and regrowth with right greater than left lateral recess stenosis, bilateral L5-S1 posterior facet and/or scar overhang.

POSTOPERATIVE DIAGNOSIS: Same, except only slight central and rightward L5-S1 annulus relaxation without definite disk herniation.

OPERATIVE FINDINGS: Prior L4 and L5 laminectomies were noted with epidural scar from L3-4 to S1, especially severe at the right L4-5 level involving the right L5 and S1 root sleeves posteriorly and laterally. There was severe regrowth of the L4 lamina and lesser regrowth of the L5 lamina with bilateral L4-5 lateral recess stenosis, right more severe than left. L3-4 annulus was flat and normal. L4-5 scar/annulus was firm and flat with minimal stepoff. There was slightly central and rightward L5-S1 annulus relaxation without definite disk herniation. No disk resection was thought indicated at L5-S1. Bilateral L3-4 lateral, recess stenosis was caused by posterior facet overgrowth, right more severe than left. Bilateral L5-S1 posterior scar and facet overgrowth caused lateral recess stenosis bilaterally.

PROCEDURE: Under general endotracheal anesthesia with legs wrapped from toes to groins with Ace wraps and with Foley catheter in the urinary bladder, the patient was turned prone on the Wilson frame and the frame flexed. Sponge rubber pads were placed under the face with great care taken to protect the eyes and to support the head so head was not dangling excessively. Arms were placed on sponge rubber pads from elbows to the hands and anterior axillas were free of the frame. Care was taken not to hyper-abduct or hyper-elevate the arms. Sponge rubber pads were placed under the knees and pillows beneath the shins. Safety strap was passed across the posterior thighs. Back was shaved, prepared and draped after marking out a midline incision excising the old lumbar scar in elliptical fashion.

Skin incision was infiltrated with a total of 18 cc's 1/2% Xylocaine with 1:200,000 Epinephrine and skin incision made sharply. Hemostasis was obtained with Bovie. Subcutaneous fat was divided in the midline and lumbodorsal fascia divided in the midline from inferior margin of residual L3 spinous process to superior tip of S1 spinous process. Kocher clamp was placed on this evident most inferior L3 spinous process, and lateral portable spine X-ray documented this to be L3.

Midline scar was then divided down to the laminar level and then scar incision extending in inverted T fashion to the lateral margins of the laminae on each side at L4 and L5. Muscle scars were stripped off L3 lamina and spinous process and off superior S1. Using sharp periosteal dissection, superior margin of S1 was freed of scar tissue and the epidural space entered laterally. Epidural scar was then cleaved upward along the L5 lamina, until lamina began to deviate medially indicating some regrowth. The L4 lamina was markedly regrown with a thin central ribbon of scar filling the residual central gap. Outer cortices of inferior L3 lamina were shaved down with heavy bone instruments and bone waxed with bone wax. Inferior margin of L3 spinous process was amputated and edge waxed with bone wax.

Review Case 5-21, *continued*

OPERATIVE NOTE - Page 2

Using a 5 mm. high speed diamond bur drill, bilateral inferior partial laminectomies were carried out at L3 with the right posterior facet noted to be more bulbous than the left. L3-4 facet capsule was stripped off the dura first on the left and then on the right. This gave access to normal dura above. Similarly, scarified dura had been exposed interiorly at the superior margin of SI. A 5 mm. diamond bur drill was then used to drill a trough connecting the exposed normal dura superiorly at L3 and the exposed scarified dura inferiorly at S1 with that trough carried down on each side through the L4 and L5 laminae where necessary and the L4-5 posterior facets. After this initial trough was placed, the binocular operating microscope was brought into the field and remainder of dissection carried out under microscopic magnification.

Using 3 mm. and then 2 mm. high speed diamond bur drills, vertical lateral channels were drilled from superior L4 to inferior L5 on each side drilling into the more lateral bone over the lateral recesses and leaving the more medial bone which was densely encased in scar and markedly adherent to dura for later removal. Central slivers of posterolateral bone were then removed after blunt and sharp dissection removing the residual bone slivers from epidural scar and from the outer aspect of the dura directly. Drilling was carried out into the inferior articulating facets at L4 and superior articulating facets of L5 to give wide lateral recess decompression. Posterior scar was sharply lysed and meticulous hemostasis obtained on posterolateral scar with bi-polar coagulation. Decompression was carried laterally and inferiorly until the L4 root sleeve was completely uncovered, from its origin at the dura to its exit point at the L4-5 foramen and the L5 root sleeve was similarly uncovered from its origin on the dura to exit at the L5-S1 foramen on each side. Particularly adherent and bulky scar was noted on the right side at L4-5. This scar was meticulously sharply dissected off the dura to allow dural expansion posteriorly and root sleeve expansion posteriorly. No dural injury was caused. A small rectangle of Gelfoam soaked in Thrombin was left in the posterior axilla of the right S1 root sleeve for scarified dural hemostasis.

Epidural explorations were carried out first on the left at L3-4, L4-5 and L5-S1 and then on the right. On the left at L3-4, annulus was firm, hard and flat. Right angle nerve hook exploration laterally and inferolaterally revealed no lateral protrusions. Dura and root sleeve were allowed to fall back in anatomic position. On the left at L4-5 annulus/scar was firm and flat with minimal palpable, stepoff. No disk re-resection was indicated. Right angle nerve hook exploration laterally and inferolaterally revealed no lateral protrusions and no lateral fragments. Dura and root sleeve were allowed to fall back in anatomic position. Exploration on the left at L5-S1 revealed annulus slightly relaxed with no definite disk herniation. No disk resection was thought indicated. Right angle nerve hook exploration laterally and inferolaterally revealed no lateral protrusions. Dura and root sleeve were allowed to fall back in anatomic position.

Exploration on the right at L3-4 revealed firm, flat annulus and widely patent foramen on right angle nerve hook exploration with no lateral or inferolateral protrusions. Dura and root sleeve were allowed to fall back in anatomic position. Exploration on the right at L4-5 revealed extensive and densely adherent epidural scar involving the L5 and S1 roots posteriorly and laterally. This was meticulously cleaved off the dura as noted and removed giving wide posterior decompression. L4-5 scar/annulus was firm and flat with minimal stepoff and no disk re-resection was thought indicated. Right angle nerve hook exploration laterally revealed no lateral protrusions. Inferolaterally there was still residual lateral adherent epidural scar. Dura and root sleeve were allowed to fall back in anatomic position. Exploration on the right at L5-S1 revealed slight central and rightward annulus relaxation with no frank herniation. Epidural hemostasis was obtained with bi-polar coagulation and this actually caused some shriveling and flattening of the slightly prominent annulus. No disk resection was thought indicated. Right angle nerve hook exploration laterally and inferolaterally revealed no lateral protrusions and no lateral fragments.

After drilling and removal of facet tissues and posterolateral scar, dura expanded markedly throughout its course essentially filling available space with thin residual slivers of epidural space between dura and lateral drill margins over the extent of the resection. At this point there was no epidural bleeding. A U-shaped piece of Gelfoam soaked in Thrombin with a transverse band at inferior L3 and a long sliver in the lateral gutter from L3 to SI was then placed in the epidural space without compression of the dura.

continued

Review Case 5-21, *continued*

OPERATIVE NOTE - Page 3

Wilson frame was taken out of flexion. Muscle self-retaining retractor blades were removed and hemostasis obtained on muscle with Bovie. A 10 mm Jackson-Pratt drain was placed in the epidural space behind the central scarified dura and brought out through a stab wound at right inferior sacral area several centimeters below the skin incision. Drain was temporarily ligated in the stab wound with 2-0 silk sutures and sutured to skin with a 2-0 silk suture. Deep scarified muscle was closed with interrupted 0 Vicryl sutures with great care taken not to entrap the drain. Scarified lumbodorsal fascia was closed with interrupted 0 Vicryl sutures with great care taken not to entrap the drain. Drain was kept at bulb suction. Fat was closed in two layers with deep interrupted inverted 0 Vicryl and superficial interrupted inverted 2-0 Vicryl sutures incorporating subcuticular tissue in the outer layer. Skin was closed with running/locking 3-0 nylon.

Adaptic 4×4 and Elastoplast with tape frame pressure dressing was applied. The patient was turned supine, extubated and transferred to the recovery room in satisfactory condition.

OPERATIVE TIME: 8 hours and 5 minutes.

ESTIMATED BLOOD LOSS: 200 cc's. The patient received 2700 cc's lactated Ringer's in the operating room.

At termination of the case she dorsiflexed ankles and toes with pin to each sole and with pin to the bottoms of the 5th toes bilaterally.

PATHOLOGY REPORT

PATIENT: Hiliary Hill

MEDICAL RECORD: 17-39-43

DOCTOR: Dr. Redi

OPERATION: BILATERAL PARTIAL L3 LAMINECTOMY, LATERAL LEFT L4-L5 DISC DECOMPRESSION L5-S1 DISKECTOMY, LAMINA, MISCELLANEOUS TISSUE, SKIN SCAR

AGE: 64

DATE: 3/14/xx

GROSS: Submitted from L5-S1 are portions of pink-tan tissue which appear to be comprised of both bone and soft tissue and together measure approximately 3.5 cm. Also present is a strip of skin and subcutaneous tissue grossly containing old scar formation. The strip measures 10.5 cm. in length x 0.5 cm. in width x 1.3 cm. in maximum depth. Representative portions of the bone are submitted for decalcification and subsequent examination. Representative portions of the soft tissue are submitted for examination.

MICRO: Sections through skin and subcutaneous tissue reveal old scar formation. Additional sections reveal trabecular bone together with fibrocartilage. The fibrocartilage reveals severe degenerative change. No nerve tissue is identified.

Skin and subcutaneous tissue with old scar formation, removed in the course of surgery.
Fibrocartilage (intervertebral disc) with severe degenerative change.
Trabecular bone and associated soft tissue, removed in the course of laminectomy.

continued

Review Case 5-21, *continued*

ICD-9-CM/ICD-10-CM diagnosis code(s): _____

ICD-9-CM procedure and ICD-10-PCS procedure code(s): _____

MS-DRG: _____

Review Case 5-22

Health Record Face Sheet

Western Regional
Medical Center

Record Number:	17-33-41
Age:	74
Gender:	Female
Length of Stay:	3 days
Service Type:	Inpatient
Discharge Status:	To Home
Diagnosis/Procedure:	Spinal Stenosis
	Lumbar Myelogram
	Bilateral partial L3 laminectomy
	Bilateral L4-5 decompression

DISCHARGE SUMMARY

ADMISSION DATE: 11/1/xx

DISCHARGE DATE: 11/3/xx

DIAGNOSIS:

1. High grade severe multi-level spinal stenosis with far lateral disk herniation L3-4.
2. Multi-level degenerative disk disease.
3. Degenerative scoliosis.

OPERATIONS & DIAGNOSTIC PROCEDURES PERFORMED: Lumbar myelogram.

HOSPITAL COURSE: 74-year-old female admitted for the above diagnostic procedure performed without difficulty or incident. Patient appeared to have little difficulty postoperatively. Had slight headache and was given a caffeine drip for this. This slowly passed.

She was discharged in stable condition to return to the office for reassessment anticipating spinal surgery in approximately 2 weeks.

COMPLICATIONS: Post myelogram spinal headache.

DISPOSITION: Caffeine drip, bed rest, fluids.

ADMISSION HISTORY & PHYSICAL

ADMISSION DATE: 11/1/xx

72-year-old female brought in at this time for diagnostic lumbar myelogram. See attached records. She is admitted primarily for diagnostic purposes. No operation is planned at this point for high grade spinal stenosis suggested by a preoperative CT scan.

IMPRESSION: Spinal stenosis, high grade, admitted for lumbar myelogram.

LUMBAR MYELOGRAM

HISTORY: Low back pain.

LUMBAR MYELOGRAM:

Correlation was made with a previous MRI study. After consent was obtained, a lumbar puncture was performed at level L1-2. Clear spinal fluid was easily obtained and sent to the laboratory for analysis. Following this, 18 cc. of 180% Iohexol was injected.

There is a fairly high grade block at L3-4. The patient was placed in an upright position for 15 minutes. Finally a small amount of contrast managed to drain down into the end of the thecal sac.

Again, there is lack of contrast from L3-4 to L5-S1. With the underlying scoliotic deformity, this is consistent with a high grade spinal stenosis. Again, the majority of block is probably at L3-4.

With the patient upright for another 15 to 20 minutes, there is a little bit better filling of the distal end of the thecal sac. At L5-S1, the configuration of the sac is grossly within normal limits. No definite extradural defects are seen at L5-S1. Again, there is very minimal if any contrast identified from the mid portion of L3 to the lower portion of L5. This is probably displaced, secondary to spinal stenosis changes.

Superiorly at L2-3, there is a very prominent central bulge. This is fairly broad based, and probably represents changes related to degenerative spurring and relaxation of the annulus. The L1-2 level is relatively intact views of the conus are within normal limits.

Patient did not have any complications after the procedure.

IMPRESSION:

High grade block at L3-4, extending past L4-5. Central bulging at L2-3, relatively unremarkable L5-S1 level.

continued

Review Case 5-22, *continued*

ICD-9-CM diagnosis code(s): _____

ICD-10-CM diagnosis code(s): _____

MS-DRG: _____

Review Case 5-23

Health Record Face Sheet

Western Regional
Medical Center

Record Number:	58-16-17
Age:	25
Gender:	Female
Length of Stay:	2 days
Service Type:	Inpatient
Discharge Status:	To Home
Diagnosis/Procedure:	Term Pregnancy Cesarean Section

Review Case 5-23, *continued*

OBSTETRIC DISCHARGE SUMMARY

Ginny Gray

Patient Name

Date of admission : *10-15-xx*

Date of discharge : *10-17-xx*

Procedures intrapartum
- ☐ Spontaneous vaginal delivery
- ☐ Vacuum assisted delivery
- ☐ Forceps assisted delivery
- ☐ Episiotomy
- ☒ Cesarean section
- ☐ Induction/augmentation of labor
- ☐ _____

Complications
- ☒ None
- ☐ _____ Perineal laceration
- ☐ (Vaginal) (Cervical) laceration
- ☐ Pelvic infection
- ☐ Urinary infection
- ☐ Pulmonary infection

Discharge diagnosis
- ☒ Term pregnancy - delivered
- ☐ False labor - undelivered
- ☐ Preterm labor - delivered/undelivered
- ☐ PROM X _____ hours _____
- ☐ PIH
- ☐ UTI
- ☐ _____
- ☐ _____
- ☐ _____

Other _____

discussed pp depression _____

Admitting diagnosis
- ☒ Active labor
- ☐ Induction
- ☐ Cesarean section
- ☐ Preterm labor
- ☐ Observation
- ☒ *Prev c/s* _____

Procedures postpartum
- ☐ None
- ☐ Rh_0(D)Ig   *RH +*
- ☐ Rubella Ig
- ☐ Tubal Ligation
- ☒ Antibiotics   *A Cord e/imp*
- ☐ _____

- ☐ Wound infection
- ☐ PIH
- ☐ Hemorrhage
- ☐ Dysfunctional labor
- ☐ _____
- ☐ _____

Discharge information
- ☐ Medications *Ib, Tylenol, PNV*
- ☐ Return visit *2 weeks*
- ☐ Activity *routine C/S*
- ☐ H & H *36*

Newborn information
- ☒ Female   ☐ Male

Weight *5-12* _____

continued

SHORT FORM
HISTORY & PHYSICAL

HISTORY		PHYSICAL	
Reason for Admit or Hx of Present Illness	Admit Date	Heent	*WNL (within normal limits)*
Previous C/S	*10-15-xx*		
Active labor		Heart & Lungs	*CTA / RRR with 2/6*
		Breast	*c/s*
		Abdomen	*Gravid - non-tender*
Surgery	*C/S, BURCH, Appy*		
		Genitourinary	*No distress or tenderness*
			Cx 2 cm, thick
Allergies	*Ingesine / PCN*	GYN	*Increased presacral tenderness*
Transfusions		Extremities	*sym*
Medications	*PNV Synthroid .125*	Neurological	*DTR 2/4*
Prior Med Hx: (Inc Immunizations for Children) *Usual*		Vascular	*c/s*
		Skin	*c/s*
Significant Family Hx: *Mom - DVT*		Lymphatic	*Mod edema*
Cancer *MGM - DVT* *Neg W/V*			
Heart *Sister- DVT*		Musculoskeletal	*c/s*
Social Hx: Smoker Alcohol			
Pertinent Review of Systems - Cardiovascular		Rectal	
BP P Lungs		Assessment *Pregnancy at term*	
WT HT		*Active Labor*	
Respiratory		Plan *Previous C/S (cesarean section)*	
COPD		Contraindications	
Asthma			
TB			
Other: Seizures		Informed Consent	
CVA			
Diabetes		*For IP Surgery On*	
Kidney		Comprehensive H & P Dictated:	
Hx of Anaesthetic or Coagulation Problems		Signature: *Dr. Smart* Date: 10/15/xx	

Review Case 5-23, *continued*

MOTHER INTRAPARTUM

MEMBRANES RUPTURED	MONITORING		DATE	TIME	COMPLICATIONS	☐ Elevated Mat. Temp _____

MEMBRANES RUPTURED
TIME_____
LOR AT DEL._____

MONITORING
☐ FSE   ☐ IUPC
☑ EXTERNAL
☐ INTERMITTENT

ONSET OF LABOR
COMPLETE DILATION
DELIVERY TIME
PLACENTA TIME

COMPLICATIONS   ☐ Elevated Mat. Temp _____
☐ ABRUPTION   ☐ PREVIA   ☐ PROLAPSE CORD
☐ STILLBORN   ☐ MULTIPLE BIRTHS X _____
☐ OTHER _____
FHR. _____

TIME	MEDICATION DOSE	RT	SITE	NURSE SIG

2ND STAGE

PRESENTATION: _____

☐ SPONTANEOUS   ☐ SHOULDER DYSTOCIA   ☑ FORCEPS   ☐ ROTATION
☐ VACUUM EXTRACTION:
EPISIOTOMY: ☐ NONE   ☐ ML   ☑ OTHER
LACERATION: ☐ NONE   ☐ PERINEAL   ☐ 1⁰   ☐ 2⁰   ☐ 3⁰   ☐ 4⁰
   ☐ SULCUS _____   ☐ CERVICAL _____
   ☐ OTHER _____
☐ URINARY CATH-TIME _____
ANESTHESIA: ☐ NONE   ☑ LOCAL   ☐ PUDENDAL   ☐ PARACERVICAL   ☐ EPIDURAL
ANESTH _____
REMARKS: _____

(handwritten diagonal: C-sect)

V A G I N A L

TIME	BP	PULSE	RESP	FUNDUS	FLOW

OBSERVATIONS: *delivery viable female*
per C/S

3RD STAGE

PLACENTA   ☐ SPONTANEOUS   ☐ MANUAL   ☐ INTACT   ☐ FRAGMENTED   ☐ CURRETAGE
ABNORMALITIES OF PLACENTA: _____
   ☐ EBL>500 CC
REMARKS: _____

TRANSFER TIME: *TO SURG 1615*

RN SIGNATURE

INFANT

APGARS	1	5
HEART RATE		
Absent 0		
Below 100 1	2	2
Over 100 2		
RESP EFFORT		
Absent 0		
Slow, 1 Irreg 1	2	2
Strong Cry 2		
REFLEX STIM		
No Response 0		
Grimace 1	2	2
Cough Sneeze 2		
MUSCLE TONE		
Flaccid 0		
Some Flexion 1	1	2
Well Flexed 2		
COLOR		
Pale Blue 0		
Body Pink w/		
Blue Extremit. 1	1	1
All Pink 2		
TOTAL	8	9

SEX: ☐ M   ☑ F
BAND# _0421_

WEIGHT _____ GMS
_6_ LBS. _12_ OZ.
LENGTH _41.0_ CM _19_ IN.
☐ VOIDED   ☐ STOOL

RESUSCITATION
SUCTION
☐ Prior-deliv. shoulders
☐ Bulb
☐ Delee _____ CC
   Color _____
☐ O₂ _blow by_
☐ Bag & Mask

☐ CORDS VISUALIZED
☐ INTUBATION
By _____

☐ ANOMALIES*

NURSE'S SIGN.: _____

INFANT INTERIM OBSERVTION

TIME	COLOR	TEMP	RESP	ACTIVITY
1313	Pink	warm	strong cry	MAE

OBSERVATIONS: *Delivery viable female per C/S - cry spontaneous lungs clear with cry. pink with cry and blow by O2 Active strong cry Double wrap to nursery per Dad's arms with nurse in attendance*

ATTENDING PHYSICIAN'S EXAM

INFANT

	NL	OTHER
HEENT		
HEART		
CHEST		
ABDOMEN		
GU		
EXTREMITIES		
REFLEXES		
Physician Sig.		

MOTHER

WAS PT MONITORED?   ☑ Yes   ☐ No
FHM PATTERN OBSERVATION:
☐ Late decels   ☐ Early decels   ☐ Variable decels
☐ Bradycardia   ☐ Tachycardia   ☑ NL/Reassuring

EVALUATION:

Physical Exam is unchanged from that recorded in the office prenatal record with the exception of term gravid uterus.

CORD	TIME	MEDICATION/DOSE	RT	STE	NURSE SIG
VESSELS: ☑ 3 ☐ 2	1350	Vit K	IM	L (leg)	
NUCHAL CORD _____					
☐ OTHER _____					
☑ CORD BLOOD SENT					
☐ CORD pH _____					
(IF INDICATED)					

Transfer Time to Nursery: *1343*

DELIVERY RECORD

continued

OPERATIVE REPORT

PATIENT NAME: Ginny Gray

DATE OF ADMISSION: 10/15/xx

ROOM #: 250

SURGERY DATE: 10/15/xx

SURGEON: Dr. Smart
ASSIST: Dr. Petty

PREOPERATIVE DIAGNOSIS: Pregnancy at term, previous cesarean section, and active labor.

POSTOPERATIVE DIAGNOSIS: Pregnancy at term, previous cesarean section, active labor, and significantly attenuated lower uterine segment.

OPERATIVE PROCEDURE:

ANESTHESIA:
ESTIMATED BLOOD LOSS: 700 cc.
IV FLUIDS: Crystalloid replacement.
DRAINS: .   Foley catheter
SPECIMENS: None.

HISTORY:
 Ginny is a 25-year-old multiparous female, status post cesarean section status post VBAC, who presented with contractions, presacral pain, and poorly presenting cephalad fetus at a high station. After reviewing options, she opted again for elective cesarean section as had been discussed in the office. After discussing pros and cons, given her previous cesarean section status and her previous Burch status, informed consent was obtained, understanding the risks of infection, bleeding, damage to associated organs, transfusion, and anesthetic risks.

INTRAOPERATIVE FINDINGS:
 Very attenuated lower uterine segment.

DESCRIPTION OF OPERATIVE PROCEDURE:
 With the patient under conduction anesthesia and in dorsal supine position she was suitably prepped and draped with left lateral tilt. Bladder drained by Foley catheter. A transverse suprapubic skin incision was made going through the previous cicatrix. This was carried through the scar to the anterior fascia, entered sharply, and transversely. This was dissected from the underlying rectus muscles, which were dissected along the midline and the abdominal cavity was entered sharply. The vesicouterine plicae was dissected inferiorly and a uterine incision was made on the scar and margins extended transversely. Fluid was clear and fetus' head was delivered through the incision and suctioned per oropharynx and nasopharynx. Body delivered, cord doubly clamped, sectioned, and neonate transferred to warmer with Dr. Adoles in attendance. Apgars were vigorous. Cord samples were obtained and placenta was delivered intact manually. The intrauterine cavity was curetted with dry lap sponges, irrigated, and the scar debrided and approximated the uterine incision with a running and locking suture of #1 Vicryl. The scar was then imbricated. All operative sites were evaluated and found to be hemostatic. The adnexa were evaluated without adhesions or abnormalities. Irrigation was carried out. All operative sites were again evaluated and when counts were correct, the rectus muscle was closed in the midline and the fascia closed with #0 PDS and the subcutaneous space approximated with absorbable sutures. The skin edges were approximated with skin staples. Dressing applied.

 The patient was placed in the lithotomy position. Cervix and vaginal vault evacuated of clots and debris. Both patient and neonate went to the Recovery Room in stable condition.

Review Case 5-23, *continued*

ICD-9-CM/ICD-10-CM diagnosis code(s): _____

ICD-9-CM procedure and ICD-10-PCS procedure code(s): _____

MS-DRG: _____

Review Case 5-24

Health Record Face Sheet

Western Regional
Medical Center

Record Number:	05-14-36
Age:	40
Gender:	Male
Length of Stay:	2 Days
Diagnosis/Procedure:	Acute Intoxication with Isopropyl Alcohol
Service Type:	Inpatient
Discharge Status:	To Home

continued

DISCHARGE SUMMARY

DATE OF ADMISSION: 12/20/xx
DATE OF DISCHARGE: 12/21/xx

PRESENT ILLNESS:

This 40-year-old man who has a long history of alcoholism was admitted to the hospital after a 30-day binge of heavy drinking terminated by drinking rubbing alcohol. Please see admission history and physical for further details.

HOSPITAL COURSE:

The patient was admitted and given IV rehydration. He had quite a bit of vomiting after ingesting the isopropyl alcohol. He was treated with IM Thiamine and given multiple vitamins. The ativan was used IM and then PO for sedation. He was treated with Amoxicillin for a bronchitis. He is a heavy smoker. The patient showed rapid improvement. The day of discharge he was feeling a lot better. He had had some nightmares the night before but no hallucinations or seizures. He was feeling well enough to go home. He was having some diarrhea, probably secondary to alcohol withdrawal and maalox therapy.

The patient was given alcohol counseling prior to discharge to discuss outpatient treatment options.

COMPLICATIONS: None.

FINAL DIAGNOSIS:

1. Acute intoxication with isopropyl alcohol.

SECONDARY DIAGNOSIS:

2. Alcoholism.
3. Bronchitis.
4. Heavy cigarette smoking.

PLAN:

The patient was discharged to stay with his mother. The patient was left up to himself to arrange for outpatient alcohol treatment. He was given written discharge instructions concerning diet, activity, medications, and follow-up. He is usually seen by Dr. Carver and was advised to see him in follow-up as needed.

DISCHARGE MEDICATIONS:

1. Zantac 150mg 1 bid #15.
2. Amoxicillin 500mg 1 tid #21.
3. Ativan 1mg 1 g 6–8 hours prn severe nervousness #10.
4. Imodium 2 stat and one after each loose stool up to 6 per day #15.

Review Case 5-24, *continued*

HISTORY & PHYSICAL

DATE OF ADMISSION: 12/20/xx

PRESENT ILLNESS:

This 40-year-old man came to the emergency room brought in by his family with a history of drinking rubbing alcohol. He has a history of chronic alcoholism going back many years. He said he had been doing reasonably well over the past 6 years although he has had a few bouts of heavy drinking. He started a drinking binge this last time 30 days ago and was using 2 fifths a day of whiskey plus 1 case of beer per day. He ran out of money and so started drinking the rubbing alcohol. He developed severe gastric distress with a lot of vomiting and so came to the hospital and wanted a "medical withdrawal" from his alcoholism. At the time of admission he was not interested in an inpatient program because of lack of funds. He said that he had been through "a dozen" inpatient alcohol programs in the past years. Last program was the County rehab program at the County facility. He said that he has had DT's when withdrawing from alcohol in the past. He thought he may have had a seizure several years ago also.

MEDICATIONS: None.
ALLERGIES: None

PAST MEDICAL HISTORY:

CHILDHOOD ILLNESSES: None unusual.
ADULT ILLNESSES: The patient says he has had PAT in the past but this hasn't apparently been a problem. He thinks it might have been related to his drinking.
PREVIOUS SURGERY: Right radial head excision and tonsillectomy.
TRAUMA: Fractured right elbow.
SMOKING: 2–3 packs per day.
ALCOHOL: As above.
SUBSTANCE ABUSE: The patient uses marijuana about once a month. Denies use of other drugs in the past including IV drugs.

FAMILY HISTORY:

His father died from an MI at age 60. There is diabetes in the family. Mother is diabetic and has had multiple surgeries. He has 2 brothers who are alcoholic.

REVIEW OF SYSTEMS:

The patient has had a cough and congestion for several weeks. The rest of the review of systems is negative.

SOCIAL HISTORY:

The patient is married for the second time. He has 3 children and his wife has 3 children. He is working as a county mill worker but hasn't actually been working for the last 30 days. That is when he started drinking. He has lived in town his entire life. He has a high school education plus a couple of years of college about 10 years ago. He is of the Catholic faith.

PHYSICAL EXAM:

At 11 o'clock on Friday I examined the patient. He was somewhat sedated since he had just gotten some IM Ativan. He was in no distress at the time and was fully oriented. He could give a reliable history.
VITAL SIGNS: See chart.
HEENT: Normocephalic, TM's are clear. Eyes – PERRL, EOM's intact without nystagmus.
MOUTH & THROAT: Negative.
NECK: Supple without masses.
CHEST: Clear to A&P. A large tattoo is present on his chest.
HEART: Regular rhythm without murmur.
ABDOMEN: Soft and nontender without masses.
GENITALIA: Normal male without hernia.

continued

Review Case 5-24, *continued*

HISTORY & PHYSICAL—PAGE 2

RECTAL: Showed no masses, and a normal prostate. Stool is present and hemoccult negative.

EXTREMITIES: No edema or deformity. The patient could stand unassisted but was a little wobbly and weak.

IMPRESSION:

1. Alcoholism with 30-day relapse.
2. Recent ingestion of isopropyl alcohol.
3. Heavy cigarette smoking.
4. Bronchitis.
5. History of PAT.

PLAN:

See orders.

EMERGENCY ROOM NOTE

Chuck is a 40-year-old white male who presents on 12/20/xx. He is a patient of Dr. Carver who has asked me to evaluate the patient. He is here primarily for alcohol withdrawal. He wants to go acute detoxification in the hospital, he does not want to be admitted to an inpatient rehabilitation program because he has been through the county program before. He cannot afford to be in an inpatient rehabilitation program. We are also concerned because today he drank 3/4 of a bottle of rubbing alcohol, that's one pint of rubbing alcohol. He has done this in the past, but now he is profoundly nauseated, he is vomiting frequently, and retching as well. He drank this at about 3:30 this afternoon. He is not sure if he had other alcohols today, but in the past 30 days he has been drinking 3–4 fifths of hard liquor, along with beer, daily. He has a history of alcoholism in the past, history of paroxysmal atrial tachycardia. Presently he is on Tranxene. Apparently this was given to him by Dr. Carver according to his family, and the family gave him one of these today. Now he is here in the emergency room requesting admission for acute detoxification. He is not aware of ever having had withdrawal seizures in the past, but says that he certainly goes through some violent alcohol withdrawal.

EXAMINATION: Presently his temperature is 98.4, pulse 96, respirations 20, blood pressure 162/84. In the emergency room he is retching and vomiting clear material, there is no blood in it. He has not vomited any blood today with all the vomiting since he ingested the rubbing alcohol. He has not had any ulcers or melanotic or black or tarry stools. Again, his ENT examination other than red faces, he does not appear to be in any acute distress when he is not vomiting. His neck is supple. Carotids are full and symmetrical. His heart has a regular rate and rhythm without murmurs or extra heart sounds. Lungs are clear to auscultation in all fields. His abdomen has epigastric tenderness but no significant masses or organomegaly. He has not had pancreatitis in the past.

The family and the patient request admission at this time. I contacted Dr. Bryner and kept him in the emergency room for a two-hour period, to make sure that he still would like to be admitted to the hospital, and at one time he indicated that he wanted to go home, but then I advised him that certainly he could do whatever he wanted to. I told him that his current road was towards a suicidal death from intoxication, and he agreed to be admitted to the hospital to Dr. Bryner's service. We gave him 2 mg. of Ativan intramuscularly in the emergency room, along with Thiamine 100 mg, started an I.V.

His lab work had been done, which included a CBC, SMAC, serum ketones and a urinalysis. He had serum and urine ketones. Otherwise he really did not have remarkable other abnormalities.

We started an I.V. of D5/half normal saline with Mag. sulfate 2 grams, to run 150 m and he was admitted to the medical floor to the care of Dr

IMPRESSION: Acute isopropyl alcohol ingestion, and chronic history of alcoholism.

continued

Review Case 5-24, *continued*

RADIOLOGY REPORT

HISTORY: Wheezing. Isopropyl alcohol ingestion.

CHEST:

The lungs are clear. There is no pneumothorax or pleural effusion.

Cardiac, hilar, mediastinal and other structures normal.

IMPRESSION:

Normal. No change since chest x-ray six months ago

DIAGNOSTIC IMAGING

ICD-9-CM/ICD-10-CM diagnosis code(s): _____

ICD-9-CM procedure and ICD-10-PCS procedure code(s): _____

MS-DRG: _____

Review Case 5-25

Health Record Face Sheet

Record Number:	09-43-18	Western Regional Medical Center
Age:	34	
Gender:	Male	
Length of Stay:	2 days	
Service Type:	Inpatient	
Discharge Status:	To Home	
Diagnosis/Procedure:	Refractory Vomiting Diabetes Insipidus	

Review Case 5-25, *continued*

DISCHARGE SUMMARY

PATIENT: Donald Deboy

ADMIT DATE: 4/14/xx
DISCH DATE: 4/16/xx

PHYSICIAN: Dr. Craig

ADMISSION DIAGNOSIS: Refractory vomiting.
DISCHARGE DIAGNOSIS: Diabetes insipidus.

HOSPITAL COURSE:

The patient is a 34-year-old white male seen in the Emergency Room for inhaling, he said, sulfuric acid. He had refractory vomiting for quite some time. He was often confabulatory and the family had noted that he has been quite ill since a head injury in 2006, where he had been run over by a roller coaster. He had been prescribed three potassium pills per day but they had not given him a clear diagnosis. Further analysis on delving into the history and talking with his family revealed that he has a history of diabetes insipidus. He has no other past medical history. Evidently his GI tract had been severely irritated.

On the second day after admission pH had dropped considerably from the original 7.73 to 7.53. Creatinine had been high originally but stabilized and decreased slowly. PC02 was originally 7.73 and went to 7.54, and 7.53 down to 7.5 just before discharge. Urine toxicity screen was negative. No other abnormalities were noted.

He was restarted on his potassium on 4/15/xx orally with good efficacy. He was taking fluids and taking oral intake well with no significant problems or diarrhea. Nausea had abated. There were no further problems noted.

DISPOSITION:

He was released to the care of his family to follow up at the Clinic in 1 week with myself.

continued

HISTORY AND PHYSICAL

PATIENT: Donald Deboy

ROOM #: 4104

ADMIT DATE: 4/14/xx

PHYSICIAN: Dr. Craig

CHIEF COMPLAINT: Inhalation of sulfuric acid fumes.

HISTORY OF PRESENT ILLNESS:

Patient is a 34-year-old white male seen here today at the Emergency Room. Parents said that he inhaled sulfuric acid earlier today and was coming in by private car. He arrived approximately one hour later, doing well, and in no apparent distress. Blood pressure 110/70, pulse 120, respiratory rate 18, 02 saturation 100%, temperature 97.6.

He was alert. Skin was normal and dry. Normal demeanor, and normal face.

PAST HISTORY:
CURRENT MEDS:
ALLERGIES: Penicillin gives him hives.
SURGERIES:
MEDICAL ILLNESS: Significant only for a head injury in 2006, evidently run over by a roller coaster, for which he received a metal plate in his head. He now has iatrogenic diabetes insipidus from this for which he takes three potassium pills per day of an unknown dose. Other past medical history reveals when he was 8 years old he had pneumonia. He was also admitted to the ICU for the head injury six years ago, and subsequent to that, about 4 years ago, was admitted to the medical floor here for an episode of vomiting similar to the one witnessed today.

SOCIAL HISTORY:

He lives at home with parents currently. Smokes one-half pack of cigarettes per day. Occasional alcohol use. Mother says he drinks a lot a beer.

FAMILY HISTORY:

Mother is 60 years old with no health problems. Father is 67 and has had a stroke, Type 2 diabetes, and hypertension. His stroke was six months ago.

REVIEW OF SYSTEMS:

As noted previously. Family notes he does have quite a few confabulatory episodes. He lies about quite a few different things and but most of the information he had given me had been fairly true, although they said there were some discrepancies which they corrected readily.

PHYSICAL EXAM:
GENERAL:
HEENT: No problems in the oropharynx or around the eye. Extraocular movements are intact. Pupils were equal, round and reactive to light. Conjunctiva are normal. Normal mucosal surfaces of the mouth and nose.

NECK: Unremarkable
CHEST: Chest is clear to auscultation bilaterally.
HEART: Regular rate and rhythm, no murmur, occasionally going up to a higher heart rate of 120 and then back down again. No abnormalities noted on the EKG or the electronic strip.
ABDOMEN: Benign.
EXTREM: Unremarkable
GU: Unremarkable
NEURO: No focal neurological deficits. Deep tendon reflexes are 2/2. No focal neurological deficits. Good strength in the hands and arms.
MENTAL: Mini-mental status examination is 28/33 with five off for memory. He also is disoriented as to time but he states this is a common occurrence.

Review Case 5-25, *continued*

HISTORY & PHYSICAL PAGE—2

LABORATORY:
>   In the Emergency Room, EKG with sinus tachycardia with mild elevations in the P waves but none outside the normal limits. Glucose 125, BUN 9, creatinine 2.5, sodium 149, potassium 3.5, chloride 101, calcium 10.3, phosphorus 2.3, pH 7.73, pCO2 20, pO2 85, bicarbonate 28, 02 saturation 98% showing chloride responsive alkalosis, probably from the vomiting, and diabetes insipidus concomitantly. White count is 7.8, H & H is 17 and 49, platelets at 300.

ADMISSION DIAGNOSIS:
>   1. Vomiting, possibly due to sulfuric acid fumes and irritation of the GI tract vital signs respiratory tract, currently refractory to Phenergan at this time.
>   2. Iatrogenic diabetes insipidus from trauma.
>   3. Mental status deficiencies not yet characterized, possibly due to head injury.
>   4. Chloride responsive metabolic alkalosis secondary to #1.

PLAN:
>   1. We will replace electrolytes, control his pH disturbance and electrolyte disturbance with normal saline and with potassium, rapidly correcting this while monitoring his fluid status and control of his vomiting should produce leveling of his metabolic deficiencies.
>   2. Further workup will be detailed as the patient comes back to normal. Hopefully he will be discharged in the morning with only minor delay.

EMERGENCY ROOM REPORT

PATIENT: Donald Deboy

DATE: 4/14/xx

TIME: 06.00 p.m.

PHYSICIAN: Dr. Craig

....

S: Patient is a 34-year-old white male seen here in the Emergency Room today for refractory vomiting. Evidently he was working with some sulfuric acid at his place of employment when he contracted a large whiff of the fumes and was breathing it at about 5:30 this morning. There were significant problems. Immediately he was removed from work and he was not able to continue. He has had significant vomiting, from that time for about 12 hours without significant relief.

O: On physical examination, patient is a thin white male. Blood pressure 110/70, pulse 20, respirations 18, 02 saturation 98%, temperature 97.6. He is evaluated between vomiting episodes in the Emergency Room. HEENT examination is within normal limits. He does have a severe scar over the frontotemporal region of his head. He says he has a lead plate in there. No clubbing, cyanosis, or edema of the extremities. Cranial nerves are intact. Neurologically he is intact. Chest is clear to auscultation bilaterally. Heart is tachycardiac at 120 bpm. He does have a very jerky affect which may be due to an electrolyte imbalance. He says that he has been on Potassium only as a medication.

A: Chemical inhalation.

P: We will admit him to the hospital at this time pending laboratory results because of the severity of his inhalation and with his history of the instability of his electrolytes. We will monitor him closely over the next few hours and see how his symptoms progress. If there is no detailed derangement we will release him in the morning.

ICD-9-CM/ICD-10-CM diagnosis code(s): _____

ICD-9-CM procedure and ICD-10-PCS procedure code(s): _____

MS-DRG: _____

SECTION THREE

Advanced Coding

In this section, students are assigned physician office charts, outpatient hospital charts, and inpatient hospital charts to code. Students are given real-world medical records and must apply what they learned in Section II to the documentation provided.

Chapter 6 **Advanced Physician Office Coding**

Chapter 7 **Advanced Outpatient Hospital Coding**

Chapter 8 **Advanced Inpatient Hospital Coding**

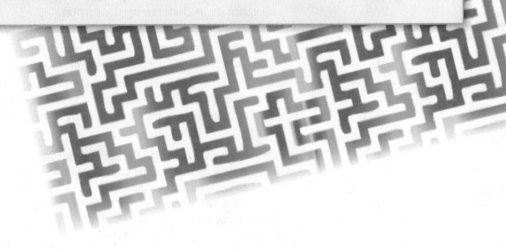

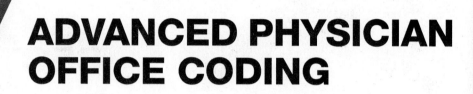

ADVANCED PHYSICIAN OFFICE CODING

6

Physician office coding is unique due to the different types of settings in which a physician may provide services to a patient. The most recognized setting is the physician's office. Other settings include, but are not exclusive to, acute care inpatient, same-day surgery, long-term care inpatient, and home health settings. A physician office professional coder must be able to code the applicable diagnoses, procedures, and evaluation and management (E/M) codes that each unique setting requires. The professional coder is also responsible for reporting modifiers and following other third-party healthcare plans according to each setting's reporting guidelines.

For all cases presented in this chapter, apply all of the coding skills and knowledge you have to do the following:

1. Assign and sequence the primary ICD-9-CM and ICD-10-CM diagnosis codes first, followed by applicable secondary diagnoses to include appropriate V-code and E-code assignment as dictated by the setting.

2. Assign and sequence the primary CPT procedure code first, followed by applicable additional procedure codes to include modifiers as appropriate. Modifiers may include CPT Level 1 and/or HCPCS Level II as dictated by the setting.

3. Utilize CMS National Correct Coding Initiative (NCCI) edits when assigning codes in this chapter. NCCI edits are utilized to promote national correct coding methodologies and to control improper coding, which leads to improper payments for Medicare Part B.

Instructions for accessing the official outpatient coding guidelines online and web links to CMS for official outpatient setting regulations and guidance appear in Appendix A of this text. Instructions for accessing the E/M guidelines online appear in Appendix C of this text. Utilize the cited resources and reference information to jump start your physician office coding tasks.

Case 6-1

Physician Office Face Sheet

Western Medical Clinic

Record Number: 05-61-74

Age: 37

Gender: Female

Patient Status: Established Patient

Diagnosis/Procedure: Acute Sinusitis

VISIT 2

S: Myra is here with a chief concern of sinus congestion and discharge. This has been going on for about the last week. She got up this morning and said that her chest hurt. She was coughing and having some difficulty breathing. She is having difficulty breathing through her nose. She was treated by Dr. Ramsey last week for a thrombosed external hemorrhoid. She continues to smoke and says that she is not ready to quit because she likes it too much.

O: VITAL SIGNS: Weight is 236. Temperature is 96.4, blood pressure 100/74. Pulse is 84, respirations 16. GENERAL: she is a pleasant woman who appears somewhat fatigued. EYES: Mild conjunctival injection, no discharge. ENT: Nasal mucosa is beefy red and swollen with green rhinorrhea. Mild posterior pharyngeal erythema. Tympanic membranes normal in color and landmarks. LUNGS: Clear to auscultation throughout. No crackles or wheezes. She is breathing comfortably. 02 saturation is 93% on room air.

A: Acute sinusitis in the setting of continuous smoking.

P: I prescribed Zithromax 500 mg daily for three days and promethazine/codeine 6.25/10 per 5 ml, 5 ml by mouth every four to six hours as needed for cough, #6 ounces with no refill. I also strongly encouraged smoking cessation, Follow-up on this issue will be for failure of symptoms to resolve or any worsening symptoms.

Electronically authenticated by: Howard Johnson, M.D.

ICD-9-CM diagnosis code(s): _____

ICD-10-CM diagnosis code(s): _____

CPT code(s) with modifier, if applicable: _____

Physician Office Face Sheet

Western Medical Clinic

Record Number: 14-31-88

Age: 68

Gender: Female

Patient Status: Physician Office

Diagnosis/Procedure: Oral Bleeding Post Tooth

SUBJECTIVE: Helen is here following her hospitalization on Saturday through Tuesday at Eastern Valley Medical Center. She had persistent oral bleeding after her upper teeth extractions. Her INR was apparently above 4 when she was hospitalized. She required two units of packed red blood cells. An oral surgeon saw her and performed some stitches with absorbable material in her mouth. She is not describing any chest discomfort, palpitations or difficulty breathing. She said she has felt a little woozy, but is doing better.

MEDICATIONS
1. Coumadin dose is 2.5 mg daily
2. She is also on Lovenox until her INR is greater than 2.5
3. Aspirin 81 mg daily
4. atorvastatin 80 mg daily
5. metoprolol 50 mg twice daily
6. lisinopril 10 mg daily
7. furosemide 40 mg daily
8. Niaspan 1000 mg each bedtime
9. Potassium chloride 10 mEq daily

OBJECTIVE: Weight is 220 1/2. Temperature is 97.1. Blood pressure 122/68. Pulse 65. Respirations 16.

GENERAL: She is a pleasant woman resting in no acute distress. Lungs are clear to auscultation. No crackles or wheezes. Cardiac regular with a mechanical heart valve closure sound. ENT, she has large sutures in place in her upper gums and there is just a small amount of oozing in the right upper suture.

ASSESSMENT: Oral bleeding after tooth extraction requiring transfusion in the setting of chronic Coumadin therapy for mechanical mitral valve.

PLAN: Repeat INR today. She needs to continue Lovenox until her INR is greater than 2.5. She will follow up though the office and the nurses to make sure that this goal is achieved and is aware that I will be out of the office until

Electronically authenticated by : Howard Johnson, M.D.

Case 6-2, *continued*

ICD-9-CM diagnosis code(s): _____

ICD-10-CM diagnosis code(s): _____

CPT code(s) with modifier, if applicable: _____

Case 6-3

Physician Office Face Sheet

Western Medical Clinic

Record Number:	56-44-58
Age:	55
Gender:	Male
Patient Status:	Established Patient
Diagnosis/Procedure:	Low Back Pain

S: Mark is here today with a chief concern of low back pain. He said that he has not had any recent back injuries, but over 20 years ago he strained his back lifting a trailer up by the tongue. He also said that over 20 years ago he had x-rays done as part of an employment situation, where he was told that he had lumbar spine arthritis. He said over the last few months that he has had worsening pain in the lumbar spine that radiates across his pelvis. He said it feels like a lot of pressure like bones are being pushed together. He says that he has intermittent numbness and tingling down both legs, though not at the same time. He denies any bowel or bladder incontinence. He said he called Dr. Grovett's office to see if he could get an appointment, but was told he needed to see his primary care doctor first. He would like a referral to Dr. Grovett.

O: VITAL SIGNS: His weight is 315 pounds, temperature 96.6, blood pressure 126/68, pulse 80, and respirations 16. GENERAL: He is a pleasant gentleman resting in no acute distress. MUSCULOSKELETAL: Low back examination shows no pain or muscle spasm with palpation. Negative straight leg raise bilaterally. No obvious motor abnormalities in his lower extremities.

A/P:
1. Low back pain. I do think that his history, especially of the paresthesias, is concerning. I have ordered a lumbar spine x-ray and a lumbar spine magnetic resonance imaging and he would like to have a referral to a neurosurgeon following that test.
2. Hypertension, currently well-controlled. I have given him a requisition to have some tests including a lipid profile, basic metabolic panel, AST, ALT, and TSH. We will also check a PSA as well.
3. Follow up will be initially by phone later this week regarding his lab tests and subsequent referral.

Electronically authenticated by: Roger Batt, M.D.

continued

Case 6-3, *continued*

Examination	**Lumbosacral Spine**
Exam Date	9/9/xx
Comparison Study	None
Clinical information	Low Back Pain. Lower Extremity Paresthesias

---

Findings: The pertinent positive and negative findings are as follows:

- AP, lateral and oblique views
- Five non-rib-bearing normal height vertebral bodies
- Disk spaces normal height
- Moderate hypertrophic degenerative changes around the anterolateral margins of the vertebral bodies
- Posterior elements intact
- Mild to moderate facet joint arthropathy in the lower lumbar spine
- Alignment unremarkable
- No recognizeable recent traumatic changes
- Faint calcification in the abdominal aorta

Impression: Moderate Multilevel Degenerative Changes

Radiologist: Paula Tipton, D.O.

Electronically authenticated by: Paula Tipton, D.O.

Case 6-3, *continued*

Examination   **MRI Lumbar Spine**
Exam Date   9/9/xx

Comparison Study   None
Clinical information   Low Back Pain with Lower Extremity Paresthesias

---

Technical Data:

- Sagital Inversion Recovery, TI and T2 weighted images
- Axial TI and T2 weighted images

Findings: The pertinent positive and negative findings are as follows:

- Vertebral bodies normal height
- Normal signal intensity in the vertebral marrow
- Disk spaces normal height
- General configuration of the bony spinal canal normal
- Spinal cord terminates normally over upper lumbar spine
- Dural sac normal configuration
- Nerve root sleeves unencumbered
- No focal disk protrusion or extrusion
- Hypertrophic degenerative changes around the anterolateral margins of the vertebral bodies
- Mild facet joint arthropathy in the lower lumbar spine
- No significant hypertrophy of the ligamentum flavum
- Paraspinous soft tissues unremarkable

Impression: Mild Multilevel Degenerative Changes

Radiologist: Paula Tipton, D.O.

Electronically authenticated by: Paula Tipton, D.O.

ICD-9-CM diagnosis code(s): _____

ICD-10-CM diagnosis code(s): _____

CPT code(s) with modifier, if applicable: _____

Case 6-4

Physician Office Face Sheet

Western Medical Clinic

Record Number: 98-00-54

Age: 1

Gender: Female

Patient Status: Established Patient

Diagnosis/Procedure: Serous Otitis Media

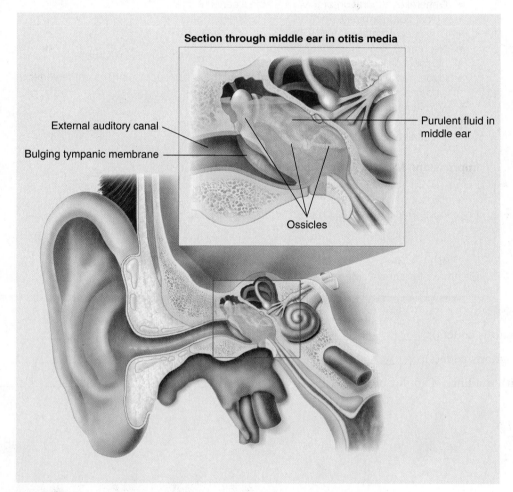

Otitis media.
Source: Pearson Education/PH College

Case 6-4, *continued*

S: Riley is here for evaluation of ear pain. Mom said that she holds her ears all the time. She is sleeping well. She does not nap, but she sleeps through the night. She is not having fever. She is kind of fussy. She really has not had a runny nose, cough, or signs or symptoms of allergies.

0: VITAL SIGNS: Her weight is 23 pounds 11 ounces. Her temperature is 98.1, pulse 110, and respirations 20.

GENERAL: She is a vigorous child in no acute distress. EYES: No conjunctival injection. No icterus. ENT:

She has profuse clear rhinorrhea. The tympanic membranes are normal in color with normal light reflex, but there is the appearance of clear fluid behind them. No significant injection or erythema. No oropharyngeal lesions, erythema, or exudate. NECK: Supple. No lymphadenopathy. LUNGS: Clear to auscultation. No crackles or wheezes. She is breathing comfortably.

NEUROLOGIC: Normal strength and tone. Age-appropriate neurologic examination.

A/P: Serous otitis media (otitis media with effusion). I explained to mom that I do not see any indication for antibiotics, but that we should try antihistamines to see if we can improve the fluid behind her ear. Mom is also going to give her a pacifier frequently to see if that will help equalize the pressure as well. Follow-up will be with me as scheduled for her next well visit sometime next week. She will return sooner if there are any problems in the interim.

Electronically authenticated by: Chris Nichols, M.D.

ICD-9-CM diagnosis code(s): _____

ICD-10-CM diagnosis code(s): _____

CPT code(s) with modifier, if applicable: _____

Case 6-5

Physician Office Face Sheet

Western Medical Clinic

Record Number:	97-14-63
Age:	15 Months
Gender:	Male
Patient Status:	Established
Diagnosis/Procedure:	Croup

continued

SUBJECTIVE: A 15-month male here with his mother and older brother with two-to-three day history of clear rhinorrhea, fevers to 101° as well as a croupy cough. No vomiting or diarrhea. Appetite is decreased. He is taking fluids well and has normal wet diapers. He has had some mild rhinorrhea recently which mother attributes to allergies. His older brother has now developed a similar barky cough. No smoke exposure. Mother works as a preschool teacher and the boys go with her and are in daycare during those timeframes. They just returned from vacation a couple of days ago.

OBJECTIVE: VITAL SIGNS: See flow sheet. Temperature 97.6. GENERAL: Alert male in no distress. EYES: No conjunctival infections. TMs are clear though there is some mild erythema along the superior aspect of the right TM though everything else is normal. Nares, some swelling with minimal amount of clear drainage. Oropharynx, mucous membranes are moist with no erythema or exudates. NECK: Supple without adenopathy. LUNGS: Clear. There is no tachypnea or respiratory distress. HEART: Regular without murmur. Skin: Warm and dry with good turgor and brisk capillary refill.

IMPRESSION: Croup

PLAN: We discussed croup with mother and we will have her continue to use humidifier and continue to push fluids. Tylenol p.r.n. We also discussed dexamethasone including that it is usually beneficial in moderate-to-severe cases though his appears to be fairly mild at this point. However, mother would like to go ahead and try the dexamethasone as he has not improved much in the last two to three days. Thus, we will treat him with a single 0.6 mg/kg dose (his weight is 28 pounds) (12.8 kilo) and thus we will treat him with 7.5 mg. Mother would also like to give him his flu shot now which is reasonable, shot is given today. Call or follow up should symptoms worsen or persist or for any other issues or problems.

Electronically authenticated by: Barbara Rudford, M.D.

ICD-9-CM diagnosis code(s): _____

ICD-10-CM diagnosis code(s): _____

CPT code(s) with modifier, if applicable: _____

Case 6-6

Physician Office Face Sheet

Western Medical Clinic

Record Number: 04-19-38

Age: 72

Gender: Male

Patient Status: Established

Diagnosis/Procedure: Anxiety
                            Left Chest Wall Pain

S: This is a 72-year-old male here to discuss some problems he had with hydrocodone pain pills. I had seen him 6 days ago for an aggravation of his left chest wall pain. Tylenol #3 had not helped prior to that, and thus I gave him hydrocodone/acetaminophen 10/500 mg (see my note from 6 days ago). He took 2 pills at a time and took several doses in the first 24 hours or so after our visit. However, he then seemed to develop some anxiety and pressure in his head and generally did not feel well. Thus he stopped the hydrocodone and took just ibuprofen alone. He then stopped the ibuprofen a day or so after that. He has felt much better in the last 2 days, and the symptoms have resolved. In looking back, he tells me the symptoms are the same as the panic attacks he used to have before he was on Lexapro (and he has been on that for over 2 years now). No fevers, chills, or cough. The discomfort in his left chest wall is much better as well. He currently rates it about a 2/10 and it is not bothersome. He is sleeping well. He had also been on ranitidine, though he stopped that last week as well.

O: VITAL SIGNS: See flow sheet. Temperature is 97.2. GENERAL: Alert male in no distress. He is not anxious currently. Mood and affect are normal. CHEST: He has some very slight tenderness over the left chest wall at about the anterior axillary line, though it is much less than last week.

A:
1. Anxiety.
2. Left chest wall pain, improving.

P: The increased dose of hydrocodone seemed to contribute to some anxiety, which is now resolved. He will continue with his Lexapro 20 mg daily, which I did refill today. He does take lorazepam 0.5 mg at bedtime—I have told him that he can take an extra dose as needed throughout the day should he have any further panic attacks, though I doubt that will be the case. If he does need the pain medication down the line, we will still likely use hydrocodone, though would use the lower 5/325 mg dose (which he had taken before last week, though it was just not quite enough for his pain). I reviewed this with him, and he understands and agrees.

Electronically authenticated by: James Jeffries, M.D.

continued

Case 6-6, *continued*

ICD-9-CM diagnosis code(s): _____

ICD-10-CM diagnosis code(s): _____

CPT code(s) with modifier, if applicable: _____

Case 6-7

Physician Office Face Sheet

Record Number:	77-08-11	Western Medical Clinic
Age:	84	
Gender:	Female	
Patient Status:	Established	
Diagnosis/Procedure:	Foot Pain DM	

Case 6-7, *continued*

S: This is an 84-year-old female here with her husband with complaints of pain in her feet and legs. She describes it as a constant dull ache, and it is worse at night. No real numbness and denies a burning quality to the discomfort. She has had the same issues off and on for many years according to her husband, though it has been worse in the past couple of weeks, as best I can tell, particularly worse in the last 2 or 3 days. No falls. No fever, chills, cough or swelling in her legs. The discomfort is not worse with walking. She does have long-standing diabetes. In reviewing her medications, she has now quit her gabapentin. She had been on that since about late April for postherpetic neuralgia. It helped quite a bit, and her neuralgia progressively improved. Thus, she stopped the gabapentin about 3 weeks ago. She has been somewhat dizzy off and on as well, and it was an issue yesterday though not at all a problem today. She was seen at the urgent care a couple of weeks ago with some shakiness and some dizziness. A repeat TSH at that point was normal at 4.24. She also had a CBC and comprehensive metabolic panel in early May which were stable, and an abnormal urine microalbumin with a subsequent 24-hour urine which showed a creatinine clearance of 40 and a glomerular filtration rate of 40 but a normal 24-hour protein. She has had some slight discomfort in her right elbow at times recently and has had some tingling and possibly slight swelling of her lower lip in the last few days.

O: VITAL SIGNS: See flow sheet. Weight is 136.4 pounds, which is stable for a visit with me in May, and blood pressure is 136/60. GENERAL: Alert female in no distress. There is no swelling or redness of her lips. LUNGS: Clear. HEART: Regular rate and rhythm, with a 3/6 systolic murmur, which is unchanged. ABDOMEN: Soft and nontender. EXTREMITIES: No edema. No skin breakdown on her feet, and feet are not cool to touch. Distal pulses are palpable in her feet. A 10-gram monofilament testing is 7/10 on the right and 6/10 on the left. No pain with palpation over her feet or legs.

A: Lower extremity/foot pain bilaterally, due to neuropathy.

P: I suspect her symptoms are due to peripheral neuropathy, due to her underlying diabetes. We talked about the options, and for now, we will have her restart the gabapentin 300 mg at bedtime for 4 days and then increase to 300 mg twice daily. She had tolerated this well when she was on it recently for the shingles. She will let me know if she has ongoing symptoms or has no benefit at all from the gabapentin. Otherwise, I have asked that she see me again in about 6 to 8 weeks, though certainly sooner for any other issues or problems as well.

Electronically authenticated by: Chris Nichols, M.D.

ICD-9-CM diagnosis code(s): _____

ICD-10-CM diagnosis code(s): _____

CPT code(s) with modifier, if applicable: _____

Case 6-8

Physician Office Face Sheet

Western Medical Clinic

Record Number: 16-46-55

Age: 50

Gender: Male

Patient Status: Established Patient

Diagnosis/Procedure: DOT Physical Examination

SUBJECTIVE: The patient is here for DOT physical. DOT form was filled out with a copy included in the patient chart. The patient is diabetic and we have not seen him in a year and a half. I kind of read him the riot act today. I told him that that is not okay to go so long without follow-up and he needs to assure consistent and regular follow-up visits to successfully manage his diabetes. The goal is to assure that the patient has good control of his diabetes. I reminded him that diabetes is the #1 cause of blindness, kidney failure and amputations.

In addition to his diabetes, he is overweight and has high blood pressure. There is not any laboratory work for him in over a year and a half, and that is just not medically okay. I reviewed all of his diabetes care with him. I encouraged him to work on weight loss as well. I made a goal for him to be down to 200 pounds by the time we see him in regular follow-up in three and a half months. The patient's blood pressure is a little high at 136/72. It has been a little high every time he comes in for the new diabetes recommendations, running in the 30s/70s. I added hydrochlorothiazide 25 mg a day to his regimen of Lisinopril 20 mg daily. I warned him this new drug would cause him to urinate a little bit more and hopefully, it will get his blood pressure down.

The patient is on an ACE inhibitor. He is taking an aspirin. He is on glipizide 10 mg twice daily, Metformin 1000 mg twice daily, and Avandia 4 mg twice daily. He received a pneumonia shot today. I encouraged him to get a flu shot every year. The patient does not smoke. He does not drink. He is married. He farms for a living, so he is very active there.

OBJECTIVE: On examination, all is listed on the D.O.T form. The patient does have an umbilical hernia, which he has had for twelve years. It does not seem to bother him. The umbilical hernia is not reducible, and I am honestly not convinced that it is a hernia. It may just be some other kind of a cyst or something around his umbilicus because it is completely non-reducible and has been non-reducible for a long time. It does not really bother him so I am just going to follow that along for now.

ASSESSMENT/PLAN:

1.   D.O.T. physical. Official form is completed.

2.   Diabetes with unknown degree of control. I ordered laboratory work on him including a hemoglobin, urine for protein, and creatinine. We will check his cholesterol, his liver test, and we will do a PSA as well and notify him of all of those results. I encouraged him to get an eye examination because he has not done that in a year. We did do a foot examination today, and he has normal sensation and good pulses. No sores on his feet. Other than that, he is on the ACE inhibitor and aspirin and good medications for his diabetes so we will follow.

3.   Hypertension. Inadequately controlled today given that he is diabetic. I am going to add hydrochlorothiazide 25 mg to his lisinopril and we will follow.

4.   Obesity. I encouraged him strongly to work on weight loss. Really at 5 foot 4 inches, he should weigh closer to 150 pounds. I encouraged him to start working on a 10-pound weight loss between now and when we see him in follow-up in approximately four months.

5.   We will see him back again in about four months, and we will go from there. I did tell him that I was not going to refill his medications for more than four months at a time so that I can use that to make him come back in here and get checked out.

Electronically authenticated by: Chris Nichols, M.D.

continued

Case 6-8, *continued*

ICD-9-CM diagnosis code(s): _____

ICD-10-CM diagnosis code(s): _____

CPT code(s) with modifier, if applicable: _____

Case 6-9

Physician Office Face Sheet

Western Medical Clinic

Record Number: 85-14-99

Age: 77

Gender: Male

Patient Status: Established

Diagnosis/Procedure: Abnormal skin lesions
Shave biopsy

S: This is a 77-year-old male here to have a lesion checked on his right forearm. He has noticed it in the last 2 months or so, and it has been growing fairly rapidly. It has not bled and does not bother him at all. No other recent skin issues. He does have a history of basal cell skin cancers on his nose and cheek back in May. He feels well and has no other issues or concerns.

O: VITAL SIGNS: Elevated blood pressure. GENERAL: Alert male in no distress. SKIN: Examination of his right forearm shows a lesion on the radial aspect of the proximal part of the forearm. It is 4 mm in size and is about 2 cm raised. It is slightly red and irritated appearing, though there is no ulceration.

A: Abnormal skin lesions right forearm, probable keratoacanthoma.

P: After verbal informed consent was obtained, the lesion was prepped with alcohol, anesthetized with 2% lidocaine with epinephrine. Shave biopsy was then performed. Hemostasis was with 35% aluminum chloride. Tolerated well. Covered with a bandage. We will contact him with the pathology results. Additionally, his blood pressure is a bit elevated today, and I have asked that he follow up with me in the next month or 2 on his medical problems.

Electronically authenticated by: Marta Greenhust, M.D.

Case 6-9, *continued*

ICD-9-CM diagnosis code(s): _____

ICD-10-CM diagnosis code(s): _____

CPT code(s) with modifier, if applicable: _____

Case 6-10

Physician Office Face Sheet

Record Number:	25-77-22	Western Medical Clinic
Age:	35	
Gender:	Female	
Patient Status:	Established Patient	
Diagnosis/Procedure:	Interstitial Cystitis	

continued

S: This is a 35-year-old female who is seen today to establish care. She needs medication refills today for her Elmiron for her interstitial cystitis, hyoscyamine for her irritable bowel problems, Nabumetone for fibromyalgia, and she uses Vivelle Dot for her artificial menopause after hysterectomy. She was diagnosed with fibromyalgia a few years ago, which she is seeing a rheumatologist for. She has no acute concerns today, other than she is out of her medications.

PAST MEDICAL HISTORY:
1. Interstitial cystitis.
2. Anxiety.
3. Depression.
4. Endometriosis.
5. IBS.
6. Fibromyalgia.
7. Surgical menopause.

ALLERGIES: Iodine, sulfa, codeine.

PAST SURGICAL HISTORY:
1. TAH/BSO
2. Ectopic pregnancy
3. C-section x 2

SOCIAL HISTORY: The patient does not use tobacco. She is divorced. She works at a bank.

CURRENT MEDICATIONS:
1. Elmiron 100 g three times daily.
2. Hyoscyamine sublingual 0.125 mg twice daily PRN.
3. Cymbalta 60 mg daily.
4. Premarin vaginal cream PRN.
5. Vivelle Dot 0.05 mg, one patch twice weekly.
6. Ambien PRN at bedtime.
7. Nabumetone 750 mg twice daily.
8. Vitamin D 1.25 mg weekly.

O: VITAL SIGNS: Weight 176 pounds. Height 64 inches. Blood pressure 110/78. Temperature 97.1. Pulse 105. Respirations 16. Saturating 97% on room air. GENERAL: Alert and oriented x 3. No acute distress.

A: This is a 35-year-old female with menopausal disorder, interstitial cystitis, irritable bowel syndrome and fibromyalgia.

P: 1. Interstitial cystitis. We will refill her Elmiron 100 mg three times daily.
2. Irritable bowel syndrome. We will refill her hyoscyamine.
3. Menopausal disorder. The patient has never had labs done to make sure that she is really in menopause. She is off of her Vivelle Dot and has been for about a month. We will check her FSH, LH, Estradiol levels. If they are in fact showing she is in menopause, she will restart her Vivelle Dot.
4. Fibromyalgia. We will refill her Nabumetone 750 mg twice daily. This keeps her fibromyalgia under good control.

Forty minutes were spent with the patient today and more than 50% of that time was spent on counseling and coordination of care.

Electronically authenticated by: Harrison Adams, M.D.

Case 6-10, *continued*

ICD-9-CM diagnosis code(s): _____

ICD-10-CM diagnosis code(s): _____

CPT code(s) with modifier, if applicable: _____

Case 6-11

Physician Office Face Sheet

Western Medical Clinic

Record Number:	18-05-44
Age:	29
Gender:	Female
Patient Status:	New Patient
Diagnosis/Procedure:	Nephrolithiasis

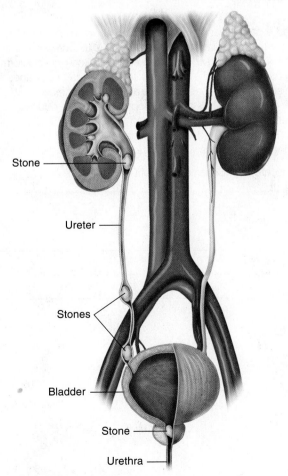

Stone

Ureter

Stones

Bladder

Stone

Urethra

Nephrolithiasis.

Source: Pearson Education/PH College

continued

Case 6-11, *continued*

S: This is a 29-year-old female seen today for a right flank pain and possible kidney stones. She has had a history of kidney stones in the past but has not had an attack since she was in the Army about 5 years ago. The pain started in the right flank and worked its way around. The pain is spasmodic in nature and currently feels like it is down in her groin area. This is very typical of kidney stone attacks she has had in the past. She does not have any burning with urination. She denies any fever, nausea, vomiting, diarrhea, or constipation. She has tried straining urine in the past to catch stone, but she has always been unable to catch any. She does not know what type of kidney stones she passes. She has never had kidney stones that required surgical intervention.

PAST MEDICAL HISTORY: PCOS, kidney stones, seasonal allergies.
SURGICAL HISTORY: Wisdom teeth.
MEDICATIONS: Glucophage 500 mg t.i.d., Yaz daily, Zyrtec p.r.n., multivitamin daily, ibuprofen p.r.n.

O: Weight 226 pounds, height 66 inches, blood pressure 128/82, temperature 98.7, pulse 100, respirations 18, saturating 99% on room air. GENERAL: Alert and oriented x 3, no acute distress. CHEST: Clear to auscultation bilaterally. CV: Regular rate and rhythm. ABDOMEN: Soft, nondistended, nontender. Right flank without tenderness.
URINALYSIS: Specific gravity of 1.005, pH 5, leukocytes 1+, nitrite negative, protein negative, blood 250.

A: This is a 29-year-old female with nephrolithiasis.

P: We have obtained a strainer and have asked her to strain her urine and try to catch the stone for us, and if so, bring that in for evaluation. She is to increase her fluid intake. Calcium oxalate stones are very common, so I have asked her to look up calcium oxalate stone diet for things to avoid. I have sent her urine for a routine UA and culture since she did have white blood cells, to make sure that she does not have any brewing infection. She is to follow up over the weekend or after hours if she has any development of fever, nausea, vomiting, or worsening pain or visible hematuria. I did give her some hydrocodone 5/325 mg 40 tablets today to use as needed. The patient declined CT with renal protocol at this time. She is fairly certain these are kidney stones, but if things worsen, she will agree to imaging at that time.

Electronically authenticated by: Chris Nichols, M.D.

ICD-9-CM diagnosis code(s): _____

ICD-10-CM diagnosis code(s): _____

CPT code(s) with modifier, if applicable: _____

Case 6-12

Physician Office Face Sheet

Western Medical Clinic

Record Number:	17-45-80
Age:	60
Gender:	Female
Patient Status:	New Patient
Diagnosis/Procedure:	Eustachian Tube Dysfunction

SUBJECTIVE: This is a 60-year-old female who presents today complaining of right ear pain. This has been going on for about a week and a half. She has a little bit of popping, but not a whole lot. She does have a runny nose and a scratchy throat and a mild cough. She denies any fevers, nausea, or vomiting. She is not having any pain in the left ear.

ALLERGIES: Codeine.

CURRENT MEDICATIONS:
1. Enalapril 40 mg daily.
2. Metoprolol 50 mg b.i.d.
3. Triamterene and hydrochlorothiazide 37.5/25 mg daily.
4. Potassium gluconate 550 mg two tablets daily.
5. Flaxseed oil 1000 mg daily.
6. Multivitamin daily.
7. Ibuprofen 200 mg three tablets q.8h.

PHYSICAL EXAMINATION:
VITAL SIGNS: Weight 331 pounds, blood pressure 144/82, temperature 97.2, pulse 88, respirations 20, and satting 97% on room air.
GENERAL: Alert and oriented x3, in no acute distress.
HEENT: Normocephalic. TMs and canals are clear bilaterally. Oropharynx is clear without erythema.
NECK: Supple, no lymphadenopathy.
CHEST: Clear to auscultation bilaterally.
CARDIOVASCULAR: Regular rate and rhythm.

ASSESSMENT: This is a 60-year-old female with eustachian tube dysfunction and otalgia.

PLAN: The patient will try Sudafed and Afrin nasal spray. She can use the Afrin nasal spray up to three to four days in a row before taking two or three days off from use. If her symptoms do not improve with these decongestants over the next one to two weeks, she can follow up in clinic and we may need to do a trial course of nasal steroids. If her symptoms worsen in the meantime, she can follow up with me in clinic.

Electronically authenticated by: Paula Tipton, D.O.

continued

Case 6-12, *continued*

ICD-9-CM diagnosis code(s): _____

ICD-10-CM diagnosis code(s): _____

CPT code(s) with modifier, if applicable: _____

Case 6-13

Physician Office Face Sheet

		Western Medical Clinic
Record Number:	38-58-22	
Age:	56	
Gender:	Male	
Patient Status:	Established Patient	
Diagnosis/Procedure:	Depression	

Case 6-13, *continued*

SUBJECTIVE: This is a 56-year-old male who is seen today for follow-up of depression and anxiety. Since switching him to Fluoxetine, his depression and anxiety have worsened and he has become very angry. His wife is here today for the first time because she is afraid of him. He says that he would never touch her physically, but she says she is not so sure because he gets so angry since he started this medication. He said he feels like he is slipping and has less control of himself. He denies suicidal thought.

PAST MEDICAL HISTORY:
1. Coronary vascular disease
2. Depression
3. Abdominal aortic aneurysm with bilateral iliac aneurysms repaired
4. Right lower extremity radiculopathy
5. Varicose veins
6. Erectile dysfunction
7. Syncope
8. Deep venous thrombosis
9. Lumbar spondylosis
10. Obstructive sleep apnea
11. Coronary artery disease

ALLERGIES: Fluoxetine intolerance anger.

CURRENT MEDICATIONS
1. Fluoxetine 40 mg daily
2. Toprol XL 25 mg twice daily
3. Plavix 75 mg daily
4. atorvastatin daily
5. Hydrocodone p.r.n.

OBJECTIVE: Height 6 feet. Blood Temperature 97.7. Pulse 98. Respirations 20. on room air.
GENERAL: Alert and oriented x3 in no acute distress.

ASSESSMENT: This is a 56-year-old male with depression, anxiety, and increasing anger on fluoxetine.

PLAN: Discontinue the fluoxetine. We will put him back on the Paxil CR 50 mg daily. I am going to add BuSpar 7.5 mg twice daily. After two or three days, he can increase that to three times per day if needed. I put in a referral to Dr. Halverson for a consultation. He has an appointment with her in two weeks. He is going to follow-up with me in the meantime if he has any worsening symptoms or problems with the medication.

Electronically authenticated by: Harrison Adams, M.D.

ICD-9-CM diagnosis code(s): _____

ICD-10-CM diagnosis code(s): _____

CPT code(s) with modifier, if applicable: _____

Physician Office Face Sheet

Western Medical Clinic

Record Number: 84-27-65

Age: 30

Gender: Male

Patient Status: Established Patient

Diagnosis/Procedure: Low Back Pain Sciatica

CHIEF COMPLAINT: Follow-up of the low back pain.

HISTORY OF PRESENT ILLNESS: He recently had some increased activity as he carried some boxes, helping a friend move. As expected, there was some increasing discomfort in the lumbar area with some right sciatica, but there is no new loss of strength or sensation of the right lower extremity, no joint pain or stiffness or swelling or redness by review of systems, and with his current use of Soma and ibuprofen, he has also by review of systems no blood in the stools, constipation, diarrhea, heartburn, nausea, stomach pain or vomiting, or blood in the urine, chest pain, shortness of breath or wheezing.

ALLERGIES: No known drug allergies.

CURRENT MEDICATIONS:
1. Paxil l0 mg daily.
2. Ativan 1.5 mg daily (both of these medications prescribed by Dr. Randolph, his psychiatrist, who has been seeing him for years).
3. Hydrocodone 5 mg/acetaminophen 325 mg twice daily PRN pain, with a limit of 15 per month. For his more frequent daily pain, ibuprofen 200 mg up to four times daily.
4. Acetaminophen 500 mg three times daily as needed, rarely uses because it does not seem to help much.
5. Soma 350 mg PO four times daily PRN.

ACTIVITY: He has been walking but not on a daily basis.
A second problem is smoking. He wants to quit now. His wife is due to deliver their baby, sometime between Christmas Day and New Year's. I provided local support group numbers and recommended tapering a little less than one-half pack per day and then setting a quit date. We did discuss possible use of medications but he prefers to quit without additional medication if possible.

ALLERGIES: No known drug allergies.

ADVERSE DRUG EFFECTS: Manic with nortriptyline.

PHYSICAL EXAMINATION: VITAL SIGNS: Weight 201 pounds. Height 74 inches. BMI 26. Blood pressure 120/88. Temperature 99.6. Pulse 75. Respiratory rate 16. 02 saturation 98% on room air. GENERAL: He is alert. BACK: No acute guarding of the back or acute distress. He is able to walk without antalgic gait. He is able to walk on the heels and on the balls of the feet, able to do five squats in a row. Forward flexion to the knees, right lateral flexion above the knees, left lateral flexion to the knees, extension about 10°. LUNGS: Resonant to percussion and clear to auscultation. CARDIAC: Exam with S1 and S2, without murmur. ABDOMEN: Soft. Bowel sounds present. Nontender. No palpable hepatosplenomegaly. EXTREMITIES: Negative straight leg raising on the left to 90° from a seated position, and on the right straight leg raising revealed some right lumbar but not sciatica discomfort. Motor strength 5/5 throughout extensor hallucis longus, tibialis anterior, quadriceps, and gastrocnemius. Light touch sensation symmetrically intact throughout lower extremities. Deep tendon reflexes 2/4 bilateral gastrocnemius and 1/4 bilateral quadriceps with augmentation. Babinski's down-going bilaterally.

IMPRESSION/PLAN
1. Low back pain with intermittent right sciatica. No new sensory or motor radiculopathy. The expected flare-up with lifting boxes, helping his friend move. He is using Soma less now, averaging about twice daily, and he notes a little slowness of the thinking with the Soma so he takes it primarily in the evening. The Soma definitely helped with some muscle spasm he has been having lately. He does have a prescription for Soma 350 mg, #50, with two refills.
2. He is staying within the guidelines of his chronic pain contract, with the hydrocodone #15 per month. Drowsiness precautions.
3. I encouraged him to continue his walking and to quit smoking as he plans. Follow-up in approximately two months.

Electronically authenticated by: Andrea Rodriguez, M.D.

continued

Case 6-14, *continued*

ICD-9-CM diagnosis code(s): _____

ICD-10-CM diagnosis code(s): _____

CPT code(s) with modifier, if applicable: _____

Case 6-15

Physician Office Face Sheet

Record Number:	95-80-55	Western Medical Clinic
Age:	34	
Gender:	Female	
Patient Status:	Established Patient	
Diagnosis/Procedure:	Pain with Intercourse	

Case 6-15, *continued*

CHIEF COMPLAINT: Pain with intercourse.

HISTORY OF PRESENT ILLNESS: The patient is a 34-year-old who states that it is very difficult for her to enjoy intercourse because her vaginal lips are so long that they fold up and they get in the way. She states this has been for the last many, many years, and this is the first time she has gotten up her courage to come and have something done about it.

PAST MEDICAL HISTORY: Status post TAH-BSO for severe endometriosis.

MEDICATIONS: Her medications at the present time are Premarin for estrogen replacement. She is on no other medicines.

ALLERGIES: She is allergic to no medicines. However, taking Tylenol makes her itch all over.

FAMILY MEDICAL HISTORY: Significant for a father with diabetes and heart disease.

REVIEW OF SYSTEMS: Otherwise within normal limits.

OBJECTIVE: Weight is 147 pounds, blood pressure is 100/64, pulse is 78, the patient is afebrile. Lungs are clear to auscultation, good breath sounds are heard. Heart has normal sinus rhythm, on murmur noted. Abdomen is soft and nontender to deep palpation. No organomegaly is present. Pelvic exam is deferred at the present time. Extremities show no edema. Deep tendon reflexes are +2.
From previous exam, vaginal lips are bilateral extremely long, with the right side being slightly longer than the left, hanging down close to 2 to 3 inches below the perineum.

ANALYSIS: Pain with intercourse due to elongated labia majora.

PLAN: Bilateral labial reduction. Pros and cons and the risks and benefits were gone over with the patient. She understands the risks which are mostly from anesthesia, infection, blood loss, and/or loss of sensitivity to the area, which might decrease her satisfaction with intercourse however, the patient states "I can't have intercourse now because I'm so unsatisfied with it." The patient understands this and still wants this done. Therefore, we will bring her into the hospital as scheduled to perform a bilateral reduction of the labia majora.

Electronically authenticated by: Patrick Ulyss, M.D.

ICD-9-CM diagnosis code(s): _____

ICD-10-CM diagnosis code(s): _____

CPT code(s) with modifier, if applicable: _____

Case 6-16

Health Record Face Sheet

Western Medical Clinic

Record Number: 03-54-12

Age: 2

Gender: Female

Length of Stay: N/A

Service Type: Emergency Room

Discharge Status: To Home

Diagnosis/Procedure: Lip Laceration
Suture Repair

Case 6-16, *continued*

EMERGENCY ROOM REPORT

PATIENT: Madison Miller
AGE: 2
RECORD NUMBER: 03-54-12
PHYSICIAN: Dr. Floyd
DATE: 8/18/xx

IDENTIFICATION: This is a 2-year-old Caucasian female.

CHIEF COMPLAINT: Lip laceration.

HISTORY OF PRESENT ILLNESS: This is a two-year-old female who fell. Mother does not know how she fell but she went to the child immediately and the child was crying. She has a through and through lip laceration. Her tetanus is up to date. She has no other complaints. No loss of consciousness.

ALLERGIES: NO KNOWN ALLERGIES

CURRENT MEDICATIONS: No current medications.

PHYSICAL EXAMINATION: Reveals an alert female with a temperature of 95, pulse 124, respirations 28, weight of 30 pounds. Skin is warm and dry. The extraocular muscles are intact. Pupils are equal, round and reactive to light and accommodation.

Exam of the lip revealed a through and through lip laceration on the lower lip, left side through the buccal surface and through the outside just at the vermillion border. It is 1 cm x 0.3 cm and is through and through. A neurololgic exam was performed on movement, strength and coordination and all are within normal limits.

IMPRESSION: LIP LACERATION.

PLAN: I discussed the repair with the mother. The mother requested suturing because the child pulls on her lips at all times. It was fairly well approximated.

SUMMARY OF PROCEDURE: The child was given some Thorazine, Vistaril, and Demerol. Under sterile procedure, three interrupted sutures were utilized to close the lip laceration.

Mother was given wound instructions. The patient will need to have the sutures out in four days. Mom is instructed to use Tylenol for pain. Any worsening of symptoms or problems with sutures, the patient is to return to the emergency department.

ICD-9-CM diagnosis code(s): _____

ICD-10-CM diagnosis code(s): _____

CPT code(s) with modifier, if applicable: _____

Health Record Face Sheet

Western Medical Clinic

Record Number:	14-78-11
Age:	27
Gender:	Female
Length of Stay:	N/A
Service Type:	Physician Office / Delivery Note
Discharge Status:	To Home
Diagnosis/Procedure:	36-week pregnancy with vaginal delivery New-onset hypertension Edema

DELIVERY NOTE

HISTORY: Patient is a 27-year-old single white female gravida 1 RH positive at approximately 36 3/7 completed weeks who presented with new onset of hypertension in the moderate range. Associated edema and mild proteinuria were noted though other lab function studies of preeclampsia were negative. Fetal lung maturity was documented per amniocentesis. Artificial rupture of membranes was performed and internal monitoring performed. Pitocin augmentation of labor was begun. Approximately 5 cm. magnesium sulfate prophylaxis was also initiated.

She progressed rapidly through labor with one hour stage two of labor without fetal monitor abnormalities. She delivered a female neonate over a midline episiotomy with nuchal cord x 1. Fluid was clear. Suction per nasopharynx and oropharynx was performed on the perineum. Apgars were vigorous with only stimulation and blow by 02. Placenta was delivered intact. Uterine atony was encountered but responded to vigorous pitocin and 250 micro units of Hemabate intramyometrially.

2 cm. fourth-degree midline perineal lacerations was encountered. The rectal mucosa was closed with a chromic suture, and mucosal spearing fashion. The perirectal fascia was re-approximated. The anal sphincter and superficial perineal muscles were re-approximated and the remainder of the episiotomy closed in the usual fashion. No mucosal lesions, rectal and no rectal vaginal defects or weaknesses in the fascia were palpated.

Both patient and neonate went to recovery in stable condition.

Will continue patient's Magnesium Sulfate and monitoring of blood pressure for at least 24–48 hours.

ICD-9-CM diagnosis code(s): _____

ICD-10-CM diagnosis code(s): _____

CPT code(s) with modifier, if applicable: _____

Case 6-18

Health Record Face Sheet

		Western Medical Clinic

Record Number: 02-55-84

Age: 27

Gender: Female

Length of Stay: N/A

Service Type: Physician Office /
Amniocentesis Report Coding

Discharge Status: N/A

Diagnosis/Procedure: Assess Fetal Lung Maturity
Amniocentesis

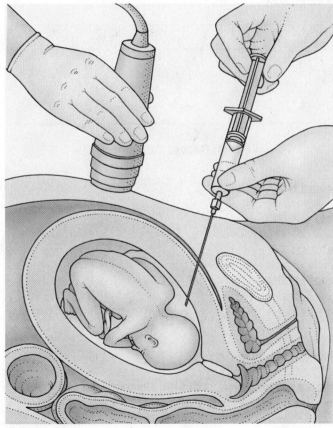

Amniocentesis.
Source: Halli Verrinder © Dorling Kindersley

continued

Case 6-18, *continued*

AMNIOCENTESIS

PATIENT: Maria Lopez
AGE: 27
RECORD NUMBER: 02-55-84
PHYSICIAN: Dr. Smith
DATE: 6/14/xx

HISTORY: Assess fetal lung maturity.

PROCEDURE: Utilizing local anesthetic a 22-gauge spinal needle was inserted into the right upper uterus and about 3 cc. of clear straw colored fluid was sent to the laboratory for assessment. Amniocentesis was performed adjacent to the lower spine and left buttock region of the fetus. There were no apparent complications. The patient tolerated the procedure well. There was good fetal activity following the procedure. No evidence of Braxton-Hick's contractions. Fetal cardiac activity was normal with a fetal heart rate of 147 bpm following amniocentesis. The proximal tibial ossification center (35 week marker) is present.

FINDINGS: Successful amniocentesis without apparent complication.

ICD-9-CM diagnosis code(s): _____

ICD-10-CM diagnosis code(s): _____

CPT code(s) with modifier, if applicable: _____

Case 6-19

Health Record Face Sheet

Record Number:	38-15-20	Western Medical Clinic
Age:	62	
Gender:	Female	
Length of Stay:	N/A	
Service Type:	Physician Office—Operative Report Coding	
Discharge Status:	To Home	
Diagnosis/Procedure:	Chronic Renal Failure DM Catheter Placement	

Case 6-19, *continued*

OPERATIVE REPORT

DATE: 2/19/xx
SURGEON: Dr. Belton
ANESTHESIA: General

PREOPERATIVE DIAGNOSIS: Chronic renal failure in a very brittle diabetic, unable to tolerate peritoneal dialysis because of loss of protein and albumin.

POSTOPERATIVE DIAGNOSIS: Same.

OPERATION: Cut down placement of permanent catheter right internal jugular and removal of peritoneal dialysis catheter.

ESTIMATED BLOOD LOSS: 50 cc.

COMPLICATIONS: None.

SUMMARY OF PROCEDURE: The patient was taken to the operating room having been put to sleep, endotracheal tube in place. She had Betadine prep of the entire neck, jaw, and upper thorax down to the nipples. She also had prep of the left lower quadrant around the permanent catheter. She had a sterile drape in both areas.

Attention was turned towards placing a permanent catheter. Initially a transverse incision was made in the skin line, distal third of the neck on the right, transverse fashion and carried down through platysma muscle. Hemostasis was obtained with a Bovie. Flaps were developed inferiorly and superiorly, sufficient to allow muscle splitting incision through anterior body sternocleidomastoid muscle. The dissection was carried straight down. Deep fascia of the neck was encountered and there was marked scarring in this location. The patient had had a previous temporary dialysis catheter long term on this side. The carotid artery was palpated and adjacent to the artery just laterally. The lateral border of the scarred, whitish colored wall of the internal jugular vein was identified. With gradual dissection over the top of this, we were able to isolate the jugular vein from the carotid artery taking care not to injure the vagus nerve. The vein was dissected free for a distance of approximately 2 cm. Vascular tape was passed without difficulty. Dissection was prolonged because of the dense tissue in this region. We were able to get around this without entering the vessel.

A #4-0 Prolene vascular purse-string was then placed in a broad fashion and once this was accomplished, the patient was placed in Trendelenburg position. Ends were placed inferiorly on the purse-string so that it could be tied directly down on the vein. The catheter was then inserted after what was felt to be the appropriate length was selected. Incision was then made so a #36 French catheter could be inserted through skin tunnel located below the clavicle on the right side and brought through a portion of the muscle to allow for adequate bend without kinking. Once this was accomplished, the internal jugular was lifted anteriorly with the Bakke pickups and a #15 blade was used to make an opening in the vein. The vein, as indicated, was scarred and sclerosed, however, an opening was made sufficient to allow placement of the catheter without difficulty. In the process, approximately 25 cc of blood was lost. The purse-string was then tied down. There was a small leak on the superior aspect and stick tie of #4—0 Vascular Prolene was then used to secure this.

X-ray was obtained and catheter was seen in the part of the superior vena cava, and it was pulled out approximately 2 cm so that the pledget regressed still just inside the skin. This was accomplished and wound was irrigated. A #2-0 Vicryl was used to approximate the deep fascial layer of the neck and platysmal muscles also approximated with #2-0 Vicryl. A #4-0 Vicryl was used subcuticular and Steri-strips were used on the skin. The wound was dressed and a tegaderm was placed over the catheter where it came out of the skin. Attention was then turned towards the peritoneal dialysis catheter. Dressings were removed off of this location and cut so we could get to where the catheter had been inserted just above the iliac crest on the left. The incision for insertion was well above where the catheter went down to. It was a good 6 cm above where the catheter failed to go. A 1/4 inch was made directly over where we thought the catheter was inserted on the lateral border of the rectus muscle. Hemostasis was obtained with a Bovie after incision was made in the skin. With blunt dissection, we were able to go down and identify the catheter, go through the abdominal wall musculature. This was identified just lateral to the edge of the rectus. The catheter was then grasped. It was cut in this location and the pledget was placed near the skin, was removed after making a 1-1/2 cm incision along the tract of the catheter. Sharp dissection was then used to follow the tract of the, catheter down to its junction with peritoneum. This was identified. The catheter was pulled back after it was removed and there was adherent omentum on the catheter in this location. This was transected after being clamped with a small clamp and the end of the omentum tied off with #2-0 silk and the omentum was tucked back into the abdominal cavity. The edges of the peritoneum and fascia which were hypertrophied were grasped with clamps and three #3-0 stick ties of #0 Vicryl were used to close this opening in the peritoneum. The wound was irrigated and the fascial layer anteriorly was then closed with #0 Vicryl.

The wound was irrigated. A #3-0 Vicryl was then used to approximate the subcuticular layer and #4-0 Prolene used to run and close skin. Accu-chek prior to coming back to the ICU approximately 30 minutes before case was over was 230. The patient had no complications during surgery. She was sent to the recovery with stable vital signs.

continued

Case 6-19, *continued*

ICD-9-CM diagnosis code(s): _____

ICD-10-CM diagnosis code(s): _____

CPT code(s) with modifier, if applicable: _____

Case 6-20

Health Record Face Sheet

Western Medical Clinic

Record Number:	13-77-42
Age:	17
Gender:	Female
Length of Stay:	N/A
Service Type:	Emergency Room
Discharge Status:	To Home
Diagnosis/Procedure:	Cervical Strain MVA

Case 6-20, *continued*

EMERGENCY ROOM REPORT

PATIENT: Gabriella Garcia
AGE: 17
RECORD NUMBER: 13-77-42
DATE: 5/28/xx

IDENTIFICATION: This is a 17-year-old Hispanic female.

CHIEF COMPLAINT: Pain in cervical spine.

HISTORY OF PRESENT ILLNESS: This is a 17-year-old woman whose vehicle struck another vehicle on the passenger's side going through an intersection. The patient had no loss of consciousness. She was unrestrained. She was ambulatory at the scene, got out of her car, and laid down on the curb. The paramedics arrived, assessed her, and found her to be hemodynamically stable but complaining of neck pain. She was placed in C spine and lumbar spine immobilization and transferred to the emergency room hemodynamcially stable. The patient's chief complaint is pain in the entire cervical spine.

ALLERGIES: NONE KNOWN

CURRENT MEDICATIONS: None.

PREVIOUS ILLNESS: None.

LMP: The patient states she does not believe she is pregnant. We have explained to her the importance in terms of attempting to determine this prior to prescribing medications.

PHYSICAL EXAMINATION: This is an alert, pleasant young lady in no acute distress. Temperature afebrile, pulse 80, respiratory rate 20, blood pressure 138/88. Head normocephalic, atraumatic. Cranial nerves II-XII are intact. TMs benign. No rhinorrhea. Good dental occlusion. She is tender over the entire nuchal musculature bilaterally and over the sternocleidomastoids. There is no bony step off of the cervical spine. There is no tenderness over the thoracic or lumbar spine. She has good breath sounds bilaterally. The heart is regular in rate and rhythm. There is a 1/6 systolic murmur present at the left lower sternal border. The abdomen is flat, soft, good bowel sounds. No peritoneal signs. The pelvis does not reveal any tenderness on compression of the pelvic rims or the public bone. The extremities are neurovascularly intact. Reflexes are 2-3+ and symmetrical. No sensory deficit. Complete range of motion with no bony deformity.

RADIOLOGY: Cervical spine films are negative.

IMPRESSION: CERVICAL STRAIN MVA.

PLAN: The collar was removed after lateral C spine was taken and found to be normal. She had no bony tenderness, only nuchal muscular tenderness. Subsequently, complete C spine was negative. She will be fitted with a soft collar. She was given Soma as a muscle relaxant and Tylenol for pain. She is not to take the Soma if she believes she is pregnant. We have explained this to her at length. Ice to the affected area. After ice for 48 hours, she is to use heat. She is given the physician referral number.

continued

Case 6-20, *continued*

ICD-9-CM diagnosis code(s): _____

ICD-10-CM diagnosis code(s): _____

CPT code(s) with modifier, if applicable: _____

Case 6-21

Health Record Face Sheet

Western Medical Clinic

Record Number: 82-19-09

Age: 27

Gender: Female

Length of Stay: 3 days

Service Type: Physician Office/
Discharge Summary
only Coding

Discharge Status: To Home

Diagnosis/Procedure: Pre-eclampsia
Term Delivery

Case 6-21, *continued*

DISCHARGE SUMMARY

PATIENT: Christina Carr
RECORD NUMBER: 82-19-09
ADMITTED: 3/14/xx
DISCHARGED: 3/16/xx
PHYSICIAN: Dr. Huerrera

DISCHARGE DIAGNOSES: Pregnancy at 39 3/7 completed weeks with moderate pregnancy induced hypertension/preeclampsia. Second degree midline perineal laceration repaired.

HISTORY: Patient is a 22-year-old single Asian A positive gravida 1 with fractionated prenatal care. Her first evaluation at 30 weeks. Mild elevated blood pressure was noted by 36 weeks, significant elevation with diastolic 98-100 noted. Patient was admitted.

HOSPITAL COURSE: Upon admission she was inducted and magnesium prophylaxis begun IV as well as anti-hypertensives. She progressed well through labor and subsequently delivered a vigorous 7 pound 3 ounce female over a second-degree laceration. Fluid was clear. Apgars reassuring. Placenta was delivered intact. Peritoneal laceration was repaired without difficulty and patient went to recovery in stable condition.

Postpartum course was uncomplicated. Review of chart shows serum magnesium levels largely within therapeutic range. CBC on admission revealed hematocrit of 38.5. Platelet count 304,000. Chemistry screen showing uric acid of 2.9, Creatinine .5. Liver function studies unremarkable. SLM clearly reassuring at 138.

DISPOSITION: Patient was discharged to home on the second postpartum day in good condition with well-controlled blood pressure on oral medications. She was given specific instructions on activities of daily living and wound care follow-up. Medications to include Procardia and Motrin and reviewed signs and symptoms of return of preeclampsia.

PROCEDURES: None.

CONSULTATIONS: None.

ICD-9-CM diagnosis code(s): _____

ICD-10-CM diagnosis code(s): _____

CPT code(s) with modifier, if applicable: _____

Health Record Face Sheet

Western Medical Clinic

Record Number:	03-14-55
Age:	62
Gender:	Male
Length of Stay:	N/A
Service Type:	Emergency Room
Discharge Status:	To Home
Diagnosis/Procedure:	Hyper Anticoagulation with Contusion

EMERGENCY ROOM REPORT

MEDICAL RECORD NUMBER: 03-14-55
AGE: 62
SEX: M

Admit Date: 6/04/xx
Admitting Physician: Dr. Brown

SUBJECTIVE: The patient comes in complaining of having a large bruise from his mid-upper arm down. He says that he bumps it occasionally on the skid loader and it is quite swollen and tender. It is swollen enough that it is causing a little bit of discomfort. There has been no injury except as described above. The patient is on Coumadin for blood clots that he has had in the past.

OBJECTIVE: LUNGS: Clear. HEART: Regular rate and rhythm. Unremarkable.
EXTREMITIES: There is a large purple ecchymosis from the mid-biceps down to the hand. Distal neurovascular checks in the hand are normal.

LABORATORY/DIAGNOSTIC: Blood work shows a protime of 37.1 with an INR of 7.5.

ASSESSMENT: Hyper anticoagulation with contusion of left arm.

PLAN: We gave him 2 ampuls of vitamin K. We will have him stop his Coumadin for 2 days and then he will start back at 2.5 mg every other day. He is to have his blood checked in one week and follow up with his regular physician.

Case 6-22, *continued*

EMERGENCY
Extremity Trauma

TRIAGE   TIME ___2010___   emergent   urgent   (non-urgent)

D.O.B. _____   AGE: ___62___   (M)   F

HISTORIAN: patient   EMT   family _____

ARRIVAL MODE: car   EMS   police _____

^IMMUNIZATIONS: current / referral _____

tetanus _____ flu _____ pneumovax _____

TREATMENT PTA   see EMS report   IV   O₂   c-collar   backboard

last blood glucose _____

VITALS

B.P. _153/90_   P _62_   RR _20_   temp _____ TM O R Ax

SaO₂ _____ RA/O₂ _____ RTS _____

PAIN LEVEL current: _4_/10   max _7_/10   acceptable _____/10

scale used _____   quality _____

CHIEF COMPLAINT ___Hit arm on skid loader___

occurred just PTA _____ hrs/days ago _last Thurs. Area is very_
bruised and swollen. Is on Coumadin.

INJURIES / PAIN

	R			L	
shldr	hip		shldr		hip
arm	thigh		(arm)		thigh
elbow	knee		(elbow)		knee
f-arm	leg		(f-arm)		leg
wrist	ankle		wrist		ankle
hand	foot		hand		foot
fingers	toes		fingers		toes

ALLERGIES (NKDA) _____

drug. PCN/ASA / sulfa / latex / codeine / iodine _____
food -

MECHANISM

fall _____ animal bite _____

twisting _____ GSW / stab wound _____

(direct blow)/crush _____ burn _____

puncture wound _____ cut with _____

_____

MEDS ___Isinopril 40 mg.___
___triam/HCTZ 78/50___
___Mexoprotol 50 1/2 day___
___Warfarin 5 mg. 1/2 q day___

PAST MEDICAL HX   negative

R/L handed / HTN / diabetes: _Insulin_ _____

past surgeries none _____

SOCIAL HX

smoker _____ ppd   drugs / alcohol _____

^TB exposure / symptoms _____

^has been physically hurt or threatened by someone close _____

LNMP _____ G _____ P _____ Ab _____ pregnant / postmenop / hyst

---

INITIAL ASSESSMENT   TIME ___2010___

GENERAL APPEARANCE

(no acute distress)   __mild / moderate / severe distress _____

(alert oriented)   __anxlous / decreased LOC _____

__disoriented to person / place / time

_____

FUNCTIONAL / NUTRITIONAL ASSESSMENT

(independent ADl)   __assisted / total care _____

__appears well   __obese / malnourished _____

nourished / hydrated   __recent weight loss / gain _____

CVS   __cool / diaphoretic _____

(skin warm & dry)   __pale / cyanotic _____

__cap refill less than 2 sec.   __cap refill greater than 2 sec. _____

KEY:	T = Tenderness	S = Swelling	E = Erythema	B = Burn
	A = Abrasion	V = Vesicles	Lac = Laceration	

UPPER EXTREMITIES   __see diagram _____

__no evidence of trauma   __active bleeding _____

(skin intact)   __deformity _____

__non-tender   __ROM limited _____

(no deformity)   __pulse deficit _____

(full ROM)   _Bruised and swollen arm_

__pulses nml   _from wrist to upper arm_

__pulses

LOWER EXTREMITIES   __see diagram _____

(no evidence of trauma)   __active bleeding _____

__skin impact   __deformity _____

__non-tender   __ROM limited _____

__no deformity   __unable to bear weight _____

__full ROM   __pulse deficit _____

__pulse nml   _____

_____

ADDITIONAL FINDINGS

continued

Case 6-22, *continued*

OXYGEN

TIME	Flow Rate	Delivery Method (Mask, N.C. etc)	SaO$_2$	INIT

IV STARTS

TIME	#	site	gauge	attempts	complications	INIT

IV / MEDICATION INFUSION RECORD

Stat Time	Solution / Med	IVPB	Rate ml/hr	Stop Time	Amount Infused	INIT
Response: no change *Improved*						
Response: no change *Improved*						
Response: no change *Improved*						

MEDICATION

TIME	Medication	Dose	Route	Site	INIT
21:05	*Vitamin K 2 amps IM* Ⓛ *hip*				
Response: no change *Improved*				
Response: no change *Improved*				
Response: no change *Improved*				
Td/TT	0.5mL	IM			
lot #: exp. date manufac				
Response no change Improved				

PROCEDURES

TIME		INIT
	__cm laceration repair to _____	
	assisted Dr. _____ with laceration repair	
	excisional debridement	
	foreign body removed assisted by:	
	assisted Dr with dislocation/fix reduction	
	shoulder elbow MTP patella	
	splint / sling applied arm leg short long	
	type	
	assessed post-procedure	
	nml color / sensation / movement	
	(lab drawn) / sent by ED tech / nurse / (lab)	
	results back	
	cleaned would applied abx ointment	
	applied dressing / Band-Aid / elastic wrap	
	crutch training w/proper return demonstration	
	to X ray for _____ w/ monitor / nurse / O$_2$ / tech	
	return to room	

VITAL SIGNS

TIME	BP	P	PR	T	SaO$_2$	GCS	Pain	Pupils	INIT
							/10		
							/10		
							/10		
							/10		

ADDITIONAL NOTES

_____

_____

_____

_____

☒ No meds or script sent. _____

☐ Script sent home with patient _____

MEDS SENT HOME WITH PATIENT

_____

_____

INTAKE _____ OUTPUT _____

__IV / saline lock discontinued: Total Amt Infused _____

_____ Time _____ Initials _____

PROPERTY TO

__patient __family

DISPOSITION

(discharged) (home) *police   nursing home   funeral home*

(verbal)/ written instructions / RX given to: patient _____

(verbalized understanding)

__ learning barriers addressed _____

__accompanied by / driver _____

__ER observe _____

__admitted / transferred to _____

☐ RN transport with ambulance _____

__report to _____ time _____

__transfer documentation completed

__notified family / police _____

__left AMA / LWBS   *signed AMA sheet   refused* _____

__physician notified of: _____

Discharge Vitals
BP _____   HR _____   RR _____   Temp _____   SaO$_2$ _____
__pain level at discharge ____ /10   *doesn't appear to be in pain*

CONDITION

__unchanged   __improved   (stable)   __other_____

Depart Time *2110* Mode:(walk) *crutches   W/C   stretcher   ambulance*

ER treatment time:

Discharge Nurse Signature

☐ Continuation Sheet

SIGNATURE	INITIAL
V. Scurraws, RN	

Case 6-22, *continued*

LABORATORY RESULTS

Sex: M
Age: 62

Prothrombin Time			Ref. Range/Male
BS			
PT	H 37.1	13.5	10.0–14.0 secs
INR	H 7.5	1.2	0.9–5.0

ICD-9-CM diagnosis code(s): _____

ICD-10-CM diagnosis code(s): _____

CPT code(s) with modifier, if applicable: _____

Case 6-23

Health Record Face Sheet

Western Medical Clinic

Record Number:	46-14-08
Age:	73
Gender:	Female
Patient Status:	Established
Diagnosis/Procedure:	Foot Pain
	HTN

continued

Case 6-23, *continued*

S: 73-year-old female here for follow-up on left foot pain. I had seen her six days ago with significant pain in the left midfoot and lateral aspect of the foot, though there had been no particular injury or trauma. The following day, her pain worsened, as did the swelling. She tells me the entire foot was quite red and warm to touch as well and that even a sheet touching it at night hurt dramatically. Her pain was so severe that she went into the emergency room on the evening of 8/22/xx. At that point, she was noted to have significant swelling and tenderness of the foot, though no evidence of cellulitis. Her uric acid level was elevated at 9.5, though her sedimentation rate and C reactive protein were normal. She was treated with a Medrol dose pack for probable gout and was asked to follow up. Her pain has improved significantly, as has the swelling. She was having difficulty walking, though that is much better now as well. She finishes the Medrol dose pack tomorrow. They also had her taking some ibuprofen, though she has cut back on the dosing and is only taking it one or two times a day now. No nausea or stomach pain with that. Of note, her uric acid levels at the health fair last fall and prior to that have been in the mid 7 range for the most part. She does have a brother who has gout and he is on daily colchicine for prophylaxis. The patient is also on hydrochlorothiazde for her blood pressure, though, she has been on that for a number of years. No other issues or concerns currently. The x-ray of her foot six days ago was unremarkable.

O: VITAL SIGNS: See flow sheet. Her blood pressure is 132/60. GENERAL: Alert female in no distress. EXTREMITIES: Examination of the left foot shows some very slight swelling over the midfoot only this is improved from our visit last week. There is no redness or warmth to touch. No tenderness over the malleoli or over the lateral Her gait is now normal.

A: Left foot pain—probable gout.

P: I agree that her symptoms are most consistent with gout. She is significantly better at this point and thus she will finish off her Medrol dose pack and stop ibuprofen in another day or two as well. We discussed gout and she has done some reading on-line. Reviewed diet and things to avoid. She does not drink much beer and she does not eat much in the way of processed meats, etc, though she will continue to limit those things. We will not change her hydrochlorothiazide at this point. However, should she have another flare up, I would consider stopping the hydrochlorothiazide. I would plan to treat any recurrent flare-ups with colchicine and I reviewed that with her. Tentatively, I have asked that she follow up with me in about three months and she will have a basic metabolic panel and a uric acid level repeated shortly before that appointment. She is to call or follow up sooner for any issues or problems.

Electronically authenticated by: Andrea Rodriguez, M.D.

ICD-9-CM diagnosis code(s): _____

ICD-10-CM diagnosis code(s): _____

CPT code(s) with modifier, if applicable: _____

Case 6-24

Health Record Face Sheet

Western Medical Clinic

Record Number:	85-17-04
Age:	47
Gender:	Male
Length of Stay:	N/A
Service Type:	Same-Day Surgery
Discharge Status:	To Home
Diagnosis/Procedure:	Neck Lump with Excision

SAME-DAY SURGERY

PATIENT: Frank Floyd
DATE: 4/02/xx
PHYSICIAN: Dr. Macadi

OPERATIVE REPORT

PREOPERATIVE DIAGNOSIS: Lump left side of neck
POSTOPERATIVE DIAGNOSIS: Lump left side of neck possible dermatofibroma

PROCEDURE: Wide excision lump left neck

HISTORY: The patient is well known to me and presents today with the complaint of a lump in his neck. The patient noticed this lump approximately three months ago. At first the lump was described as approximately the size of a watermelon seed. The lump has grown and he is seeking treatment. The patient has an area of induration approximately 1.5 cm in diameter below his left jawline. The decision was made to excise the lump and send to pathology for identification. The patient was given information regarding the procedure and consent was given from the patient to proceed.

PROCEDURE:
The patient was taken to the surgical suite and after general anesthesia was prepped and draped for wide excision of a lump on the left neck. The lump was identified on the left neck just below the jawline. A wide excision of the 1.5 cm lump was performed. After the excision, the lump appeared to be a dermatofibroma. Closure was attained with interrupted 4-0 Vicryl and Dermabond to seal the skin edges. Routine wound care was given. The patient tolerated the procedure well with no complications and was taken to recovery room in good condition.

PATHOLOGY REPORT returned with the confirmed diagnosis of dermatofibroma. The patient was notified of the diagnosis.

continued

Case 6-24, *continued*

ICD-9-CM diagnosis code(s): _____

ICD-10-CM diagnosis code(s): _____

CPT code(s) with modifier, if applicable: _____

Case 6-25

Physician Office Face Sheet

Record Number: 01-14-10

Age: 68

Gender: Female

Patient Status: New Patient

Diagnosis/Procedure: Ventral Wall Hernia

Western Medical Clinic

Case 6-25, *continued*

REASON FOR VISIT: Referral from Dr. Vectus.

REASON FOR REFERRAL: Referred concerning a ventral hernia.

HISTORY OF PRESENT ILLNESS: This is a 68-year-old white female who had an emergency laparotomy for an incarcerated paraesophageal diaphragmatic hernia with both stomach and large bowel trapped within it. She had this reduced and the diaphragm was primarily repaired with sutures and a gastrostomy was performed to tack the stomach down.

Since that time, she has developed a marked bulging in her abdominal wall. She denies any symptoms from this. Her bowels move normally. She has no problem with eating. No nausea or vomiting. No crampy abdominal pain. No signs of bowel obstruction. However, she is a little concerned about the large bulge that she has in her abdomen.

PAST MEDICAL HISTORY:
1. Hypertension.
2. Macular degeneration.
3. Osteoarthritis.

PAST SURGICAL HISTORY:
1. Hysterectomy.
2. Mastoidectomy.
3. Left total knee.
4. Above-mentioned surgery.

SOCIAL HISTORY: She smoked for many years, but she quit 20 years ago. She is retired. She is a native here and spends the winters in Florida.

PHYSICAL EXAMINATION:
ABDOMEN: Pertinent findings were limited to the abdomen. There is a midline abdominal scar, which has healed well. There is a large defect estimated at 9-10 cm on physical examination and corroborated by a computed tomography scan. This reduces spontaneously when supine. There is no abdominal tenderness and no other masses visible.

ASSESSMENT: Large ventral wall defect secondary to surgery in February.

PLAN: I had a long discussion with the patient. She is completely asymptomatic. I advised her if she wants that she can wear a girdle for cosmetic purposes and, since she is asymptomatic, there is no pressing need to fix this. Should the situation change, she is certainly welcome to return for reevaluation. This defect is large enough that I would consider an open repair with relaxing incisions in the lateral rectus rather than a laparoscopic repair, especially considering that she has had a gastrostomy tube and her stomach will be stuck to the abdominal wall and making placement of a patch extremely difficult.

ICD-9-CM diagnosis code(s): _____

ICD-10-CM diagnosis code(s): _____

CPT code(s) with modifier, if applicable: _____

Case 6-26

Physician Office Face Sheet

Western Medical Clinic

Record Number: 18-27-77

Age: 17

Gender: Male

Patient Status: Established Patient

Diagnosis/Procedure: Sports Physical

SUBJECTIVE: Jacob is now 17 years old. He presents today for a sports physical before he goes to play football. He has had a couple of concussions in the past. He did have to miss some of the season I believe of his freshman year. Since then, he really has not had a lot of trouble. The only problem that he is having is that he had one episode of left shoulder subluxation by history while he was lifting weights this summer. He has had no history of seizures. No history of sudden death in his family. He has been worked up for heart disease in the past due to a family history and his echocardiogram was negative. He is healthy. He has no exercise induced asthma. No chronic medical problems.

OBJECTIVE: His physical examination was unremarkable including his joint examination. Please see his physical examination form.

ASSESSMENT: Sports physical.

PLAN: We will go ahead and see him back prn.

ICD-9-CM diagnosis code(s): _____

ICD-10-CM diagnosis code(s): _____

CPT code(s) with modifier, if applicable: _____

Case 6-27

Physician Office Face Sheet

Western Medical Clinic

Record Number: 82-77-16

Age: 34

Gender: Female

Patient Status: Established Patient

Diagnosis/Procedure: Normal Postpartum Visit

SUBJECTIVE: This is a 34-year-old G5P5, status post-normal vaginal delivery. She is doing well. She initially had some breastfeeding issues, but she is no longer having any problems. Nursing is going fine. She said that she bled faintly for six weeks. She describes it as tapering off overtime. It is usually brown in color and occasionally it is a little bit red. She has not had any gushes since the two week mark other than last week she does say she had a little bit heavier flow and it felt like a period. She denies any vaginal odor or itching. She initially had some constipation and hemorrhoids, but those have since resolved. Early on, she had some postpartum blues, but now she just feels tired and is better overall. For contraception, she and her husband are thinking that he will have a vasectomy performed.

OBJECTIVE: VITAL SIGNS: As per chart. ABDOMEN: Soft and nontender. The uterus is not palpable trans-abdominally. GENITOURINARY: Normal external genitalia. The cervix was visualized. No vaginal discharge and no blood in the vaginal vault. The cervix was visualized and a Pap smear was obtained. A pelvic examination was performed. Her uterus is normal in size and contour. No adnexal masses or tenderness.

ASSESSMENT: 34-year-old G5P5 here for a normal postpartum visit.

PLAN: 1. Pap today

                2. I cautioned her to call me if her bleeding picks up at all.

                3. We will notify her of her Pap results.

ICD-9-CM diagnosis code(s): _____

ICD-10-CM diagnosis code(s): _____

CPT code(s) with modifier, if applicable: _____

Health Record Face Sheet

Western Medical Clinic

Record Number:	62-18-08
Age:	15
Gender:	Female
Length of Stay:	N/A
Service Type:	Emergency Room
Discharge Status:	To Home
Diagnosis/Procedure:	Pink Eye

EMERGENCY ROOM REPORT

CHIEF COMPLAINT: This patient is a 15-year-old white female with a chief complaint of pink eye.

HISTORY OF PRESENT ILLNESS: She awoke two days ago with both eyes stuck shut from discharge and was unable to describe the color of this discharge. That day she went to summer school and her teachers complained that her eyes looked quite red and sent her to the school nurse who sent her home with the instructions to obtain medication before she returned to school. Yesterday morning she awoke with the left eye glued shut with discharge and this morning the right eye. She complains of mild tenderness in the eyes with some itch. She has also had some sneezing. No history of hayfever or allergies. She denies any changes in vision or photophobia. She denies fever, chills, nausea, vomiting or diarrhea.

PAST MEDICAL HISTORY: Negative.

CURRENT MEDICATIONS: None.

ALLERGIES: NONE KNOWN.

PHYSICAL EXAM:

GENERAL: Alert, white, thin female in no acute distress. Vital signs: BP 116/68, temp 97, pulse 84, respirations 16.

HEENT: Head is normocephalic and atraumatic. The TMs are normal bilaterally. Eyes, PERRLA. EOMI. Sclerae are nonicteric. They are slightly injected. The limbus is spared. The discs are flat. She has no photophobia. Sinuses are nontender to palpation. The pharynx is clear.

NECK: Supple and nontender without lymphadenopathy or thyromegaly.

ASSESSMENT: CONJUNCTIVITIS, POSSIBLY BACTERIAL.

PLAN: Sodium Sulamyd drops 1 in each eye q 3-4 hours until better. Follow up prn.

Case 6-28, *continued*

ICD-9-CM diagnosis code(s): _____

ICD-10-CM diagnosis code(s): _____

CPT code(s) with modifier, if applicable: _____

Case 6-29

Health Record Face Sheet

Western Medical Clinic

Record Number:	48-12-05
Age:	24
Gender:	Male
Length of Stay:	N/A
Service Type:	Emergency Room
Discharge Status:	To Home
Diagnosis/Procedure:	Motorcycle Accident

continued

Case 6-29, *continued*

EMERGENCY ROOM REPORT

CHIEF COMPLAINT: The patient is a 24-year-old male who was in a motorcycle accident. He was the driver and ran into a pick-up truck, rear-ended it and was brought in. He was not wearing a helmet. He does not know if he had a loss of consciousness. He does not remember the events of the accident. He is not complaining of a headache. He complains of right elbow abrasions and bilateral knee abrasions. He denies neck pain. He denies chest pain. He denies abdominal pain, pelvic pain, any pain in his extremities except as above. He denies headache.

PAST MEDICAL HISTORY: He has had problems with his right knee and is on Naprosyn for that.

ALLERGIES: NONE KNOWN. Last tetanus shot is unknown, more than 10 years.

PHYSICAL EXAM:	The patient is awake and alert. Temp is 98.6, BP is 150/77, pulse 78, respirations 16.
HEENT:	He has a laceration, 3 cm, midline forehead, vertically oriented through the skin into the subcutaneous tissue but it does not penetrate the galia. EOMI. PERRLA. TMs are normal.
NECK:	Supple, completely nontender. It is in a Philadelphia collar.
CHEST:	Wall is nontender. Breath sounds are equal and clear.
ABDOMEN:	Soft and nontender.
PELVIS:	Stable and nontender.
EXTREMITIES:	No bony tenderness at all. He has some abrasions over both knees and over his left elbow but there is no bony tenderness or joint tenderness at all and ROM is normal.
NEURO:	He has CN II-XII intact. No peripheral or motor sensory deficits.

X-RAYS: C-spine x-rays are taken despite the fact that he had no pain and they are read by me as completely normal.

DIAGNOSIS:	MOTORCYCLE ACCIDENT WITH ABRASIONS AND FOREHEAD CONTUSION.

ED COURSE AND TREATMENT: The patient was initially evaluated. Initially his C-spine was cleared and a primary survey revealed that there was no indication for bony x-rays of the areas where he had the abrasions. His mental status was very good. He was awake, alert and answered questions real appropriately and I did not feel that head CT scanning was indicated. I am going to send him home with head instructions, but I feel pretty comfortable that he has not had a concussion. He has no headache and his mental status is real good. Once his C-spine was cleared, I went ahead and palpated his neck and checked and made sure range of motion was okay and there were no problems with that. I removed the C-collar, then went ahead and repaired the laceration of his forehead. This was done with primary closure. The wound was infiltrated with Marcaine mixed with 2% Lidocaine with epinephrine and then irrigated with saline, prepped with Hibiclens and then closed in a single layer with 6-0 Ethilon, 10 simple continuous sutures were placed and then I used two simple interrupted sutures in between a couple of sutures to give good approximation. The wound approximated real nicely and should heal up with minimal scarring unless he has some sort of accelerated idiopathic scarring process.

The patient is going to return in 5 days for suture removal and is going to watch for infection. I had a talk with his wife and she is going observe him tonight for any evidence of head injury and will wake him up a couple of times. Tetanus shot was also given.

Case 6-29, *continued*

ICD-9-CM diagnosis code(s): _____

ICD-10-CM diagnosis code(s): _____

CPT code(s) with modifier, if applicable: _____

Case 6-30

Health Record Face Sheet

Western Medical Clinic

Record Number:	05-18-42
Age:	7
Gender:	Male
Length of Stay:	N/A
Service Type:	Emergency Room
Discharge Status:	To Home
Diagnosis/Procedure:	Femur Fracture

continued

Case 6-30, *continued*

EMERGENCY ROOM REPORT

CHIEF COMPLAINT: This is a 7-year-old white male who presents to the ER after being involved in a bicycle accident. The patient was hitting a good rate of speed, headed down the road when he came upon a fire hydrant at the same speed. The leg absorbed his energy. He is now complaining of leg pain. There was no loss of consciousness. The patient denied having a helmet on.

PAST MEDICAL HISTORY: Unremarkable.

FAMILY HISTORY: Is noncontributory. Vaccinations are up-to-date.

ALLERGIES: NONE KNOWN.

SOCIAL HISTORY: He lives with his mother.

REVIEW OF SYSTEMS: Is negative for chest pain, headache, sore throat, otalgia, loss of consciousness, cough, abdominal pain, urinary retention, numbness or tingling.

PHYSICAL EXAM:	BP 105/60, respirations 22, pulse 105, temp 99. Glasgow Coma Score 50, Trauma Score 11.
HEENT:	EOMI. Pupils are equal, round and reactive to light and accommodation.
NECK:	Supple. TMs are without hemotympanum. Conjunctivae were white.
CHEST:	No pain on AP lateral compression of the chest or pelvis.
LUNGS:	Clear.
HEART:	Has a regular rate and rhythm.
ABDOMEN:	Soft. Bowel sounds are present. No organomegaly. No pain on AP lateral compression of the pelvis.
EXTREMITIES:	All extremities were normal except for the right lower extremity where there was an excoriation of the distal medial aspect of the femur and behind the popliteal area. Distal pulses and sensation were intact.

X-RAYS: X-ray of the area revealed a horizontal, closed, nonangulated 5% displaced femur fracture, 5 cm proximal to the epiphysis.

TREATMENT: Dr. Hilt was called and notified of all of the above and requested that we splint the patient and he will see the patient on Tuesday.

With the mother's permission the area was cleaned and dressed. It was then padded and a splint was placed.

Approximately ten minutes later while I was doing a bladder tap on another patient, I heard some screaming in the room. We went into the room and the patient was complaining of burning in his leg. We immediately took the splint off the child's leg and noticed that it was quite warm. It was on a plastic pillow. We noticed that his leg was pink. We reexamined the leg one half hour later. It still remained mildly hyperemic. We were somewhat concerned about a first-degree burn although it was unclear whether it would actually be a first-degree burn. There were no signs of skin damage at this time. The splint was reapplied. The mother was given precautions on wound precautions, burn precautions, splint precautions, cast precautions. The child was given some Tylenol with codeine elixir. He will see Dr. Hilt on Tuesday. The mother was warned that if he has any difficulties whatsoever to call us in the ER.

DIAGNOSIS:	1. FEMUR FRACTURE.
	2. POSSIBLE MINOR BURN TO THE LEG.

Case 6-30, *continued*

EMERGENCY DEPARTMENT TRAUMA FLOW RECORD

| | | Time 2000 | Conducted By: R. Griffin, R.N. |

PRE-HOSPITAL INFORMATION   ☐ SCENE   ☐ INTERHOSPITAL

Via: ☐ Car   ☐ _____
☐ Helicopter   ☐ Ambulance

MECHANISM OF INJURY
☐ Auto
  ☐ Seatbelt
  ☐ Driver
  ☐ Passenger
  ☐ Front
  ☐ Back
☐ Pedestrian
☒ Fall
☐ Crush
☐ GSW
☐ Motorcycle, ATV
☒ Bicycle
  ☐ Helmet
☐ Blunt Assault
☐ Stabbing
☐ Other

Site of Accident   *home*
Time of Accident   *1930*
Description of Incident
_____
_____
_____
_____
_____
_____
☐ Unconscious Minutes ___ Ø

Chief Complaint
Fell onto Rt leg p̄ running
into a fire hydrant
while riding his bike

Allergies   Ø

Medical History   Ø

| Last TT *current* | Last Ate *1730* | Height *?* | Weight *60?* | LNMP Ø |

Siderails: ☐ L   ☐ S   ☐ NA
Calf Light: ☐ Yes   ☐ NA
Restraints: ☐ Arms   ☐ Legs

INTRAVENOUS FLUIDS:
TIME _____
I.V. STARTED BY _____
FLUID _____ AMT. _____
NEEDLE _____
SITE _____

TIME _____
I.V. STARTED BY _____
FLUID _____ AMT. _____
NEEDLE _____
SITE _____

TIME _____
I.V. STARTED BY _____
FLUID _____ AMT. _____
NEEDLE _____
SITE _____

MEDICATIONS PRIOR TO ARRIVAL

☐ Oral Airway   ☐ Nasal
☐ Oxygen ____ L/m _____
☐ Suctioning _____
☐ Endotracheal Intubation
☐ ___ Nasal ___ Oral ___ mm
☐ Assisted Ventilation
☐ Hyperventilation
☐ Control Bleeding
☐ Spinal Immobilization
  ☐ C-Collar
  ☐ Backboard
☐ Splints _____
☐ Traction _____
☐ Foley
☐ NG Tube _____
☐ Restraints _____
☐ Monitor _____
☐ Mast Trousers
  ☐ Legs Inflated
  ☐ Abdomen Inflated
☐ Other _____
_____

GLASGOW COMA SCALE

EYE OPENING	Spontaneously	④
	To speech	3
	To pain	2
	None	1
VERBAL RESPONSE	Oriented	⑤
	Confused	4
	Inappropriate	3
	Incomprehensible	2
	None	1
MOTOR RESPONSE	Obeys Commands	⑥
	Localizes Pain	5
	Withdraws	4
	Flexion to pain	3
	Extension to pain	2
	None	1

Total GLASGOW **15**

TRAUMA SCORE

RESPIRATORY RATE	10 — 24	4
	25 — 35	3
	more than 35	2
	less than 10	1
	0	0
RESPIRATORY EXPANSION	Normal	1
	Shallow/Retroactive	0
SYSTOLIC BLOOD PRESSURE	more than 90	4
	70 — 90	3
	50 — 70	3
	less than 50	1
	0	0
CAPILLARY REFILL	Normal less than 2 sec.	2
	Delayed more than 2 sec.	1
	None	0

Total TRAUMA

Modified Glasgow Scale For Children (4)

Eye Opening	
Spontaneous	4
To speech	3
To pain	2
None	1
Best Verbal Response	
Coos Babbles	5
Irritable cries	4
Cries to pain	3
Moans to pain	2
None	1
Best Motor Response	
Normal spontaneous movements	6
Withdraws to touch	5
Withdraws to pain	4
Abnormal flexion	3
Abnormal extension	2
None	1

TOTAL

INITIAL ASSESSMENT/OBSERVATION:

TIME		NA	WNL	ABN	DETAILS OF ABNORMALITIES
	AIRWAY BREATHING		✓		
	CIRC/ RHYTHM		✓		
	NEURO		✓		☐ Lethargic ☐ Uncooperative ☐ Confused ☐ Combative ☐ Hysterical ☐ AOB
	PUPILS		✓		☐ Pinpoint ☐ Responding ☐ Dilated ☐ Fixed
	SKIN		✓		☒ Pale ☐ Diaphoretic ☐ Cyanotic ☐ Hot ☐ Cold ☐ Cool
	HEAD		✓		
	NECK		✓		
	CHEST		✓		
	ABDOMEN		✓		
	PELVIS				*Denies pain*
	BACK		✓		
	ARMS				*Moving well.*
	LEGS				*Rt thigh pain. Rt knee pain, ⊕ pedal abrasion inner anterior thigh. ⊕ blanching. Rt knee swelling*

Nursing Diagnoses

Initial Vital Signs
T *99.7*   P *105*   R *22*   BP *105/60*

continued

Case 6-30, *continued*

TRAUMA FLOW RECORD

Date	Patient Name	ED Number

Time

Graphic Code ∨ ∧ Systolic Diastolic BP Doppler BP ▼	Temp											
	106	240										
	105	220										
	104	200										
	103	180										
	102	160										
	101	140										
	100	120										
✗ Pulse Black	99	100										
	98	80										
● Oral T	97	60										
	96	40										
⊙ Rectal Temp	95	30										
	94	20										
○ Resp	93	10										
	92	0										
	SaO₂											
	GCS											

(Graph column at 2145 shows plotted points: X at 100, ● at 99/100, X at 60, ○ at 20)

TIME	PLAN-EVALUATION
2010	Rt leg is bent at knee. Pt is on Rt side. States he can't move his leg. Positive pedal pulse, positive tibial pulses. Ice to leg.
2020	Exam per Dr. Beck. Mother at bedside. Review findings with patient and mother. Pulses and refill remain intact.
2145	Good relief with med and sedation. Pt is arousable. Wound dressing changed with adapter and 3 x 5 around area cleansed.
2200	Applied splint to leg - mom

TIME	MEDICATIONS
2110	Mepergan 25/25 IM, Lt Quad

Valuables

☐ None ☐ With Patient ☐ Home/Family ☐ Valuables Envelope To Security

Type

DISPOSITION	TIME NOTIFIED	TIME OUT
☐ Floor _____		
☐ ICU _____		
☐ OR _____		
☐ Morgue/Coroner _____		2300
☑ Home _____		
☐ Report Given _____		
To: _____		

Via: ☐ Stretcher ☐ W/C | Identification Band on? | Organ donor?
☐ Bed ☐ Ambulatory ☐ Carry | ☐ Yes ☐ No | ☐ Yes ☐ No

Case 6-30, *continued*

RADIOLOGY REPORT

AP AND LATERAL RIGHT FEMUR:

CLINICAL DATA: Pain after trauma.

FINDINGS:

Without comparison films. There is nondisplaced fracture of the distal right femur proximal to the epiphyseal growth plate and not extending into the growth plate, the distal fragment is angulated relative to the proximal fragment, approximately 5°, with the apex of angle directed posteriorly. No other abnormalities are identified.

IMPRESSION: SIMPLE MINIMALLY. ANGULATED DISTAL RIGHT FEMORAL SHAFT FRACTURE NOT EXTENDING INTO THE EPIPHYSEAL GROWTH PLATE, AS DESCRIBED.

ICD-9-CM diagnosis code(s): _____

ICD-10-CM diagnosis code(s): _____

CPT code(s) with modifier, if applicable: _____

Case 6-31

Health Record Face Sheet

Western Medical Clinic

Record Number:	51-09-26
Age:	35
Gender:	Male
Length of Stay:	4 days
Service Type:	Inpatient
Discharge Status:	To Home
Diagnosis/Procedure:	AV Fistula

continued

Case 6-31, *continued*

OPERATIVE REPORT

PREOPERATIVE DIAGNOSIS: Right Arteriovenous Fistula.
Seizure disorder
Hypertension

POSTOPERATIVE DIAGNOSIS: Right Arteriovenous Fistula.
Seizure disorder.
Hypertension

OPERATION: Craniotomy
Resection Right Arteriovenous Fistula.

PROCEDURE:

The patient was brought to the operating room, with general anesthesia was placed in the supine position. The right side of his head was prepped and draped in sterile fashion. The transverse sinus and lesion were clearly identified on the scalp via preoperative CT scan. A U-shaped, inverted flap was surgically created to accommodate containment of the lesion. The flap also allowed access below the transverse sinus.

Incision was made down to bone. Dissection carried down to the periosteum utilizing cautery to contol bleeding. The scalp flap was reflected inferiorly and tacked into place after Raney clips were applied. Four bur holes were surgically created. Two bur holes were created above the transverse sinus and two bur holes were created below the transverse sinus. Great care was taken to confirm sinus location by image guidance intraoperatively. The dura was dissected free underneath the bone and then the Midas B1 bit was used to cut out a craniotomy flap in this area. Craniotomy flap was set aside for replacement at the end of the procedure. Small arterialized feeders to the right posterior margin of the bone were identified with bipolar coagulation utilized.

The bone flap was elevated and revealed normal appearing dura. The transverse sinus was appreciated. A C-shaped flap was made in a small fashion below the transverse sinus with the base on the transverse sinus overlying the cerebellum. Cut was extended through the dura with small arterialized feeders taken from the surface of the cerebellum to the dural AV fistula. The entire dorsal surface of the cerebellum was freed from the tentorium and transverse sinus. Another C-shaped flap was then created above the transverse sinus with the base on the transverse sinus overlying the inferior parietal lobe. The vein of Labbé was visualized. Small pial and dural arterialized vessels were controlled with bipolar coagulation without difficulty or significant bleeding. The base of the fistula revealed a large group of arterial vessels entering a cortical vein which was adjacent to the transverse sinus. This was coagulated with bipolar coagulation and divided sharply. The entire inferior parietal area was elevated off the transverse sinus. A small anastomotic portion of the vein of Labbé was also taken to allow for removal of the transverse sinus as pretermined with preoperative angiography. Preoperative angiogram revealed occlusion of the lateral transverse sinus.

Once the parietal lobe and cerebellum were lifted free off the tentorium, large clips were applied to the transverse sinus. Careful incision through the anterior and posterior margins of the transverse sinus accomplished a resection that extended just medial to the transverse sinus along the tentorium and around to the posterior margin of the resection. No significant bleeding was encountered. The remaining portion of the inferior parietal lobe adjacent, which contained a large venous varix, was surgically removed. A cordicotomy was created in a circular fashion surrounding the nidus. Surgical specimens and AV fistula were sent to pathology for confirmatory identification.

Bipolar coagulation of the remaining surface of the brain was accomplished along with application of Gelfoam. No significant bleeding was encountered. The rest of the brain surface was normal. Important to note that intraoperatively the median nerve somatosensory-evoked potentials which did not change throughout the surgery.

Closure was achieved with a piece of bovine pericardium being utilized to sew in the defect in the lateral dura, using a running 4–0 Vicryl stitch. The craniotomy bone flap was reattached using a small cranial plating system. The galea and muscle were closed using inverted 2–0 Vicryl sutures, followed by staples for the skin. Sterile dressings were applied.

Estimated blood loss was 300 cc. Sponge and needle counts were correct. Patient was sent to recovery room in stable condition.

Case 6-31, *continued*

ICD-9-CM diagnosis code(s): _____

ICD-10-CM diagnosis code(s): _____

CPT code(s) with modifier, if applicable: _____

Case 6-32

Health Record Face Sheet

Western Medical Clinic

Record Number:	70-49-08
Age:	53
Gender:	Male
Length of Stay:	3 days
Service Type:	Inpatient
Discharge Status:	To Home
Diagnosis/Procedure:	Cardiomyopathy
	Heart Catheterization

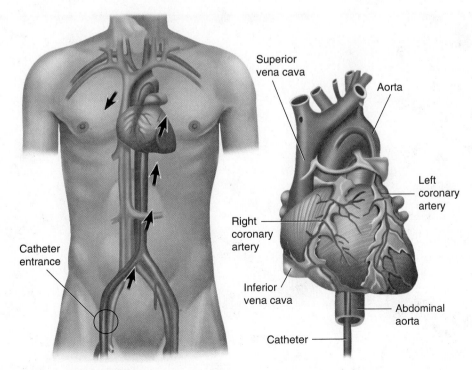

Cardiac catheterization.

Case 6-32, *continued*

DISCHARGE SUMMARY

ADMISSION DATE: 9/9/xx

DISCHARGE DATE: 9/11/xx

HISTORY OF PRESENT ILLNESS: The patient is a 53-year-old male admitted for evaluation of grossly abnormal Thallium test.

LABORATORY DATA: Glucose 106, BUN 11, Creatinine 1.1, liver function tests are all normal. Albumin 4.2, Sodium 141, Potassium 4.8, Cholesterol 166, Triglycerides 122, Iron 82. White count 6900, Hemoglobin 17.2, MCV 95, Platelets 136,000.

Resting MUGA ejection fraction is performed. This shows an ejection fraction of 4.7%.

The patient is admitted to the hospital and taken to the cardiac catheterization lab. The patient's hemodynamics showed right atrial pressure 4, pulmonary artery 32/14, pulmonary capillary wedge is 6, cardiac output is 6.5, pulmonary vascular resistance is 186, oximetry is unremarkable. Coronary arteries are all perfectly normal. There is no mitral regurgitation. Left ventricle is quite dilated. Ejection fraction angiographically is 46%. All walls are hypokinetic except for the anterobasilar wall which is normal.

This is felt to be due to an idiopathic cardiomyopathy with normal hemodynamics.

A resting MUGA scan was obtained as a baseline. The patient was discussed with Dr. Wright. The patient was discharged on 9/11/xx to be admitted on Thursday for myocardial biopsy.

DISCHARGE MEDICATIONS: Enteric Aspirin 5 grains once a day and Capoten 12.5 mg 1 1/2 tablets q 12 hours.

He is to follow up with me in a couple of weeks.

DISCHARGE DIAGNOSIS:

1. Idiopathic dilated cardiomyopathy, uncertain etiology.
2. Left bundle branch block.

Case 6-32, *continued*

HISTORY & PHYSICAL

DATE OF ADMISSION: 9/9/xx

HISTORY OF PRESENT ILLNESS:

The patient is a 53-year-old white male receiving primary care from Dr. Thomas with a grossly abnormal thallium treadmill test admitted now for heart catheterizatian.

The patient really has minimal symptoms, He presented to the health care system recently for a complete physical just to make sure that everything was going fine. Dr. Abbott noted that the patient was having some fatigue, and that he had a left bundle branch block. After discussing the case with Dr. Wright, a Thallium treadmill test was ordered which was quite abnormal as noted below.

The patient works in a factory doing fairly manual labor. He notes no exertional chest discomfort, neck discomfort, etc. of any type. He says that his exertional capacity and his exertional dyspnea is worse than it was 10 years ago, but feels that it is the same as it was 3 months ago and that it is the same as it was about a year ago. Apparently he had an upper respiratory infection with productive cough, runny nose, sneezing, etc. this fall, but feels that he recovered satisfactorily from that. He does recall several episodes of epigastric discomfort manifest as a pressure sensation lasting perhaps a day at a time. He says he ignored it and it went away, and wondered whether he might have some gallbladder trouble. This never seemed to particularly get worse with exertion.

The patient has no orthopnea, PND, or edema. He has used 2 pillows on his bed at night under his head for a long time. He has occasional heart racing but no light-headed spells, near syncope, or syncope. The patient smoked 1 1/2 packs of cigarettes daily for 30 years stopping 2 weeks ago. There is no history of hypertension, hyperlipidemia, diabetes, congenital heart disease, rheumatic fever, heart murmur, or MI. The patient is adopted and has no knowledge of his blood relatives.

He takes absolutely no medications. He has no allergies. His general review of systems in detail is unremarkable. His only surgery is minor surgery on his knee. He does not use alcohol at all and never has. He uses 1 caffeinated beverage a day. He has no GI distress. He denies history of drug abuse, eye problems, cancer, liver disease, emphysema, thyroid problems, gout, asthma, hay fever, hives, migraine headaches, TIA's, stroke, deep venous thrombosis, pulmonary embolism, kidney stones, etc.

PHYSICAL EXAMINATION:

BP 128/94, pulse 96, respirations 20, temp 97.9. No jugular venous distension.
LUNGS: Clear.
HEART: S1, S2 within normal limits with no murmurs, gallops, rubs or clicks.
ABDOMEN: Unremarkable. There is no peripheral edema.
SKIN: Is warm and dry.

ELECTROCARDIOGRAM: Complete left bundle branch block, with frequent PVC' s. Axis is +90°. Borderline right atrial enlargement.

EXERCISE THALLIUM TEST:

The patient exercised 5 minutes 37 seconds on a Bruce Protocol elevating his heart rate to 178 (107% predicted maximum), and blood pressure to 174/84. He was stopped because of fatigue. The patient's heart rate increased rapidly with exercise and at the end of 3 minutes of exercise his heart rate was already 165. At the end of 2 minutes of exercise it was 157. He remained in left bundle branch block throughout and there were no significant ST changes and no arrhythmias. He had no chest discomfort. The images showed a dilated left ventricle with hypoperfusion of the anterior wall, septal wall, and posterior wall. There was some redistribution of the anterior and anteraseptal aspects of the heart. There was no redistribution of the inferior aspect.

continued

Case 6-32, *continued*

HISTORY & PHYSICAL—PAGE 2

ECHOCARDIOGRAM:

The test is technically limited, but shows severely reduced left ventricular function with normal chamber dimensions. Left atrium is at 3.9 cm. E point to septal separation is 1.4.

ASSESSMENT:

1. High-risk thallium scan with reduced LV function on echocardiogram in patient with left bundle branch block and no symptoms.
2. Unknown family history.
3. Heavy smoking history.

PLAN:

Admit for heart catheterization.

CARDIAC CATHETERIZATION LABORATORY

PROCEDURE REPORT:

PATIENT: Jacob Tulley

Study Date: 9/10/xx

Referring Physician: Dr. Wright

PROCEDURE: Right and left heart catheterization, selective coronary angiography and left ventriculography.

PROCEDURE NOTE: The patient is brought to the cardiac catheterization lab, and the right inguinal area is prepped and draped in the usual manner. Using Seldinger technique, both the right femoral artery and right femoral vein are cannulated, and sheath introducers are placed in each vessel. All catheter manipulations are done using a guidewire and under fluoroscopic control. A fiberoptic Swan-Ganz catheter is positioned in the right heart. A pigtail catheter is positioned in the ascending aorta. Hemodynamic pressure measurements are made. The aortic valve is crossed in a retrograde manner. Hemodynamic pressure measurements are made. Thermodilution cardiac output is measured. Oximetry is measured in the right and left heart. The Swan-Ganz catheter is removed.

Left ventriculography is performed in the RAO projection and is recorded on 35-mm cineangiographic film. The catheter is then pulled back across the aortic valve while pressure measurements are being made.

The catheter is then exchanged over a guidewire for a Judkins left coronary catheter, and left coronary cineangiography is performed in multiple projections in the usual manner. The catheter is then exchanged over a guidewire for a Judkins right catheter, and right coronary cineangiography is performed in the usual manner.

At the conclusion of the case hemostasis is obtained after catheters were pulled. There are no complications.

HEMODYNAMIC FINDINGS: Right atrial pressure mean is 4 mm. of mercury. X and Y descent appear to be normal. The right ventricular end diastolic pressure is equal to the left ventricular end diastolic pressure. These two pressure wave forms are superimposed throughout diastole. Pulmonary artery pressure is 32/14, mean 21. Pulmonary capillary wedge mean is 6, with a normal V wave. Left ventricular pressure is 125/8. Aortic pressure is 125/65, mean 86. There is no gradient across the mitral valve during diastole or across the aortic valve during systole. Thermodilution cardiac output is 6.46 liters per minute. Systemic vascular resistance is 1015. Pulmonary vascular resistance is 186. Oximetry on blood samples shows saturation as follows: pulmonary artery 65%, right ventricle 64%, right atrium 64.7%, vena cavae 65%. Room air blood gas in the left ventricle 7.45, P02 62, PC02 37, Bicarb. 26, Saturation 89%.

Case 6-32, *continued*

CARDIAC CATHETERIZATION LABORATORY—PAGE 2

LEFT VENTRICULOGRAM: There is no mitral regurgitation. The anterobasilar wall moves normal. All other walls of the ventricle are hypokinetic. The left ventricle is moderately dilated, with an end diastolic volume of 321 cc's (upper limits of normal for his body surface area is 257 cc's). Ejection fraction is measured on several beats and ranges between 42 and 52%.

CORONARY ANGIOGRAPHY: The coronary arteries are perfectly smooth and within normal limits. The LAD gives rise to a moderate sized first diagonal branch and a moderately large second diagonal branch. There is a large bifurcated ramus intermedius branch. There are two moderately large posterolateral branches of the circumflex. The right coronary artery gives rise to the posterior descending artery and one posterolateral branch.

CONCLUSIONS:
1. Normal coronary arteries.
2. Dilated hypocontractile left ventricle with no mitral regurgitation.
3. Normal hemodynamics and cardiac output.
4. Normal oximetry.
5. Mild resting hypoxia.

This picture is consistent with an idiopathic dilated cardiomyopathy.

ICD-9-CM diagnosis code(s): _____

ICD-10-CM diagnosis code(s): _____

CPT code(s) with modifier, if applicable: _____

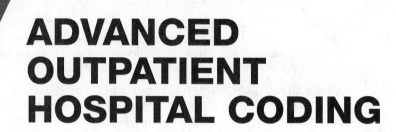

ADVANCED OUTPATIENT HOSPITAL CODING

7

Hospital outpatient coding comprises a majority of hospital coding because many hospital outpatients are seen on a daily basis. The hospital outpatient coder is responsible for assigning codes for patients seen in the emergency department and those seen for same-day surgeries, observations, and ancillary departments, such as dialysis, oncology, hyperbarics, radiology, the laboratory, and physical therapy, to name a few.

For all cases presented in this chapter, apply all of the coding skills and knowledge you have to do the following:

1. Assign and sequence the primary ICD-9-CM and ICD-10-CM diagnosis codes first, followed by any applicable secondary diagnoses to include appropriate V-code and E-code assignments as dictated by the setting.

2. Assign and sequence the primary CPT® procedure code first, followed by any applicable additional procedure codes to include modifiers as appropriate. Modifiers may include CPT Level 1 and/or HCPCS Level II codes as dictated by the setting.

3. Assign APC assignments.

It might be helpful to review the ICD-9-CM and/or ICD-10-CM *Official Guidelines for Coding and Reporting* for outpatient coding (refer to Appendix A for instructions for accessing the guidelines online) as you start to assign codes to these case studies. Remember, facility E/M ER levels are not assigned in this text because these are based on each facility's own coding guidelines.

Health Record Face Sheet

Western Regional
Medical Center

Record Number:	15-06-78
Age:	20
Gender:	Male
Length of Stay:	Not Applicable
Diagnosis/Procedure:	Multiple Drug Ingestion
Service Type:	Emergency Room
Discharge Status:	Transfer to Psychiatric Facility

continued

EMERGENCY ROOM REPORT

ALL EKGs, X-RAY REPORTS AND LABORATORY TESTS NOTED IN DICTATION ARE THE INTERPRETATION OF THE DICTATING PHYSICIAN UNLESS SPECIFICALLY NOTED OTHERWISE. ALL CONSULTS WITH PHYSICIANS AS LISTED IN DICTATION ARE <u>BY TELEPHONE</u> UNLESS OTHERWISE SPECIFIED.

PATIENT	PHYSICIAN	DATE OF SERVICE
Emmett Ernest	Dr. Bates	12/26/xx

CHIEF COMPLAINT: MULTIPLE INGESTION.

HISTORY OF PRESENT ILLNESS: This 20-year-old presents to the ED very irritated, yelling, somewhat combatively. When I am able to finally calm him down, he states that he and a girl-friend have a bond, and she gave a key back today that kind of set this all off and he became very upset, disgruntled, and wanted to kill himself. He subsequently ingested a mouthful of regular gasoline, some car wax, some hydrogen peroxide, and about 15 mg of what he states are Doral tablets, at least what was reported, this is somewhat unclear and unable to be substantiated although we do have a bottle of quasopam here with him. He then tried to use a knife and injure himself, however his brother stopped him, and the police by this time had arrived. I understand the patient did have kind of an upset stomach, and he called dispatch and subsequently the police were sent to the home. He was brought in by the authorities now for evaluation and admission.

PAST MEDICAL HISTORY: He tells me it is one for admission in hospital, even though he states he was given no diagnosis. He states he has had some liver enzymes elevated in the past but denies hepatitis or other medical problems.

CURRENT MEDICATIONS: None.

<u>MEDICATION ALLERGIES:</u>   **<u>NONE KNOWN.</u>**

SOCIAL HISTORY: This patient is not married, lives here in the west-side area.

PHYSICAL EXAM: The patient initially refused vitals, but ultimately we received permission. They include BP 113/76, P 76, R 16, afebrile.

HEENT: Nonfocal.

NECK: Supple.

LUNGS: Clear.

HEART: Showed regular rate and rhythm.

ABDOMEN: Soft and benign.

EXTREMITIES: Unremarkable.

NEURO: He is very baseline, intact, pupils are not pinpoint, they are mid reactive at this point, he remains stable.

CONTINUED

EMERGENCY ROOM REPORT

ALL EKGs, X-RAY REPORTS AND LABORATORY TESTS NOTED IN DICTATION ARE THE INTERPRETATION OF THE DICTATING PHYSICIAN UNLESS SPECIFICALLY NOTED OTHERWISE. ALL CONSULTS WITH PHYSICIANS AS LISTED IN DICTATION ARE <u>BY TELEPHONE</u> UNLESS OTHERWISE SPECIFIED.

PATIENT	PHYSICIAN	DATE OF SERVICE
Emmett Ernest	Dr. Bates	12/26/xx

PAGE TWO

EMERGENCY DEPARTMENT COURSE: The poisondex and poison control was reviewed, it was decided not to charcoal this gentleman or NG or lavage this patient because of risk of gasoline ingestion. He will be observed here closely in the ED. He was admitted at 2220, remained stable throughout his ED stay until subsequent discharge at 0115.

LABORATORY: CBC and SMAC were reviewed and very normal at this time. His urine tox screen was only positive for marijuana, negative for everything else at this point.

ASSESSMENT: MULTIPLE DRUG INGESTION, APPEARS MINOR.

PLAN: This patient was transferred by the police to West Valley Health Facility for further psychiatric evaluation, he will be closely observed for tonight, and he was discharged from the ED with appropriate transfer papers in stable and satisfactory condition.

Dr. Bates
_____

continued

Case 7-1, *continued*

E.D.#: 15-06-78

MEDICAL RECORDS

EMERGENCY TREATMENT RECORD

ARRIVAL DATE: *12/26/XX*　　TIME: *22:20*　　AM.

PATIENT NAME: *Emmett Ernest*

PHYSICIAN: *Dr. BATES*

AGE *20Y*　　SEX *M*

BIRTH DATE: *09-14-XX*

CHIEF COMPLAINT

　Ingested Gasoline, Carwax, Meds

ACTIVITY LEVEL

PHYSICIAN'S NOTES

R　　　L

DISABILITY
　Estimated No. of Days _____

☒ Chart Dictated　　☐ Not Dictated

DIAGNOSIS: *Drug Ingestion Suicide attempt*

DISCHARGE CONDITION:
☒ Stable　　☐ Unchanged　　☐ Transferred　　☐ Improved　　☐ AMA
☐ Admitted　　☐ Expired　　☐ Not Seen By Physician

P.A., F.P. RESIDENT SIGNATURE

E.D. PHYSICIAN SIGNATURE

CONSENT FOR TREATMENT

　CONSENT FOR TREATMENT: I am presenting myself for inpatient and/or outpatient care at Western Regional Medical Center and I voluntarily consent to the rendering of such care including diagnostic procedures and medical treatment by authorized agents and employees of Western Regional Medical Center and by its medical staff or their designees as in their professional judgment may be deemed necessary. I acknowledge that no guarantees have been made to me as to the result of examination or treatment in this hospital.

PATIENT OR REPRESENTATIVE SIGNATURE

　　　　　　Emmett Ernest

DATE	TIME	IF REPRESENTATIVE, INDICATE RELATIONSHIP
WITNESS SIGNATURE		DATE
WITNESS SIGNATURE		DATE

PHYSICIAN'S ORDERS

E.D.#

PATIENT NAME: *Emmett Ernest*

DATE	TIME	1	2	3	ORDERS
12/26	10:45 pm				CBC, SMAC, UA
					UA TOX SCREEN

Case 7-1, *continued*

ICD-9-CM diagnosis code(s): _____

ICD-10-CM diagnosis code(s): _____

CPT code(s) with modifier, if applicable: _____

APC: _____

Case 7-2

Health Record Face Sheet

Western Regional
Medical Center

Record Number:	46-11-08
Age:	87
Gender:	Male
Length of Stay:	Not Applicable
Diagnosis/Procedure:	Contusion of Left Ischial Tuberostiy
Service Type:	Emergency Room
Discharge Status:	To Home

EMERGENCY ROOM REPORT

IDENTIFICATION: THIS IS AN 87-YEAR-OLD CAUCASIAN MALE.
CHIEF COMPLAINT: BACK INJURY.

HISTORY OF PRESENT ILLNESS: The patient states that he has had difficulty with his gait for the last six months. He stumbled and fell at around 10:00 yesterday morning and landed on his left side. The patient did not suffer any loss of consciousness or light-headedness or head injury. The patient states that when he woke up this morning, he had difficulty getting out of bed because of soreness over the left buttock area. The patient now presents for evaluation and would like to get an x-ray of the area of soreness.

ALLERGIES: NONE.

CURRENT MEDS: Digoxin.

PREVIOUS ILLNESSES: History of atrial fibrillation.

PHYSICAL EXAMINATION: Temp. 97.8° orally, pulse 86 and irregular, resp. 22, BP 162/92. Pleasant, elderly, Caucasian male in no acute distress. On lower extremity exam, the patient had no evidence of external rotation or shortening of the hip. The patient had normal flexion and extension of the hip and no pain on rotation of the left hip passively. Palpation of the patient's lumbar spine revealed there was no significant tenderness. The patient had +2 tenderness over the left ischial tuberosity. Straight leg raising was negative bilaterally. The patient was able to flex both hips without difficulty. DTRs knee jerks could not be elicited. Babinski and downgoing toes bilaterally. X-ray of the pelvis showed no evidence of fracture or dislocation. Some degenerative changes in both hips were noted.

IMPRESSION: CONTUSION OF THE LEFT ISCHIAL TUBEROSITY.

PLAN: The patient was reassured. He is to take Tylenol 10 grams po q4h prn pain and follow up here prn. The patient is to follow up with Dr. Smalls.

continued

Case 7-2, *continued*

			MEDICAL RECORDS	

E.D. #: 46-11-08	**EMERGENCY TREATMENT RECORD**	ARRIVAL DATE: *9/14/xx*	TIME: *14:00 A.M.*

Patient Last Name	First Name	Middle Initial	AGE	SEX	BIRTH DATE
Ellis	*Ernie*		*87 Y*	*M*	*5/15/xx*

CHIEF COMPLAINT	ACTIVITY LEVEL
BACK INJ	

PHYSICIAN PROGRESS NOTES

Difficulty with gait x 6 months

No LOC

No Light head

R   *Fell at 10 am onto L hip*

This AM hard to get up

See Abd - 39

No shrinking

spine no tenderness

No Set

nl EAROM

+2 tender ribs post

No pain on rotation

Tx check tubules

DISABILITY

Estimated No. of Days _____   ☒ Chart Dictated   ☐ Not Dictated

DIAGNOSIS

Contusion Left ischial tuberosity

DISCHARGE CONDITION:

☒ Stable   ☐ Unchanged   ☐ Transferred   ☒ Improved   ☐ AMA
☐ Admitted   ☐ Expired   ☐ Not Seen By Physician

P.A., F.P. RESIDENT SIGNATURE

E.D. PHYSICIAN SIGNATURE

CONSENT FOR TREATMENT

CONSENT FOR TREATMENT: I am presenting myself for inpatient and/or outpatient care at Western Regional Medical Center and I voluntarily consent to the rendering of such care including diagnostic procedures and medical treatment by authorized agents and employees of Western Regional Medical Center and by its medical staff or their designees as in their professional judgment may be deemed necessary. I acknowledge that no guarantees have been made to me as to the result of examination or treatment in this hospital.

PATIENT OR REPRESENTATIVE SIGNATURE

Ernie Ellis

DATE	TIME	IF REPRESENTATIVE, INDICATE RELATIONSHIP
WITNESS SIGNATURE		DATE
WITNESS SIGNATURE		DATE

PHYSICIAN'S ORDERS

E.D. #				PATIENT NAME: *Ernie Ellis*

DATE	TIME	1	2	3	ORDERS
9/14/xx	1445				*Pelvis X-ray*
9/14/xx	1455				
					Tylenol V po q 4 hr prn.
					ORDERED DRAWN RETURNED TO X-RAY RETURN

Case 7-2, *continued*

DEPARTMENT OF RADIOLOGY AND MEDICAL IMAGING

ER

AP PELVIS,

CLINICAL DATA: Pain.

IMPRESSION: NO HIP FRACTURES. MILD DEGENERATIVE CHANGES APPROPRIATE FOR AGE.

VASCULAR CALCIFICATIONS.

ROUNDED MARKED DENSITY RIGHT PELVIS OF UNCERTAIN ETIOLOGY AND/OR POSITION. WOULD REQUIRE CT SCAN FOR FURTHER DEFINITION.

NO PELVIC FRACTURES.

ICD-9-CM diagnosis code(s): _____

ICD-10-CM diagnosis code(s): _____

CPT code(s) with modifier, if applicable: _____

APC: _____

Case 7-3

Health Record Face Sheet

Western Regional
Medical Center

Record Number:	95-04-13
Age:	59
Gender:	Female
Length of Stay:	Not Applicable
Diagnosis/Procedure:	Radial Fracture
Service Type:	Emergency Room
Discharge Status:	To Home

continued

Case 7-3, *continued*

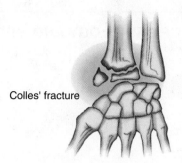

Colles' fracture

A break in the distal portion
of the radius.
Source: Pearson Education/PH
College

EMERGENCY ROOM REPORT

CHIEF COMPLAINT: INJURY TO RIGHT WRIST.

HISTORY OF PRESENT ILLNESS: This 59-year-old tripped over her water hose this morning, sustaining injury to the right wrist. No other injury. She is in here for evaluation.

PAST MEDICAL HISTORY: Remarkable for surgical thyroidectomy.

MEDICATIONS: Include thyroid supplement.

ALLERGIES: **NONE KNOWN.**

PHYSICAL EXAM:
GENERAL: This is a 59-year-old white female with some swelling to the right wrist area. Her MCP, PIP and DIP joints are otherwise WNL, with full ROM of the right elbow. She is tender over the distal right radius.

X-ray demonstrated a comminuted fracture of the distal right radius, with joint space involvement, however, her fragments appear in good position at this time. She did have a chip off the ulna styloid as well. No other fracture is appreciated.

HOSPITAL COURSE: A bivalve fiberglass splint was placed, and she will follow up with Dr. Redi who I initially tried to contact via phone, however, he was in the OR and a message was left for him that this patient will be following with him in the office this next week.

ASSESSMENT: RIGHT DISTAL RADIUS FRACTURE AND ULNA STYLOID FRACTURE.

PLAN: Bivalve splint, ice, elevate. She was offered something for pain, but felt she did not require it. She will follow up with Dr. Redi this next week, and return for any marked worsening symptoms or problems and/or prn.

Case 7-3, *continued*

MEDICAL RECORDS

| E.D. # 95-04-13 | **EMERGENCY TREATMENT RECORD** | ARRIVAL DATE: *07-15-xx* | TIME: *11:50 A.M.* |

| NAME: *Iris Itle* | PHYSICIAN: *Dr. Gregson* | AGE: *59 Y* | SEX: *F* | BIRTH DATE: *03/14/xx* |

CHIEF COMPLAINT
 INJ RIGHT WRIST

ACTIVITY LEVEL

PHYSICIAN'S NOTES

R   L

DISABILITY
 Estimated No. of Days _____ ☒ Chart Dictated ☐ Not Dictated

DIAGNOSIS:
Right Radius Fx/Ulna Styloid Fx.

DISCHARGE CONDITION:
☒ Stable ☐ Unchanged ☐ Transferred ☐ Improved ☐ AMA
☐ Admitted ☐ Expired ☐ Not Seen By Physician

PHYSICIAN'S ORDERS

| E.D. # | | | | PATIENT NAME: Iris Itle |

DATE	TIME	1	2	3	ORDERS
7/15/xx	12:10 pm				*Right Wrist*

| | | | | | | ORDERED | DRAWN | RETURNED | TO X-RAY | RETURN |

continued

Case 7-3, *continued*

RADIOLOGY REPORT

RIGHT WRIST:

Comminuted fracture involving the distal radius. Fracture line extends into the radiocarpal joint space. Small avulsion fracture of the ulnar styloid. The carpal row appears intact.

IMPRESSION: COMMINUTED FRACTURE WITH EXTENSION INTO THE RADIOCAR-PAL JOINT DISTAL RADIUS.

AVULSION FRACTURE ULNAR STYLOID.

ICD-9-CM diagnosis code(s): _____

ICD-10-CM diagnosis code(s): _____

CPT code(s) with modifier, if applicable: _____

APC: _____

Case 7-4

Health Record Face Sheet

		Western Regional Medical Center
Record Number:	18-40-56	
Age:	29	
Gender:	Male	
Length of Stay:	N/A	
Diagnosis/Procedure:	Epigastric Pain	
Service Type:	Emergency Room	
Discharge Status:	To Home	

Case 7-4, *continued*

EMERGENCY ROOM REPORT

ALL EKGS, X-RAY REPORTS AND LABORATORY TESTS NOTED IN DICTATION ARE THE INTERPRETATION OF THE DICTATING PHYSI-
CIAN UNLESS SPECIFICALLY NOTED OTHERWISE. ALL CONSULTS WITH PHYSICIANS AS LISTED IN DICTATION ARE <u>BY</u> <u>TELEPHONE</u>
UNLESS OTHERWISE SPECIFIED.

PATIENT	PHYSICIAN	DATE OF SERVICE
Frank Fuller	Dr. Bates	4/15/xx

ID AND CHIEF COMPLAINT: This 29-year-old male comes in with abdominal pain.

HISTORY OF PRESENT ILLNESS: He has a one-month history of epigastric pain associated
with eating heavy foods such as pizza. He describes a burning sort of sensation in the epigastrium. Sometimes it radiates through to his back. He has had no nausea or vomiting. He states
that the pain sometimes lasts as long as 4-5 hours. This morning, it woke him up at about 3 or
4 a.m. It has been very uncomfortable, and he has been unable to get back to sleep. It seems
to be less of a problem if he doesn't eat so late in the day and if he eats very mild foods. He
has tried antacids, but this doesn't seem to have helped at all.

ALLERGIES: NONE KNOWN.

CURRENT MEDICATIONS: Mylanta.

PAST MEDICAL HISTORY: Significant for hypertension in the family. Otherwise negative.

PHYSICAL EXAM:	BP 152/110, temp 97, pulse 56, resp 12.
GENERAL:	This adult male appears in mild discomfort. His color is good, skin is warm and dry.
HEENT:	TMs, nose, and throat are clear. PERRLA.
NECK:	Supple without adenopathy.
LUNGS:	Clear to auscultation.
HEART:	Normal.
BACK:	No CVA tenderness.
ABDOMEN:	Soft, there is mild epigastric pain, and there is tenderness in the right upper quadrant, particularly when he takes a deep breath. Bowel sounds are normally active in all quadrants, and there are no masses. No rebound or guarding.

EMERGENCY DEPARTMENT COURSE: The patient was given a GI cocktail, and he says it
seems to give him some mild relief, but it certainly doesn't completely relieve the discomfort.
However, he states that he has gradually gotten a lot more comfortable over the last hour or
so. I ordered a CBC and SMAC. His white count is 5,600 with 39 polys, 45 lymphs, 1 atypical
lymph, 10 monos, 1 eo, and 4 basos. Hemoglobin is 16.9, hematocrit 49.8, platelet count
258,000. SMAC is completely within normal limits in all parameters.

ASSESSMENT: EPIGASTRIC PAIN ASSOCIATED WITH EATING HEAVY FOODS,
                   BUT THE EXACT ETIOLOGY IS UNDETERMINED AT THIS TIME. IT
                   MAY BE EITHER GALLBLADDER OR GASTRITIS OR ESOPHAGEAL
                   SPASM.

PLAN: We will try a few days of Tagamet 400 mg bid. Also, will schedule him for gallbladder
ultrasound, and it will be done tomorrow, and he will follow up with Dr. Williams sometime
toward the end of the week. If he gets acutely worse, he may return any time.

continued

Case 7-4, *continued*

MEDICAL RECORDS

E.D. # 18-40-56	**EMERGENCY TREATMENT RECORD**	ARRIVAL DATE: *04/15/xx*	TIME: *0450 A.M.*

PATIENT NAME: *Frank Fuller*	PHYSICIAN: *Dr. Bates*	AGE: *29 Y*	SEX: *M*	BIRTH DATE: *1/9/xx*

CHIEF COMPLAINT

STOMACH PAIN

ACTIVITY LEVEL

PHYSICIAN'S NOTES	**DISABILITY**

1 mo hx of epigastric pain P̄

eating heavy food such as pizza.

A burning in the epigastric on right

R   L

Estimated No. of Days _____   ☐ Chart Dictated   ☐ Not Dictated

DIAGNOSIS:

Abdominal pain ? Etiology

DISCHARGE CONDITION:

☒ Stable   ☐ Unchanged   ☐ Transferred   ☐ Improved   ☐ AMA
☐ Admitted   ☐ Expired   ☐ Not Seen By Physician

P.A., F.P. RESIDENT SIGNATURE

E.D. PHYSICIAN SIGNATURE

CONSENT FOR TREATMENT

CONSENT FOR TREATMENT: I am presenting myself for inpatient and/or outpatient care at Western Regional Medical Center and I voluntarily consent to the rendering of such care including diagnostic procedures and medical treatment by authorized agents and employees of Western Regional Medical Center and by its medical staff or their designees as in their professional judgment may be deemed necessary. I acknowledge that no guarantees have been made to me as to the result of examination or treatment in this hospital.

PATIENT SIGNATURE

Frank Fuller

DATE	TIME	IF REPRESENTATIVE, INDICATE RELATIONSHIP
WITNESS SIGNATURE		DATE
WITNESS SIGNATURE		DATE

PHYSICIAN'S ORDERS

E.D. #					PATIENT NAME: Frank Fuller

DATE	TIME	1	2	3	ORDERS
4/15/xx	5:05				*CBC, SMAC*
					Schedule for G.B. ultrasound on Mon. or Tues.
					F/u with Dr. Williams
					Tagament 4 BID
					GI Cocktail
					ORDERED DRAWN RETURNED TO X-RAY RETURN

Case 7-4, *continued*

ICD-9-CM diagnosis code(s): _____

ICD-10-CM diagnosis code(s): _____

CPT code(s) with modifier, if applicable: _____

APC: _____

Case 7-5

Health Record Face Sheet

Western Regional
Medical Center

Record Number:	30-03-46
Age:	75
Gender:	Male
Length of Stay:	N/A
Diagnosis/Procedure:	Chest Wall Syndrome
Service Type:	Emergency Room
Discharge Status:	To Home

EMERGENCY DEPARTMENT VISIT

SUBJECTIVE: By history the patient is a 75-year-old male with a history of angina, hypertension and diabetes. The patient states that he has been in his usual state of health until awakened from sleep about an hour ago. He was awakened by pain in his right thoracic back in the intrascapular area. There is no radiation of the pain. No associated shortness of breath or diaphoresis. He denies any anterior chest discomfort. The pain is described as a steady achiness. He is unaware of any injury to the area. The pain is not in any way similar to angina or any other particular pain he has had. The pain was apparently quite severe but it has subsided slightly. The pain is not pleuritic nor is there any other specific activity which aggravates the pain.

OBJECTIVE: The patient is alert. His color is good. He is in no acute distress. The neck is supple and full range of motion does not aggravate his pain. The lungs are clear to auscultation. Cardiac exam reveals a regular sinus rhythm. There is a grade 2/6 systolic murmur; the patient is hypertensive at 172/88. His other vital signs are normal. The chest wall is quite tender locally in the right interscapular back. There is no flank or CVA tenderness and the abdomen is benign. An EKG and chest x-ray are obtained which show no significant change from previous records.

ASSESSMENT: Chest wall syndrome.

PLAN: The patient will be treated with Nalfon 600 mg three times daily. He is also given six tablets of Tylenol with Codeine #3 which he may take 1 or 2 every four hours as needed for pain. Follow up will be with Dr. Hart at his earliest convenience.

continued

Case 7-5, *continued*

RADIOLOGY REPORT

EXAM: Chest

CHEST:

Two views of the chest are compared with AP portable recumbent film about 3 years ago. No significant change has taken place. The lungs are free of infiltrates. Heart size is borderline enlarged. There is a little soft tissue density in the left cardiophrenic angle probably secondary to a small hiatus hernia. I can only see it on the PA view. The patient has had a previously documented hiatus hernia. Mediastinum and thoracic cage are otherwise unremarkable. There is a little calcification in the left upper lobe which is stable. Some minor degenerative end plate changes in the dorsal spine can be seen as well as some mild atheromatous plaqueing in the aortic knob.

Pulmonary flow pattern is within normal range.

IMPRESSION:

Stable borderline cardiomegaly.

HISTORY: Chest pain.

DIAGNOSTIC IMAGING

ICD-9-CM diagnosis code(s): _____

ICD-10-CM diagnosis code(s): _____

CPT code(s) with modifier, if applicable: _____

APC: _____

Case 7-6

Health Record Face Sheet

Record Number:	38-14-51	Western Regional Medical Center
Age:	36	
Gender:	Female	
Length of Stay:	N/A	
Diagnosis/Procedure:	Chest Pain	
Service Type:	Emergency Room	
Discharge Status:	To Home	

Case 7-6, *continued*

ALLERGIES		TETANUS STATUS
CURRENT MEDS		LMP

HISTORY & PHYSICAL   T: P: R: BP: SaO$_2$: WT: BY (INIT)

TIME OF MD
INTIAL ASSESSMENT

R   L

LABS		
☐ ABG on _____ *l*		
☐ Admit Packet		
☐ Amylase		
☐ Cardiac Packet		
☐ CBC		
☐ CBG on _____ *l*		
☐ Chem Profile _____		
☐ CPK/ISO		
☒ EKG		
☐ Glucose		
☐ HGD ☐ SERUM ☐ URINE		
☐ Lytes		
☐ PT/PTT		
☐ Trauma Packet		
☐ Type & Screen		
☐ Type & Cross _____		
☐ UA		
☐ CSF		
☐ Culture _____		

DICTATED ☒ Yes ☐ No

TIME	TREATMENT ORDERS	X-RAYS
2020	Viscous Xylocaine 15 cc + Mylanta 30 cc p.o.	☐ Chest
		☐ C-Spine
		☐ Flat Plate/Upright (ABD)
		☐ CT ☐ HEAD ☐ ABD

DIAGNOSIS:
   Probable Reflux Esophagitis

DISCHARGE TIME *2220*	DISCHARGE INSTRUCTIONS

(1) Zantac 150 mg bid # 30
(2) Carofate given qid 1/2 hr AC/HS

EMERGENCY DEPARTMENT RECORD

continued

Case 7-6, *continued*

PG _____ OF _____

MEDICAL RECORDS

ETA _____   MR# 38-14-51

DATE: 03/14/xx   □ EMERGENT □ URGENT ☑ NON URGENT

| PATIENT NAME: Jamie Johnson | AGE 36 | □ M ☑ F | ED NO: 38-14-51 | PVT MD | | MODE OF ARRIVAL | □ Rescue/Amb. □ Wheelchair ☑ Ambulatory □ Air □ Carried |

HISTORY / CHIEF COMPLAINT

Anterior chest pain

MVA - RESTRAINED   □ YES □ NO
MORTORCYCLE - HELMET   □ YES □ NO
REPORTABLE INJURY   □ YES □ NO

REPORTED TO: DATE   TIME

TRIAGE
MENTAL STATUS: alert   COLOR: good
RESPIRATIONS: even   SKING TUGOR: good

□ O₂   □ Elevate   □ MED. _____
□ Splint □ Dressing   □ MED. _____
□ Ice   □ _____   TRIAGE NURSE

PTA GCS CRAMS   □ BACKBOARD □ C-COLLAR □

| **ALLERGIES** | *Ampicillin* | | **TETANUS** |

CURRENT MEDICATIONS   Ø

☑ CURRENT   □ R
□ NOT CURRENT   □ L
□ TT □ Td   □ DEL
□ DT □ DPT   □ TH

PMH   *Hypokalemia*

ASSESSMENT

(NEURO, CARDIAC, RESPIRATORY, GI, GU, SKIN, INCIDENT TIME)

LOT #

Presents to ER c/o pain in anterior chest rediating through to back, sharp between shoulders. Denies radiation to arms. Pt states when pain began was diaphoretic, felt very weak. Shaky, blurry eyesight. Feels like needles in R arm

VISUAL ACUITY
OD _____
OS _____
OU _____

WT

LMP

TIME	TEMP	P	R	BP	SaO₂ O₂	TIME	MEDICATION/DOSE	ROUTE	SITE	SIGNATURE
2020	988	79	18	116/79	—0	2055	Mylanta / 30 cc	PO		
2100	984	91	18	121/86	0	2105	Visc Lidocaine / 15cc	SQ		
				/						
				/						
				/						

TIME	IV FLUID/AMOUNT	MEDICATION ADDED	RATE/HR	SIZE	SITE	TIME Dc'd	AMT INFUSED	SIGNATURE

TIME	PROBLEM/CHANGE	INTERVENTION	PATIENT RESPONSE / EVALUATION
2055		Med as above	
2100		EKG	

SIGNATURE/ TITLE X   *A. Smith, R.N.*

SIGNATURE/ TITLE X

□ SEE ADDENDUM ED NURSES FLOW SHEET

DISCHARGE TIME: *3:45 PM*

DISPOSITION ☑ Discharged □ AMA
□ Admit/Transfer _____
Report Given To: _____
CONDITION ON DISCHARGE/TRANSFER ☑ Stable
□ Stabilized   □ Improved   □ Expired
DISCHARGE MODE: ☑ Ambutatory
□ Wheelchair □ Stretcher □ Carried
Accom. by _____

PATIENT BELONGINGS	BAG	ON PT.	NONE
Clothing _____	□	□	☑
Wallet/Purse _____	□	□	☑
Money _____	□	□	☑
Jewelry _____	□	□	☑
Glasses _____	□	□	☑
Dentures _____	□	□	☑

DISPOSITION: ☑ Not Disrobed □ Patient □ Family
□ Security □ SEE BELONGINGS LIST

Case 7-6, *continued*

EMERGENCY ROOM HISTORY AND PHYSICAL

The patient is a 36-year-old female who comes in to the emergency room at this time complaining of some pain in her anterior chest. She states this pain radiates directly through to her back. She also experiences some pain down her right arm. She notes the pain is quite intense at this time between her shoulder blades. She notes that at one point in time, when the pain began, she was quite sweaty. She has been feeling weak and shaking. She states she has been under a great deal of stress from marital and family problems. She is allergic to ampicillin. She has a history of hypokalemia.

EXAMINATION: Physical examination at this time includes a blood pressure of 116/79, respirations 18, pulse 79, temperature 98.8. Exam of the patient reveals her head to be normal cephalic. Ears: Tympanic membranes are intact and within normal limits bilaterally. Pharynx: No erythema or exudates noted. Neck is supple and non-tender. No adenopathy noted. Lungs are clear to auscultation and percussion. Heart: Normal S1 and S2, without murmur or gallop noted. Abdomen: Soft with normal bowel sounds. No masses, tenderness, organomegaly palpable. Back: No CVAT, no edema.

An EKG obtained tonight shows a sinus rhythm with normal QRST configuration. The patient was given viscous Xylocaine 15 cc plus Mylanta 30 cc p.o. and noted moderate relief with this medication.

ANALYSIS: Probable reflux esophagitis.

PLAN: Will treat with Zantac 150 mg p.o. b.i.d. plus Carafate one gram q.i.d. dissolved in liquid and taken one half hour before meals and at bedtime. The patient is to return for a recheck if getting worse or if not improving.

ICD-9-CM diagnosis code(s): _____

ICD-10-CM diagnosis code(s): _____

CPT code(s) with modifier, if applicable: _____

APC: _____

Case 7-7

Health Record Face Sheet

Western Regional
Medical Center

Record Number:	06-58-95
Age:	91
Gender:	Female
Length of Stay:	Not Applicable
Diagnosis/Procedure:	Congestive Heart Failure
Service Type:	Emergency Room
Discharge Status:	Home

EMERGENCY ROOM REPORT

MR Number: 06-58-95   Age: 91   Sex: F

S: The patient comes in stating that her legs are swollen and tender to touch. She has had a little bit of shortness of breath and just has not been feeling normal.
PAST MEDICAL HISTORY: Congestive heart failure, hypertension, gastritis.
MEDICATION: Warfarin, potassium, Lasix, clonazepam, metoprolol, Dilantin, and omeprazole.
ALLERGIES: PENICILLIN.

O: VITAL SIGNS: As noted. 02 saturations 88%.
GENERAL: Alert and oriented.
HEENT: Unremarkable. LUNGS: There are a few crackles in the lungs.
HEART: Regular rate and rhythm.
EXTREMITIES: There is edema.
LABORATORY/DIAGNOSTIC: Normal CBC. Comprehensive panel shows a BUN that is slightly elevated, otherwise unremarkable. Her BNP is high at 442.

A: Congestive heart failure. Peripheral edema.

P: We will have her double up her Lasix taking 2 a day and potassium 2 a day for the next 5 days and then go back to her regular medications. If she is still having swelling problems she is to let us know.

ICD-9-CM diagnosis code(s): _____

ICD-10-CM diagnosis code(s): _____

CPT code(s) with modifier, if applicable: _____

APC: _____

Case 7-8

Health Record Face Sheet

Western Regional
Medical Center

Record Number:	17-20-29
Age:	70
Gender:	Male
Length of Stay:	N/A
Diagnosis/Procedure:	Acute Urinary Retention
Service Type:	Emergency Room
Discharge Status:	To Home

continued

EMERGENCY ROOM REPORT

ALL EKGS, X-RAY REPORTS AND LABORATORY TESTS NOTED IN DICTATION ARE THE INTERPRETATION OF THE DICTATING PHYSI-
CIAN UNLESS SPECIFICALLY NOTED OTHERWISE. ALL CONSULTS WITH PHYSICIANS AS LISTED IN DICTATION ARE <u>BY TELEPHONE</u>
UNLESS OTHERWISE SPECIFIED.

PATIENT : Gage James	PHYSICIAN : Dr. Urey	DATE OF SERVICE : 3/18/xx

CHIEF COMPLAINT: URINARY RETENTION.

INFORMANT: The patient.

HISTORY OF PRESENT ILLNESS: The patient had a catheter removed at approximately 3:00
this afternoon by Dr. Urey and by 5:00 he was starting to feel like he was having difficulty
voiding. He was able to void a bit initially but then he could tell that he was beginning to
obstruct again.

REVIEW OF SYSTEMS: He is complaining primarily of low suprapubic pain. He has not passed
any clots today. He has not had any rigors or fever. He is having no nausea or vomiting.

PAST MEDICAL HISTORY: Several biopsy procedures recently done by Dr. Urey for cancer
of the prostate. Most recently a week ago, he had biopsy done via cystoscopy. He has had a
catheter in now for approximately five days. They have been irrigating at home any clots, however it had improved enough that they felt that they could remove the catheter this afternoon.

SOCIAL AND FAMILY HISTORY: Noncontributory.

CURRENT MEDICATIONS: Bactrim.

ALLERGIES: NONE KNOWN.

PHYSICAL EXAM: Blood pressure 167/95, temperature 96.3, pulse 96, respiratory rate
                    24. Color is a bit pale. Skin is warm and dry.
CHEST: Lung and heart exams are normal.
ABDOMEN: Showed marked tenderness in the mid suprapubic area. He was not
                    noticeably distended however. He had 850 cc of residual urine that
                    looked quite clear.

DIAGNOSIS: ACUTE URINARY RETENTION.

TREATMENT: Foley catheter is placed with the 850 cc of urinary residual. I discussed the case
with Dr. Urey He would like the urine cultured. The patient will follow up tomorrow with Dr. Urey
He is welcome to follow up here if further problems arise.

Case 7-8, *continued*

MEDICAL RECORDS

E.D. # 17-20-29	**EMERGENCY TREATMENT RECORD**	ARRIVAL DATE: 3/18/xx	TIME: 5:50 P.M.

PATIENT NAME: Gage Grimes	PHYSICIAN: Dr. Urey	AGE: 70 Y	SEX: M	BIRTH DATE: 01/15/xx

CHIEF COMPLAINT

URINARY RETENTION

ACTIVITY LEVEL

PHYSICIAN'S NOTES

Patient presents difficulty with urine retention.

Patient underwent a cystoscopy with biopsy approximately 1 week ago. Catheter utilized since cystoscopy. Patient has had Foley catheter replaced three times since procedure. Cath placed on Friday.

Cath placed on Saturday. Cath was plugged and was irrigated. Dr. Urey did the irrigation.

Catheterization just pulled at 3 p.m. today. A few hours later started having difficulty voiding.

Personal History: Prostate cancer. Social History:

Married.. Family History: Father – 96 died with heart problems. Mother died heart issues at age

41. Two healthy brothers.

R   L

DISABILITY

Estimated No. of Days _____   ☑ Chart Dictated ☐ Not Dictated

DIAGNOSIS

Acute Urinary Retention

DISCHARGE CONDITION:

☑ Stable   ☐ Unchanged   ☐ Transferred   ☐ Improved   ☐ AMA

☐ Admitted   ☐ Expired   ☐ Not Seen By Physician

P.A., F.P. RESIDENT SIGNATURE

E.D. PHYSICIAN SIGNATURE

Dr Urey

CONSENT FOR TREATMENT

CONSENT FOR TREATMENT: I am presenting myself for inpatient and/or outpatient care at Western Regional Medical Center and I voluntarily consent to the rendering of such care including diagnostic procedures and medical treatment by authorized agents and employees of Western Regional Medical Center and by its medical staff or their designees as in their professional judgment may be deemed necessary. I acknowledge that no guarantees have been made to me as to the result of examination or treatment in this hospital.

PATIENT OR REPRESENTATIVE SIGNATURE

Gage Grimes

DATE	TIME	IF REPRESENTATIVE, INDICATE RELATIONSHIP
WITNESS SIGNATURE		DATE
WITNESS SIGNATURE		DATE

PHYSICIAN'S ORDERS

E.D. #					PATIENT NAME: Gage Grimes	

DATE	TIME	1	2	3	ORDERS	
3/18/xx	18:15				Urine C&S	
3/18/xx	19:00				Cipro 500 mg now & 500 mg in am	
					ORDERED / DRAWN / RETURNED / TO X-RAY / RETURN	

continued

Case 7-8, *continued*

ICD-9-CM diagnosis code(s): _____

ICD-10-CM diagnosis code(s): _____

CPT code(s) with modifier, if applicable: _____

APC: _____

Case 7-9

Health Record Face Sheet

Western Regional
Medical Center

Record Number:	04-19-36
Age:	77
Gender:	Female
Length of Stay:	N/A
Service Type:	Emergency Room
Discharge Status:	Direct Admit
Diagnosis/Procedure:	Proximal Tibial Fracture

Case 7-9, *continued*

EMERGENCY DEPARTMENT VISIT

Mrs. Jackson is a 77-year-old female. She was brought to our emergency room by ambulance. She was involved in a pedestrian auto accident in which the car that she just got out of and she was going to walk in front of drove forward and struck her, primarily on the left side, and she significantly injured her right knee. She fell to the ground and was unable to bear weight. The ambulance was called and she was brought to our emergency room. She remained stable through her hospital transport and even in the emergency room with a blood pressure of 110/78 and a pulse of 66. She complains only of right knee pain and left buttocks pain. She did, however, strike her head although there was no loss of consciousness. She has a contusion and abrasion on the occipital scalp which has been bleeding very minimally. She has no complaints of significant headache or neck pain. She has no complaints of back pain, other than the left buttocks. Her right knee is slightly deformed with a little varus deformity at the knee with a large effusion and swelling about the knee. She has no complaints of hip or ankle or foot pain on the right side and her lower extremity is atraumatic. She has a small abrasion on the right elbow and a contusion on the left medial epicondyle of her left elbow. She has no abdominal pain, no chest pain. Again, her vital signs remained stable in the emergency room. We updated a Dip-Tet. Her head to toe examination showed that her ENT examination is essentially normal. She has full range of motion of her head and cervical spine without complaints of any neck pain. Her clavicles are not tender. Her heart has an irregularly irregular rhythm. She has a history of a pacemaker and underlying history of cardiovascular disease. She has an S3 and S4 gallop rhythm. Her lungs remain clear to auscultation in all fields. Her chest is not tender. Abdomen is soft, flat, and not tender. There are no masses or organomegaly. Femoral pulses are present and symmetrical. We log-rolled her gently onto her right side and she has a large left hematoma of the left buttocks which is more on the medial aspect with a medial contusion. Again, this is a large subcutaneous hematoma which is quite indurated at this time and I marked off the boundary where the induration started with this hematoma so we could monitor any development in the next few hours. Her upper extremities, other than the abrasion and contusion as mentioned above, are not remarkable. The right knee is significantly swollen. The left lower extremity is not remarkable. X-ray of her right knee shows a transverse fracture of the proximal tibia along with a lateral tibial plateau fracture. There appears to be also a non-displaced fracture of the proximal fibular head. Otherwise the knee is not remarkable. We x-rayed her pelvis which is not remarkable to radiographic examination. I contacted Dr. Nicols at the patient's request. The patient was admitted to Dr. Nicols service and he will evaluate the patient later on this day to consider surgical repair or further treatment of the right knee injury. In the meantime we will have nursing monitor neurovascular checks to the right lower extremity as well as enlargement of the right buttocks' hematoma.

IMPRESSION:

1. Proximal right tibial fracture with associated right tibial plateau fracture.
2. Fractured right proximal fibula.
3. Large hematoma of the left buttocks.
4. Contusion and abrasions of the upper extremities.

ICD-9-CM diagnosis code(s): _____

ICD-10-CM diagnosis code(s): _____

CPT code(s) with modifier, if applicable: _____

APC: _____

Case 7-10

Health Record Face Sheet

Western Regional
Medical Center

Record Number: 43-65-16

Age: 27

Gender: Male

Length of Stay: N/A

Service Type: Emergency Room

Discharge Status: To Home

Diagnosis/Procedure: Nasal Fracture
Closed-Head Injury

Case 7-10, *continued*

EMERGENCY ROOM REPORT

This is a 27-year-old white male who presents to the emergency department with some facial injuries. Informant is the patient and his significant other.

HISTORY OF PRESENT ILLNESS: The patient apparently stated he was sleeping after he had some alcohol. He was awakened by a police officer and struck in the face with a night stick. He does not really recall whether he was knocked out or not. He is complaining of some right face pain, occasional diplopia. He has no problem with difficulty breathing. He is also complaining of some tinnitus and some right cheek pain. The rest of the review of systems is negative.

PAST MEDICAL HISTORY: Unremarkable.

TETANUS STATUS: Up to date.

FAMILY HISTORY: Noncontributory.

PHYSICAL EXAM: Reveals an alert male in mild distress. Blood pressure of 124/76, temperature 98, pulse 66, respirations 18. Skin is warm and dry.

HEENT: Extraocular muscles are intact. Pupils are equal, round, and reactive to light and accommodation. He has a large subconjunctival hematoma on the right. He also has some mild skin lacerations across the bridge of his nose. TMs were normal. There is no pain over the frontal sinuses nor over the maxillary sinuses. There is on septal hematoma. There is no pain over the TMJs.

NECK: Supple. The rest of the physical exam is normal.

TREATMENT: While here the patient had a CAT scan of his head along with some facial bones. The patient had a nasal fracture, nondisplaced, nonangulated. He also had a 21 x 22 right maxillary polyp. He also had some obscuration of his frontal and maxillary sinuses and possibly his ethmoid.

CAT scan of the head did not reveal any bleeds, subdurals, epidurals, or intracerebral difficulties.

IMPRESSION: 1. NASAL FRACTURE.

2. CLOSED-HEAD INJURY.

3. FACIAL CONTUSION.

4. NASAL LACERATION,

5. MAXILLARY POLYP.

PLAN: The patient was given six Empirin #3 to go and a prescription for 22. He is instructed with head injury instructions, wound instructions. He is also given the number of Dr. Entol if he has a problem with his nose and we discussed that or if he wants to get his maxillary polyp extracted. We discussed the difficulties with polyps including infection and death. The patient will follow up with Dr. Entol. Any worsening, he is welcome to return to the emergency department.

continued

Case 7-10, *continued*

RADIOLOGY REPORT

NASAL BONE FILMS:

CONCLUSION: NORMAL. NO FRACTURE SEEN.

CT BRAIN SCAN:

MIDLINE: No shift.

VENTRICLES: Normal size.

SULCI: Normal.

CONTRAST: Not given.

FINDINGS:

No focal area of parenchymal abnormality or intracranial mass effect is identified.

IMPRESSION: NORMAL NONCONTRAST CRANIAL CT SCAN.

FACIAL BONE CT:

CLINICAL DATA: Patient struck at bridge of nose. Rule out facial bone fractures.

TECHNIQUE: Serial computerized axial tomographic images are obtained at 5-mm intervals through the facial bones.

FINDINGS:

The patient has a large slightly greater than 20-mm polyp in the right antrum. At least one opacified right ethmoid air cell and opacified right frontal sinuses. No fractures.

IMPRESSION: FINDINGS OF SINUSITIS.
               NO FRACTURES.

ICD-9-CM diagnosis code(s): _____

ICD-10-CM diagnosis code(s): _____

CPT code(s) with modifier, if applicable: _____

APC: _____

Case 7-11

Health Record Face Sheet

Western Regional
Medical Center

Record Number:	16-25-09
Age:	52
Gender:	Female
Length of Stay:	N/A
Serviced Type:	SDS
Discharge Status:	To Home
Diagnosis/Procedure:	Adhesive Capsulitis Right Knee Manipulation under Anesthesia

continued

Case 7-11, *continued*

HISTORY AND PHYSICAL

PATIENT: Kay King

MR NUMBER: 16-25-09

ROOM #: 201

ADMIT DATE: 5/12/xx

PHYSICIAN: Dr. Redi

CHIEF COMPLAINT: Adhesive capsulitis right knee.

HISTORY OF PRESENT ILLNESS:

Ms. King is admitted to the same-day surgery suite for manipulation of her right knee under anesthesia. History reveals that the patient was in a skiing accident and had a rather severe injury to her knee where she tore the ACL and also the medial collateral ligament of the right knee. She underwent surgery on 4/15/xx with repair of the above. She has been in physical therapy but has had some loss of motion in the knee. She did not respond to physical therapy so we decided to treat her with manipulation.

PAST MEDICAL HISTORY:

CURRENT MEDS: None

ALLERGIES: **CODEINE**

SURGERIES: Relatively noncontributory other than that on the knee done.

MEDICAL ILLNESS: Unremarkable

PSYCHOSOCIAL HISTORY: Unremarkable

FAMILY HISTORY: Unremarkable

REVIEW OF SYSTEMS:

HEENT: No history of headaches, blurred vision, double vision, or loss of vision. No history of frequent sore throats, nosebleeds, or neck pain.

CHEST: She denies shortness of breath, diaphoresis, palpitation, or chest pain.

ABDOMEN: No history of nausea, vomiting, diarrhea, or weight loss.

GU: No history of frequency, hesitancy, urgency, hematuria, or dysuria.

PHYSICAL EXAM:

GENERAL: Alert and cooperative female who appeared to be in good health.

HEENT: Head was normocephalic. Pupils are equal and react to light and accommodation. Extraocular muscles are intact. Oropharynx and nasopharynx are within normal limits.

NECK: Supple. No evidence of any lymphadenopathy.

CHEST: Clear.

HEART: Regular rate and rhythm. No murmurs.

ABDOMEN: Soft, no masses.

GU: Deferred.

EXTREM: Examination of the knee revealed she only has about 70 degrees of flexion of the right knee, which is passive range of motion. The active is less than that.

NEURO:

ADMISSION DIAGNOSIS: Adhesive capsulitis right knee.

PLAN: 1. The patient will be admitted to the hospital for manipulation under anesthesia.

2. The procedure, sequelae, alternatives, and complications discussed.

Case 7-11, *continued*

OPERATIVE REPORT

PATIENT: Kay King

MR NUMBER: 16-25-09

ROOM: 201

ADMIT DATE:

DATE OF SURGERY: 5/12/xx

SURGEON: Dr. Redi

ASSIST: Dr. Nicols

PREOPERATIVE DIAGNOSIS: Adhesive capsulitis post-op right knee surgery.

POSTOPERATIVE DIAGNOSIS: Adhesive capsulitis post-op right knee surgery.

OPERATIVE PROCEDURE: Manipulation of right knee under anesthesia with injection of 80 mg. of Depo-Medrol and 10 cc. of 0.5% Marcaine with epinephrine.

GROSS FINDINGS: Prior to manipulation she had 0–70 degrees of motion. Postoperatively she had 0–120 degrees of motion. The keloid had broken open on the midline incision. With so many adhesions, he had broken open in two small places just proximal to the kneecap.

DESCRIPTION OF OPERATIVE PROCEDURE:

The patient was taken to the Operating Room and placed on the operating table in the supine position. After she was adequately anesthetized using general inhalation anesthesia, her knee was gently manipulated over time until we obtained 0–120 degrees of motion. After this, the knee was injected with 0.5% of Marcaine with epinephrine, 10 cc., as well as 2 cc. of Kenalog. She was then sent to the Recovery Room in satisfactory condition where she will be placed on a CPM.

ICD-9-CM diagnosis code(s): _____

ICD-10-CM diagnosis code(s): _____

CPT code(s) with modifier, if applicable: _____

APC: _____

Case 7-12

Health Record Face Sheet

Western Regional
Medical Center

Record Number: 87-14-12

Age: 45

Gender: Female

Length of Stay: N/A

Serviced Type: Same-Day Surgery

Discharge Status: To Home

Diagnosis/Procedure: Rotator Cuff Impingement
Acromioplasty/Decompression

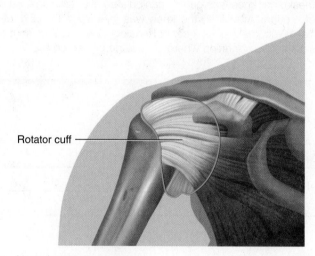

Rotator cuff

Normal rotator cuff anatomy.

Case 7-12, *continued*

HISTORY AND PHYSICAL

PATIENT: Khloe Kruz

MEDICAL RECORD NUMBER: 87-14-12

ROOM #: 204

ADMIT DATE: 6/2/xx

PHYSICIAN: Dr. Mayer

CHIEF COMPLAINT:
   Partial tear of the supraspinatus tendon and possible subacromial decompression and acromioplasty.

HISTORY OF PRESENT ILLNESS:
   History reveals that the patient was working in the kitchen at the Country Cafe. She had pain while lifting a pot above her shoulders. She was seen about a week later because she continued to have pain and to be examined. She was placed on Ibuprofen and physical therapy. She has been working with Physical Therapy but has discomfort and therapy feels that she has some problems that could not be repaired by or helped with physical therapy and she was referred to me. We examined her and a MRI that revealed a partial tear and severe impingement of the shoulder. She is admitted to the hospital for surgery.

PAST MEDICAL HISTORY:
   CURRENT MEDS: Zoloft and hormones.
   ALLERGIES: **DENIES.**
   SURGERIES: Denies.
   MEDICAL ILLNESS: Unremarkable.

PSYCHOSOCIAL HISTORY: Unremarkable.

FAMILY HISTORY: Unremarkable.

REVIEW OF SYSTEMS:
   HEENT: No history of headaches, blurred vision, double vision, or loss of vision. No history of frequent sore throats, nosebleeds, or neck pain.
   CHEST: She denies shortness of breath, diaphoresis, palpitation, or chest pain.
   ABDOMEN: No history of nausea, vomiting, diarrhea, or weight loss.
   GU: No history of frequency, hesitancy, urgency, hematuria, or dysuria.

PHYSICAL EXAM:
   GENERAL: Alert and cooperative female who appeared to be in no acute distress.
   HEENT: Head was normocephalic. Pupils are equal and react to light and accommodation. Extraocular muscles are intact. Oropharynx and nasopharynx are within normal limits.
   NECK: Supple. No evidence of any lymphadenopathy.
   CHEST: Clear.
   HEART: Regular rate and rhythm. No murmurs.
   ABDOMEN: Soft, no masses.
   GU: Deferred

ADMISSION DIAGNOSIS:
   Partial tear of the supraspinatus tendon and possible subacromial decompression and acromioplasty.

PLAN:
   1. The patient will be admitted to the hospital for acromioplasty, subacromial decompression, and possible repair of the anterior glenoid labrum.
   2. The procedure, sequelae, alternatives, and complications were discussed.

continued

Case 7-12, *continued*

OPERATIVE REPORT

PATIENT: Khloe Kruz

MEDICAL RECORD NUMBER: 87-14-12

ROOM: 204

DATE OF SURGERY: 6/2/xx

SURGEON: Dr. Mayer

ASSIST: Dr. Tilley

PREOPERATIVE DIAGNOSIS:	Rotator cuff impingement and tear of the near superior glenoid labrum of the right shoulder.
POSTOPERATIVE DIAGNOSIS:	Rotator cuff impingement and tear of the near superior glenoid labrum of the right shoulder.
OPERATIVE PROCEDURE:	Acromioplasty and subacromial decompression and repair of the anterior glenoid labrum tear using a 2.1 Mitek anchor.
GROSS FINDINGS:	There was a tear of the anterior glenoid labrum. There was also rotator cuff tendinitis secondary to impingement.

DESCRIPTION OF OPERATIVE PROCEDURE:

The patient was taken to the Operating Room and placed on the operating table in the supine position. After she was adequately anesthetized using general inhalation anesthesia, her right shoulder was prepped with Betadine and properly placed sterile drapes.

Attention was turned to the right shoulder where a skin incision was made over the anterior distal border of the acromion extending to the coracoid process and then extending down into the deltopectoral groove. The subcutaneous tissue was incised along the skin incision with hemostasis obtained with clamp and cautery. The deltoid was then detached from the acromion and a portion of the anterior clavicle and then split in the deltopectoral groove. It was carried down until the anterior capsule could be visualized and anterior capsulotomy was performed. We inspected the joint and there were no loose bodies or advanced degenerative disease but there was a tear of the anterior glenoid labrum. This area was freshened up with a curette and then a 2.2 Mitek was used to anchor the anterior glenoid labrum along with suture. After this, it was inspected and found to be satisfactory. The anterior capsule was then repaired using #0 Ethibond simple interrupted sutures.

Attention was turned to the supraspinatus and subacromial area where there was impingement on the supraspinatus tendon. The anterior aspect of the acromion was removed and subacromial decompression was performed with an egg-shaped bur. After this, the wound was infiltrated with 0.5% Marcaine with epinephrine using 10 cc. The deltoid was reattached to the remaining acromion with #0 Ethibond simple interrupted sutures and the split in the deltoid with #0 Vicryl simple interrupted sutures. The skin was then closed using 3-0 Ethilon vertical mattress suture. Sterile dressing was placed on the patient and the patient was sent to the Recovery Room in satisfactory condition.

Case 7-12, *continued*

ICD-9-CM diagnosis code(s): _____

ICD-10-CM diagnosis code(s): _____

CPT code(s) with modifier, if applicable: _____

APC: _____

Case 7-13

Health Record Face Sheet

Western Regional
Medical Center

Record Number:	56-09-13
Age:	57
Gender:	Female
Length of Stay:	N/A
Service Type:	Emergency Room
Discharge Status:	Expired
Diagnosis/Procedure:	MVA Cardiac Arrest

continued

EMERGENCY DEPARTMENT VISIT

SUBJECTIVE: This 57-year-old woman was brought to the emergency room from a motor vehicle accident in full arrest. We were notified about five minutes before her arrival by paramedics that they had a middle-aged female involved in a two-car motor vehicle accident on the highway near the state border. The patient apparently did not have a pulse. They were requesting use of a mass suit and were intubating the patient at the time they notified us. The patient was apparently unconscious from the time of their arrival. She was making some respiratory efforts, however, they were quite shallow upon their arrival. The patient was extricated using a cervical collar and a KED. Her pupils initially were reactive, however, they were unable to palpate any peripheral pulses. They were also uncertain as to whether or not there was a carotid pulse present. Upon hooking the patient up to the monitor the monitor showed a bradycardia of about 40, again, with no detectable peripheral pulses. In route the patient was intubated with slight difficulty as she had vomited several times. Initially her teeth were clenched and there was some emesis in the air way. The patient was then ventilated with a bag mask and 100% oxygen. Several attempts at a peripheral in route were unsuccessful. This was even after the mass suit had been inflated with all three compartments. Further history from the police and paramedics indicate that this patient's vehicle travelled across the center line on the Highway, it apparently was not going at a high rate of speed, but it crossed into oncoming traffic lane. The oncoming vehicle, a van, saw the vehicle in the wrong lane, began slowing down and pulling to the right, and was almost at a complete stop at the time of impact. Additionally, however, the paramedics and police report that the patient's vehicle had significant secondary impact with the steering wheel being bent. Upon arrival in the emergency department, the full code team was present in the emergency room. The patient was noted to be in full arrest with no peripheral pulses, ventilation in progress. Checking the placement of the ET tube revealed good breath sounds on the left, decreased breath sounds on the right. The tube was withdrawn about three-quarters of an inch and good breath sounds were heard bilaterally. The patient was immobilized on a long back board with KED and cervical collar in place. Her pupils were mid-point and unreactive.

OBJECTIVE: Physical exam reveals a middle-aged female. She is extremely pale. The monitor, initially, showed a flat line consistent with asystole. No peripheral IV was in place and several attempts at peripheral IVs were made by the nursing staff while I proceeded to place a central line in the right subclavian region. This line was inserted without difficulty six minutes after the patient's arrival. Exam of the patient's head revealed a laceration on her chin. This was a fairly deep, long laceration, just parallel to her lower lip. The laceration was not bleeding at all upon her arrival. Tympanic membranes were clear bilaterally with no evidence of blood. Chest wall revealed several ecchymoses, particularly about the left breast, however, both chest walls were bruised. The patient's abdomen actually was quite soft as soon as an NG tube was inserted and was quite protuberant, but did not feel distended, as soon as the NG tube was placed and the stomach was decompressed. The patient's neck was never fully evaluated with cervical films, however, the cervical collar was left in place at least throughout the initial portion of this resuscitation. Lower extremities did not reveal any significant trauma. The patient's back was eventually evaluated and showed no evidence of significant trauma or injuries. Returning to the resuscitation, the patient was given 2 mg of epinephrine. The first one was given via the endotracheal tube. Again, cardiac activity was noted in the form of a wide QRS ventricular type of complex, but no peripheral pulses were palpable. CPR was continued throughout this time. Repeat doses of epinephrine was given as well as one milligram of atropine. Eventually, a total of seven milligrams of epinephrine were administered in the central line with no significant improvement in peripheral pulses and no detectable peripheral pulses. Several attempts at arterial blood gasses were made. These were presumably venous gasses as the pH was reported at 6.61, PCO2 of 117, PO2 of 21. Again, the patient's ventilation was checked and she was being ventilated well with bag endotracheal ventilations. A portable chest x-ray was obtained. This revealed the presence of several fractured ribs on the left, but no evidence of significant pneumothorax or hemothorax. There was no evidence of mediastinal widening and the heart shadow actually appeared fairly small for supine film. One attempt was made at pericardicentesis before the chest film was returned, using an 18-gauge spinal needle. Five cc of dark blood was obtained presumably this blood was from the ventricle. No further pericardicentesis was done, however, after the chest film was reviewed. An old record was eventually obtained which indicated the patient was diabetic. At this time, she was given 1 amp of D-50, again, through the subclavian catheter with, again, no significant improvement. Resuscitation attempts were continued for a total of 35 minutes in the emergency department. The patient's pupils were 4 mm and unreactive to light at this point in time. This is in addition to approximately 20 minutes of down time in the pre-hospital setting. The resuscitation attempt was discontinued at 10:00 a.m. with the patient expiring. The coroner was notified and the family additionally was notified. The family was present in the emergency room. I did suggest to the family and to the coroner that a post-mortem examination, at least of the heart, would be very helpful in this setting to clarify the exact etiology or mechanism of her demise.

FINAL IMPRESSION:

1. Cardiac Arrest

2. Chin laceration

3. Rib fractures

4. MVA

Case 7-13, *continued*

RADIOLOGY REPORT

Port. Chest

Chest Portable Chest X-ray

HISTORY: MVA.

PORTABLE CHEST:

The heart and other mediastinal structures are normal. NG tube, ET tube and central venous catheters are in satisfactory position.

Lungs are clear. There, are fractures of the lateral aspects of the left 6th and 7th ribs, but no complication of these fractures seen.

IMPRESSION:

Fractured ribs. Otherwise negative chest.

ICD-9-CM diagnosis code(s): _____

ICD-10-CM diagnosis code(s): _____

CPT code(s) with modifier, if applicable: _____

APC: _____

Case 7-14

Health Record Face Sheet

Western Regional
Medical Center

Record Number:	19-88-54
Age:	40
Gender:	Male
Length of Stay:	Not Applicable
Diagnosis/Procedure:	Chronic Sinusitis Caldwell-Luc Procedure
Service Type:	Same-Day Surgery
Discharge Status:	To Home

continued

Case 7-14, *continued*

HISTORY & PHYSICAL

ADMISSION DATE: 10/11/xx

This 40-year-old has a long history of chronic pressure pain symptoms involving the left side of the face. He also has chronic cough and generalized malaise. He has been found to have a totally opacified left maxillary sinus which has not resolved with prolonged and adequate medical treatment. He has misshapen sinuses bilaterally secondary to a congenital mid face deformity. He is presently admitted for a left Caldwell-Luc procedure.

PAST MEDICAL HISTORY: Otherwise reasonably benign. Patient takes Centrax occasionally for anxiety and is currently still on Ceftin as an antibiotic. He denies allergies.

FAMILY HISTORY: Non-contributory.

REVIEW OF SYSTEMS: Negative.

EXAM: Well-developed male in no acute distress.

EYES: Clear.

EAR CANALS & DRUMS: Within normal limits.

NOSE: Reveals a nasal septal deviation with a spur deformity to the left which is not obstructive to the nasal airway but may very well obstruct the middle meatus.

ORAL CAVITY: Clear.

NECK: Negative.

CHEST: Clear to percussion and auscultation.

HEART: Regular rate and rhythm without murmurs or gallops.

ABDOMEN: Benign.

EXTREMITIES: Within normal limits.

DIAGNOSIS: Chronic left maxillary sinusitis.

PLAN: Caldwell Luc procedure. The patient wants to proceed with nasal surgery for the septal spur.

OPERATIVE NOTE

DATE OF PROCEDURE: 10/11/xx

PREOPERATIVE DIAGNOSIS: Chronic left maxillary sinusitis.

POSTOPERATIVE DIAGNOSIS: Same

PROCEDURE PERFORMED: Left Caldwell-Luc

DESCRIPTION:

The patient was brought to the operating room and induced into general oral tracheal anesthesia. He was positioned, prepped, and draped in the standard fashion. 1% Xylocaine with 1:100,000 Epinephrine was infiltrated locally into the left sublabial canine fossa. 5% Cocaine on cottonoids was placed in the nostrils bilaterally. A sublabial incision was made and carried down to bone. The antrum was entered with a gouge and mallet and the enterotomy was enlarged with a Kerrison rongeur. Sinus was full of extremely thick inspissated mucous which required a pituitary forceps to remove as it was much too thick to be suctioned. A culture was obtained. Interestingly, aside from a few very small sessile polyps along the left lateral wall, the sinus mucosa appeared reasonably healthy. A large nasal antral window was then created by egg shelling the bone over the medial wall of the sinus and creatinine an inferiorly based flap of nasal mucosa which was turned into the sinus. Hemostasis was achieved with electrocoagulation. No packing was necessary. The sublabial wound was closed with interrupted 4-0 chromic.

The patient tolerated the procedure well. His throat was thoroughly suctioned and he was awakened, extubated and taken to the recovery room in satisfactory condition and there were no complications.

Case 7-14, *continued*

PHYSICIAN'S ORDERS & PROGRESS RECORD

DATE	ORDERS	✓	DATE	PROGRESS
				DATE: *10/11/xx*
				DIAGNOSIS: *Chronic ⓁL max sinusitis*
				PLANNED PROCEDURE: *Ⓛ Caldwell-Luc*
				INFORMED CONSENT: *yes*
				PREOPERATIVE REVIEW OF BODY SYSTEMS
				Cardiovascular *Ok*
				Pulmonary *Ok*
				Other *Ok*
				Regular Medications: *Central*
				Allergies: *NKA*
				Bleeding/Clotting Disorders *None*
				Detailed H & P dictated? *Yes*

PHYSICIAN'S ORDERS	Another brand of drugs identical in form and content may be dispensed unless checked.	**PROGRESS RECORD**

continued

Case 7-14, *continued*

PHYSICIAN'S ORDERS & PROGRESS RECORD

DATE	ORDERS	✓	DATE	PROGRESS
10/11/xx	VS per RR normal Diet & Activity as tolerated. Elevated HOB 30 degrees.		10/11/xx	ⓁCaldwell-Luc without complications.
	IV - D5O.2NS @125 cc/hr			
	D/C IV when tol po fluids well			
	Vicodin 250 mg po q4h prn pain			
	Droperidol 1/2 cc IV q 4 hr prn N&V			
	Fentanyl 2cc IV q6h prn severe pain			
	Discharge Dispense Vicodin #15 200 mg po q 4h prn pain			Doing well No bleeding No swelling

PHYSICIAN'S ORDERS	**PROGRESS**

ICD-9-CM diagnosis code(s): _____

ICD-10-CM diagnosis code(s): _____

CPT code(s) with modifier, if applicable: _____

APC: _____

Case 7-15

Health Record Face Sheet

Western Regional
Medical Center

Record Number: 46-11-08

Age: 74

Gender: Male

Length of Stay: Not Applicable

Diagnosis/Procedure: Rectal Polyp with Colonoscopy

Service Type: Same-Day Surgery

Discharge Status: To Home

OUTPATIENT SURGERY

LAST NAME:	FIRST NAME:	MIDDLE:	AGE:	BIRTHDATE:	DATE:	TIME:
Itle	Ivan	L	74	1/02/XX	3/31/XX	0700

TIME	BP	TPR	NURSING REMARK
0715	124/78	97.7	OPS—Colonscopy—Pre OP teaching done. IV started R hand with
			20 gauge cath / D5 1/2 NS TKO side rails up
0910			Return from colonoscopy per cart with rack up. Oriented Ox per NC on 02 sat still down
	IV TKO		
1030			DCd IV 7.50 cc infused 05 1/2 NS
1640	128/82	98.6	602 DC's Went to rest room voided large amount

LIST ANY ALLERGIES OR OTHER SPECIAL INFORMATION: NURSE'S SIGNATURE   PATIENT CONDITION ON DISCHARGE:

NKA   J. Martinez, R.N.   Good

PHYSICIAN'S REPORT

DOCTOR

1145 130/88-84-16 - Patient verbalized understanding discharge
instructions and ambulated under own power from OPS.

DIAGNOSIS:

TREATMENT:

DISPOSITION:

AUTHORIZATION FOR MEDICAL and/or SURGICAL TREATMENT: X   Ivan Itle

continued

Case 7-15, *continued*

COLONOSCOPY REPORT

DATE OF PROCEDURE: 3/31/xx

INDICATIONS: 74-year-old male with a history of a rectal polyp five years ago treated with fulguration. Recently he underwent a flexible proctosigmoidoscopy and was found to have a sigmoid polyp. He has undergone a Go-Lyte prep and comes for total colonoscopy.

EXAMINATION: Following informed consent, he was sedated with Demerol 50 mg, Phenergan 25 mg and Versed 1 mg IV. Prior to any sedation, his 02 sat. was in the mid-80's and nasal 02 was placed. He has a history of congestive failure and is on a diuretic and presumably Digoxin. Digital rectal exam was unrevealing. An Olympus OES type CF1T10L colonoscope was introduced and advanced to the cecum. Ileocecal valve was visualized. The bowel prep was adequate but moderate lavage was required to remove semi-fluidic stool. The scope was withdrawn with detailed circumferential inspection of the mucosa. In the ascending colon, a diminutive sessile polyp was identified. This was biopsied and ablated with hot forceps. The only other finding of note was that of a 3/4-cm. semi-pedunculated sigmoid polyp. This was removed by snare electrocautery. The burn site was inspected and there was good hemostasis. The polyp was aspirated on the scope tip but ultimately came into the channel and required the cleaning brush to remove it. No other lesions were identified and he tolerated the procedure well.

FINAL IMPRESSION: Two polyps as described.

PLAN: Home when ambulatory. Avoidance of Aspirin or other nonsteroidal anti-inflammatory drugs for 10 days.

ICD-9-CM diagnosis code(s): _____

ICD-10-CM diagnosis code(s): _____

CPT code(s) with modifier, if applicable: _____

APC: _____

Case 7-16

Health Record Face Sheet

Western Regional
Medical Center

Record Number:	30-55-14
Age:	64
Gender:	Male
Length of Stay:	Not Applicable
Diagnosis/Procedure:	Heartburn with EGD
Service Type:	Same-Day Surgery
Discharge Status:	To Home

Case 7-16, *continued*

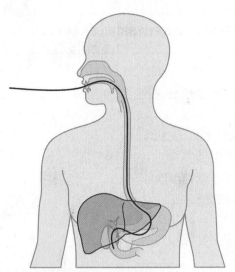

Esophagogastroduodenoscopy.
Source: © Dorling Kindersley

<table>
<tr><td colspan="4"></td><td colspan="1" align="center">OUTPATIENT SURGERY</td></tr>
</table>

TIME	BP	TPR	NURSING REMARK
0720	130/80	96.3 68-16	OPS–EGD Pre op teaching done.
0745	130/80	80-20	IV started L forearm with 20 guage, LR TKO 1 mg versed IVP per
			Dr. Ashaye with side rails up.
0825			Return from OPS in cart with side rails up.
			Oriented mo. c/o pain. IV infusing well
0900			DC I.V. 300 cc when tolerating fluids well
			OOB dressed. States no discomfort.
0915	130/80	72-18	Discharged ambulating to car with wife driving him home

LIST ANY ALLERGIES OR OTHER SPECIAL INFORMATION: NURSE'S SIGNATURE   PATIENT CONDITION ON DISCHARGE:

NKA   J. Martinez, R.N.   Good

continued

Case 7-16, *continued*

HISTORY & PHYSICAL EXAMINATION

Chief Complaint   *Severe Heart Burn for 6 months*

Hx of Present Problem   *No melena. AYID not helping*

Past Medical History   *ASPVD*

Family/Social History   *Unremarkable*

Previous Surgery   *Back 11 years ago*

Previous Illness   *None recent*

ALLERGIES   *Unremarkable*

Present Medications   *AXID*

Review of Systems   *Neg clear*   *Admit for EGD*

HEENT   *Neg normal limits*   *NPO*

Cardiovascular   *Neg RSR*   *IV - RR @ 100/h*

Respiratory   *Even*   *Versed 1 mg prior to surgery*

Abdominal   *No masses*

GYN   *N/A*

GU   *Regular*

Neurological   *Normal*

Skeletal   *Normal*

Lymphatics   *Normal*

DISCHARGE NOTE

Hospital Course   *Tolerated EGD without problems*

Procedures   *EGD—Versed 2 mg IV. No complications*

Findings: HH with chronic change. Mild duodenitis

Discharge Instructions

Diet   *Reg*

Activity   *activities as tolerated*

Follow-up   *My office in 3 weeks*

Medications   *Zantac 150 mg q4hrs po bid x 30 days*

PRINCIPAL DIAGNOSIS   *HH with chronic esophagitis. Mild duodenitis*

Discharge Date: 8/14/xx

Case 7-16, *continued*

ESOPHAGOGASTRODUODENOSCOPY

DATE OF PROCEDURE: 8/14/xx

INDICATION OF PROCEDURE:

6-month history of epigastric tenderness and burning, unresponsive to conservative management with H2 blockers.

DESCRIPTION OF PROCEDURE

With the patient having had the posterior pharynx sprayed with 10% oral xylocaine, having been given Versed IV with the patient in left lateral decubitus position the Olympus gastroscope was passed using video technique. The esophagus appeared normal throughout except at the EG junction where he had a sliding hernia. There was chronic change present at the EG junction. There was no evidence of mass, no bleeding and no acute ulceration of the stomach which distended normally. Retroflex view of the cardia and EG junction was normal. The antrum, body, and incisura were not normal. The pylorus was not scarred. The duodenal bulb, however, had moderate erythema present. There was no ulcer. The scope was advanced to the distal segment of the duodenum which was entirely normal. The scope was retrieved. They were removed. The esophagus again visualized and no additional findings noted. The procedure was terminated and the patient sent to recovery with stable and normal vital signs.

IMPRESSION:

Hiatal hernia with chronic esophagitis and mild duodenitis of the bulb.

ICD-9-CM diagnosis code(s): _____

ICD-10-CM diagnosis code(s): _____

CPT code(s) with modifier, if applicable: _____

APC: _____

Case 7-17

Health Record Face Sheet

Western Regional
Medical Center

Record Number:	07-17-09
Age:	25
Gender:	Female
Length of Stay:	Not Applicable
Diagnosis/Procedure:	Chronic Pelvic Pain Laparoscopy Lysis of Adhesions
Service Type:	Same-Day Surgery
Discharge Status:	To Home

continued

Case 7-17, *continued*

DISCHARGE SUMMARY

PATIENT: Leeza Lopez

ADMIT DATE: 11/21/xx
DISCH DATE: 11/22/xx

PHYSICIAN: Dr. Smith

DIAGNOSIS: Abdominal pain status postoperative laparoscopy with lysis of adhesions, appendectomy, ovarian biopsy (interval appendicitis versus unilateral PID).

The patient was discharged to home with instructions in follow-up. She will be discharged with saline lock and maintenance to follow up in the Emergency Room tomorrow for an additional dose of Rocephin and have the saline lock discontinued at that time. She will continue on Vibramycin, 100 mg b.i.d., and follow up with me in the clinic in one week. Instructions were given on activities, bowel care and precautions.

HISTORY: The patient is a 25-year-old female with persistent right lower quadrant pain. She underwent IV antibiotic therapy approximately two and a half weeks ago with incomplete resolution and subsequent return of her pain. She underwent laparoscopy, at which time adhesions of the right lower quadrant involving the cecum, appendix, small bowel, right ovary, fallopian tube and omentum were encountered. Adhesiolysis was performed, appendectomy performed, right ovarian biopsy. She was maintained on IV antibiotics for 24 hours and subsequently discharged to home as listed above.

HISTORY AND PHYSICAL

PATIENT: Leeza Lopez

ADMIT DATE: 11/21/xx

PHYSICIAN: Dr. Smith

CHIEF COMPLAINT: Abdominal adhesive disease, probable right salpingitis versus chronic interval appendicitis.

HISTORY OF PRESENT ILLNESS:
This is a 25-year-old female with a history of persistent right pelvic pain. She had initial flare approximately three weeks ago and was given five days of IV antibiotic followed by a week of p.o. antibiotic and had near but not complete resolution of her pain. It was associated with some GI complaints, though not notable. Ultrasound was performed which showed a generous sized right ovary consistent with oophoritis or normal variant. The patient is quite large. Appendix was not visualized. She is now status post operative laparoscopy with lysis of adhesions, appendectomy, ovarian biopsy, tubal dye perfusion. She tolerated it well but because of previous infection and likelihood of involved infection she is kept for further observation for antibiotic therapy.

PAST HISTORY:
CURRENT MEDICATIONS-Proventil inhaler p.r.n., Voltaren, 50 mg, one to two q. six hours, Lortab and Vibramycin.
ALLERGIES-NKDA.
SURGERIES-Cesarean section 5 years ago
MEDICAL ILLNESS-Chronic hypertension, obesity.

SOCIAL HISTORY: She smokes greater than one pack per day, denies significant use of alcohol or recreational drugs.

FAMILY HISTORY: Significant for malignancy of her father, specifics unknown, as well as some hypertension.

REVIEW OF SYSTEMS:

PHYSICAL EXAM:

GENERAL: Alert and appropriate. Blood pressure 140/90. She is afebrile. Skin is clear.
HEENT: Unremarkable.
NECK: Unremarkable.
CHEST: Lungs are clear to auscultation with decreased pulmonary excursion secondary to habitus.
HEART: Regular rate and rhythm.
ABDOMEN: Soft. Bowel sounds are normal. Incisions are dry.
EXTREMITIES: Unremarkable.

continued

OPERATIVE REPORT

PATIENT: Leeza Lopez

DOB: 6/14/xx

DATE: 11/22/xx

SURGEON: Dr. Smith

ASSIST: Dr. Manows

HISTORY:

Patient is a 25-year-old female with chronic pelvic pain. Status post trial of IV antibiotics.

PREOPERATIVE DIAGNOSIS: Persistent right pelvic pain.

POSTOPERATIVE DIAGNOSIS: Abdominal pelvic adhesive disease. Chronic interval appendicitis versus chronic P.I.D. versus endometriosis.

PROCEDURE: Laparoscopy with lysis of adhesions, right ovarian biopsy, tubal dye perfusion, and appendectomy.

ESTIMATED BLOOD LOSS: Less than 50 cc.

COMPLICATIONS: None

DRAINS: None

SPONGES/NEEDLES/TOWEL COUNT: Correct

INTRAOPERATIVE FINDINGS:

The right ovary was large and boggy, approximately 6 cm. in greatest dimension. It was swollen, lacking superficial convolutions. The appendix was involved with fat wrapping and adhesions to the pelvic brim which also included distal right fimbria, large and small bowel, as well as omentum. The left ovary was normal size, consistency, normal convolutions, stigma of ovulation. Left fallopian tube was normal as was the uterus, vesicouterine plicae, and peritoneum of the pelvis including the ovarian fossa bilaterally. Upper abdominal sweep was unremarkable.

PROCEDURE:

With patient under general anesthetic and in dorsal lithotomy position, suitably prepped and draped with bladder drained with straight catheter, a Kroner uterine manipulator was placed. A pneumoperitoneum was created and trocar placed. Additional trocars in the suprapubic bilateral space were placed under direct visualization. The upper abdominal sweep showed findings as listed at the right pelvic brim. The patient was placed in gentle Trendelenburg and left tilt. Adhesiolysis was carried out until the base of the appendix was freed. The right fallopian tube was also freed as was the right ovary. A right ovarian wedge biopsy was carried out and specimen submitted. An endo GIA was used to perform an appendectomy with sharp and blunted adhesiolysis to the appendiceal stump and a single white endostaple placed across the appendiceal stump. Hemostasis was immediate. Copious irrigation was undertaken. Additional adhesiolysis involving large and small bowel to normalize anatomy and mobility. The left ovary and remainder of pelvis was visualized and peritoneum again was noted to be normal. No alterations or distortions of the superficial vasculature. No scarring throughout the cul-de-sac, anterior vesicouterine plicae. Tubal dye perfusion was then performed and easy spill noted bilaterally. Irrigation was again carried out. Inferior trocars were removed and remained hemostatic. Abdominal trocar was removed. Pneumoperitoneum was allowed to escape. Sutures were placed in the fascia on the 10 or greater trocar sites and subcuticular stitches of 4-0 undyed Vicryl used to approximate the skin. Instrumentation was removed from the vagina. Dressings were applied. Patient was taken to the Recovery Room in stable condition.

Case 7-17, *continued*

TISSUE REPORT

PATIENT: Leeza Lopez
DATE: 11/22/xx
SEX: F   DOB: 6/14/xx
DOCTOR: Dr. Smith
TISSUE: R ovarian   bx
              Appendix

HISTORY: None

Gross: The tortuous appendix is 11 cm in length, 5 mm in width, and blends with abundant mesoappendix. The serosal surface of the appendix is smooth; the wall is firm: the lumen contains firm brown fecal material.

The specimen labeled ovarian biopsy consists of two irregular portions of light grey or dark red hemorrhagic tissue, the larger 25 x 10 x 5 mm. three blocks

MICROSCOPIC: DONE

DIAGNOSIS: 1.   APPENDIX, NORMAL

                          2.   SEGMENT, OVARY, NORMAL, RIGHT SIDE

COMMENT: The entire appendix was examined microscopically and there is no evidence of an acute, subacute appendicitis. There is also no evidence of a periappendicitis such as one might expect to find in pelvic inflammatory disease.

The ovarian biopsy simply reveals normal ovarian stroma containing a few primordial follicles.

ICD-9-CM diagnosis code(s): _____

ICD-10-CM diagnosis code(s): _____

CPT code(s) with modifier, if applicable: _____

APC: _____

Case 7-18

Health Record Face Sheet

Western Regional
Medical Center

Record Number: 11-84-96

Age: 9

Gender: Female

Length of Stay: Not Applicable

Diagnosis/Procedure: Fracture of Arm
                                    ORIF

Service Type: Same-Day Surgery

Discharge Status: Home

continued

Case 7-18, *continued*

9-year-old; fall on trampoline with pain and deformity Left arm

PAST MEDICAL HISTORY:

YES	NO		YES	NO	
	✓	WEAR CONTACTS		✓	LUNG DISEASE/ASTHMA
	✓	SMOKE		✓	STOMACH/INTESTINAL
	✓	DRINK ALCOHOL		✓	JAUNDICE/LIVER DISEASE
	✓	PREGNANT		✓	KIDNEY DISEASE/STONES
	✓	DIABETES		✓	NEUROLOGICAL PROBLEMS
	✓	HEART DISEASE		✓	ANEMIA/BLOOD DYSCRASIA
	✓	HYPERTENSION		✓	FAMILY HX SERIOUS ILLNESS
	✓	EPILEPSY		✓	HX OF ANESTHETIC PROBLEM
	✓	BLEEDING TENDENCIES			OTHER ILLNESS (EXPLAIN)

ALLERGIES TO MEDICATIONS ___*NKDA*___

TAKE MEDICINE OR DRUGS ___*None (pain meds)*___

OPERATIONS ___*None*___

PHYSICAL EXAMINATION:

ABN	WNL		ABN	WNL	WA	
	✓	HEART			PELVIC	*Pain intact digits*
	✓	LUNGS	✓		EXTREMITIES	*slight decrease sensation*
	✓	HEENT	✓		NEUROLOGICAL	*arm splinted pink and BID*
	✓	ABDOMEN				*EPL/FPL/Int Fixation*

COMMENTS: ___*X-Ray FX displaced mid shaft*___

LABS: *None*

	HCT
	CBC
	UA
	BLOOD GLUCOSE

	POTASSIUM
	MISC LABS
	ECG
	CHEST XRAY

ASSESSMENT AND PLAN: *Closed versus Open reduction and IM flexible*

PHYSICIAN'S SIGNATURE: ___*Dr. Brackel*___

DATE: 7/21/xx

Case 7-18, *continued*

SURGEON: Dr. Brackel

ASSISTANT: Dr. Redi

PREOPERATIVE DIAGNOSIS: Left both-bone forearm fracture, closed.

POSTOPERATIVE DIAGNOSIS: Grade 1 open fracture of midshaft radius and closed ulna fracture.

OPERATION: Irrigation and debridement of open fracture with open reduction internal fixation with intramedullary flexible nails.

ANESTHESIA: General LMA.

OPERATIVE DATA: Implants: Synthes titanium flexible nails, 2.0 mm and 2.5 mm. Tourniquet: Not inflated. Estimated blood loss: 10 mL. IV fluids: 300 mL.

INDICATIONS: The patient is a 9-year-old female with history of fall off trampoline last evening. She was seen in the emergency room last night. This provider was contacted by the nurse practitioner on duty.

The patient reportedly had a both-bone forearm fracture, reported to be closed. The patient was splinted and instructed to follow up n.p.o. this morning after review of x-rays on the Internet revealed a displaced midshaft radius fracture and an angulated ulna fracture. The patient presented on the morning of surgery to the orthopedic clinic and indicated for and consented for closed versus open reduction and internal fixation. The risks and benefits, indications and alternatives were discussed with the patient to include malunion, nonunion, infection, loss of motion, need for removal of hardware, and damage to local structures. The patient and the parents were counseled at length and elected to proceed.

DESCRIPTION OF PROCEDURE: The patient was identified in the preoperative holding area by voice and by armband, and the left upper extremity was identified as the operative extremity, confirmed by operative consent. The patient was then taken to the operating room where general LMA anesthesia was administered; after which, the splint was removed, and examination of the volar forearm showed a 3–4 mm skin laceration on the volar wrist and radial aspect, a suspected open fracture grade 1 with no significant contamination seen. The procedure was halted while this provider discussed with the parents the findings underneath the splint, as previous examination had been performed with the splint on. Indications for open irrigation and debridement of the wound. The parents were counseled on incidents of infection on open fractures and difference of open fracture versus closed fracture treatment. They demonstrated understanding and elected to proceed. The limb was then prepped and draped in the usual sterile orthopedic fashion.

An extension of the wound both proximally and distally on the forearm was performed. The wound track was easily identifiable; the blood stained fat down to the fascia with a rent in the fascia. The fascia was then incised both proximally and distally to allow delivering and identification of the fracture. Fracture ends were delivered through the wound and curetted and irrigated. There was no significant contamination seen. After several liters of irrigation, high flow and low pressure, the fracture was then reduced using reduction maneuver. An incision was made on the dorsal radial radius. Care was taken to be proximal to the epiphysis, which was seen on fluoroscopy scan, which also confirmed reduction. The 2.0 mm wire was then introduced into the dorsal wrist and tapped proximally until good fracture reduction was completed and the fracture stabilized. Attention was then turned to the ulna. The ulna was approached from the proximal ulna underneath the flexor mass. A stab incision was performed and the introducer awl used to make a cortical perforation; after which the 2.5 mm nail was placed intramedullary in the ulna. Fracture reduction was confirmed and fracture stabilization was confirmed, both on the AP and lateral radiographs.

After completing fracture stabilization, the pins were cut and tapped down juxtacortically, and the wounds were then irrigated and closed in a layered fashion with absorbable suture 3-0 and 4-0 Monocryl. Steri-Strips were placed, a Xeroform dressing, and a bulky sugar-tong splint. The patient tolerated the procedure well and was taken in stable condition to the PACU.

Postoperative, the patient will be managed in a bulky splint. Will follow up in ten days for wound check and placement in a long-arm cast. The patient was to be discharged to home after an additional two doses of antibiotics.

continued

Case 7-18, *continued*

OPERATIVE REPORT

Pre-Op Diagnosis___ *Irrigation & debridement* ___

Operation___ *Open fx L arm ORIF* ___

Post-Op Diagnosis

Anesthesia given H
General ☒   Regional ☐
Spinal ☐   Local ☐
Enter OR___ 0930 ___   Leave OR___ 1145 ___

Anesthesia Start_____   Finish_____

Incision Time___ 1005 ___   Finish___ 1122 ___

SURGICAL POSITIONING

Supine ☒   Prone ☐

B = Bovie
S = Safety Straps
P = Prep
X = Padding
T = Tourniquet

BODY POSITION
Jackknife ☐   Lateral ☐   Lithotomy ☐   Legs uncrossed ☒
Other_____

TRANSPORTATION TO HOLDING AREA
Via Patient Bed   ☐   Via Wheelchair   ☐
Via Cart   ☒   Carried   ☐
SPECIMEN TO LAB   Yes ☐   No ☒
Culture Site_____
WOUND CLASSIFICATION   ① 2   3

COUNT PROCEDURES

Type	Correct	Incorrect
Lap	yes	
Raytec	yes	
Kittner	NA	
Tonsil	NA	
Instrument	yes	
Needle	yes	
Blade	yes	

OPERATIVE CHECKLIST

Pre-op orders on chart—dated & noted	☑
Identification band correct	☑
Lab reports on chart	☑
Surgical Permit signed	☑
Consent Form agrees with surgery schedule	☑
Allergies noted on Chart	☑
Confirmation surgical site and side (patient response)	☑
History and Physical Done	☑

In-Patient ☐   Out-Patient ☒
Behavior Observed
Cooperative   ☒   Restless   ☐
Crying   ☐   Resistive   ☐
Withdrawn   ☐   Combative   ☐
Talkative   ☐   Other

GENERAL APPEARANCE	Pre-operative
No Problem	x
Flushed	
Pale	
Cyanotic	
Jaundiced	
Diaphoretic	
Rash	
Bruise	
Reddened Area	
Mottled	

SURGICAL SKIN PREP
Betadine Scrub ☐   Betadine Paint ☐   Other_____
IRRIGATION
N.S. ☒   Sterile water ☐   Sorbitol ☐   Other_____
Additives_____
POSITIONING AIDS
Pillow ☐ Foam Pads ☒ Sandbag ☐ Stirrups ☐ Chest roll ☐
X-ray Taken   Yes   ☒ No   ☐

DRAINS OR PACKING		SIZE	LOC
Hemovac	Hemovac 2		
Penrose			
Jackson Pratt			
Nasal Gastric			
Foley			

Case 7-18, *continued*

RADIOLOGY REPORT

XR FOREARM 2V LT

Reason for Procedure: LT FX POST OP

FINDINGS

Long intramedullary rods are present, extending from the distal left radial and ulnar metaphysis into the proximal diametaphysis of the radius and ulna. These intramedullary rods extend across fractures involving the left mid radial shaft and left mid to slightly distal ulnar. Alignment of the fracture fragments is near anatomic.

IMPRESSION

1. Status post open reduction internal fixation with intramedullary rods of left radial and ulnar shaft fractures with near anatomic alignment.
2. These images are obtained through fiberglass splint.

ICD-9-CM diagnosis code(s): _____

ICD-10-CM diagnosis code(s): _____

CPT code(s) with modifier, if applicable: _____

APC: _____

Case 7-19

Health Record Face Sheet

Western Regional
Medical Center

Record Number:	46-72-01
Age:	26
Gender:	Male
Length of Stay:	N/A
Serviced Type:	ER
Discharge Status:	To Other Short-Term Facility
Diagnosis/Procedure:	Suicidal Thoughts

continued

Case 7-19, *continued*

EMERGENCY ROOM REPORT

This 26-year-old male was brought in by police because he has had some suicidal thoughts for about one week. He thought of jumping off the bridge, was the major thought. He did not really think about overdosing. He is a paranoid schizophrenic plus he has some depression. He named several different counselors, but his most recent psychiatrist has been Dr. Norman, although he has sometimes seen Dr. Wazel, and it sounds like he is a Region IV patient. It has been about one week since he was feeling suicidal. When he was seven years old, he jumped off some high object and broke his ribs and had fairly serious injuries. He has not tried suicide since. He has had long-standing psychiatric programs and about five years ago, he was in Valley Medical Center. He claims he is taking his current medicines. They deliver them one week at a time in a carousel reminder box and he takes 10 mg of Prolixin in the morning and 40 at night. He takes Anafranil 25 mg at hs plus Cogentin bid. He denies any other major health problems. General health is otherwise good. He, right now, has a very sore throat and a cough, little or no chills, nonproductive cough. He is a 1/2 to 3/4 pack a day smoker. No history of asthma, gastrointestinal problems, kidney problems. Vital signs are stable and he is afebrile. The police have put him on a 24 hold and Mental Health has already seen him.

PHYSICAL EXAM: Vital signs are stable. He is afebrile. TMs are clear. Pharynx is quite red and injected with minimal exudate. Slightly tender cervical nodes. No nuchal rigidity.

CHEST: Sounds are clear.

HEART: Tones are clear.

ABDOMEN: Fine.

DIAGNOSES: SUICIDAL THOUGHTS FOR A WEEK OR MORE. PHARYNGITIS.

TREATMENT: He will be turned over to Mental Health and the police to go to Valley Medical Center, but I am starting him on Biaxin samples, three days worth. Valley Medical Center can continue for a complete dose.

ICD-9-CM diagnosis code(s): _____

ICD-10-CM diagnosis code(s): _____

CPT code(s) with modifier, if applicable: _____

APC: _____

Case 7-20

Health Record Face Sheet

Record Number:	02-99-81	Western Regional Medical Center
Age:	57	
Gender:	Male	
Length of Stay:	Not Applicable	
Diagnosis/Procedure:	Melanoma Wide Excision and Graft	
Service Type:	Same-Day Surgery	
Discharge Status:	To Home	

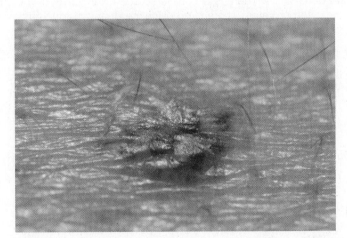

Melanoma.
Source: D. Kucharski & K. Kucharska/Shutterstock

continued

Case 7-20, *continued*

HISTORY & PHYSICAL

DATE OF ADMISSION: 6/22/xx

HISTORY:

This is a 57-year-old male who for 1 1/2 years had noted a lesion which had been changing over the right upper sideburn area on the right. This was excised and was a superficial spreading melanoma .8mm depth level 2 Clark's classification. There are some dysplastic changes at the margin and the patient presents for a wide excision with most likely a graft for coverage.

PAST HISTORY:

Right knee surgery. Otherwise no serious illnesses. (He has had a cardiovascular workup by Dr. Hart which was essentially normal except for an accelerated beat.)

PRESENT MEDICATIONS: Calan and a gout medication.

FAMILY HISTORY: Negative for cancer and diabetes.

REVIEW OF SYSTEMS:

In recent good and stable health in regards to respiratory, cardiovascular, GI, or GU systems. The patient is scheduled to have back surgery in 2 weeks.

PHYSICAL EXAMINATION:

Alert and oriented.

HEENT: Within normal limits. There is a transverse scar at the level of the superior helix on the right in the side-burn area. There is no evidence of any residual tumor. There is no adenopathy or swelling either over the parotid or neck region.

CHEST: Clear anteriorly and posteriorly with equal breath sounds.

CARDIOVASCULAR: Regular sinus rhythm without murmur.

ABDOMEN: No abnormal masses.

EXTREMITIES: Within normal limits.

NEUROLOGIC: No deficits noted.

IMPRESSION:

Melanocarcinoma of right side of face, Clark's level II, Breslow .8mm.

PLAN:

Wide excision and graft.

A very thorough discussion with the patient regarding the pros and cons of wide excision with graft versus wide excision with graft and an incontinuity parotidectomy and neck dissection were ensued also with the patient's wife. The pros and cons of both were clearly pointed out and he was offered the more extensive procedure but has decided on the wide excision with graft which is certainly an acceptable way to go.

Risks and complications of the procedure including bleeding, infection, nontake of the graft. The area of donor site and the supraclavicular or postauricular area were discussed as well as anesthetic complications.

Case 7-20, *continued*

OPERATIVE NOTE

DATE OF PROCEDURE: 6/22/xx

PREOPERATIVE DIAGNOSIS: Melanocarcinoma of the right side of the face.

POSTOPERATIVE DIAGNOSIS: Same.

OPERATIVE PROCEDURE: Wide excision of melanocarcinoma of the right side of his face with supraclavicular full-thickness skin graft.

SURGEON: Dr. Lucia

ASSISTANT: Dr. Fabios

INDICATIONS: This 57-year-old male had a superficial spreading melanoma Breslow level .8 mm, Clark's level II, excised from the sideburn area of his face on the right. He presents for a wide excision and a full-thickness skin graft.

OPERATIVE PROCEDURE: After satisfactory induction under general endotracheal anesthesia, the entire right side of the face and neck were prepped and draped in the usual sterile manner. The central portion of the wound was measured and a distance of approximately 2 1/2 cm. around the entire area was outlined with methylene blue.

An incision was made and dissection carried down to the underlying subcutaneous level. At this level the resection was performed, taking care to not damage the underlying frontal branch to the forehead. This specimen was appropriately marked with a long nasal suture and a shorter inferior suture and sent to pathology for permanent section. All gloves and instruments used in the first portion of the procedure were discarded. Hemostasis was established with a coagulating current on the Bovie. The defect measured about 6 x 6 cm.

An area in the supraclavicular region was outlined with an ellipse paralleling the clavicle. The incision was made and the full-thickness graft taken. Hemostasis was established, undermining performed and then closure of the defect performed with 2 and 3-0 Vicryl suture in the dermal layer and a subcuticular 4-0 Prolene suture for the skin. Steri-Strips were applied. Adaptic dry dressing and Elastoplast support dressing was applied.

The skin graft was then defatted and contoured to match the defect. With hemostasis established the graft was sutured in with 4-0 Novafil stents running the edges with a 6-0 Prolene suture.

Adaptic and a cotton stent were used over which the sutures were then tied.

The entire procedure was tolerated well by the patient who was sent to the recovery area in satisfactory condition.

continued

PATHOLOGY REPORT

PATIENT: Krammar Kruz   AGE: 57

RECORD NO: 02-99-81   DATE: 6/22/xx

DOCTOR: Dr. Lucia

OPERATION:

WIDE EXCISION MELANOMA, RIGHT SIDE OF FACE
SHORT SUTURE INFERIOR MARGIN, LONG SUTURE NASAL MARGIN

GROSS: Submitted is a somewhat rounded portion of skin and subcutaneous tissue which measures 5.0 × 5.0 × 0.5 cm. There is old scar formation present measuring to approximately 3.5 cm. in length. It is well healed. There is a long suture at one border indicated as nasal margin. The inferior margin is marked with a short suture. The entire peripheral margin is marked with India ink. With the inferior margin in the inferior position and the nasal margin to the right, the specimen is bisected through its mid portion from the nasal margin to the posterior margin. The upper section then is serially sectioned from right to left and submitted as A through I. The bottom specimen is serially sectioned from right to left keeping the original orientation and submitted in its entirety for examination as J through R.

MICRO: Sections reveal portions of skin and subcutaneous tissue without evidence of residual melanoma. In one section, there is identified a compound nevus which is unrelated to the previously diagnosed melanoma.

FINDINGS: Wide excision, superficial spreading melanoma, no residual tumor present. Compound nevus, excised.

ICD-9-CM diagnosis code(s): _____

ICD-10-CM diagnosis code(s): _____

CPT code(s) with modifier, if applicable: _____

APC: _____

Case 7-21

<u>**Health Record Face Sheet**</u>

Western Regional
Medical Center

<u>**Record Number:**</u>	44-09-56
<u>**Age:**</u>	59
<u>**Gender:**</u>	Male
<u>**Length of Stay:**</u>	Not Applicable
<u>**Diagnosis/Procedure:**</u>	Balanitis and Fibrosis Foreskin Circumcision
<u>**Service Type:**</u>	Same-Day Surgery
<u>**Discharge Status:**</u>	To Home

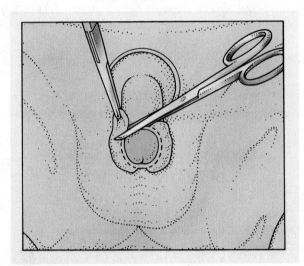

Circumcision.
Source: © Dorling Kindersley

continued

Case 7-21, *continued*

HISTORY AND PHYSICAL

DATE: 2/19/xx

HISTORY: The patient came in referred by Dr. Green on Monday. He has been fighting a problem with his penis since Spring. His general health is pretty well okay, except he did have a double bypass and hip surgery in the past. He has had two heart attacks before that time. The only medications that he takes are occasional Aspirin.

ALLERGIES: None.

ILLNESSES: None.

Social history, psychiatric history unremarkable.

REVIEW OF SYSTEMS: Skin and lymphatics normal. HEENT normal. Chest clear to auscultation. Cor regular sinus without problems. Abdomen negative. GI negative. Back and extremities negative. Neurological negative. Hematological negative. Endocrine negative.

FAMILY HISTORY: Negative as evaluated for this particular procedure.

PAST MEDICAL HISTORY: Operations - as noted on the bypass. Developmental history normal. Immunizations many years ago.

PHYSICAL EXAMINATION: Skin and lymphatics normal. Temperature normal. Pulse 72 and regular. Blood pressure normal. Respirations 16 and regular. Head normocephalic. Ears - TMs normal, hears well in left and right. Eyes - pupils equal, and reactive to light and accommodation. Back and extremities normal. Neurological normal. EOM normal. Nose, mouth and throat normal. Neck is supple. Chest is clear to auscultation. Cor regular sinus rhythm, no murmurs. Abdomen is soft without masses, organomegaly, tenderness, or bruits. Back and extremities normal. Genitalia normal. Rectal exam demonstrated a normal prostate gland.

FINAL IMPRESSION: Irritation of the penis underneath the foreskin, no evidence of any significant abnormality today.

PLAN: Is to do a circumcision. This is scheduled for the hospital.

OPERATIVE REPORT

DATE: 2/21/xx

PREOPERATIVE DIAGNOSIS: Balanitis and fibrosis of the foreskin.

POSTOPERATIVE DIAGNOSIS: Same.

OPERATION: Circumcision.

COMPLICATIONS: None.

SURGEON:

BLOOD LOSS: Minimal.

PROCEDURE: The patient was placed supine on the operating table. His penis was prepped and draped. I then made a circumscribed incision about the shaft of the penis just proximal to the glans. I then made a circumscribed incision in the mucosa proximal to the glans. These two were connected. The strip of skin was removed, bleeders were cauterized or tied using #3-0 chromic suture, then used #4–0 interrupted sutures to close the mucosa to the skin catching some subcutaneous tissues as well around the penis entirely, also placed one stitch at the frenulum, mattress type suture. He tolerated the procedure well and was returned to the recovery room in good condition.

PATHOLOGY REPORT

PATIENT: Larry Larson   AGE: 59

RECORD NO: 44-09-56   DATE: 2/21/xx

DOCTOR: Dr. Urey

OPERATION: CIRCUMCISION
              FORESKIN

GROSS: The specimen consists of a roughly rectangular piece of wrinkled, brown skin that is up to 5.6 x 3.0 x 0.7 cm. Representative sections are processed.

MICRO: The specimen in section shows skin covered by folded, well differentiated, stratified, squamous epithelium. There is brown granular pigmentation in the basal epithelial layer. Subjacent connective tissue is vascular and focally congested. All portions are well differentiated.

FINDINGS: Foreskin, circumcision procedure.

continued

Case 7-21, *continued*

PHYSICIAN'S ORDERS & PROGRESS RECORD

INSTRUCTIONS:—NOTE PROGRESS OF CASE, COMPLICATION, CHANGE IN DIAGNOSIS, CONDITION ON DISCHARGE, INSTRUCTIONS TO PATIENT.

DATE	ORDERS	✓	DATE	PROGRESS
1	Routine p.o. V.S. then q shift.		2/21/xx	P.O. circumcision
2	DC IV when alert			Complication – none
3	Discharge			
4	Vicodin check			
5	Keflex Check			
6	Appointment at 9 am in the ER tomorrow to remove his dressing.			

PHYSICIAN'S ORDERS	Another brand of drugs identical in form and content may be dispensed unless checked.	**PROGRESS RECORD**

Case 7-21, *continued*

ICD-9-CM diagnosis code(s): _____

ICD-10-CM diagnosis code(s): _____

CPT code(s) with modifier, if applicable: _____

APC: _____

Case 7-22

Health Record Face Sheet

Western Regional
Medical Center

Record Number:	13-40-05
Age:	59
Gender:	Male
Length of Stay:	Not Applicable
Diagnosis/Procedure:	Bile Duct Stricture ERCP
Service Type:	Same-Day Surgery
Discharge Status:	To Home

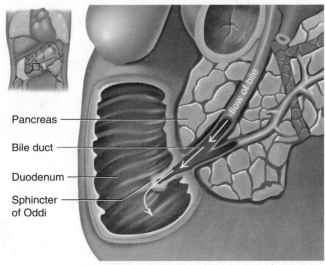

Pancreas

Bile duct

Duodenum

Sphincter of Oddi

flow of bile

Flow of bile.

continued

ENDOSCOPIC RETROGRADE CHOLANGIOPANCREATOGRAPHY:

DATE OF PROCEDURE: 12/1/xx

INDICATIONS:

59-year-old male with metastatic adenocarcinoma of the colon. He had a segmental resection of the lesion about a year ago and received chemotherapy. The CEA time has been normal up until recently. Over the past week he has had progressive jaundice. A CT scan of the abdomen demonstrates 2 nodules in the liver but there is also common bile duct dilatation. His bilirubin is 11, his alk phos is in the mid 200 range. He is beginning to have some pruritis. Palliative interventions have been discussed including surgery and stent placement. We are unable to place a stent locally but on talking with Dr. Sericati, the gastroenterologist at the University Medical Center, he prefers that a cholangiogram be obtained prior to transferring the patient there for stent placement. He has received Cefobid 2 grams IV.

EXAMINATION:

Following informed consent, sedated with Demerol 50mg and Versed 1mg IV. Oral pharyngeal anesthesia with Cetacaine spray was administered. An Olympus OES type JF1T10 side viewing duodenoscope was introduced. The ampulla was easily identified and cannulated with the patient in the prone position. A selective cholangiogram was obtained. Only the distal 4-5cm of common duct could be filled. There was a tight stricture which was asymmetrical. Despite moderate pressure, dye could not be introduced beyond the proximal side of the stricture. He tolerated the procedure well. No attempt was made at pancreatography.

IMPRESSION:

Tight stricture of the distal common bile duct as described.

PLAN:

The patient has been given the options of surgical bypass or an attempt at endoprosthesis placement elsewhere. He will be discharged to home ambulatory.

Case 7-22, *continued*

EXAM:

ERCP

HISTORY: Carcinoma of the colon, metastatic to the liver. Increasing bilirubin. Recent CT scan shows dilated proximal biliary tree. Evaluate obstruction.

ERCP:

After informed consent and sedation, the duodenoscope was inserted into the oropharynx and advanced through the stomach to the ampulla. We cannulated the ampulla of Vater. Contrast was injected retrograde filling the distal 3-4 cm. of the common duct. Above this the duct narrowed eccentrically. No contrast could be passed into the more proximal biliary tree. The eccentric narrowing would be compatible with extrinsic obstruction from carcinoma of the colon, metastatic to nodes in the porta hepatis or to a pancreatic lesion.

IMPRESSION:

Obstructed common bile duct 3-4 cm. above the ampulla of Vater.

James Holt, M.D.
_____
RADIOLOGIST

DIAGNOSTIC IMAGING

continued

Case 7-22, *continued*

PHYSICIAN'S ORDERS & PROGRESS RECORD

INSTRUCTIONS: — NOTE PROGRESS OF CASE, COMPLICATION, CHANGE IN DIAGNOSIS, CONDITION ON DISCHARGE, INSTRUCTIONS TO PATIENT.

DATE	ORDERS	✓	DATE	PROGRESS
				DATE: _12/1/xx_
				DIAGNOSIS: _obstructive jaundice_
				PLANNED PROCEDURE: _ERCP_
				INFORMED CONSENT: _received_
				PREOPERATIVE REVIEW OF BODY SYSTEMS
				Cardiovascular_____
				Pulmonary_____
				Other_ _metastatic adenocarinoma of colon_
				Regular Medications:_ Ø _
				Allergies: _morphine_
				Bleeding/Clotting Disorders _ Ø _
				Detailed H & P dictated?_ Ø _
				Signature_ Dr. Wise _

PHYSICIAN'S ORDERS

Another brand of drugs identical in form and content may be dispensed unless checked.

PROGRESS RECORD

Case 7-22, *continued*

ICD-9-CM diagnosis code(s): _____

ICD-10-CM diagnosis code(s): _____

CPT code(s) with modifier, if applicable: _____

APC: _____

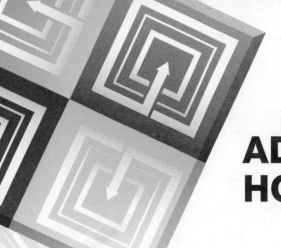

ADVANCED INPATIENT HOSPITAL CODING

8

Inpatient hospital coding traditionally has been the most complicated type of coding. The reason why inpatient coding is typically more difficult is because inpatient accounts reflect the higher level of care and treatment (i.e., the hospitalization) required by an inpatient over that required by an outpatient. Inpatient coders typically have a greater amount of data to review because inpatient hospital records can have multiple pages for each day of a patient's stay.

An inpatient coder becomes an expert on many different types of patients and the departments they access, such as cardiac, respiratory, orthopedic, urology, gynecology, obstetrics, pediatric, and newborn, to name a few. Due to the variety of patient types, inpatient coders will probably be those most impacted by the future implementation of the ICD-10-CM and ICD-10-PCS coding systems. Inpatient coders will also be the only coders who are responsible for assigning ICD-10-PCS codes.

For all cases presented in this chapter, apply all of the coding skills and knowledge you have to do the following:

1. Assign and sequence the principal ICD-9-CM and ICD-10-CM diagnosis codes with POA indicators first, followed by any applicable secondary diagnoses with POA indicators, to include appropriate V-code and E-code assignments as dictated by the setting.

2. Assign and sequence the principal ICD-9-CM and ICD-10-PCS procedure codes first followed by applicable additional procedure codes.

3. Calculate the correct MS-DRG.

It might be helpful to review the ICD-9-CM and/or ICD-10-CM *Official Guidelines for Coding and Reporting* for inpatient coding (refer to Appendix A for instructions for accessing the guidelines online) as you start to assign codes to these case studies. It also might be helpful to review the POA guidelines (for which online access instructions are also located in Appendix A). Remember that CPT® codes are not assigned by hospital inpatient coders.

Case 8-1

Health Record Face Sheet

Record Number:	12-01-11	*Western Regional Medical Center*
Age:	79	
Gender:	Female	
Length of Stay:	12 days	
Diagnosis/Procedure:	Colon CA with Partial Colectomy	
Service Type:	Inpatient Surgical	
Discharge Status:	Skilled Nursing Facility	

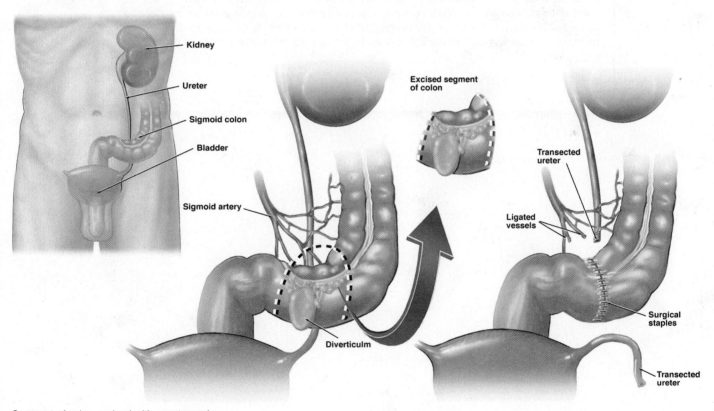

Segment of colon excised with anastomosis.
Source: © Nucleus Medical Art Inc/Alamy

continued

DISCHARGE SUMMARY

DATE OF ADMISSION: 1/2/xx
DATE OF DISCHARGE: 1/3/xx

ADMITTING DIAGNOSIS:
1. ABDOMINAL PAIN.

FINAL DIAGNOSIS:
1. COLON CANCER, SPECIFICALLY ADENOCARCINOMA WITH THE PATIENT UNDERGO-
   ING PARTIAL COLECTOMY.

HOSPITAL SUMMARY: The patient is a 79-year-old white widow who was admitted to the hospital for workup of some abdominal pain. She had been having trouble for several weeks and been going downhill. Her appetite had been bad. She was brought into the hospital initially for workup and part of that workup included a barium enema which showed a constricting annular lesion of the colon. At that point, the patient was seen by Dr. Minut who evaluated the patient and after transfusing some blood to build up her hematocrit, she was taken to surgery electively and underwent a partial colectomy for treatment of this condition. Her postpoerative course was excellent and was under the direction of myself. She was able to be discharged temporarily to a nursing home to continue her recovery. Please see Dr. Minut's full operative dictation for complete details of the surgical procedure.

Case 8-1, *continued*

HISTORY AND PHYSICAL EXAMINATION

ADMISSION DATE: 1/2/xx

CHIEF COMPLAINT: ABDOMINAL PAIN AND FULLNESS.

HISTORY OF PRESENT ILLNESS: Mrs. Neal is a 79-year-old white female who has been ill for the past several days with abdominal pain and bloating, even some diarrhea on the day prior to admission. She thought that maybe she just had the stomach flu, but when she did not get better, she was brought to the office for an examination. At that time, the patient looked pale and she was admitted to Short Stay initially for workup. The patient had been known to be anemic recently and been taking some iron pills for that. She denied any blood in the stool or any blood in the urine or any place else.

PAST MEDICAL HISTORY: MEDICAL PROBLEMS:

1. History of anemia.
2. She has a history of obstructive hydrocephalus that was due to an arachnoid cyst and she did undergo ventriculoperitoneal shunt placement for that.
3. She also has a history of psoriasis.

SURGERY: She has had a hysterectomy, appendectomy and the shunt placement as mentioned above for the hydrocephalus. She also had a laminectomy for spinal stenosis 10 years ago. I believe the shunt placement in her head was in 1999 earlier in the year. MEDICATIONS: Besides some topical ointment for psoriasis and iron for the anemia, she is not on any medications. ALLERGIES: NO KNOWN DRUG ALLERGIES. HABITS: She does not smoke or drink. She used to smoke, but quit about 30 years ago.

SOCIAL HISTORY: The patient is a widow. She lost her husband to heart problems in about

REVIEW OF SYSTEMS: She has lost some weight over the past several months. She is not sure exactly how many pounds. She has been progressively getting weaker in the past several months as well.

PHYSICAL EXAMINATION

GENERAL: She presents as a pale-appearing white elderly female. She is in no acute distress.

VITAL SIGNS: Normal with a temperature of 98.8°, blood pressure 124/60. Pulse is 74 and regular.

HEENT: Negative, excepting pale mucous membranes of the eyes and oral mucosa.

NECK: Supple with no masses.

CHEST: Lungs are clear.

CARDIOVASCULAR: Heart is regular. No murmurs or gallops.

BREASTS: Not examined at this time.

ABDOMEN: Soft. It is tender to palpation in all quadrants. No definite mass is felt to palpation.

EXTREMITIES: Extremities show no cyanosis, clubbing or edema.

INITIAL IMPRESSION: ABDOMINAL PAIN OF UNKNOWN CAUSE. I HAVE A SUSPICION THAT THIS PATIENT MAY HAVE SOME SORT OF OCCULT MALIGNANCY WITH THE WEIGHT LOSS AND ANEMIA, SPECIFICALLY COLON CANCER.

PLAN: Admission and workup of these problems.

continued

OPERATIVE REPORT

OPERATION DATE: 1/4/xx

PREOPERATIVE DIAGNOSIS: ADENOCARCINOMA OF THE HEPATIC FLEXURE OF THE COLON, CHOLECYSTITIS AND CHOLELITHIASIS.

POSTOPERATIVE DIAGNOSIS: SAME.

PROCEDURE PERFORMED: Right hemicolectomy, cholecystectomy.

SURGEON: Dr. Minut

ASSISTANT: Dr. Ricardo

ANESTHESIA: GENERAL

DESCRIPTION OF PROCEDURE: The patient was brought to the Operating Room with IV infusing. Perioperative antibiotics had been administered. General anesthesia was induced and a nasogastric tube and Foley catheter were inserted. The abdomen was prepped with Betadine sterilely.

Skin marker was used to outline a transverse upper abdominal incision beginning in the right mid abdomen laterally and extending toward the epigastrium. Skin incision was made with a #10 blade and carried through subcutaneous tissue to expose fascia. Bleeding was controlled with electrocautery. Oblique muscles were divided with electrocautery as is the rectus muscle exposing the peritoneum. The peritoneum was identified and entered. Manual and visual exploration of the abdominal cavity reveals tumor in the hepatic flexure of the colon without obvious extension into pericolonic tissues. The gallbladder is chronically inflamed and contains stones. Buchwalter retractor was positioned. With traction on the fundus of the gallbladder, the peritoneum overlying the hepatoduodenal ligament is incised. By blunt dissection, the cystic duct is skeletonized, doubly clipped and divided. Similarly, the cystic artery is bluntly dissected, doubly clipped and divided. With traction on the divided duct, the gallbladder is dissected from the liver bed with the use of the electrocautery. Specimen is submitted for pathologic evaluation. Pack in placed into the liver bed and removed after approximately 10 minutes and there is no evidence of bleeding from this surface.

Attention is then turned to the colon section. The lateral peritoneal reflection is incised with Metzenbaum scissor and the colon is reflected medially. By blunt dissection, the mesentery is elevated from the retroperitoneum. The right ureter is identified and preserved. Point of division is chosen in the distal ileum and a GIA stapler is passed and fired. Similarly a point in the mid transverse colon is chosen for division and a GIA stapler passed and fired. Peritoneum overlying the mesentery is incised with the Metzenbaum scissor. Mesentery is then divided between clamps and 2-0 silk ties and the right colon is submitted for pathologic evaluation. Area of dissection is irrigated and examined carefully for hemostasis prior to anastomosis. The small bowel was juxta opposed against the transverse colon and secured in place with 0 muscular 2-0 silk interrupted suture. An enterotomy is made in the small bowel and colon and the GIA stapler is passed and fired forming the anastomosis. Enterotomy is then closed in two layers. The first layer is a running 3-0 chromic full-thickness suture and the second is an interrupted 0 muscular 3-0 silk suture. Mesentery is then closed using a running 2-0 Vicryl suture. The area of dissection is examined carefully for hemostasis prior to closure. Following correct sponge, needle and instrument counts the abdomen is closed. Posterior fascia is approximated using a running suture of #1 Vicryl. The anterior rectus sheath and external oblique muscles are approximated using a running #1 Vicryl suture reinforced at intervals with #1 Prolene. Subcutaneous layer was irrigated and examined for hemostasis. Scarpa's fascia was then approximated using interrupted 2-0 Vicryl suture. Skin is approximated with skin stapler. Dry sterile dressings were applied. The patient tolerated the procedure well and was transferred to the Recovery Room in stable condition.

Case 8-1, *continued*

TISSUE REPORT

PATIENT: Nancy Neal
DATE: 1/4/xx
SEX-AGE: F 79   **DOB:** 6/14/xx
DOCTOR: Dr. Minut
ORIGIN: INPATIENT
TISSUE: 1. Gallbladder   2. Right side of colon & terminal ileum

HISTORY: CA of colon

Gross: 1. is a gallbladder .7 × 4 × 2 cm. The surface of the gallbladder is smooth; the wall appears to be slightly thickened, the mucosa is green, the lumen contains about 10 cc of bile and numerous mulberry green gallstones, the largest 5 mm in diameter, one block

2. consists of the right side of the colon including attached terminal ileum and right side of colon without the appendix. The terminal ileum is 10 cm in length. It has a fairly smooth but granular serosal surface, a firm wall, a mucosa that is folded and light green. The segment of colon is 35 cm in length, includes cecum, ascending and transverse segments of the colon. In the ascending portion of the colon there is a somewhat pedunculated irregular polyp 55 × 40 × 30 mm; the surface is folded and light grey but the center is superficially ulcerated, granular and light grey. The cut section of this lesion reveals it appears to be confined to the mucosa although In the center there is a suggestion that the lesion infiltrates into the muscle coat. 5 cm distal to this polypoid lesion in the region of the transverse segment of the colon there is a 7 cm in length 4 cm in width circumferential penetrating and perforating polypoid tumor that extends to the muscle coat and into the serosal adipose tissue. The margins around the area of penetration are thickened, granular, polypoid, grey to red injected. On cut section of the mesentery in this region it also infiltrates into the attached mesenteric adipose tissue. 6 cm distal to this lesion and approximately 3 cm from the distal resection margin there is an additional pedunculated polyp 15 × 5 × 3 mm. The cut section of the mesentery reveals eleven firm light grey lymph nodes several of which appear to be obviously replaced by firm light grey tumor. The lymph nodes are more or less discrete, the largest 15 mm in diameter.
Slide key:

A sections of terminal ileum one block
B sections of the most proximal polypoid lesion three blocks
C sections of large penetrating lesion six blocks
D sections of most distal polypoid lesion one block
E sections of mesenteric lymph nodes four knocks
TM:k

MICROSCOPIC: 1. The gallbladder reveals changes of chronic cholecystitis.

2A reveals normal terminal ileum

2B, the most proximal polypoid lesion, reveals a tubulovillous adenoma the center of which reveals a well-differentiated adenocarcinoma that has infiltrated into the muscle coat.

2C 5 cm distal to the polypoid area reveals a poorly differentiated adenocarcinoma composed of malignant epithelial cells having vacuolated cytoplasm arranged in cords and nests or solid sheets having provoked a rather prominent desmoplastic response extensively infiltrating the muscle coat into the serosal surface and the attached mesenteric adipose tissue. The mesenteric adipose tissue immediately adjacent to the area where the lesion has infiltrated into the mesenteric adipose tissue reveals areas thickened by proliferated fibrous connective tissue containing lymphocytes. No definite involvement in these areas can be Identified.

see page 2   **DOCTOR'S COPY**

continued

S98.000639   **TISSUE REPORT**

PATIENT: Nancy Neal
DATE: 1/4/xx
SEX-AGE: F 79   **DOB:** 6/14/xx
DOCTOR: Dr. Minut
ORIGIN: INPATIENT
TISSUE: 1. Gallbladder   2. Right side of colon & terminal ileum

CONTINUED:

2D the most distal polyp reveals a benign tubulovillous adenoma.

The sections of the 11 mesenteric lymph nodes 2E reveal basically hyperplastic lymph nodes without any evidence of metastases. Sinusoids contain plasma cells or a few giant cells.

DIAGNOSIS: CHOLECYSTITIS, CHRONIC
                    A. CALCULUS, MULTIPLE

        RIGHT SIDE OF COLON AND TERMINAL ILEUM
                A. ADENOCARCINOMA, POORLY DIFFERENTIATED, PROXIMAL
                   PORTION, TRANSVERSE SEGMENT OF COLON
                    1. LESION INFILTRATES INTO THE SEROSAL SURFACE AND
                       THE MESENTERIC ADIPOSE TISSUE
                B. ADENOCARCINOMA, WELL DIFFERENTIATED, MUCOSA, AS-
                   CENDING PORTION OF THE COLON
                    1. ADENOCARCINOMA INFILTRATES INTO THE SUPERFICIAL
                       MUSCLE COAT
                C. POLYP, ADENOMATOUS OR TUBULAR TYPE, DISTAL PORTION,
                   TRANSVERSE SEGMENT OF THE COLON
                D. LYMPH NODES, HYPERPLASTIC, MULTIPLE (11), MESENTERY,
                   RIGHT SIDE OF THE COLON
                E. SEGMENT, TERMINAL ILEUM, NORMAL

COMMENT: This 79-year-old female in the proximal transverse segment of the colon has a 7 cm in length 4 cm in width circumferential penetrating and perforating polypoid lesion that extended right to the serosal surface and the adipose tissue. On microscopic examination this is a poorly differentiated adenocarcinoma of colonic mucosa. 11 adjacent lymph nodes were isolated and are free of metastases. In addition proximal to this adenocarcinoma there was a 55 mm polyp in the ascending portion of the colon the center of which reveals development of an early well-differentiated adenocarcinoma of colonic origin infiltrating into superficial muscle coat.

Pathological stage: T3 NO MO, modified Dukes B2

DOCTOR'S COPY

Case 8-1, *continued*

ICD-9-CM/ICD-10-CM diagnosis code(s): _____

ICD-9-CM procedure and ICD-10-PCS procedure code(s): _____

MS-DRG: _____

Case 8-2

Health Record Face Sheet

Western Regional
Medical Center

Record Number:	05-23-99
Age:	34
Gender:	Female
Length of Stay:	4 Days
Diagnosis/Procedure:	Hemorrhoids with Excision
Service Type:	Inpatient Surgical
Discharge Status:	To Home

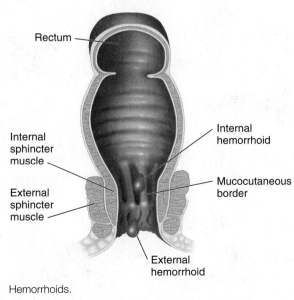

Hemorrhoids.

Source: Pearson Education/PH College

continued

DISCHARGE SUMMARY

ADMISSION DATE: 4/14/xx

DISCHARGE DATE: 4/17/xx

ENTERING COMPLAINT: Severe hemorrhoids.

PERTINENT LAB & X-RAY DATA: All essentially normal.

PROCEDURES & HOSPITAL COURSE: The patient underwent a hemorrhoidectomy and had an uneventful course. At the time of discharge the operative site was healing nicely, her bowels were moving and she was up and about without problems.

DISPOSITION & REMARKS: Home and office.

CONDITION: Recovered.

FINAL DIAGNOSIS: Severe internal and external hemorrhoids.

OPERATION DONE: Hemorrhoidectomy.

Case 8-2, *continued*

HISTORY & PHYSICAL

DATE OF ADMISSION: 4/14/xx

HISTORY: This 34-year-old woman has developed hemorrhoids. They came on gradually but have been especially prominent over the last year or so. They have increased dramatically in size and have become increasingly symptomatic. We treated her conservatively with sitz baths and stool softeners and so forth and she has done well for awhile but recently they have again begun bleeding and protruding and causing considerable pain. They are very marked hemorrhoids and so she has elected to have surgery and she enters now for that.

PAST HISTORY: Her health has always been good. She has had a hysterectomy with no other operations. She is on no medication now and has no allergies.

REVIEW OF SYSTEMS:

HEENT: Negative.

CARDIORESPIRATORY: She smokes but has no shortness or breath nor lung symptoms. She has never had any heart problems.
GI: Negative other than in present illness.
GU, GYN & REST: Not remarkable.

Her personal, social, and family histories are normal.

PHYSICAL EXAM:

She is a normal-appearing young woman who was in no distress and had normal pulse and blood pressure.
SKIN: Negative.
HEENT: Showed no abnormalities.
NECK: Supple without masses.
LUNGS: Clear to auscultation and percussion.
HEART: Regular rhythm without murmur.
ABDOMEN: Soft and flat with no masses or tenderness.
PELVIC: Not done as she has no symptoms referable to that area.
RECTAL: Shows severe circumferential internal and external hemorrhoids.
EXTREMITIES & NEUROLOGICAL: Normal.

INITIAL IMPRESSION:

Severe internal and external hemorrhoids.

continued

Case 8-2, *continued*

OPERATIVE NOTE

DATE OF PROCEDURE: 4/15/xx

SURGEON: Dr. Alvarez

PREOPERATIVE DIAGNOSIS: Severe internal and external hemorrhoids.
POSTOPERATIVE DIAGNOSIS: Same

OPERATION DONE: Hemorrhoidectomy.

PROCEDURE:

We established satisfactory general anesthesia and placed the patient up in the dorsal li-thotomy position. I did insert a rigid sigmoidoscope and advanced it to 7 or 8cm but there encountered a large amount of stool. I saw nothing in the distal rectum.

We then prepped and draped the entire rectal area and I inserted a speculum and inspected the area. She had the hugest area of hemorrhoids right at about between 6 and 7 o'clock, posteriorly. This was a huge area that had a surface that was completely eroded off and was very red and inflamed. There was a small area immediately adjacent to it at 4 or 5 o'clock. The lateral edges were okay. Anteriorly at about between 11 and 12 o'clock there was another huge hemorrhoid with a smaller one just to the left of that. I initially placed a Pean clamp around the one at 7 o'clock and then placed a suture in the mucosa up in the rectum above it. I then incised under the clamp and lifted the hemorrhoid up and then tied the stitch around the base of it and amputated it. This left a bare area in which I achieved hemostasis with one 2-0 chro-mic cat gut stitch and then electrocautery. I then placed the Pean clamp on the hemorrhoid about 5 o'clock immediately adjacent and excised it in the same way. I did leave a small rim of mucosa in between the two. I then went anteriorly and the very large hemorrhoid there I placed a Pean clamp on and incised under the clamp and then placed a 2-0 chromic cat gut stitch through the base of the hemorrhoid up in the rectum and removed that hemorrhoid. I removed a smaller one immediately adjacent to the left of it also leaving some mucosa between. In each of the bare areas I achieved hemostasis with 3-0 plain cat gut stick ties but mostly with electro-cautery. After hemostasis was secured we infiltrated the entire area with 0.25% marcaine with Epinephrine and then applied a dressing. She tolerated the procedure well.

PATHOLOGY REPORT

OPERATION: HEMORRHOIDECTOMY

GROSS: Submitted are multiple, polypoid-like structures which appear grossly to be com-prised of anal mucosa and submucosa. Within the submucosa are numerous, dilated, and congested blood vessels. The specimen in its entirety measures to approximately 3.0 cm. Representative portions are submitted for examination.

MICRO: The specimen reveals fragments of anal mucosa and submucosa. Within the submu-cosa are numerous dilated and congested blood vessels.

IMPRESSION: External and Internal hemorrhoids.

Case 8-2, *continued*

DATE	ORDERS	✓	DATE	PROGRESS
4/14/xx	Admit to Surgical Floor. CBC, SMAC, UA R/o Dr.		4/14/xx	For elective hemorrhoidectomy
4/15/xx	NPO until ambulatory Follow until change to clear liquids po - reg diet. Routine po v.s. q 2 hr up bathroom with help		4/15/xx	General Anesthesia Hemorroidectomy
	PCA 1 dose 1 mg Compazine 10 mg			
	Straight cath prn inability to void E.S. Tylenol every 4 hrs prn headache			
4/16/xx	Keep IV running 50-75 After oral diet decrease to BKO Remove dressing and start sitz baths qid 3 mins. Colac 100 mg		4/16/xx	Afebrile - alert Continue sitz baths. Move on diet as tolerated.
4/17/xx	DC IV and PCA Demerol 75-100 mgs IV q 3 hrs as needed for pain Tylox (two tabs) q 3 hrs as needed pain May have sitz after bm		4/17/xx	Doing well. Tolerating sitz baths well. No change yet.
4/17/xx	Home Office in one week Colace and Tylenol 3		4/17/xx	Had BM Sitz ok.

continued

Case 8-2, *continued*

ICD-9-CM/ICD-10-CM diagnosis code(s): _____

ICD-9-CM procedure and ICD-10-PCS procedure code(s): _____

MS-DRG: _____

Case 8-3

Health Record Face Sheet

Western Regional
Medical Center

Record Number:	12-49-33
Age:	77
Gender:	Female
Length of Stay:	10 Days
Diagnosis/Procedure:	Ulcerative Colitis Right Hemi Colectomy
Service Type:	Inpatient Surgical
Discharge Status:	To Home

Case 8-3, *continued*

DISCHARGE SUMMARY

DATE OF DISCHARGE: 12/10/xx

ENTERING COMPLAINT: Chronic ulcerative colitis.

LAB/X-RAY: Her SMAC showed her blood sugar to be 120. Her SGPT was 28. Her sodium was 139. Her urinalysis was not remarkable. Her CBC on a number of occasions was normal. Her last hemoglobin was 13.6. The one on admission was normal. The rest of her lab data was normal.

PROCEDURES/HOSPITAL COURSE: The patient underwent a bowel prep and then a total abdominal colectomy with proctectomy and an end ileostomy. Her postoperative course was amazingly uneventful. The nasogastric tube was removed in 48 hours. When her ileostomy functioned and bowel function resumed, we started her on a diet. Her perineal drains were gradually advanced. At the time of discharge, they were out and that area was doing well. There was no drainage. Her incision looked good. Her ileostomy was functioning well and she had learned how to take care of it satisfactorily. She was on a regular diet and up and about without problems.

DISPOSITION/REMARKS: Home and office.

CONDITION: Recovered.

FINAL DIAGNOSIS: Chronic ulcerative colitis.

OPERATION: Total abdominal colectomy with total proctectomy and end ileostomy.

Case 8-3, *continued*

HISTORY AND PHYSICAL

DATE OF ADMISSION: 12/1/xx

HISTORY: This 77-year-old woman has had ulcerative colitis for at least 20 or 25 years. It has been more or less active most of the time as treating her has been extremely difficult. She has been on Azulfidine and Prednisone off and on, but feels that these medications react with her and has really not taken her medication as ordered. Dr. Gregson relates that she has been difficult in that sense that she doesn't always do what she is told to do. She is on a new current medication for ulcerative colitis and that is all at the present time. She is symptomatic all the time with cramps and bloody diarrhea. She has recently had colonoscopy done and biopsies of a couple of pseudo polyps showed dysplastic changes and they were definite pre-malignant. We discussed the situation with her. In view of her age and attitude, she probably would not be a candidate for any type of pull through operation. In view of the dysplastic changes and the propensity to develop carcinoma, she should have her colon ablated. She agreed to a total colectomy and an end ileostomy. She enters at the present time for bowel prep and that procedure.

PAST HISTORY: Her general health has been good. She is allergic to Penicillin. Her only current medication is the one for ulcerative colitis. Her only operation was a cholecystectomy a few years ago.

REVIEW OF SYSTEMS: HEENT is negative. Cardiorespiratory - she does not smoke. She has never had any shortness of breath nor lung problems. She has never had any chest pain or known heart problems nor hypertension. GI is negative except for her present illness. GU/GYN/Remainder is not remarkable.

Personal, social and family histories are not contributory.

PHYSICAL EXAMINATION: She is a normal-appearing elderly woman who was in no distress and had normal vital signs. Skin is negative. HEENT showed no abnormalities. Her neck was supple without masses. Lungs were clear to auscultation and percussion. Heart had a regular rhythm without murmur. Abdomen is soft and flat with no masses or tenderness. Pelvic was not done as she has no symptoms there. Rectal was deferred because we were going to take it out anyway. Extremities and neurological are not too remarkable.

INITIAL IMPRESSION: Chronic ulcerative colitis with dysplastic changes present in the pseudo polyps.

Case 8-3, *continued*

OPERATIVE REPORT

DATE OF OPERATION: 12/2/xx

SURGEON: Dr.Otto

PREOPERATIVE DIAGNOSIS: Chronic ulcerative colitis with dysplasia in the pseudo polyps.

POSTOPERATIVE DIAGNOSIS: Same.

OPERATION: Total colectomy, proctectomy with end Brooke ileostomy.

PROCEDURE: We established satisfactory general anesthesia and prepped and draped the entire abdomen. I made a midline incision from just underneath the xiphoid down to the symphysis pubis and extended it down through linea alba, through the peritoneum and into the abdominal cavity. There were a large number of adhesions in the upper abdomen from her previous operation. I had to dissect all of these out and completely free up the omentum from the anterior abdominal wall. We then went down and I freed up some adhesions between the sigmoid colon and the lateral pelvic wall. I could not feel her liver because of adhesions, but her stomach felt normal. The small bowel all looked normal. Her uterus was normal. The right ovary was very atrophic. The left had a large cyst which I just ruptured. The rest of the exploration was not too remarkable. I initially divided the middle sigmoid colon and then began dividing the sigmoid meso-colon going distally. I stayed close to the colon and did leave a considerable amount of sigmoid meso-colon posteriorly. I then incised the peritoneum on each side of the sigmoid colon around to the peritoneal reflection again staying close to the colon so I would have enough peritoneum to reperitonealize the pelvic floor. I then dissected the rest of the sigmoid meso colon and divided it and tied it off going down into the sacrum. I then went into the hollow of the sacrum and completely freed up the recto-sigmoid posteriorly very easily down to beyond the coccyx. I then went anteriorly and freed up the rectum anteriorly dissecting underneath the symphysis pubis. I dissected it down until I was clear past the symphysis pubis. This just left a lateral attachment. I divided these between clamps all the way down to the lower most end of the dissection. We tied off all of these with #2-0 silk. This completely freed up most of the rectum and the entire rectal sigmoid. I then transected the rectum down about at the peritoneal reflection, tying it off with an umbilical tape. The upper portion was removed. We left a lap sponge in there and washed out the pelvis with Cefadyl solution and then reperitonealized. I closed the peritoneum over it with a continuous #2-0 Vicryl to completely reperitonealize the floor. We then incised the peritoneal reflection along the left gutter and completely mobilized the descending colon. I then went over in midline and went through the gastro-colic omentum about in midline and then divided the gastro-colic omentum laterally over past the spleen.

I left the omentum attached to the colon. We tied off all of these with #2-0 silk. I then divided the mesentery of the descending colon and divided the left side of the mesentery of the transverse colon, staying fairly close to the back wall of the abdomen. We tied these off with #2-0 silk. We then over the right gutter and I incised along the right gutter and mobilized the cecum. I incised the peritoneum of the appendix and the terminal ileum to totally immobilize it. We then went up and I divided the right side of the gastro-colic omentum and freed up all of the attachments between the right colon and the liver. I then by blunt dissection completely mo-bilized the right colon. I then divided the right side of the transverse meso-colon and then divided the mesentery of the right colon, tying all of these off with #2-0 silk. I then transected the ileum right at the ileocecal valve with a GIA stapler and then removed the specimen from the field. I had the pathologist check the end and it was okay as far as disease was concerned so I knew we could do the ileostomy any place. I transected the terminal ileum straight across, but it did not have good blood supply and I had to go back about 1–1/2 inches. We had our enterostomal therapist, mark the place for the ileostomy. I excised a button of skin there and then excised a portion of the anterior rectus sheath and then opened the hole clear through into the abdominal cavity. I then freed up the terminal ileum leaving as much mesentery as I could. I pulled it out through the abdominal wall and had a sufficient length out there. I then doubled it back on itself and did a Brooke ileostomy. The ileostomy itself was about an inch long. This was after I doubled it back. I sutured the edge of the mucosa as I doubled it back to the bowel and then to the skin holding it in place. The blood supply appeared satisfactory and it looked good when we finished. I went inside and then sutured the ileum to the anterior abdominal wall with interrupted #4-0 silk. I then closed the right gutter by suturing the mesentery to the peritoneum with interrupted #4-0 silk. We then washed out the abdominal cavity with two liters of Cefadyl solution. The small bowel was replaced in its normal position and the abdominal wall closed. This was done with continuous #1 Vicryl on the fascia, #2 nylon stay sutures and staples on the skin. We then placed the patient up in dorsal lithotomy, and prepped and draped the entire perineum. I sutured the anus shut with an #0 silk. I then made an incision around the anus staying fairly close to it and not making a large incision. I then dissected in staying right on the wall of the rectum and after a very short period of time entered the pre-sacral space posteriorly. We dissected down so low it was easy to remove the rectal stump. I then dissected the lateral levators off the rectum and then dissected the rectum off the underside of the vagina and completely freed it up and removed it. We achieved hemostasis with electrocautery. I then placed four Penrose drains up in the pre-sacral space and brought these out through the incision.

I closed the levators loosely over the drains with a few interrupted #0 Vicryl sutures and closed the skin down with a few inter-rupted #3-0 nylon sutures. A pressure dressing was then applied there. She tolerated the procedure well.

continued

Case 8-3, *continued*

PATHOLOGY REPORT

OPERATION: TOTAL PROCTOCOLECTOMY
#1 COLON
#2 PIECES OF COLON, RECTUM, SIGMOID
ULCERATIVE COLITIS, PSEUDOPOLYPS, CHECK TERMINAL ILEUM FOR DISEASE

GROSS: Specimen #1 is a rim of terminal ileum, cecum with attached appendix, ascending, transverse, and descending colon. The specimen, after fixation, measures 50 cm. in length. The rim of terminal ileum measures to approximately 0.5 cm. in length. A representative portion of the terminal ileum is submitted for Frozen Section. FROZEN SECTION DIAGNOSIS: Terminal ileum with lymphoid hyperplasia but no evidence of ulcerative colitis. There are scattered segments of the colon with linear areas of erosion and flattening with numerous, small polypoid structures present ranging in size from 1.5 to 0.4 cm. Representative portions of the cecum are submitted as 1A and of the vermiform appendix as 1A. Representative portions from the site of the rim of terminal ileum are submitted as 1B, of the ascending colon as 1C, of the transverse colon to include areas of polypoid change as 1D and 1E, and of the descending colon as 1F, 1G, and 1H. Specimen #2 is the sigmoid, anus, and rectum. The sigmoid measures 17.5 cm. in length. There is flattening of the mucosa with polypoid structures arising from the mucosa. One measures 1.5 cm. in greatest dimension. The other measures 1.4 cm. in greatest dimension. The anal rectal segment measures 6.5 cm. in length. There are no distinct gross abnormalities noted except for some flattening of the mucosal surface in the proximal portion of the specimen. Representative portions of the specimen to include the polypoid structures are submitted for examination. A small, ovoid portion of skin and subcutaneous tissue is also present measuring to 2.3 cm. in greatest dimension. A representative portion is submitted for examination. A segment of small bowel is present measuring to 2.5 cm. in length. A representative portion is submitted for examination.

MICRO: Sections through the vermiform appendix reveal luminal fibrosis. Sections through the bowel reveal an acute and chronic inflammatory exudate with marked eosinophilia within the lamina propria and extending superficially into the submucosa. In many areas, there is lymphoid hyperplasia. Within the cecum adjacent to the ileocecal valve, there is minimal inflammation present with inflammation increasing as one progresses distally. Crypt abscesses are present within many areas. Areas of dysplasia of the nuclei are noted. Areas of pseudopolyps are present with erosion over portions of the surfaces. Within these pseudopolyps, there is more intense inflammation together with small capillary and fibroblastic proliferation. Within the sigmoid colon, there are areas of abscess formation within the submucosa. Sections through the rectum and anus reveal inflammation similar to that described in the more proximal colon.

IMPRESSION: Chronic ulcerative colitis involving the colon and rectum with formation of inflammatory pseudopolyps, focal dysplasia, and focal submucosal abscess formation.

Terminal ileum, free of disease.

ICD-9-CM/ICD-10-CM diagnosis code(s): _____

ICD-9-CM procedure and ICD-10-PCS procedure code(s): _____

MS-DRG: _____

Case 8-4

Health Record Face Sheet

Western Regional
Medical Center

Record Number: 40-43-29

Age: 59

Gender: Male

Length of Stay: 3 Days

Diagnosis/Procedure: Cholecystitis Cholelithiasis
                              Cholecystectomy

Service Type: Inpatient Surgical

Discharge Status: To Home

DISCHARGE SUMMARY

ADMITTED: 3/23/xx
DISCHARGED: 3/25/xx

DISCHARGE DIAGNOSIS: Cholelithiasis, cholecystitis.

REASON FOR ADMISSION: Mr. Nelson is a 59-year-old African-American male who was admitted for cholecystectomy for cholelithiasis and cholecystitis. The patient had no admitting lab or x-ray, it had all been done as an outpatient and was all normal.

HOSPITAL COURSE: The patient was taken to surgery where an attempt was made at laparoscopic cholecystectomy. This could not be accomplished because of severe adhesions and an inability to distinguish anatomy in the area. The patient, therefore, underwent an open cholecystectomy. His postoperative course was entirely uncomplicated and he is being discharged to be seen in follow up in my office in one week.

DISCHARGE DIAGNOSIS: Cholelithiasis, cholecystitis.

DISCHARGE DIET: Regular.

DISCHARGE ACTIVITY: As tolerated except for heavy lifting or straining.

DISCHARGE MEDICATIONS: As before.

DISCHARGE WOUND CARE: Nil. He may bathe or shower and pat his incision dry.

DISCHARGE INSTRUCTIONS: The patient is to report any nausea, vomiting, diarrhea, fever, or chills, redness or swelling of his incision. He is not to drive if he takes pain pills.

DISCHARGE CARE: The patient is being discharged in the care of his wife.

HISTORY & PHYSICAL

ADMISSION DATE: 3/23/xx

CHIEF COMPLAINT: Abdominal pain.

HISTORY OF PRESENT ILLNESS: Mr. Nelson is a 59-year-old African-American male who has had known gallbladder disease for five years with multiple episodes of severe right upper quadrant pain with penetration through to the back accompanied by diarrhea and belching. He has also had intolerance of fatty foods. Symptoms have been getting progressively worse and he is now being admitted for a cholecystectomy.

PAST MEDICAL HISTORY: Usual childhood diseases. Medical Diseases: He had an MI approximately 14 years ago. No other medical diseases. Previous surgery was an appendectomy and a coronary artery bypass. He has had multiple small bone fractures. He denies any allergies.

MEDICATIONS: He takes Lopressor, Pepcid and Aspirin.

He has had no transfusions.

FAMILY HISTORY: Mother is alive with diabetes and three MI's. His father died of pulmonary embolism. No other history of familial diseases.

SOCIAL HISTORY: The patient is disabled because of back problems. He is married. Does not drink or smoke.

REVIEW OF SYSTEMS: Negative and non contributory.

PHYSICAL EXAMINATION: Demonstrates a well-nourished, well-developed 59-year-old African-American male.

HEENT: Normal.
NECK: Supple. Trachea midline. Thyroid is normal. There are no nodes, masses or bruits in the neck. The supraclavicular and infraclavicular regions are clear.
THORAX: There is normal anterior posterior diameter to the thorax.
BREASTS: Undeveloped without masses.
LUNGS: Clear to auscultation and percussion.
HEART: Regular rhythm without murmur. S1, S2 are normal. No S3, S4.
ABDOMEN: Soft. Bowel sounds are normal. No megaly, mass, hernias, bruits.
SPINE: Straight. No CVA tenderness.
RECTAL: Demonstrates a normal sphincter and no masses.
EXTREMITIES, NEUROLOGICAL & VASCULAR EXAMINATIONS: Normal.
IMPRESSION: Cholelithiasis and cholecystitis.
PLAN: Laparoscopic cholecystectomy.

OPERATIVE NOTE

DATE OF PROCEDURE: 3/24/xx

PREOPERATIVE DIAGNOSIS: Cholelithiasis and cholecystitis.

POSTOPERATIVE DIAGNOSIS: Same.

OPERATION:
1. Laparoscopy.
2. Cholecystectomy with operative cholangiography - open.

ANESTHESIA: General.

PROCEDURE: After adequate sedation the patient was brought to the operating room and placed in the supine position on the operating table. Anesthesia was induced with intravenous Pentothal, endotracheal tube was passed and the patient was maintained on endotracheal anesthesia.

After obtaining proper anesthesia, the patient was prepped and draped in the usual fashion.

An infraumbilical incision was made and the Verres needle introduced and satisfactory pneumaperitoneum obtained. The 10 mm. trochar was then placed through the infraumbilical incision and the camera introduced after which a second 10 mm. and two 5 mm. ports were placed.

Laparoscopy was performed in the usual fashion and except for a large amount of adhesions to the gallbladder, no pathology was identified. Using sharp and blunt dissection, an attempt was made to free the adhesions from the gallbladder. The patient's colon was stuck in this area and in spite of an extensive attempt it was felt unsafe to proceed any further trying to separate the colon from the gallbladder. It was therefore elected to do the procedure open. A standard subhepatic incision was accomplished, carried down through subcutaneous tissue. The anterior rectus fascia was divided with a knife, the rectus muscle with a Bovie. The posterior sheath and peritoneum were divided with a knife and the peritoneal cavity entered. Exploration of the peritoneal cavity was normal. The adhesions to the gallbladder were all carefully taken down after which cystic duct was identified. A clip was placed on its junction with the gallbladder and operative cholangiography performed in the usual fashion and read by the radiologist and myself as being normal. The gallbladder was then taken down in retrograde fashion. Hemostasis was obtained with a Bovie. The cystic artery was clipped twice proximally and once distally and then divided. The gallbladder was then excised. A 10 mm. Jackson-Pratt drain was placed. The wound was irrigated with antibiotic solution. Hemostasis was checked and found to be satisfactory after which the posterior sheath and peritoneum were approximated with continuous #1 Vicryl. The anterior sheath was approximated with continuous #1 Vicryl. The wound was irrigated with antibiotics, injected with Marcaine after which the skin was approximated with staples. Sterile dressings were applied. The patient was allowed to wake up, was extubated and taken to recovery where he arrived in satisfactory condition.

continued

Case 8-4, *continued*

PATHOLOGY REPORT

OPERATION: CHOLECYSTECTOMY

GROSS: Submitted is a gallbladder with a slightly thickened wall. The specimen has been opened prior to submission into Pathology. Contained within the lumen is an ovoid, yellowish-green stone measuring 2.2 cm. in greatest dimension. There is cholesterolosis present over the mucosal surface. The mucosa is otherwise greenish-yellow and velvety. Representative portions of the wall and cystic duct are submitted for examination.

MICRO: Sections through the gallbladder reveal multiple areas of mucosal erosion. There are scattered lymphocytes and plasma cells present within the submucosa and extending into the wall. There is mild serosal thickening and edema as well as mild thickening of the muscularis.

IMPRESSION: Chronic cholecystitis and cholelithiasis.

INTRAOPERATIVE CHOLANGIOGRAM

There is a filling of the biliary tree. There is spillage of the contrast into the duodenum. No filling defects are noted. No obstructive changes.

IMPRESSION

Negative intra-operative cholangiogram

ICD-9-CM/ICD-10-CM diagnosis code(s): _____

ICD-9-CM procedure and ICD-10-PCS procedure code(s): _____

MS-DRG: _____

Case 8-5

<u>**Health Record Face Sheet**</u>

Western Regional
Medical Center

<u>**Record Number:**</u>   05-77-06

<u>**Age:**</u>   74

<u>**Gender:**</u>   Female

<u>**Length of Stay:**</u>   8 Days

<u>**Diagnosis/Procedure:**</u>   Elective Hip Replacement

<u>**Service Type:**</u>   Inpatient Surgical

<u>**Discharge Status:**</u>   To Home

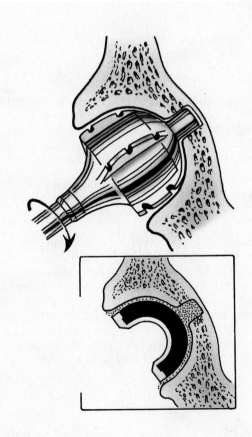

Hip replacement.
Source: © Dorling Kindersley

continued

DISCHARGE SUMMARY

DATE OF ADMISSION: 8/18/xx
DATE OF DISCHARGE: 8/25/xx

DIAGNOSIS:

1. Advanced severe degenerative arthritis left hip.
2. Postoperative complete 3rd-degree heart block.
3. Mild pre and postoperative anemia secondary to preoperative autologous blood donation and postoperative blood loss.
4. History of aclasia with esophagitis.

OPERATIONS & DIAGNOSTIC PROCEDURES PERFORMED:

1. Left cemented total hip replacement utilizing PCA cemented acetabular replacement 29mm external diameter and 54mm external diameter cemented acetabular replacement 15° poly ethylene acetabular insert.
2. #2 sized proximal femoral replacement with standard femoral neck length, 32 mm external diameter femoral head.
3. Administration of postoperative Sulcatrans postoperative auto transfusion × 2 administrations.
4. Administration 2 units preoperative autologous blood transfusion.

SURGEONS: Dr. Redi and Dr. Mayer
ANESTHESIA: Spinal isobaric.

LABORATORY DATA: Is attached on chart.

Admission WBC 9,600, hemoglobin 10.7, hematocrit 31.2. last hematocrit performed on 8/24/xx 31.3, hemoglobin 10.6, WBC 6700.

Admission T3 130, normal for this laboratory.

Admission UA benign. Specific gravity 1.008, appearance clear. pH 6.0, no protein, bile, bilirubin, or blood noted per high power field. Admission PT 11.5, PTT 23.8. Postoperative routine prothrombin times were performed with prophylactic anticoagulation. On 8/19/xx, PT at 13.3. Baseline room air arterial blood gas 7.45, PC02 36, P02 68, 02 saturation 92. Multiple cultures were taken of the hip at the time of surgery. All were negative.

EKG normal. Mean QRS axis -15°, QRS interval 0.09, QT interval 0.40. Admission chest x-ray stable left ventricular hypertrophy. Otherwise unremarkable. Mediastinum and thoracic cage benign.

HOSPITAL COURSE:

74-year-old female who had mild hypertension and LVH on preoperative chest x-ray, who had no problems with her operative course. Postoperatively as the patient was being turned, the patient developed what appeared to be complete 3rd-degree heart block and she was observed by Dr. Hart. Nothing was given for this. The patient had 2 other episodes for this and was observed in the intensive care unit. This subsequently resolved without evidence of vital signs being abnormal. The patient had no postoperative problems whatsoever thereafter. She was transferred back to the ward, progressively ambulated to a point of independence, prophylactically anticoagulated with subcutaneous Heparin and aspirin containing compounds initially. These were discontinued and switched to oral Coumadin as a prophylactic anticoagulant which we will continue for approximately 3 months.

DISCHARGE MEDICATIONS: Vicodin tabs #60, Darvon N100 #40, Coumadin 5mg as needed for 30 days.

DRAINS: 2 hemovacs removed 48 hours postoperatively after the administration of several units of autologous Sulcatrans postoperative wound drainage and filtered blood.

COMPLICATIONS: Complete heart block postoperatively primarily

Case 8-5, *continued*

HISTORY AND PHYSICAL

DATE OF ADMISSION: 8/18/xx

DATE OF DISCHARGE: 8/25/xx

PRESENT ILLNESS: This is a 74-year-old female who has otherwise been in good health with a history of peptic ulcer disease, versus esophagitis in the past, comes in at this time for elective hip replacement.

She is otherwise in good health with non-significant medical problems. She has not had a heart attack or stroke in the past.

Attached are records. These are detailed and self-explanatory.

Dr. Hart has recently seen the patient in consultation. Her notes should be reviewed.

Attached are records which are self-explanatory.

IMPRESSION:

1. Advanced degenerative arthritis left hip.
2. Otherwise healthy female for age.
3. Status post remote history of hysterectomy.

DISPOSITION: She is admitted for left hip replacement at this time on an elective basis understanding full well the risks, complications, alternative methods of care, the possibility of death, infection, failure of surgery to eliminate her condition. She understands that loosening may occur and she may have to have revision in the future.

---

continued

OPERATIVE REPORT

DATE: 8/20/xx

PREOPERATIVE DIAGNOSIS: Advanced degenerative arthritis left hip.

POSTOPERATIVE DIAGNOSIS: Same.

OPERATION:

1. Left cemented total hip replacement utilizing PCA cemented acetabular replacement 29 millimeter internal diameter and 54 millimeter external diameter, cemented acetabular replacement with #15 degree polyethylene acetabular insert.
2. #2 size proximal femoral replacement with standard femoral neck length, 32 millimeter external diameter femoral head, cemented, femoral component.
3. Administration of Sulcatrans postoperative auto transfusion.

SURGEONS: Dr. Redi and Dr. Mayer

ANESTHESIA: Spinal, isobaric.

PROCEDURE: Supine position, turned to left side up decubitus position, spinal block, Betadine prep, alcohol rinse, prophylactic antibiotics of 1 gram Ancef and 500 mg of Vancomycin and sterile drape. A posterior approach was made to the hip incising the gluteal fibers and splitting them in the direction of their fiber. Posterior capsulectomy performed and the hip dislocated and osteotomized according to our guide. Acetabulum was retracted and visualized. Acetabulum was reamed to accept a 54 millimeter external diameter acetabular cup. Because of osteoporosity, we decided to cement the acetabulum. Four drill holes were placed, two in the ileum, one in the ischium, and one in the pubic bone. Cement was mixed and the acetabular cup was inserted. Cement was allowed to harden. Excess cement was trimmed. The permanent 15-degree polyethylene insert hood was applied. The acetabulum was isolated in the proximal femur approach. Cancellous bone was removed from the proximal femur. A #2 sized femoral broach seemed to be adequate for the femur. Two packs of Methyl Methacrylate cement were mixed. The cement was placed with a cement gun over the top of a distal femoral silastic plug. The proximal femur was then pressurized with the prosthesis, a #2 prosthesis inserted and placed in approximately 20 to 25 degrees of femoral anteversion.

The hip was located, found to be stable and we decided upon a standard neck prosthesis as it appeared to most comfortably parallel the position of the hip. Leg lengths remained normal. The hip was stable and no over-lengthening was sustained. The wound was irrigated thoroughly with Ancef and saline solution, totally approximately 20 liters throughout the procedure. Estimated blood loss 200 cc, replacement of one unit of autologous blood. Two deep Sulcatrans drains were placed in the hip for postoperative auto transfusion. The patient appeared to tolerate the procedure well.

continued

Case 8-5, *continued*

PAGE 2

The hip was closed over two deep Hemovacs, approximating the deep tensor fascia with #1 interrupted absorbable Vicryl, subcutaneous tissue with #2–0 interrupted absorbable Vicryl and the skin with stainless steel skin staples. Sterile clear plastic Opsite dressing was applied. The patient was then turned to her back initially in stable condition, but became quite hypotensive and lost peripheral pulse when she was turned to a supine position. She had been given one unit of autologous blood intraoperatively. It was probably a quick shift in peripheral blood pool. She was observed, pulses came back, no vasal pressors were given and no anti-arrhythmics. Shortly thereafter the pulse resumed and blood pressure was 130 systolic. An abduction brace was placed between the legs and the patient returned to her bed in stable condition, transferred to the recovery room in stable condition without apparent problem.

ESTIMATED BLOOD LOSS: 200 cc.

DRAINS: Two deep Sulcatrans drains.

COMPLICATIONS: Mild transient hypotension with turning of the patient from the decubitus to the supine position.

SPONGE/NEEDLE/INSTRUMENT/PATTY COUNT: Correct at termination of the procedure.

PATHOLOGY REPORT

PATIENT: Patty Perez   AGE: 74

HOS. NO: 05-77-06   DATE: 8/20/xx

DOCTOR: Dr. Redi

OPERATION   LEFT TOTAL HIP
                   DEGENERATIVE ARTHRITIC LEFT HIP

GROSS: Femoral head is asymmetrical. The articular surface is irregularly eroded, roughened, and grey-tan to yellow-brown to yellow-tan. It measures 5.4 × 5.0 × 4.7 cm. Representative sections are processed. Also included are multiple fragments and pieces of grey-tan to red-tan soft tissue, bone, and cartilage. These pieces measure up to 4.0 cm. and when piled together measure 7.0 × 6.0 × 2.0 cm.

MICRO: Cartilaginous tissues are superficially eroded. There is chondrocyte clustering as well as focal fibrous repair reaction. Cortical and trabecular bone have normal lamination and distribution of ostecytes. Intertrabecular spaces contain small patches of marrow with normal appearing myeloid and erythroid activity. Loose body consists of nodular and irregular chondromatous pattern. There is prominent chondrocyte clustering and increased chondrocyte population.

FINDINGS: Severe cartilaginous erosion and degeneration with focal fibrous repair reaction, osseocartilaginous tissues, left total hip procedure.
Osseochondromatous loose body, left hip, with chondroid hyperplasia and degeneration.

continued

Case 8-5, *continued*

RADIOLOGY REPORT

HISTORY: Pre-op hip replacement

CHEST:

Two views of the chest are compared with films about 5 years ago. No significant interval change has taken place. The lungs are free of infiltrates. Heart size is mildly enlarged with a little prominence to the left ventricle. Mediastinum and thoracic cage appear stable and intact.

IMPRESSION:

Stable mild LVH.

ICD-9-CM/ICD-10-CM diagnosis code(s): _____

ICD-9-CM procedure and ICD-10-PCS procedure code(s): _____

MS-DRG: _____

Case 8-6

Health Record Face Sheet

Western Regional
Medical Center

Record Number:	14-63-01
Age:	27
Gender:	Female
Length of Stay:	3 Days
Diagnosis/Procedure:	OB Premature Delivery
Service Type:	Inpatient
Discharge Status:	To Home

Case 8-6, *continued*

DISCHARGE SUMMARY

PATIENT: Polly Pierce

ADMIT DATE: 10/1/xx
DISCH DATE: 10/3/xx

PHYSICIAN: Dr. Johansen

PRINCIPAL DIAGNOSIS: Pregnancy at 36 3/7 completed weeks with moderate pregnancy induced hypertension/preeclampsia. Fourth-degree midline perineal laceration. Nuchal cord x one. Postpartum uterine atony.

PRINCIPAL PROCEDURE: Amniocentesis, documentation of fetal lung maturity. Prostaglandin cervical ripening, pitocin induction of labor, magnesium sulfate therapy.

Patient was discharged to home on the second postpartum day in good condition with well-controlled blood pressure on oral medications. She was given specific instructions on activities of daily living and wound care follow-up. Medications to include Procardia and Motrin and reviewed signs and symptoms of return of preeclampsia.

Patient is a 27-year-old single white A positive gravida 1 with fractionated prenatal care. Her first evaluation at 30 weeks. Mild elevation blood pressure was noted by 36 3/7 weeks, significant elevation with diastolic 98-100 were noted. Amniocentesis was performed which demonstrated fetal lung maturity, patient was admitted, induction begun and magnesium prophylaxis via peripheral vein was started as well as anti-hypertensives. She progressed well through labor and subsequently delivered a vigorous 5 pound 3 ounce female over a fourth-degree midline extension with circum nuchal cord × 1. Fluid was clear. Apgars reassuring. Placenta was delivered intact. Primary uterine apnea ensued. Was treated appropriately with good results. Peritoneal laceration was repaired without difficulty and patient went to recovery in stable condition.

Postpartum course was uncomplicated, she was continued on magnesium sulfate for approximately 24 hours. Diuresed well and was subsequently discharged as listed above. Review of chart shows serum magnesium levels largely within therapeutic range. CBC on admission revealed hematocrit of 38.5. Platelet count 304,000. Chemistry screen showing uric acid of 2.9, Creatinine .5. Liver function studies unremarkable. SLM clearly reassuring at 138.

continued

Case 8-6, *continued*

	GRAVIDA/	G	P	A	L	EDC	WKS. GEST
Patient Name: Polly Pierce	PARITY	1	0	0	0		36 1/2

MARITAL STATUS	**ALLERGIES**	*Chlorapheramine*	☐ DO NOT PUBLSIH
☐ M ☒ S ☐ D ☐ SEP			☐ NO INFORMATION

REASON FOR ADMISSION

☐ 1. ACTIVE LABOR
☐ 2. QUESTIONABLE LABOR
☒ 3. INDUCTION
☐ 4. C. SECTION _____
☐ 5. OBSERVATION

☐ 6. PROM
☐ 7. PREMATURE LABOR
☐ 8. DELIVERED PRIOR TO ADMISSION
☐ 9. BLEEDING
☐ 10. REFERRAL FROM: _____
☐ 11. OTHER _____

LABOR HISTORY
LABOR ONSET: DATE _____ TIME _____
MEMBRANES: ☒ INTACT ☐ QUESTIONABLE
☐ RUPTURED DATE _____ TIME _____
☐ CLEAR ☐ MECONIUM ☐ BLOODY ☐ FOUL
NITRAZINE: ☐ POSITIVE ☐ NEGATIVE

PRENATAL RECORD	☐ REVIEWED ☒ NOT AVAIL ☐ NO PRENATAL CARE	**PRENATAL CLASS**	☐ CURRENT PREGNANCY _____ ☐ PREVIOUS PREGNANCY ☒ NONE	BLOOD TYPE A+	ANTEPARTUM RHOGAM ☐ Y ☒ N ☐ NA
PATIENT REQUESTS	☒ BREAST FEEDING ☐ SHORT STAY	☒ BOTTLE FEEDING ☐ TUBAL LIGATION ☐ OTHER _____		**PLANS FOR ANESTHESIA**	☒ EPIDURAL ☐ NATURAL ☐ OTHER _____

BASELINE ASSESSMENT
BP _150_ | _107_ T _97.3_ P _92_ R _20_ HT _5 1-1/2_ WT _158_ WT GAIN _____ FHR _140-150_
CERVICAL DILATION _1_ EFFACEMENT _____ STATION _____ CONTRACT. FREQ. _Q4_ PRESENTATION _VTX_
REFLEXES/CLONUS _3+/0_ UP TO LAB _Ø_ EDEMA _1+_ ☐ BETA STEP SCREEN DONE (IF ORDERED)

OBSTETRICAL

CURRENT PREGNANCY

☐ NO PROBLEMS
☐ PREMATURE LABOR
☐ MULTIPLE GESTATION
☐ VAGINAL BLEEDING
  ☐ 1ST ☐ 2ND ☐ 3RD TRIMESTER
☐ CERCLAGE
☐ Rh SENSITIZED
☐ OTHER _P/H_

PREVIOUS PREGNANCIES

☐ NO PROBLEMS
☐ PRETERM LABOR *N/A*
☐ PLACENTA PREVIA
☐ PLACENTA ABRUPTION
☐ MALPRESENTATION _____
☐ INCOMPETENT CERVIX
☐ Hx INFERTILITY
☐ Hx PP HEMORRHAGE
  ☐ BLOOD REPLACEMENT
☐ Hx TERM INFANT <5#
☐ Hx INFANT >9#
☐ Hx STILLBIRTH >20 WEEKS
☐ Hx INFANT CONGENTAL ANOMALIES

_____
☐ >12 MO. FROM LAST DELIVERY
☐ Hx PIH
☐ Hx PREV. C. SECTION
☐ OTHER _____
☐ Hx PREV. C. SECTION
  REASON: _____

SURGICAL HISTORY

Right knee surgery at age 16

MEDICATION DURING PREG.

☒ VITAMINS   ☒ Fe
Proventil _____
_____
_____
_____
_____

INFECTIOUS DISEASES

☒ NO PROBLEMS IDENTIFIED
☐ GROUP B STREP
☐ HEPATITIS B
☐ HIV _____
☐ HERPES _____
☐ STD _____
☐ RECENT ILLNESS _____

CARDIOVASCULAR

☐ NO PROBLEMS IDENTIFIED
☐ HYPERTENSION
  ☐ CHRONIC ☐ ACUTE
☒ ANEMIA *DUE TO PREG*
☐ VARICOSE VEINS
☐ CHEST PAINS
☐ PALPITATIONS
☐ Hx THROMBOPHLEBITIS
☐ Hx HEART DISEASE
☐ OTHER _____

RESPIRATORY

☐ NO PROBLEMS IDENTIFIED
☐ S.O.B.
☐ COUGH
☐ CYANOSIS
☐ SMOKER PK/D _____
☒ ASTHMA
☐ Hx LUNG DISEASE
☐ OTHER _____

SKIN

☒ NO PROBLEMS IDENTIFIED
☐ OTHER _____
_____

GASTROINTESTINAL

☐ NO PROBLEMS IDENTIFIED
LAST B.M. _____
LAST SOLIDS
LAST FLUIDS
☒ HEARTBURN
☒ NAUSEA
☐ VOMITING
☐ DIARRHEA
☐ CONSTIPATION
☐ HEMORRHOIDS
☐ ABD PAIN OTHER THAN LABOR
☐ ULCERS
☐ OTHER _____
_____
_____

URINARY

☒ NO PROBLEMS IDENTIFIED
☐ PAIN   ☐ PROTEIN
☐ BURNING   ☐ GLUCOSE
☐ UTI   ☐ KETONES
☐ RENAL DISEASE
☐ OTHER _____
_____

MUSCULAR/SKELETAL

☒ NO PROBLEMS IDENTIFIED
☐ ARTHRITIS
☐ OTHER _____

NEUROLOGICAL

☒ ORIENTED
☐ CONFUSED
☐ CONVULSIVE DISORDER
  ☐ ASSOC. WITH PREG.
☐ HEADACHES
☐ VISUAL DISTURBANCE _____
☒ GLASSES FOR DRIVING
☐ CONTACTS IN
☐ HEARING IMPARED
☐ OTHER _____

METABOLIC

☒ NO PROBLEMS IDENTIFIED
☐ DIABETIC
  ☐ GESTATIONAL
  ☐ INSULIN DEPENDENT
☐ THYROID DYSFUNCTION
☐ OTHER _____

PSYCHOSOCIAL

☒ NO PROBLEMS IDENTIFIED
☐ LANG. BARRIER
☐ FAMILY CONFLICT
☐ RELINQUISHING BABY
☐ FINANCIAL CONCERNS
☐ Hx ALCOHOL USE
☐ Hx RECREATIONAL DRUG USE
☐ OTHER
☒ SUPPORT PERS
☐ RELATIONSHIP
☐ REFERALS

Case 8-6, *continued*

MOTHER INTRAPARTUM

WKS. GESTATION _36 3/7_	MONITORING		DATE	TIME	COMPLICATIONS	☐ Elevated Mat. Temp _____
	☒ FSE ☐ IUPC	ONSET OF LABOR		1400		

MEMBRANES RUPTURED

TIME ___2030___

COLOR AT DEL. _clear_

MONITORING:
☒ FSE ☐ IUPC
☐ EXTERNAL
☐ INTERMITTENT

	DATE	TIME
ONSET OF LABOR		1400
COMPLETE DILATION		1010
DELIVERY TIME		1035
PLACENTA TIME		1048

COMPLICATIONS   ☐ Elevated Mat. Temp _____
☐ ABRUPTION   ☐ PREVIA   ☐ PROLAPSE CORD
☐ STILLBORN   ☐ MULTIPLE BIRTHS X _____
☒ OTHER _PIH (pregnancy induced hypertension)_
FHR. _____

2ND STAGE

PRESENTATION: _____ _Vtx_

☒ SPONTANEOUS   ☐ SHOULDER DYSTOCIA   ☐ FORCEPS   ☐ ROTATION

☒ VACUUM EXTRACTION:

EPISIOTOMY: ☐ NONE   ☒ ML   ☐ OTHER _____

LACERATION: ☐ NONE   ☐ PERINEAL: ☐ 1⁰   ☐ 2⁰   ☒ 3⁰   ☐ 4⁰

☐ SULCUS _____NA_____   ☐ CERVICAL _____

☐ OTHER _____

☒ URINARY CATH-TIME _1145 18 French Foley_

ANESTHESIA: ☐ NONE   ☒ LOCAL   ☐ PUDENDAL   ☐ PARACERVICAL   ☐ EPIDURAL

ANESTH: _1% Zxylocaine_

REMARKS: _____

TIME	MEDICATION/DOSE	RT	SITE	NURSE SIG
1048	300 Pit 100ccLR	IV		
1053	Hemabatc 250 mg	IM		
1110	25 mg Phenergan	IV		

TIME	BP	PULSE	RESP	FUNDUS	FLOW
1055	130/92			U/3	heavy
1110	112/88	127	34	U/2	mod

OBSERVATIONS:
18 Fr foley inserted. FF V2
with mod light lochia flow

3RD STAGE

PLACENTA: ☒ SPONTANEOUS   ☐ MANUAL   ☒ INTACT   ☐ FRAGMENTED   ☐ CURRETAGE

ABNORMALITIES OF PLACENTA: _____

☐ EBL >500 cc

REMARKS: _____

TRANSFER TIME: _1150_

(VAGINAL — vertical label)

INFANT

APGARS	1	5
HEART RATE		
Absent 0	1/2	1/4
Below 100 1		
Above 100 2	2	2
RESP EFFORT		
Absent 0		
Slow, Irreg 1	1	
Strong Cry 2		2
REFLEX STIM		
No Response 0		
Grimace 1		
Cough Sneeze 2	2	2
MUSCLE TONE		
Flaccid 0		
Some Flexion 1		
Well Flexed 2	2	2
COLOR		
Pale Blue 0	0	
Body Pink w/		
Blue Extremit. 1		
All Pink 2		1
TOTAL	7	9

SEX: ☐ M ☒ F

BAND# _____

WEIGHT _2353_ GMS

_5_ LBS. _5_ OZ.

LENGTH _45.7_ CM _18_ IN.

☐ VOIDED   ☐ STOOL

RESUSCITATION

SUCTION
☑ Prior deliv. shoulders
☑ Bulb
☐ Delee _____ cc
   Color _____
☑ O₂ _6 l prn mask 15 min_
☐ Bag & Mask

☐ CORDS VISUALIZED
☐ INTUBATION
By _____

☐ ANOMALIES* _____

INFANT INTERIM OBSERVTION

TIME	COLOR	TEMP	RESP	ACTIVITY
1031	blue	36.4	24	good flexion
1045	pink	36.2	84	resting
1055	pink	36.8	80	resting
1110	pink	36.9	72	resting

OBSERVATIONS:
Small female infant with lusty cry. Lots of vernix.
Reactive and alert at 30 min. of life.
Pink skin with dusky extremities. VS stable.

ATTENDING PHYSICIAN EXAM

INFANT

OTHER

HEENT
HEART
CHEST
ABDOMEN
GU
EXTREMITIES
REFLEXES
Physician Sig.

MOTHER

WAS PT MONITORED?   ☑ Yes   ☐ No
FHM PATTERN OBSERVATION:
☐ Late decels   ☑ Early decels   ☑ Variable decels
☐ Bradycardia   ☐ Tachycardia

CORD	TIME	MEDICATION/DOSE	RT	STE

VESSELS: ☑ 3   ☐ 2
☑ NUCHAL CORD _X1_

☐ OTHER _____

☑ CORD BLOOD SENT
☐ CORD pH _____
(IF INDICATED)

Transfer Time to Nursery:
_1115_

DELIVERY RECORD

continued

Case 8-6, *continued*

ICD-9-CM/ICD-10-CM diagnosis code(s): _____

ICD-9-CM procedure and ICD-10-PCS procedure code(s): _____

MS-DRG: _____

Case 8-7

Health Record Face Sheet

Western Regional
Medical Center

Record Number: 10-08-19

Age: 54

Gender: Female

Length of Stay: 3 Days

Service Type: Inpatient Surgical

Discharge Status: To Home

Diagnosis/Procedure: Disc Herniation C-5
                          C-6 Discectomy

Case 8-7, *continued*

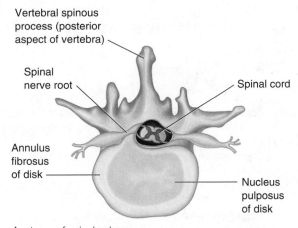

Anatomy of spinal column.
Source: Pearson Education/PH College

continued

DISCHARGE SUMMARY

DATE OF ADMISSION: 9/04/xx
DATE OF DISCHARGE: 9/07/xx

DIAGNOSIS:

1. Degenerative disc disease C5–C6 with degenerative disc bulge and multiple free fragment herniation into vertebral joint eccentrically placed on right with radicular pain right upper extremity.
2. Weakness of biceps and external rotators right arm secondary to #1.
3. Otherwise unremarkably healthy female by history.

OPERATIONS & DIAGNOSTIC PROCEDURES PERFORMED:

1. Anterior cervical microscopic diskectomy C5–C6, removal of degenerated disc into zygapophyseal joint right, decompression of C5 nerve roots bilaterally, greater on right than left, partial neural foraminotomy.
2. Takedown 50% right side posterior longitudinal ligament exploration of epidural space for free fragment, none found.
3. Harvesting right iliac crest bone donor graft.
4. Anterior interbody fusion C5–C6 with Bailey Robinson Keystone technigue with fusion.

SURGEON: Dr. Mayer
ASSISTANT: Dr. Frankos
ANESTHESIA: General by endotracheal intubation.

LABORATORY DATA:

Admission UA - benign, specific gravity 1.013, slightly hazy, pH 7.5, no cells of significance noted per high power field. Admission WBC 5600, hemoglobin 15.5, hematocrit 40.3, platelet count 281,000. Westergren sedimentation rate 4mm per hour. Admission SMAC - glucose 120, BUN 12, slight elevation cholesterol 205, other parameters entirely within normal limits.

Chest x-ray showed mild interstitial fibrosis, otherwise unremarkable.

EKG unremarkable. No evidence of an abnormal record appreciated.

HOSPITAL COURSE:

54-year-old female undergoing the elective procedure because of chronic and persistent neck and radiating right arm pain and weakness of the biceps and external rotators. She has tried a protracted course of conservative measure and underwent the above surgery understanding full well the risks, complications, alternative methods of care, the possibility of infection, failure of surgery to eliminate the condition, etc. Her postoperative course is totally unremarkable and drains were removed on the 2nd postoperative day. The patient was maintained on prophylactic subcutaneous minidose heparin and prophylactic antibiotics throughout her hospitalization.

Immediate resolution of the right arm pain and weakness of the external rotators and biceps was noted postoperatively with amelioration of the pain that brought her into the hospital. No neurologic deficit could be appreciated post surgery.

She is mobilized to a point of reasonable independence and will be discharged in stable condition to return to the office in approximately 2 weeks for x-rays and sutures.

DISCHARGE MEDICATIONS: Tylox.tabs #40, Vicodin tabs #60, Dalmane 30mg #20.

She is to remain in the rigid external mobilization and collar which was adjusted to her fit during the hospitalization. She is not to remove the collar except for dressing change. She is to bathe and shower in the collar.

COMPLICATIONS: None noted.
DISABILITY: Estimated 6 months postoperative.

ADMISSION HISTORY & PHYSICAL

ADMISSION DATE: 9/04/xx

PRESENT ILLNESS: 54-year-old female whose records are attached in the chart and should be reviewed by interested parties. She comes in at this time for operative intervention with an extradural defect C5–C6 consistent with disc herniation extending to the nerve root entrapping the right C5–C6 nerve root. She has significant radicular pain into the right upper extremity and weakness of the biceps and external rotators ipsilaterally on the right side. Attached are records which are otherwise detailed.

PREVIOUS SURGERIES: Tonsillectomy, appendectomy, cholecystectomy and back surgery

PRESENT MEDICATIONS: Darvocet.

ALLERGIES: None.

HEENT: PERRLA, EFROM.
NECK: Supple. Full range of nonpainful motion. No neck masses.
CHEST: Clear to P&A.
CARDIAC EXAM: Unremarkable.
ORTHOPEDIC EXAM: As attached.

IMPRESSION:

1. Eccentric disc herniation C5–C6 by recent cervical myelogram and post myelogram CT scan eccentrically to the right C5–C6 level.
2. Grade 1 1/2 to grade 2 weakness of biceps and external rotators right side consistent with #1.

DISPOSITION: Patient comes in at this time for operative intervention anticipating anterior cervical microscopic discectomy and interbody fusion C5–6. Patient understands the risks, complications, alternative methods of care, the options available to her, the possibility of death, paralysis, failure of surgery to eliminate the condition, the possibility of repeat surgery from behind with a posterior onlay back fusion. I believe she appreciates this and consents to surgery on a timely basis having been given all reasonable informed advice and consents to the operation as outlined.

continued

Case 8-7, *continued*

OPERATIVE NOTE

DATE OF PROCEDURE: 9/05/xx

PREOPERATIVE DIAGNOSIS:

1. Degenerative disc disease with neuroforaminal encroachment or free fragment disk herniation C5-C6 as evidenced by preoperative cervical myelogram and post myelogram CT scan findings.
2. Partial paralysis biceps and external rotators right upper extremity Grade 2 weakness both motor groups.
3. Otherwise unremarkably healthy female for age.

POSTOPERATIVE DIAGNOSIS: Same.

OPERATION PERFORMED:

1. C5-C6 anterior cervical microscopic discectomy and decompression of free fragment disk into uncovertebral joints but no evidence of extra-annular disc migration into neuroforamina.
2. Harvesting right iliac crest donor bone graft.
3. Bailey-Robinson anterior interbody fusion C5-C6 keystone technique.

SURGEON: Dr. Mayer
ASSISTANT: Dr. Frankos
ANESTHESIA: General by endotracheal intubation.

INDICATIONS: 54-year-old female who for the last 6 months has had increasing discomfort and pain in her neck and radiating right arm pain. Attached are records which are detailed and otherwise self-explanatory. She comes in at this time because of persistent pain and disability and now wishes to proceed with operative intervention as outlined and understands the risks, complications and alternative methods of care of death, paralysis, failure of surgery to stabilize or improve the pain. She understands the possibility of non union, the possibility of repeat surgery on down the line with a posterior onlay bone graft as needed if the bone graft does not heal satisfactorily.

To my knowledge I've been very blunt, frank and straightforward with the patient regarding these potential risks, options and alternative methods of care and I believe she and her husband are fully understanding of these and consent to elective operation at this time.

FINDINGS: The posterior longitudinal ligament was taken down from the midline eccentrically to the right of midline so we could see the nerve root and dura. I could identify no evidence of any free fragment disk migration into the extra-annular area although I did see a rent in the posterior longitudinal ligament prior to removing it. We probed in the epidural space and along the nerve root with a blunt nerve hook around the bodies and around the neuroforamina and the exiting nerve root and could find no evidence of any free fragment of disc. Excellent visualization of it was afforded by the magnification.

There were multiple small pieces of disc that had wedged themselves out of the uncovertebral joint and by preoperative X-rays there was a significant degree of uncovertebral degenerative change.

We decompressed this with a curet decompressing the extrinsic compression of the neuroforamina. Multiple free fragments of disc were wedged into the uncovertebral joint perhaps aggravating the condition of recess stenosis. The disc itself was markedly degenerated.

PROCEDURE: Supine position, Betadine prep, alcohol rinse after 5 lb. sandbag placed between the shoulder blades and a 5 lb. sandbag beneath the right iliac crest. A 2" oblique incision was made at mid-neck level and the carotid sheath, and tracheoesophageal interval was dissected and expanded.

Case 8-7, *continued*

OPERATIVE NOTE - PAGE 2

Making Keith needles were placed at C5–6 and C6–7 for appropriate localization. Having localized the point of attack, we made an anterior excision of the longitudinal ligament decompressing a portion of the longus coli muscles. The free fragments of disc were removed and the moderately degenerative disk material was removed without difficulty in a piecemeal fashion with curet and pituitary rongeur. The above findings appreciated. I could not find any evidence of extra-annular free fragment of disc and the problem appeared to be all intra-annular disc bulging into the neuroforamina. There was a significant degree of degenerative disc material which had wedged into the uncovertebral joint. This was decompressed and likewise bone spurs removed from both neuroforamina to widely decompress these areas as preoperative films had revealed significant bony encroachment into the neuroforaminal area.

Bone was taken from the right iliac crest while X-rays were being developed showing appropriate level of surgical approach in the neck. A tri-cortical full-thickness graft was obtained from the hip area in routine fashion. The wound was irrigated thoroughly. Care was taken to avoid injury or penetration of the pelvic contents. The deep fascia was approximated over dry Gelfoam which had been packed into the donor defect site and one single drain had been placed for postoperative hematoma evacuation. The deep fascia approximated with #1 interrupted absorbable Vicryl, subcutaneous tissue with 2-0 interrupted Vicryl and the skin with stainless steel skin staple. Clear plastic Op-Site dressing was placed on the hip wound for postoperative wound observation, and attention then totally returned to the neck area. After appropriate discectomy microscopically under fiberoptic illumination and micro instrumentation, micro curet and micro pituitary grabbers, we took down 50% of the posterior longitudinal ligament midline to the right side exploring for possible free fragment of disc and none was really found as outlined above. The disc was widely decompressed and thoroughly curetted off the end spaces. The neuroforamina were decompressed of the neuroforaminal encroachment and degenerative disc material.

Wounds were irrigated thoroughly with Ancef and saline solution and at termination of this, the disc spaces were thoroughly curetted down to raw bleeding cancellous bone about C5-C6 interval. Bone was fashioned, cut with a micro oscillating saw to be accepted in the interspace and an anterior Bailey-Robinson interbody cervical fusion performed with a keystone appearance of the graft itself. With the neck placed in 50 lbs. of longitudinal traction and hyperextension, we were able to interpose the bone fragment between the bodies and then disconnected the traction allowing the neck to collapse back on this and solid fixation was secured by observation. This wound was irrigated thoroughly throughout the procedure and deep platysma was approximated over a 10 mm. Jackson-Pratt drain with 3-0 inverted absorbable Vicryl. Subcutaneous tissues with a similar suture, and the skin with a subcuticular 4-0 Prolene. Sterile bulky dressing was applied to the neck area and over this a neck orthosis Swanson collar. The patient was awakened, extubated and returned to recovery in stable condition without noted complication.

SPONGE, NEEDLE & INSTRUMENT COUNT: Correct at termination of procedure.

COMPLICATION: None noted.

BLOOD LOSS: Nil.

At termination of procedure the patient was tested in recovery area and found to have full strength returned to the right upper extremity including the biceps which preoperative was down 1.5 to 2 grades and external rotator strength appeared to be normal as well which was down 1.5 to 2 grades noted preoperatively.

continued

PATHOLOGY REPORT

PATIENT: Queenie Qualls   AGE: 54

HOS. NO: 10-08-19   DATE: 9/5/xx

DOCTOR: Dr. Mayer

OPERATION: C5–C6 DISCECTOMY

GROSS: Received in formalin in a container labeled C5-6 disc are multiple fragments of fluffy pink-white fibrous tissue which measures in aggregate 3.2 x 2.8 x 1.3 cm. No necrosis or tumor is seen grossly. Representative sections are submitted in a single carrier.

MICRO: The specimen in section consists of cartilaginous fragments and pieces with marked vacuolization, degeneration, and chondrocyte clustering. All portions are well differentiated.

Severe cartilaginous degeneration, cartilaginous fragments and pieces, C5-C6 discectomy procedure.

Case 8-7, *continued*

RADIOLOGY REPORTS

EXAM: OR Lat. C-Spine

HISTORY: Cervical spine surgery.

OR LATERAL CERVICAL SPINE:

A single film taken in surgery shows needles superimposed over the C5–6 and C6–7 disc spaces.

EXAM: Chest

HISTORY: Pre-op for cervical spine surgery.

CHEST:

The heart and other mediastinal structures are normal. There are no infiltrates or masses. There is some minor interstitial scarring in the lungs. Hemidiaphragms and bony structures are normal.

IMPRESSION:

Mild interstitial fibrosis. Otherwise negative chest.

ICD-9-CM/ICD-10-CM diagnosis code(s): _____

ICD-9-CM procedure and ICD-10-PCS procedure code(s): _____

MS-DRG: _____

Health Record Face Sheet

Western Regional
Medical Center

Record Number:	17-07-88
Age:	80
Gender:	Male
Length of Stay:	3 Days
Service Type:	Inpatient Surgical
Discharge Status:	To Home
Diagnosis/Procedure:	Rotator Cuff Tear with Repair

DISCHARGE SUMMARY

ADMISSION DATE: 3/28/xx

DISCHARGE DATE: 3/30/xx

This 80-year-old white male was admitted relative to his right shoulder. He had incurred a severe and chronic rotator cuff disruption. He was taken to surgery on the day of admission where he was found to have rupturing of the rotator cuff including the subscapularis, supraspinatus and infraspinatus tendons. There was marked fraying of the biceps as well as the adjacent rotator cuff tendon. This was debrided and re-sutured into a groove in the proximal humerus. A distal acromionectomy as well as shoulder decompression including partial acromionectomy and coracoacromial ligament excision was carried out. The bursa was likewise excised as it was quite thickened and inflamed.

Postoperatively he ran a totally benign course and at the time of discharge he was ambulatory in a Velpeau sling. His family has been instructed in passive forward elevation of the shoulder keeping the arm internally rotated to prevent tension on the suture lines. He is not to lift this against gravity himself.

He was given Vicodin to take as necessary for pain and will be seen back in the office in follow-up a week from Thursday.

cc: office

HISTORY & PHYSICAL

ADMISSION DATE: 3/28/xx

PRESENT ILLNESS: This 80-year-old white male is admitted for right rotator cuff repair. The attached office notes should be referred to for present illness.

PAST MEDICAL HISTORY, SOCIAL HISTORY, FAMILY HISTORY & REVIEW OF SYSTEMS: Other than World War II trauma, this man is relatively healthy. He has been a heavy smoker for many years.

PHYSICAL EXAM:

VITAL SIGNS: See admission record.
GENERAL: This is an alert white male, slight hard of hearing. Appears his stated age. In no acute distress.
HEENT: Decreased air conduction bilaterally with mild otosclerosis. Bilateral arcus senilis. Plates upper and lower. Has previously had jaw bone grafting type surgery with asymmetry of the face because of that due to old war injuries.
CHEST: Clear to auscultation and percussion. Slightly hyper-resonant to percussion. There is a lipoma in the mid right thoracic area which is freely moveable posteriorly.
HEART: Regular rate and rhythm, no murmurs.
ABDOMEN: Scaphoid, soft, no organomegaly. Normal bowel sounds. He has a slightly anteriorly curved xiphoid.
GENITALIA & RECTAL: Deferred.
EXTREMITIES: With regard to the right shoulder, see attached notes.
NEUROLOGIC: Oriented x 4. Cranial nerves 2–12 intact. Deep tendon reflexes symmetrical.

IMPRESSION: Right rotator cuff tear.

EXAMINATION: On exam, he had symmetrical elevation to about 165. Internal rotation was to T7. External rotation was about 45 degrees. He maybe lacks about ten degrees less external rotation on the right side than the left. There is crepitance with elevation and rotation. Musculature shows mild fi brillation and he has some wasting of muscles. Glenohumeral joint shows no crepitation. AC joint is prominent with some osteophyte formation.

X-RAY: Standard shoulder films as well as the arthrogram were reviewed. These films are consistent with rotator cuff disruption. The dye extravasates extensively but I think considering the motion that he has this probably represents a vertical tear rather than a distraction type of disruption.

PLAN: At this time the patient is admitted because of increasing pain and disability in the right shoulder for repair of his rotator cuff which has been proven with arthrogram. There appears to be no contraindication to surgery or anesthesia. The operation as well as risks and potential complications have been outlined for the patient. With his age, anesthesia is a consideration and that was discussed as well as infection. He also has been advised that he will probably have to sleep in a semi-upright position for a period of time and go through a fairly vigorous therapy program to avoid stiffening and frozen shoulder complications.

continued

OPERATIVE NOTE

DATE OF PROCEDURE: 3/28/xx

PREOPERATIVE DIAGNOSIS: Rotator cuff tear right shoulder.

POSTOPERATIVE DIAGNOSIS: Severe chronic rotator cuff tear right shoulder with impingement.

PROCEDURE PERFORMED:
1. Mumford distal claviculectomy.
2. Partial acromionectomy and excision of coracoacromial ligament.
3. Chronic rotator cuff repair and reconstruction.

WHAT WAS DONE:

The patient was taken to the operating room and following administration of general anesthesia the patient was placed in a beach chair position and the right shoulder was prepped and draped in the usual sterile fashion. A shoulder strap curvilinear incision extending from immediately posterior to the AC joint to the deltopectoral groove was made, deepened through subcutaneous tissues with reflection of skin flaps at the fascial plain. The anterior 3rd raphe was identified and a deltoid on type approach was made with reflection of the deltoid muscular subperiosteally from the acromion and over the AC joint. Distal dissection on the clavicle was carried out and then after placement of Hohmann retractors using a small micro-oscillating saw the distal half inch of the clavicle was excised without difficulty. There was efflux of joint fluid from the shoulders through the AC joint at this point.

Next, the anterior portion of the acromion was excised along with the coracoacromial ligament which was removed in total. The underlying bursa was markedly thickened and indurated. Approximately 90% of that bursa was removed. The undersurface of the acromion was beveled and shaved in the usual fashion after Neer. This brought into view a massive underlying rotator cuff tear that extended from the subscapularis tendon to the teres minor. This was grossly frayed but could be pulled back down into a relatively good approximated position. All of the frayed and degenerate tissue was excised along with a goodly portion of the frayed tendon around the biceps tendon. A trough was developed in the proximal humerus and then using numerous #1 Ethibond sutures the cuff was gathered, pulled distally and anchored into the trough. It should be noted that the cuff was somewhat attenuated over the area of the supraspinatus but was repairable. The entire area was oversewn using #1 Vicryl suture. The arm could be placed at the side without tearing out of sutures. Once this had been accomplished the area was copiously irrigated. Drains were placed in the depths. The deltoid was approximated in the anterior 3rd raphe using #1 Vicryl and then using #1 Ethibond the proximal fascial portion was reattached to the acromion in a through bone technique. The area over the AC joint was imbricated and sutured using #1 Vicryl. Superficial tissues were irrigated. Sub Q closed with 2–0 Vicryl, skin closed with 3–0 intracuticular stainless steel wire.

Xeroform, 4X4's, and elastoplast were applied for dressing. A Velpeau sling was applied to the arm and the patient was awakened and transferred to recovery in a 45° head up position.

PATHOLOGY REPORT

PATIENT: Norman Newton   AGE: 80

HOS. NO: 17-07-88   DATE: 3/28/xx

DOCTOR: Dr. Yanzat

OPERATION: REPAIR RIGHT ROTATOR CUFF
                  BURSA, DISTAL CLAVICLE, ACROMION

GROSS: Submitted in the course of right rotator cuff repair are multiple fragments of bone and soft tissue which together measure approximately 5.0 cm. Representative portions of the bone are submitted for decalcification and subsequent examination. Representative portions of the soft tissue are submitted for examination.

MICRO: Sections reveal multiple fragments of synovium with marked reactive change. There is thickening of the villi as well as some flattening of the villi together with increased capillary proliferation. Portions of fibrocartilage are present within moderate degenerative change. Additional sections reveal trabecular bone surrounded by fibrocartilage with severe degenerative change. Non-inflammatory reactive synovium is also present. The marrow spaces have been replaced by adipose tissue. Some fibrous proliferation is present with bony repair change.

FINDINGS: Trabecular bone with associated soft tissue, removed in the course of surgery. Reactive, non-inflammatory synovium.
Fibrocartilage with moderate degenerative change, removed in the course of surgery.

continued

Case 8-8, *continued*

ICD-9-CM/ICD-10-CM diagnosis code(s): _____

ICD-9-CM procedure and ICD-10-PCS procedure code(s): _____

MS-DRG: _____

Case 8-9

Health Record Face Sheet

Western Regional
Medical Center

Record Number:	04-22-01
Age:	60
Gender:	Male
Length of Stay:	6 Days
Diagnosis/Procedure:	Cervical Spine Fractures
Spinal Fixation
Service Type:	Inpatient Surgical
Discharge Status:	To Home

DISCHARGE/TRANSFER SUMMARY

DATE OF TRANSFER/ADMISSION ORTHOPEDIC SERVICES: 2/1/xx
DATE OF DISCHARGE/TRANSFER REHAB SERVICES: 2/7/xx

DIAGNOSIS:

1.　Multiple laminar fractures posterior spine.
2.　Fracture posterior spinous process C7, Tl, T2, and T3.
3.　Jump locked impacted facet T2–T3 left.
4.　Fractured facet T3–T4 bilateral.
5.　Fracture posterior lamina C7, Tl, T2, and T3 on right side only.
6.　Neurologically intact individual.
7.　Multiple rib fractures secondary to crush syndrome.
8.　Mild exogenous obesity.

OPERATIONS & DIAGNOSTIC PROCEDURES PERFORMED:

1.　Exploration of cervical thoracic spinal fractures as noted above with anticipation of internal fixation with rods and sublaminar wire fixation which was aborted and local in situ fusion C7–T1, T1–T2, T2–T3, T3–T4, T4–T5 (6 levels).
2.　Harvesting of left iliac posterior autologous bone graft for fusion.

SURGEON: Dr. Redi
CONSULTANTS: None.

LABORATORY DATA:

SMAC 22, glucose 94, BUN 11, slight elevation of alk phos 180, all other parameters normal. Electrolytes 138, sodium and potassium 3.7. Electrolytes remained normal throughout post-operative hospitalization. On 2/2/xx, glucose 161 with IV in place. BUN 17, slight elevation alk phos at 236, sodium 134. Postoperative hematocrit stabilized in the mid low 30 to upper 20 area and on 2/6/xx hematocrit 29, hemoglobin 9.9.

Baseline room air arterial blood gas pH 7.44, PC02 36, P02 131, 02 saturation 95.

The patient was prophylactically anticoagulated and on 9/4/xx, had a protime of 17.5. The patient was given 2 units of homologous blood transfusion postoperatively for a crit that was documented down to 25 on 9/5/xx with a WBC of 10,300.

continued

continued

DISCHARGE SUMMARY

A single x-ray was obtained with hospitalization admission, lateral review localizing the posterior spinous processes for appropriate operative approach.

HOSPITAL COURSE:

60-year-old male who was thrown from a car the last week of January. Initially seen in the county hospital and was then transferred to the valley rehabilitation unit under the care of Dr. Jones and Dr. Keatley. Dr. Mayer was asked to see the patient in consultation along with Dr. Tilley, who felt that the patient had sustained a relatively unstable fracture subluxation of thoracic spine with a 50% compression fracture T4 by X-ray in addition to 50% anterior subluxation T3 on T4 by outside films. Preoperative CT scans were reperformed and compared to those obtained in January. Fractures were not fully visualized on either of the two CT scans and we were quite frankly surprised to see the multiple fractures at the time of the exploration of the thoracic spine at the time of surgery. The multiple fractures and laminar instabilities made intervention with internal fixation virtually impossible with stabilization of the spine with sublaminar technique or hook technique we would have had to hooked into C6 with either sublaminar wire or Harrington hook and we did not feel comfortable doing so. Therefore, we felt that an onlay spinal fusion and the treatment of an external orthosis was best indicated based upon the multiple fractures and fractures of the posterior spinous processes and laminar fractures, facet fractures. The patient did exhibit a fracture impaction subluxation of a T2–T3 facet not appreciated on preoperative CAT scans X 2 and because of this instability we considered taking down the facet and relocating this impacted jump locked facet without fracture but we did not feel comfortable doing so because the patient was neurologically intact and we essentially fused it in situ. The patient's postoperative course was unremarkable. The Medical Brace Shop was employed to manufacture a body shell with SOMI neck extension. The patient was progressively mobilized to a point of comfort and independence and will be transferred back to the rehabilitation unit for progressive rehabilitation and for home disposition and for further anticoagulation by the rehabilitation specialist on Thursday. His orthopedic care was stable and he did quite fine with surgery.

DISABILITY: Estimated 1 year

I will see him back in the office in approximately a month for reassessment. Sutures will be removed on the Rehabilitation Unit in the back and the hip area prior to his discharge.

Prior to his transfer back to the rehabilitation unit he was started on prophylactic anticoagulation. He was initially treated with minidose Heparin, TED stockings, pneumatic boots, and aspirin containing compounds. These were essentially discontinued when prothrombin times were adequate and transfer prothrombin time on 2/6/xx 17.1 seconds after initial loading doses of Coumadin.

RESULT OF TREATMENT: Improved.

COMPLICATIONS: None.

Case 8-9, *continued*

CONSULTATION REPORT

DATE: 2/3/xx

PRESENT ILLNESS: This is a 60-year-old male who apparently was involved in a single-car rollover accident sustaining what appears to be a complicated fracture involving compression fracture of T2 and T3 by recent x-rays.

In addition he appears to have jump locked impacted facets at T2–T3. He neurologically is intact. I was asked by Dr. Brabhoyt to see him in medical consultation, that consultation should be reviewed.

We feel that his lower cervical spine and upper thoracic spine have significant potential for instability and feel that he is best served at this time with a thoracolumbar orthosis and cervical extension. In addition, I would recommend instrumentation or at least spine fusion of his affected areas to minimize further difficulty or neurologic deficit. The patient is a laborer, but is reasonably cognizant. The patient is otherwise in reasonably good health, does smoke 1–1/2 pack a day. He denies any allergies, denies any significant prior injuries as well.

Because of his potential instability, I do recommend strongly that fusion be proceeded with and I have asked Dr. Aury to see him in medical evaluation as well for his neurologic assessment. I can demonstrate no evidence of any neurologic damage or deficit.

By preoperative x-rays it appears that he has a fracture subluxation T3–T4 with 80% compression fracture of T4 with retropulsion of vertebral fragments into the spinal canal by tomogram.

In addition it would appear that he has fractured the left pedicle of T3 and fractured the right lamina of T3 indicating a significant probability of instability.

IMPRESSION:

1. Cervical thoracic spine fractures indicated above with potential potentially unstable T3-T4 with 80% subluxation T3 on T4 without significant neurologic compromise or obvious neurologic deficit.

DISPOSITION: I have discussed with the patient in detail the options and care. I would strongly recommend that this be fused and stabilized. If we can wire the vertebral bodies together, even place Harrington fixation rods, this should be done.

If nothing else, then an external orthosis utilizing a cervical thoracic orthosis should be considered for stabilization. I believe the patient understands the potential instability of his fracture and because of his livelihood as a laborer, he wishes to proceed with operative intervention and stabilization and consents to utilization of an external orthosis for six months or so postoperatively. I have been very blunt, frank and straightforward with the patient indicating to him the options and alternative methods of care and I do believe that he wishes to proceed with operative intervention on an elective basis.

I will ask if Dr. Nicols will assist in surgery and neurologic assessment as well.

The patient consents to this as well.

continued

Case 8-9, *continued*

OPERATIVE NOTE

PRE OPERATIVE DIAGNOSIS:

1. Multiple laminar fractures posterior spine.
2. Fracture posterior spinous process C7, TI, T2, and T3.
3. Jump locked impacted facet T2–T3 left.
4. Fractured facet T3–T4 bilateral.
5. Fracture posterior lamina C7, TI, T2, and T3 on right side only.
6. Neurologically intact individual.
7. Multiple rib fractures secondary to crush syndrome.

POST OPERATIVE DIAGNOSIS: Same

PROCEDURE: 1. Exploration of cervical thoracic spinal fractures as noted above with anticipation of internal fixation with rods and sublaminar wire fixation which was aborted and local in situ fusion C7–T1, T1–T2, T2–T3, T3–T4, T4–T5 (6 levels).
2. Harvesting of left iliac posterior autologous bone graft for fusion.

SURGEON: Dr. Redi

He was mobilized and sent to the Rehabilitation Unit recently for attempted rehabilitation because he found it increasingly difficult to mobilize secondary to his rib and thoracic spine fractures. Because of the concern of potential instability of the thoracic spine, Dr. Neungen was asked to see him in consultation. He recognized the significant potential of instability and I was asked to see the patient on 2/3/xx. My consultation notes should be reviewed.

It appeared that he had, by outside films, a 50% subluxation T3 on T4 with an 80% compression fracture of T4 with a fracture of the left pedicle T3 and a fracture of the right lamina T3.

These appeared to be isolated injuries as best as I could tell to the spine itself. He is brought into surgery for attempted either sub-laminar wiring and rodding and/or Harrington rodding of the thoracic spine for stabilization and rapid mobilization in addition to fusion.

However, when we entered the spine for exploration, the below findings were noted.

Preoperatively the patient was understanding of the risks, complications, technical limitations, the alternative methods of care and the reasons for consideration of stabilization of his spine. We do feel that the spine is potentially significantly unstable and patient really does merit exploration and attempted stabilization to prevent paraplegia. I believe he was understanding of this preoperatively and consented to surgery.

FINDINGS: With exploration of the thoracic spine fracture, very unusual findings were appreciated which essentially prevented the insertion of Harrington rods or sub-laminar wires for Luque type rods. When we explored the spine fracture, we found that the posterior spinous processes from C7, TI, T2, and T3 were all fractured and grossly unstable. In addition, laminar fractures extended down into the base of the transverse processes at all of these levels bilaterally with extension of the laminar fracture into the mid portion of the body of the lamina at C7, TI, T2 and T3 making sub-laminar wiring or even hook fixation virtually impossible. If stabilization were required, we would have had to have hooked under or wired beneath C6 and we did not feel comfortable doing so.

I could not identify any frank subluxation of the spine although there was an impacted jumplocked facet which was not identified on the preoperative CT scans x 2 at the T2–T3 level on the left. This did not appear to be a fracture of the facet but rather simply an impacted jump locked facet. Because the patient was neurologically negative and because no significant instability could be appreciated by this by simply pulling on the fracture, we fused this in situ. We did not feel that significant spinal stability could be achieved by the internal fixation devices as between the spinous processes and the laminar fractures, extensive fusions would have been necessary up into the lower mid cervical spine and to the upper mid thoracic spine. We did not feel comfortable putting internal fixation hardware at these levels, so therefore the spine was fused in situ and we'll go with external fixation im-mobilization to prevent further spinal instability.

PROCEDURE: Supine position, endotracheal intubation, Foley catheter, pneumatic boots. Very carefully turned to a prone posi-tion face down with 3-point tong head supports, Hibbs back frame, pneumatic boots, prophylactic antibiotics 1 gram Ancef and 500 mg Vancomycin.

The neck and back were prepared routinely with shaving and prepping for approximately 25 minutes as the patient could not receive preoperative preparation for skin on the ward.

Dr. Redi approached the back and exposed the spine while Dr. Nicols obtained the bone graft. Dr. Nicols' notes should be reviewed for details.

A curvilinear incision was made about the left iliac crest area going through approximately 3-4 inches of fat and adipose tissue down to the hip area. Bone graft was obtained. The bone was moderately osteoporotic secondary to age and recumbency for 3 weeks.

continued

Case 8-9, *continued*

OPERATIVE NOTE

Cortical cancellous strips were obtained in routine fashion with single-thickness graft available. The wounds were irrigated thoroughly, bone wax applied to the raw bleeding cancellous surfaces after adequate bone graft was obtained and a large piece of dry Gelfoam placed in the donor site area.

This was copiously irrigated throughout the procedure with Ancef and saline solution. Two deep Hemovac drains placed in the left iliac wound. The fascia approximated with #1 absorbable interrupted Vicryl, subcutaneous tissues in multiple layers with 2-0 interrupted Vicryl and the skin with stainless steel skin staples.

Attention was then diverted from the hip wound to the neck area where Dr. Nicols and Dr. Redi approached the upper thoracic and low cervical spine and evaluated the spine for internal fixation.

Our preoperative anticipation and assessment had been to fuse from T1 to T5 or 6 utilizing sub-laminar wires and/or Harrington rods and hooks. However, with evaluation of the spine it became apparent that there was no stable element any lower than C6 to which we could utilize sub-laminar wiring or hook fixation. We could not even wire the posterior spinous processes together as they had all been fractured from C7 to T3.

This was an unexpected finding as it had not been evident on our preoperative X-rays or CT scans taken x 2.

We did note the jump locked facet without fracture at T2-T3 on the left. We evaluated this for possible takedown but because the patient was neurologically intact and dealing with the thoracic spinal canal, I felt that fusion was best indicated in situ because internal fixation could not be obtained if we removed the inferior facet at T3 to reduce the fracture subluxation impaction. Therefore, the spine was cleansed of its posterior fascial attachments. A Cibatome drill was utilized to drill cooling all points with copious irrigation decorticating the posterior elements and an onlay posterior bone graft was performed from C7 to T5 over a 6-level segment.

Bone was tamped securely into position. Two deep Hemovac drains inserted in the subfascial plane. The back fascia approximated with #1 interrupted absorbable Vicryl with the drains free. Subcutaneous tissue was approximated with 2-0 absorbable Vicryl and the skin with stainless steel skin staples. Sterile clear plastic Op-Site dressing was applied to the skin and hip areas. Thoracic brace orthosis with a SOMI attachment was reapplied.

The patient was awakened, extubated and returned to ICU in stable condition with noted complication.

SPONGE, NEEDLE, INSTRUMENT & PADDY COUNT: Correct at termination of procedure.

OPERATIVE TIME: Slightly less than 3 hours.

COMPLICATIONS: None noted.

BLOOD LOSS: Estimated less than 500 cc's between the hip and back areas. No blood replacement was administered. No Solcotrans postoperative auto transfusion was utilized.

ICD-9-CM/ICD-10-CM diagnosis code(s): _____

ICD-9-CM procedure and ICD-10-PCS procedure code(s): _____

MS-DRG: _____

Case 8-10

Health Record Face Sheet

Record Number:	07-13-96	Western Regional Medical Center
Age:	7	
Gender:	Male	
Length of Stay:	8 Days	
Diagnosis/Procedure:	Parietal Lobe Lesion Craniotomy with Excision Biopsy	
Service Type:	Inpatient	
Discharge Status:	To Home	

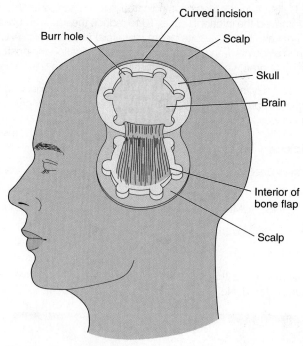

Curved incision

Burr hole

Scalp

Skull

Brain

Interior of bone flap

Scalp

Craniotomy.
Source: Pearson Education/PH College

Case 8-10, *continued*

DISCHARGE SUMMARY

HISTORY: This is a seven-year-old boy who about three years ago had new onset of tonic-clonic seizures. At that time, he was evaluated with an imaging study. The imaging study revealed a lesion over the left occipital region. Because the patient had a closed head injury at that time, it was the thought that this may represent a stroke. However, a follow-up scan revealed enlargement of this lesion. Because of the characteristic findings, it was felt that this represented a tumor rather than a parietal lesion resulting from a trauma. Subsequently, the decision was made to have the patient admitted to undergo stereotactic localization and resection of this lesion.

Past medical history was as above. Allergies were to Tegretol. Medications at the time of admission included Depakote 500 mg q.a.m. and 600 mg q.p.m., Dilantin 50 mg q.a.m. and 100 mg q.p.m.

Family and social history were unremarkable.

PHYSICAL EXAMINATION: The patient was afebrile. His vital signs were stable. In general, he was a well-nourished and hydrated, well-developed male in no acute distress. The patient neurologically showed no evidence of deficit on a detailed examination. There was no visual field cut or difficulty with visual acuity on examination. HEENT evaluation was unremarkable. Neck was supple. Lungs were clear to auscultation bilaterally. Heart was a regular rate and rhythm without murmurs, gallops or rubs. Abdominal examination was unremarkable without masses or hepatosplenomegaly. Extremities were normal.

HOSPITAL COURSE: Upon admission, the patient underwent magnetic resonance imaging scan for stereotactic localization. On 6/1/xx he was taken to the operating room where he underwent a left occipital craniotomy for excision of this lesion. Frozen section obtained intra-operatively showed a possible low-grade astrocytoma versus ganglioma. Pathology report returned as benign astrocytoma, brain, occipital lobe.

Please refer to the patient's operative note for details of the procedure.

The patient tolerated the procedure and was taken to the surgical intensive care unit for further monitoring and management. The patient's stay was uneventful and he did quite well. Subsequently the next day, he was transferred to a regular surgical ward for supportive management. The patient's hospital stay was otherwise uneventful. He gradually began ambulating independently and was tolerating p.o. well. After the results on the decision was made to discharge him to home follow-up on an outpatient basis. Prior to discharge, the patient underwent a computerized tomogram scan of the head for postoperative check and follow-up. Furthermore, a magnetic resonance imaging scan for baseline and follow-up was obtained. The latter scan revealed evidence of some hemorrhage of the tumor resection bed. This had no mass affect or midline shift associated with it. On discharge, the patient was neurologically intact without any focal deficits. His general examination was unremarkable. His surgical wound was healing well without any evidence of infection.

DISPOSITION: Follow-up evaluation was scheduled with Dr. Hollister in clinic in about three weeks. The patient will return as per schedule for removal of his surgical stitches. Discharge medications included Depakote 500 mg q.a.m. and 625 mg q.a.m. Dilantin 50 mg q.a.m. and 100 mg q.p.m. and Tylenol with Codeine 1 p.o. q. 4h to 6 hr p.r.n. The parents were given the diet instructions for the patient as tolerated and his activities were asked to be limited to those the patient could tolerate. Technically, he should stay away from strenuous activities at this time.

DISCHARGE DIAGNOSES:

1. Left occipital tumor.

2. Status post resection.

3. Seizure disorder.

PROCEDURES PERFORMED

1. Magnetic resonance imaging stereotactic localization with resection of a left occipital tumor.

2. Left occipital craniotomy.

3. Magnetic resonance imaging scan of the head.

4. Computerized tomogram scan of the head.

continued

Case 8-10, *continued*

OPERATION REPORT

PREOPERATIVE DIAGNOSIS: Right parietal lesion.

POSTOPERATIVE DIAGNOSIS: Right parietal lesion.

OPERATION PERFORMED: Stereotactic localization of right parietal lesion. Right parietal craniotomy with excisional biopsy of right parietal lesion.

Estimated blood loss: 40 cc.
Drains: None.
Complications: None.

INDICATIONS: The patient is a 7-year-old boy who has had a history of seizures. He has had previous MRIs, which showed a lesion in the right parietal area. It was felt to be a possible area of infarct, or an old area of trauma, but the lesion has increased in size, and is therefore, now felt to be a tumor. Consequently, surgery was planned to excise the lesion.

PROCEDURE: After satisfactory induction of general endotracheal anesthesia, the patient was placed in the prone position, in the BRW frame head holder. The child previously had had an MR for stereotactic localization, and using the coordinates obtained from the markers on the head, the lesion was targeted, and the entry point was obtained. The frame was partially removed. The hair was shaved, and the skin was prepped with Betadine, and the child was draped in the usual sterile fashion.

A linear incision was made in the parietal occipital region, on the right side, and retractors were placed in the skin area. The incision had been made with the stealth Bovie, and, therefore, Raney clips were not necessary. A hole was placed in the bone and the dura was stripped.

Using the Midas-Rex drill, a bone flap was removed. Wire-pass holes were placed in the cranium, and dural tack-up stitches were placed in the dura. The dura was then opened with a #11 blade, and the Mickey Mouse dissector was inserted. The dura was then opened, in a cruciate fashion, using this dissector. The dura was retracted. The stereotactic frame was replaced, and a Becker drain was passed stereotactically into the lesion and cut off at the level of the cortex. The frame was then artificially removed, again.

The microscope was brought into the field, and using microdissection, we followed the catheter down to the level of the lesion. The tissue appeared rubbery and grayish and was definitely abormal. This was biopsied, and the frozen sections returned as low grade astrocytoma versus ganglioglioma.

We took further sections for permanent pathology. We then proceeded to take out the lesion, and again, took another a bit further into the lesion. This was, again, returned with the diagnosis. We then sent more permanent sections from this area, frozen section same.

Using the bipolar electrocautery and suction, we continued to take out the tumor tissue, until normal tissue was encountered in all areas. Once we felt we had a good margin, and there was no further tumor visualized, the area was cauterized with the bipolar electrocautery, as was necessary, and Gelfoam and cotton balls were placed in the tumor bed and left for five minutes. These were then removed.

The wound was irrigated. Hemostasis was obtained with the bipolar electrocautery. The tumor bed looked quite dry; all the cotton balls and Gelfoam had been removed. Surgicel was placed in the tumor bed to line it. The scope was then removed from the field.

The dura was reapproximated, and closed with 4-0 Vicryl in a running fashion. The bone flap was returned to its normal position, and secured with microplates and screws.

The wound was copiously irrigated. The subcutaneous tissue was then closed with 3-0 Vicryl in a simple, interrupted fashion, and the skit was closed with 3-0 nylon in a running interlocking fashion. A fully perforated Jackson-Pratt drain was placed over the bone, and brought out through a separate stab-wound incision prior to closing the skin.

The child tolerated this procedure well, and was taken to recovery in stable condition.

Case 8-10, *continued*

RADIOLOGY REPORT

ADMIT DIAGNOSIS: **BRAIN TUMOR**

Coronal and sagittal Ti-weighted images were obtained as well as axial T2 images. Coronal and axial Ti-weighted images were obtained following the administration of Gadolinium. Surgical changes with blood are evident in the left posterior parietal area at the site of the patient's previously described tumor. Other than the bone and dural changes, as well as the parenchyma changes, no other abnormalities are noted within the brain, specifically the ventricles are normal. The gray white interface remains normal.

Following the administration of Gadolinium, best appreciated on the coronal images, is evidence of some Gadolinium enhancement around the blood. Small focal areas of enhancement could represent large vessels following the administration of Gadolinium, but in my opinion, may represent residual tumor. However, note should be made that on the patient's prior images, there was no evidence of Gadolinium enhancement of this tumor.

IMPRESSION: **POSTOP REMOVAL OF A LEFT POSTERIOR PARIETAL TUMOR.**

BLOOD IS PRESENT AT THE SURGICAL SITE. THERE DOES APPEAR TO BE SOME ENHANCEMENT AROUND THE BLOOD. THIS COULD REPRESENT LARGE VESSELS OR NOW ENHANCING RESIDUAL TUMOR.

ICD-9-CM/ICD-10-CM diagnosis code(s): _____

ICD-9-CM procedure and ICD-10-PCS procedure code(s): _____

MS-DRG: _____

Case 8-11

Health Record Face Sheet

Record Number:	98-44-12	Western Regional Medical Center
Age:	Newborn	
Gender:	Male	
Length of Stay:	2 Days	
Service Type:	Inpatient	
Discharge Status:	To Home	
Diagnosis/Procedure:	Newborn Male Twin Respiratory Problems at Birth	

continued

Case 8-11, *continued*

APGARS: _2_ & _8_   BIRTH WEIGHT: _4_ LB _13_ OZ   DISCHARGE WEIGHT: _4_ LB _4_ OZ

     _{1 MIN} _{5 MIN}

GESTATIONAL AGE BY DATES: _35_ WKS.   GESTATIONAL AGE BY EXAM: _34-35_ WK

PKU Stamper: **PKU DONE**   CIRCUMCISION: ☐ YES ☒ NO

	NL	PHYSICIAN EXAMINATION ON DISCHARGE
Skin	✔	COMMENTS/IMPRESSIONS:
HEENT	✔	
Chest	✔	*wt (weight) 4# 4oz (up 1/2 oz) VS PE normal A/P 1 premie gaining*
Lungs	✔	*on po Ready for discharge.*
Heart	✔	
Abdomen	✔	
Genitalia	✔	
Anus	✔	
Back	✔	
Extremities	✔	
Hips R L	✔	
Neurological	✔	
Other		

DATE	TIME	CONDITION ON DISCHARGE/INSTRUCTIONS:	BLOOD TYPE-MATERNAL:	INFANT

Circumcision : Note	☐ gomco	☐ plasti bell	☐ mogan
Complications/Infections :		☐ NORMAL NEWBORN	

Case 8-11, *continued*

NEWBORN ASSESSMENT:

HEART 132/min.
- ☑ NORMAL
- ☐ Murmur
- ☐ Capillary refill >3 seconds
- ☐ ....

RESPIRAT. 44/min.
- ☐ NORMAL
- ☐ BS Moist
- ☑ Grunting
- ☑ Nasal Flaring
- ☑ Retracting
- ☐ Breath sounds asymmetrical
- ☐ ....

SKIN
- ☑ NORMAL
- ☐ Peeling
- ☐ Pale
- ☐ Plethoric
- ☐ Meconium stained
- ☐ Central Cyanosis
- ☐ Jaundiced
- ☐ Marked acrocyanosis
- ☐ Birthmarks
- ☐ Mongolian spot(s)

HEAD
- ☑ NORMAL
- ☐ Molding
- ☐ Caput
- ☐ Cephalohematoma
- ☐ Sutures separated
- ☐ Anterior fontanelle large, bulging
- ☐ Posterior fontanelle
- ☐ ....

EYES
- ☑ NORMAL
- ☐ ....

EARS
- ☑ NORMAL
- ☐ Abnormal shape & position
- ☐ Canals not patent
- ☐ ....

NOSE
- ☑ NORMAL
- ☐ Nares not patent
- ☐ ....

MOUTH
- ☑ NORMAL
- ☐ Cleft lip
- ☐ Cleft palate
- ☐ Excessive saliva
- ☐ ....

NECK
- ☑ NORMAL
- ☐ Masses
- ☐ Restricted ROM
- ☐ ....

ABDOMEN
- ☑ NORMAL
- ☐ Enlarged liver
- ☐ Masses
- ☐ Umbihernia
- ☐ Absence of bowel sounds
- ☐ ....

GENITALIA
- ☑ NORMAL BOY
- ☐ NORMAL GIRL
- ☐ Hypospadius
- ☐ Hernia
- ☐ Undesc. tes. R L

ANUS
- ☑ PATENT
- ☐ Imperforate
- ☐ ....

SPINE
- ☑ NORMAL
- ☐ Sacral dimple
- ☐ ....

EXTREMITIES
- ☑ NORMAL
- ☐ Hip Click ☐ R ☐ L
- ☐ Femoral pulses weak or absent
- ☐ Extra digits
- ☐ ....

REFLEXES
- ☐ NORMAL
- ☑ Suck weak or absent
- ☐ Palmar grasp abnormal
- ☐ Plantar grasp abnormal
- ☐ Moro absent
- ☐ Moro asymmetrical

CRY
- ☑ NORMAL
- ☐ High pitched
- ☐ Hoarse
- ☐ Weak

MUSCLE TONE
- ☐ NORMAL
- ☑ Hypotonic
- ☐ Hypertonic

ACTIVITY
- ☑ NORMAL
- ☐ Lethargic
- ☐ Irritable
- ☐ Tremulous

ADDITIONAL FINDINGS
- ☑ NONE
- ☐ Forceps marks
- ☐ Vacuum marks
- ☐ Bruising
- ☐ Arm weakness
- ☐ Laceration
- ☐ Abrasion
- ☐ Facial weakness
- ☐ Fracture................
- ☐ Scalp lead lesion

COMMENTS:

Placed under O2 with mist. O2 at 40%. Oximeter on. Oxy-hood. IV started at 1130 in right foot. 24 gauge cath used. IV at 1000/hr. IMED pump used.

Father present at delivery and remains at bedside.

R.N. ASSESSMENT COMMENTS: *see above comments*

	NL	PHYSICIAN EXAMINATION COMMENTS/IMPRESSIONS:
Skin	✔	
HEENT	✔	
Chest		*retracting grunting Rhonchi RR=60*
Lungs		
Heart	✔	
Abdomen	✔	
Genitalia	✔	
Anus	✔	
Back	✔	
Extremities	✔	
Hips R L	✔	
Neurological	✔	

DATE	TIME	PROGRESS NOTES	BLOOD TYPE-MATERNAL:	INFAENT:
5/23/xx	*0700*	*Twin A from C/S, Apgars 2/8. Respiratory Distress 2-HMI Plar O2. IV fluids See progress notes*		

NEWBORN ASSESSMENT

continued

Case 8-11, *continued*

PROGRESS NOTES

4-13 male 1st of twins (twin B male 5-9) born
by C/Section to 29 year old G-5 P-6 mom, breech
presentation, Apgars 2/8, respiratory bagging for
decreased HR and apnea.

Amniocentesis today showed lung maturity
EGA = 34 weeks (36 weeks by dates). Grunting
and hypotonic in nursery with RR 45-60,
respirating moderaterly mild flaring. Rhonchi
bilaterally. Heart - nl.

Abd-nl. Exn - nl. Genit: testes descended
ENT- WNL RR

WBC - 11.4 Hct 4-.3%
Glucose - 60 (cont)
Stable overnight.

RR - 68 with much less grunting, less retracting.
ABG's on 35% O2: ph 7.39 PCo2: 38 PO2 140 O2
sat 98.9%

CXR read by Dr. Holt as primarily
retained fluid, repeat today.

Plan: Decrease FO2 to maintain O2 sats 95-98%.

CXR much improved, fluid resolving, no signs
of SRDS. Taper off. O2 as tolerated.

ABGs on 50% O2:
ph 7.259 pCo2 46.9
Po2 125.9 O2 sat: 97.94
BE - 6.5
CXR: Hazy increased density
R>L
Imp: Mild IRDS
Plan: IV fluids, monitor O2 sats and ABGs.

RR - 65, still some grunting and retracting.
O2 sat's 97-98% on 35% O2
Plan: Monitor sat's and respiratory effort.
ABGs in a.m.

RR - 60 on 25% O2, beginning to suck well on
D5W and breast milk feeding.

S: Has weaned off o2 overnight.
on Amp 1 gent for R/O sepsis x 48 hr.

O: wt 4# 10 oz
AF, VSS RR 30-49 SAT 97%
PE - normal premie
Lungs - clear no retractions
Abd - positive BS. ftN7 ND
LAS Na 140 BC x negative
A/P: 1. Premie 34-35 week
mild HMD resolved
Will stop Abx tomorrow if culture neg.
po/og feeds will begin weaning IUP

Case 8-11, *continued*

Progress Note

S: No problems

O: wt 4# 9 oz, VSS

PE - normal

LAS - Na 149 cultures negative

A/P: 1. premie 34-35 weeks

Doing well on room air

on increasing po/og feeds

Will stop abx.

Progress Note

S: No problems. Taking 25 cc po over approx 20 min.

No residuals

IV fell out this a.m.

O: wt 4# 4 oz (w/IV out)

VSS, PE - AF flat

sclera white, lungs clear

CV-Res WNL ABd positive BS Soft NTND

No HSM pulses 2 plus Femo

A/P: Premie 34-35 wk. Doing well. Will increase

po feeds as tolerated. Wean to crib.

S: No problems. Taking 30 cc in about 20 min.

O: AF, VSS wt 4# 2 oz

PE - normal

A/P: 1. Premie 34 - 35 weeks. Doing well

taking po feeds. Will try to room in tonight

w/parents. Discharge tomorrow.

S: No problems.

O: AF VSS PE SFML

A/P: 1. Premie po feeding well. Parents to

room in.

continued

Case 8-11, *continued*

PHYSICAN ORDERS

Check residual before each feeding. Feed no more than 2 oz per feeding.

Prefer breastmilk, but may feed Infamil. Notify Dr. if > 10 cc

residual. Guaiac all stools.

1. May change VS to qzh, in a.m. change q4h.

2. continuous oximetry - record q 4h

3. guaiac stool qd or if stool abnormal in appearance.

4. Feeding schedule po/og breast mil or Enfamile w/iron

IVF's D5 1/4 NS w/20 mlg KC

10cc q 3h x 3 feeds	5.8cc/hr
15cc q 3h x3 feeds	4.2cc/hr
20cc q 3h x 3 feeds	2.5cc/hr
25cc q 3h x 3 feeds	0.8cc/hr
30cc q 3h	heplock IVFs

NA in a.m., Bilirubin if eyes yellow

glucose in a.m.

May d/c Ampicillin d/c gentamicin

change feeding schedule

15cc q3h po/og x 3	IVF's 5cc/hr
20cc q3h x 3	IVF's 3.9cc/hr
25cc q3h x 3	IVF's 2.2cc/hr
30cc q 3h	heplock IVFs

Case 8-11, *continued*

1. heplock IVFs d/c IV

2. stop stool guaiac

3. stop residual checks- notify for heavy spitting

4. continous oximetry when sleeping - may come off if held or observed closely.

5. please encourage mom/dad to do feedings.

6. If parents wish to stay may move to room on floor.

7. wean to open crib.

1. d/c oximeter. po Ad 1 B feed minimum 30cc q 3h

2. May move to room with parents - RmIn

3. Need a.m. wt on pt.

Resume oximeter when asleep or unobserved.

RADIOLOGY REPORT

NAME: BABY BOY, TWIN A

AGE: NB
HOSPITAL NO: 98-44-12
DOCTOR: Dr. Moulie

CHEST:

HISTORY: Difficulty breathing.

FINDINGS: A few increased lung markings are present. The lungs are well inflated. The heart and mediastinum are unremarkable. The liver and
bowel gas pattern are normal in appearance. There is mild thickening of the major fissures.

OPINION: Probable mild retained fetal lung fluid. Pneumonia is felt to be un-
likely but cannot be entirely excluded. Otherwise negative.

continued

Case 8-11, *continued*

ICD-9-CM/ICD-10-CM diagnosis code(s): _____

ICD-9-CM procedure and ICD-10-PCS procedure code(s): _____

MS-DRG: _____

Case 8-12

Health Record Face Sheet

Western Regional
Medical Center

Record Number:	73-00-11
Age:	56
Gender:	Male
Length of Stay:	2 Days
Diagnosis/Procedure:	Tibia Fibula Fracture Open Reduction Internal Fixation
Service Type:	Inpatient
Discharge Status:	To Home

Case 8-12, *continued*

DISCHARGE SUMMARY

DATE OF ADMISSION: 5/22/xx

DATE OF DISCHARGE: 5/24/xx

DIAGNOSIS:

1. Closed spiral unstable fractures tibia and fibula, right involving mid and distal one-third junctions right tibia.
2. History of chronic obstructive lung disease in smoker.

OPERATIONS & DIAGNOSTIC PROCEDURES PERFORMED:

1. Open reduction internal fixation right tibia with insertion 9-hole in-bored ASIF medium sized compression plate.
2. Three compartment anterior, lateral, and posterior fasciotomies, right leg.
3. Application short leg cast.

SURGEON: Dr. Tilley

LABORATORY DATA: Glucose 85, BUN low at 6, LDH slightly elevated 196, Cholesterol slightly elevated 235 upper limits of normal at 200; all other parameters entirely within normal limits. Admission Urinalysis, specific gravity 1.004, pH 6.0, 0–1 WBC's, 0–1 RBC's noted per high power field. Admission WBC 18,300, hemoglobin 16.0, hematocrit 43.8, platelet count 359,000, differential unremarkable. Admission chest X-ray, no cardiopulmonary infiltrate noted. EKG was taken but the results are yet to be obtained on this chart.

HOSPITAL COURSE: 56-year-old male admitted for the above injury after being knocked over by his horse at home. Neurovascular was intact. Pulses were intact prior to surgery.

The surgery was carried out without difficulty or incident. Two deep drains were placed, removed at 24 hours. Patient will be progressively mobilized and ambulated by physical therapy to a point of independence and discharged on crutches, non weight bearing, to return to the office in 2 1/2 to 3 weeks for staple removal and cast and dressing change to allow early weight bearing at that point.

DISCHARGE MEDICATIONS: Tylox tabs #30, Vicodin tabs #60, Velosef .5 gr. po qid #8. Prophylactic antibiotics and prophylactic anticoagulation mini dose heparin and aspirin containing compounds were administered postoperatively and patient will also be maintained on 2 aspirin a day postoperatively to minimize the risk of deep venous blood clots or pulmonary embolization.

RESULT OF TREATMENT: Improved.

PROGNOSIS: Reasonably good.

COMPLICATIONS: None noted.

DISABILITY: 3–6 months postoperatively.

continued

Case 8-12, *continued*

CONSULTATION/HISTORY & PHYSICAL

DATE OF ADMISSION: 5/22/xx

PRESENT ILLNESS: This is a 56-year-old male who was on his ranch, apparently a horse backed up and he twisted and torqued on his right tibia, sustaining a spiral displaced slightly angulated fracture of the mid shaft distal one-third junctions, right tibia, in addition to a spiral slightly comminuted fracture of the distal fibula.

He was seen initially by Dr. Halverston in the emergency room, splinted, and comes in at this time for operative intervention.

I've given him the options, risks, alternative methods of care, the various forms of treatment vs. traction immobilization, pins and plaster, external immobilization, long leg cast with manipulation vs. short leg cast with open reduction internal fixation. I've indicated to him that he'll be probably better served by an internal fixation with plate. Because of his oblique spiral fracture rod fixation with segmental screw fixation through the rod is really not a reasonable consideration at this point.

He comes in for operative intervention, understanding full well the risks, complications, alternative methods of care, the possibilities and hazards and risks of infection, paralysis, failure of surgery, infection, alternative means of therapy and his treatment will be required for 3–4 months before reasonable healing can be sustained.

I believe he understands the options, alternative methods of care, and wishes to proceed at this time with operative intervention.

ALLERGIES: None.

PRESENT MEDICATIONS & DRUGS: None.

I think he probably drinks a little bit and he does smoke 1 pack per day.

BP: 118/70.   RESP: 20.   PULSE: 80.   TEMP: 97.8.   WT: 140.   HT: 66".
HEENT: PERLA, EFROM.
NECK: Supple, full range of nonpainful motion. No neck masses.
CHEST: Clear to P&A.
CARDIAC EXAM: Benign.
ORTHOPEDIC EXAM: As attached.

IMPRESSION:

1.   Closed spiral displaced fracture, right tibia with comminuted distal fibular fracture.
2.   Chronic obstructive lung disease and history of heavy smoking.
3.   Otherwise reasonably healthy male in no acute distress with neurovascular intact.

DISPOSITION: Options have been given of care in terms of closed vs. open treatment, long leg vs. short leg cast, weight bearing vs. non weight bearing, external vs. internal fixation. I believe the patient has been reasonably versed on the options available to him. He wishes to consider open reduction internal fixation so as to allow rapid weight bearing and more appropriate rotational control of the fracture site. To my knowledge he understands the risks, complications, alternative methods of care, these options and care, and now wishes to proceed with operative intervention.

cc: Office

Case 8-12, *continued*

EMERGENCY DEPARTMENT VISIT

SUBJECTIVE: This 56-year-old male was brought to the emergency room by his family unable to bear weight on his right leg. The patient was working with a young horse. The horse turned around to kick him and as he attempted to dodge the horse, he felt and heard a loud snap in his right leg. He was unable to bear weight on this leg from this time on. The patient denies any significant medical problems. He is a smoker. He takes no medications regularly. He denies any prior history of problems with his leg. The patient notes he has had several drinks today.

OBJECTIVE: Physical exam reveals a well-developed, well-nourished male. He is alert and oriented and in moderate discomfort. Vital signs are within normal limits. Exam of his right lower extremity reveals a markedly rotated ankle and foot. It is deviated about 60 degrees laterally. He has a good dorsalis pedis pulse. He has normal sensation in his toes and is able to move his toes. The deformity is in the distal tibia. An x-ray was obtained which shows a sharply angulated, somewhat shortened tib-fib fracture of the distal tibia. Additionally, a chest x-ray was obtained which appears within normal limits. Further exam of the patient reveals his lungs are clear. Abdomen is soft.

HEART: Regular sinus rhythm.

ASSESSMENT: Fractured right tib-fib.

PLAN: Consultation was obtained with Dr. Tilley, the orthopedic surgeon on call. The patient will be admitted to his service and prepared for surgical repair. Laboratory studies, including a CBC, SMAC, urinalysis, and an EKG were ordered. They are not available at this time. The patient's right lower extremity was gently distracted and the foot was aligned with the knee. The patient was placed in a posterior long leg splint. He was also given Demerol and Phenergan intravenously for pain. The patient was then admitted to the orthopedic service.

continued

Case 8-12, *continued*

OPERATIVE NOTE

DATE OF PROCEDURE: 5/23/xx

PREOPERATIVE DIAGNOSIS: Closed spiral unstable fracture mid distal one-third fracture right tibia and comminuted spiral unstable fracture distal fibula.

POSTOPERATIVE DIAGNOSIS: Same.

OPERATION PERFORMED:

1. Open reduction internal fixation utilization of medium sized ASIF in-bored compression plate, right tibia, 9-hole with 9-screw fixation through plate and one screw interfragmental compression technique.
2. Anterior and posterior lateral compartment fasciotomy (3-compartment fasciotomy).
3. Application short leg cast.

ANESTHESIA: Spinal isobaric.

INDICATIONS: 56-year-old male who is retired and was on his ranch taking care of the horse, the horse backed up causing him to torque or twist as it bumped him, and he sustained an oblique unstable spiral fracture of the tibia and fibula. He was initially seen and evaluated by Dr. Halverston in the emergency room, placed in a posterior splint, has been evaluated preoperatively and options been given in care in terms of closed vs. open, external vs. internal fixation.

I believe the patient is understanding of these options and alternative forms of care and wishes to proceed at this time with operative intervention.

PROCEDURE: Supine position, Betadine prep, alcohol rinse, elevation, sterile drape, sterile scrub was given for 15 minutes prior to the prep and an additional Betadine prep.

Vancomycin and Ancef were given on a prophylactic intravenous basis prior to inflation of tourniquet.

The leg was elevated, exsanguinated, and tourniquet inflated to 400 mm mercury and kept there for approximately 60 minutes while the above procedure was performed. The fracture site was identified. Anterior, posterior and lateral compartment fasciotomies were performed sharply.

The fracture was identified by subperiosteal dissection and by gentle sharp technique. The fracture was mobilized. It was necessary to dissect a fair portion of the periosteum posterior to allow mobilization of the fracture and reduction. The fracture was reduced anatomically, held in position by a lateral to medial interfragmental compression screw. This maintained rotation so that a plate could be applied. A plate was molded, bent and contoured and torqued to allow coaptation to the medial side of the tibia. Compression technique was utilized and four holes placed distally, five holes proximally. Fixation was satisfactory and good rotational control obtained. A single cortical screw was placed in the most proximal hole in the 9-hole plate. The wounds were irrigated thoroughly with Ancef and saline solution. Two deep Hemovac drains were applied. Subcutaneous tissue was approximated with #1 absorbable Vicryl, and skin with stainless steel skin staple. A sterile bulky Robert-Jones compression dressing with short leg cast was applied.

The patient awakened and returned to recovery in stable condition without noted complication. Pulses were intact at termination of procedure with excellent capillary refill. I should note the pulses were intact prior to inflation of tourniquet as well.

Sponge, needle, and instrument count correct.

BLOOD LOSS: Minimal.

cc: Office

Case 8-12, *continued*

RADIOLOGY REPORT

EXAM: Rt. Ankle to include tib fib

HISTORY: Trauma.

RIGHT LEG:

Views of the right leg in two projections include the knee and ankle joints. There is a spiral fracture of the distal tibial shaft ending about 6 cm above the ankle joint. The distal fracture fragment is laterally positioned about 5 mm but is not displaced, in the lateral projection. There is an associated distal fibular neck fracture which is essentially nondisplaced with the distal fracture fragment moved posteriorly about the width of the cortex. The upper leg appears normal. Ankle joint is preserved. Some mild soft tissue swelling is seen over the fracture area particularly medially.

AP SUPINE CHEST:

The lungs are clear of an active inflammatory process. The heart size is normal. The mediastinum and thoracic cage appear intact.

IMPRESSION:

Chest negative for active disease.

DIAGNOSTIC IMAGING

ICD-9-CM/ICD-10-CM diagnosis code(s): _____

ICD-9-CM procedure and ICD-10-PCS procedure code(s): _____

MS-DRG: _____

Case 8-13

Health Record Face Sheet

Western Regional
Medical Center

Record Number:	44-09-19
Age:	47
Gender:	Male
Length of Stay:	2 Days
Service Type:	Inpatient
Discharge Status:	Direct Admit
Diagnosis/Procedure:	Loose Bodies Knee

DISCHARGE SUMMARY

DATE OF ADMISSION: 11/16/xx
DATE OF DISCHARGE: 11/18/xx

DIAGNOSIS:
1.   Advancing degenerative change lateral compartment right knee secondary to remote history of anterior cruciate lesion, status post anterior cruciate intra-articular repair with extra-articular substitution.
2.   History of lateral meniscectomy with advancing degenerative change lateral femoral condyle and lateral compartment.
3.   Multiple loose bodies symptomatic right knee.
4.   Status post ACL intra-articular repair left knee.

OPERATION PERFORMED:
1.   Examination and manipulation right knee under general anesthesia.
2.   Diagnostic arthroscopy.
3.   Miniarthrotomy and removal of 3 large loose bodies and osteotomy of marginal peripheral osteophytes lateral femoral condyle right knee.

SURGEON: Dr. Mayer
ANESTHESIA: General by endotracheal intubation.

LABORATORY DATA:

Admission UA – specific gravity 1.023, pH 6.0, no cells, protein, bile, bilirubin, or blood noted per high power field. Admission WBC 7400, hemoglobin 16.5, hematocrit 47.3, platelet count 229,000. Sedimentation rate 2 mm per hour. Admission RA test is negative. ANA test negative at 1:40 dilution. Admission SMAC – glucose 146, BUN 17, uric acid 7.4, moderately elevated. Other parameters totally within normal limits.

HOSPITAL COURSE:

47-year-old male undergoing the above procedure without difficulty or incident. Postoperative course expected to be unremarkable. He will be mobilized to a point of independence and discharged as an outpatient to return for drain removal in 24 hours.

RESULT OF TREATMENT: Improved.

PROGNOSIS: Reasonably good by expectation.

COMPLICATIONS: With hospitalization, none appreciated.

DISCHARGE MEDICATIONS: Tylox #40, Vicodin tabs #60, Velosef .5 gram, po qid #12.

HISTORY & PHYSICAL

DATE OF ADMISSION: 11/16/xx

PRESENT ILLNESS:

47-year-old male comes in at this time for arthroscopy examination of the right knee under anesthesia expecting loose body removal.

Attached are records which are detailed and otherwise self-explanatory. He underwent a major intra and extra articular ligamentous repair about 12–13 years ago. Has done well with this up until about the last 3–4 months he has noted some loose bodies catching in the knee joint. His knee joint is stable and he doesn't really have any pain overall. He has advancing degenerative change consistent with his old ACL tear and a loss of lateral meniscus. He comes in at this time for examination under anesthesia, debridement, removal of 1 or 2 loose bodies that are catching in the lateral compartment of his knee secondary to his degenerative change.

ALLERGIES: None.

PRESENT MEDICATIONS: None.

OUTSTANDING PAST MEDICAL HISTORY: Otherwise negative and noncontributory.

VITAL SIGNS: BP 122/80, respirations 16, pulse 60, temp 97, height 6'1", weight 225.
HEENT: PERRLA, EFROM.
NECK: Supple, full range of nonpainful motion. No neck masses.
CHEST: Clear to P&A.
CARDIAC: Benign.
ORTHOPEDIC: As attached.

IMPRESSION:

Internal derangement right knee with loose bodies secondary to advancing degenerative change right knee, status post remote history anterior cruciate ligament repair lateral meniscectomy intra and extra articular repair. The knee is stable to stress but he does have evidence of degenerative change secondary to the old removal of lateral meniscus. I think he understands the options, alternative methods of care and now wishes to proceed with operative intervention for loose body removal.

continued

Case 8-13, *continued*

OPERATIVE NOTE

DATE OF PROCEDURE: 11/16/xx

PREOPERATIVE DIAGNOSIS:

1. Loose bodies right knee secondary to degenerative arthritis advancing, status post ACL tear, intra and extra articular repair with lateral meniscectomy, remote past.
2. Status post contralateral intra-articular ACL repair, stable doing well.
3. Otherwise healthy male for age.

POSTOPERATIVE DIAGNOSIS: Same.

OPERATION PERFORMED:

1. Examination and manipulation right knee under general anesthesia.
2. Diagnostic arthroscopy.
3. Arthrotomy and removal of multiple loose bodies right knee and debridement of hypertrophic peripheral osteophyte lateral femoral condyle by osteotomy right knee.

SURGEON: Dr. Mayer
ANESTHESIA: General by endotracheal intubation.

INDICATIONS:

47-year-old male who approximately 12–13 years ago underwent major ligament repair of his right knee with intra and extra articular repair. Has done well with this. No major pain. The knee has been stable. He has progressive degenerative change of the knee secondary to remote lateral meniscectomy. He comes in at this time for operative intervention because of palpable loose bodies that are catching within the knee joint and can be demonstrated by preoperative x-ray.

He understands the risks, options, and alternative methods of care and wishes to proceed at this time. He understands that he is developing progressive degenerative change of the knee joint.

FINDINGS:

The medial compartment was reasonably well maintained. The medial meniscus was benign. The old ACL tear was reasonably intact after intra-articular repair. There is hypertrophy and overgrowth of the intercondylar notch. The lateral meniscus was surgically absent with secondary degenerative change noted which was fairly extensive, and lateral femoral condyle and lateral tibial plateau loose bodies were found attached. They were not free floating but rather attached to the synovium about the lateral compartment and 3 relatively large loose bodies were removed. It was necessary to open the knee joint through a very mini arthrotomy and do an osteotomy of the peripheral osteophytes of the lateral femoral condyle whose views were overgrown and catching about the extra-articular Macintosh repair. The knee was irrigated thoroughly. No other loose bodies were found and no evidence of any free loose bodies were noted. All three large loose bodies removed were all attached to the synovium.

PROCEDURE:

Supine position, Betadine prep, alcohol rinse, prophylactic 1 gram IV Ancef antibiotic. The above procedure was performed through medial and lateral arthrotomy portals and arthroscopic portals, arthrotomy performed through a 1" lateral miniarthrotomy to remove hypertrophic overgrowth and osteophyte.

The above findings noted with examination of the knee joint. The knee was found to be stable to anterior and posterior stability. No varus or valgus instability. No pivot shift and no Lachman noted. The above procedure performed initially by insertion of arthroscope inferolaterally. The above procedure performed with removal of 3 relatively large loose bodies through the arthroscopic portals.

continued

Case 8-13, *continued*

I did do a miniarthrotomy thereafter because I felt that I could still feel a mobile loose body. In fact, the loose body was hypertrophic scar that was popping, and snapping over the hypertrophic lateral femoral condyle and peripheral marginal osteophytes. These were removed and symptoms were ablated.

I think his main problem was the large loose bodies in the lateral compartment. These were all attached to the synovium and had to be actually cut away from the synovium before they could be removed. They were sent to pathology. Retropatellar articular surface was reasonably well maintained. He had had a previous lateral retinacular release which had salvaged the retropatellar area.

His only major problem is that of advancing degenerative change of the lateral compartment secondary to remote history of lateral meniscectomy. The knee joint was irrigated thoroughly with Ancef and saline solution and likewise similar irrigation after arthrotomy.

The admitting arthrotomy approximated with #1 absorbable Vicryl and skin staples. Medial portal likewise approximated. The incisions were injected with 0.5% Marcaine for postoperative analgesia. A bulky sterile Robert Jones type compression dressing was applied. The patient returned to recovery in stable condition and after extubation.

PATHOLOGY REPORT

OPERATION: RIGHT ARTHROSCOPY
LOOSE BODIES RIGHT KNEE, MENSICUS

GROSS: Submitted from the right knee are fragments of soft tissue together with osseocartilaginous fragments. The specimen in its entirety measures to approximately 4.0 cm. Representative portions of the soft tissue are submitted for examination. Representative portions of the bone are submitted for decalcification and subsequent examination.

MICRO: Sections reveal fragments of fibrocartilage with moderate degenerative change. Non-inflammatory reactive synovium is also present. Additional sections reveal osseocartilaginous loose bodies with degenerative change. Trabecular bone is present with the marrow spaces replaced by adipose tissue.

IMPRESSION: Fibrocartilage (meniscus) with moderate degenerative change. Non-inflammatory synovium, fibrovascular connective and adipose tissue, removed in the course of surgery.

Osseocartilaginous loose bodies.

ICD-9-CM/ICD-10-CM diagnosis code(s): _____

ICD-9-CM procedure and ICD-10-PCS procedure code(s): _____

MS-DRG: _____

Health Record Face Sheet

Western Regional
Medical Center

Record Number:	33-01-19
Age:	53
Gender:	Female
Length of Stay:	4 Days
Service Type:	Inpatient
Discharge Status:	Direct Admit
Diagnosis/Procedure:	LAVH

continued

Case 8-14, *continued*

HISTORY AND PHYSICAL

PT NAME: Quadeara Quadel

ADMIT: 8/12/xx
DISCH: 8/16/xx
ATTN PHYS: Dr. Allafson

HISTORY:

This is a 53-year-old female with a history of heavy irregular menses for the last year. In addition, she has had irregulur Pap smears over the last several years. The patient underwent an endometrial biopsy which showed disordered endometrium and her last Pap smear was a repeat. The patient had a LEEP procedure last year for squamous dysplasia. She now returns with her second abnormal Pap and after discussing the risks, benefits, and alternatives it was felt by the patient that she would like to have a hysterectomy and because of her age also have her ovaries removed.

The plan is to do a laparoscopic assisted vaginal hysterectomy and bilateral salpingo-oophorectomy. The procedure, risks, benefits, and alternatives have been discussed with her and she understands these as well as the usual outcome and recovery.

PAST MEDICAL HISTORY:
No prior serious medical illnesses. She had a laparoscopic cholecystectomy.
ALLERGIES: Prilosec.
MEDICATIONS:
Accupril 20 mg daily for hypertension which was diagnosed 3 years ago.
She is also on Wellbutrin SR 150 mg which she takes only every other day
and Premphase which was started for her disorder in the endometrium.

FAMILY HISTORY:
Father is an 81-year-old with borderline diabetes. The patient's mother died secondary to vulvar cancer at age 89. The family history is otherwise negative. No anesthesia problems known in the family.

SOCIAL HISTORY:
No alcohol, tobacco, or drug use. The patient is a full-time teacher at the fifth-grade level. There is no history of domestic abuse.

REVIEW OF SYSTEMS: Unremarkable.

PHYSICAL EXAMINATION:

HEENT: Unremarkable. Neck: No thyroidmegaly or lymphadenopathy. Chest: Clear bilaterally. Cardiovascular: Regular rate and rhythm with no murmurs. S1, S2 sounds are normal. Breasts: No palpable masses. Abdomen: No palpable organomegaly or masses noted. Pelvic: External genitalia of the vagina and cervix are normal except that she does have loss of the posterior urethrovesical angle and the cervix pulls down slightly. The uterus is anterior and small. Adnexal examination is unremarkable. Rectal: Negative for guaiac. Extremities: Unremarkable. Neurologic: Unremarkable.

DIAGNOSIS: Menometrorrhagia, recurrent cervical dysplasia and stress urinary incontinence.

PLAN: Laparoscopic assisted vaginal hysterectomy and bilateral salpingo-oophorectomy.

continued

Case 8-14, *continued*

DATE	HISTORY	
8/12/xx		

REASON FOR ADMIT OR BRIEF HPI:

53-year-old G4 P4 female who has a history of irregular Paps over the last several years and some irregular menstrual flow for over a year. Patient underwent a recent endometrial biopsy which showed disordered endometrium and her last Pap showed ASCUS. She had a LEEP procedure last year for squamous dysplasia, She now returns with two abnormal Paps. After discussing the risks, benefits, and alternatives, it was felt by the patient that she desired a hysterectomy and due to her age also remove the ovaries. The plan is to do a laparoscopic-assisted vaginal hysterectomy and bilateral salpingo-oophorectomy. The procedure, risks, benefits, and alternatives have been discussed with her and she understands these as well as the usual outcome and recovery.

Significant Lab:_____

PRIOR MEDICAL HISTORY:

Immunizations (Children)

Med: No serious illness or injuries.

Surg: Laparoscopic cholecystectomy in

Allergies: Prilosec.

Transfusions: None.

Medications: Accupril 20 mg daily for hypertension which she has had for three years, Wellbutrin SR 150 mg which she is only taking every other day, and Premphase which she was started on for her disordered endometrium.

SIGNIFICANT FAMILY HISTORY:

Father with borderline diabetes. Father is still alive at age 81. Mother died secondary to vulvar cancer at age 89. Family history is otherwise negative. No anesthesia problems known in the family.

SIGNIFICANT SOCIAL HISTORY:

No tobacco, alcohol, or drug use. The patient is a full-time teacher at the 5th-grade level. There is no history of domestic abuse.

PERTINENT REVIEW OF SYSTEMS:

Cardiovascular: Unremarkable.
Respiratory: Unremarkable.

Hx of Anesthesia or Coagulation Problems:
          Negative.

Neck: No thyromegaly or lymphadenopathy.

Heart / Lungs: Regular rate and rhythm, no murmurs; S-1, S-2 sounds are normal. Lungs are clear bilaterally.

Breast: No palpable masses.

Abdomen: No palpable organomegaly or masses noted.

Genitourinary / Rectal / GYN: External genitalia and vagina appear normal. She does have loss of the posterior urethrovesical angle. Cervix pulls down only slightly. Uterus itself is anterior and small. Adnexal exam is unremarkable. Rectal exam is negative with negative guaiac.

Neurological / Extremities: Unremarkable.

Impression or DIAGNOSIS: Menometrorrhagia, recurrent cervical dysplasia, and stress urinary incontinence.

Planned Procedure: Laparoscopic-Assisted Vaginal Hysterectomy and Bilateral Salpingo-Oophorectomy.

Planned Anesthesia:

SEDATION ☐   As per ANESTHESIA ☑
                    LOCAL ☐

THE PATIENT IS AN APPROPRIATE CANDIDATE TO UNDERGO THE PLANNED PROCEDURE, SEDATION AND ANESTHESIA.
          ☑ Yes   ☐ No
INFORMED CONSENT WAS DISCUSSED WITH THE PATIENT INCLUDING RISKS, BENEFITS, POTENTIAL COMPLICATIONS AND ANY ALTERNATIVE OPTIONS ASSOCIATED WITH THE PLANNED PROCEDURE AND POSSIBLE USE OF BLOOD. ☑

OPERATIVE REPORT

PROCEDURE PERFORMED: Laparoscopic assisted vaginal hysterectomy and bilateral salphingo-oophorectomy.

PREOPERATIVE DIAGNOSIS: Menometrorrhagia and recurrent cervical dysplasia.

POSTOPERATIVE DIAGNOSIS: Menometrorrhagia and recurrent cervical dysplasia.

SURGEON: Dr. Allafson
ASSISTANT: Dr. Smith

DESCRIPTION OF PROCEDURE:
Under adequate general anesthesia the patient was placed in the semi-lithotomy position using Allen stirrups. The patient was prepped and draped in a sterile manner. A speculum was placed in the vagina and a single-toothed tenaculum on the cervix. The cervix was then circumscribed with a knife from 9 o'clock anteriorly around to 3 o'clock and then the bladder dissected with sharp and blunt dissection from the cervix. A sponge was left in place and a Valtchev uterine manipulator inserted. A Foley catheter was then inserted. A periumbilical incision was then made and this was carried to the level of the fascia. The fascia was tied with 2-0 Silk suture and then the fascia divided and the peritoneum easily entered under direct vision. Blunt trocar was then introduced and pneumoperitoneum obtained. No abnormalities were noted in the abdomen except for some minimal adhesions and the pelvis was visualized. The fallopian tubes and ovaries appeared normal. Uterus appeared normal. There were some adhesions between the sigmoid and left adnexa which were lysed. Two additional 5 mm trocar sites were made inferior and lateral to the umbilicus. The Endo-GIA was then placed along the left infundibulopelvic ligament. The staples were then applied and the pedicle divided. Two additional loads used on this side. The same procedure was carried out on the right. Again, ureters appeared normal in caliber and peristalsis during this and the staple line appeared well away from the ureters. The sponge was identified in the anterior cul-de-sac and then the peritoneum divided over the sponge.

A Deaver was then inserted transvaginally into the peritoneal cavity through this incision. Attention was then turned to the vaginal portion of the procedure and the sponge was removed as was the Valtchev uterine manipulator. The uterus was then delivered anteriorly in the Doderlein fashion with Leahey clamps. The remaining pedicles were clamped with curved Heaney clamps, divided and tied with 0 Vicryl suture removing the uterus, cervix, fallopian tubes, and ovaries. There was no bleeding noted from any of the pedicles. The peritoneum was then closed with an 0 Vicryl pursestring suture and the cuff closed with interrupted 0 Vicryl figure-of-eight sutures. There was minimal bleeding throughout the entire procedure. The pelvis was re-inspected with the laparoscope and there was no blood noted in the cul-de-sac or the pelvis. The staple lines were all clear of any blood or clot and no irrigation was required. The lower trocars were removed under direct vision. There was no bleeding from these sites intraoperative and the pneumoperitoneum released and the laparoscopic trocar removed. The incisions were then closed with 2-0 silk suture in the fascia and 4–0 Vicryl in the skin. Sponge count, needle count, and instrument counts correct.

ESTIMATED BLOOD LOSS: Less than 100 cc.

continued

Case 8-14, *continued*

PATHOLOGY REPORT

PATIENT NAME: Quadeara Quadel   Age: 53

MEDICAL RECORD NUMBER: 33-01-19   DATE: 8/12/xx

CLINICAL HISTORY: None provided.

Specimen: LAVH - BSO
        UTERUS, OVARIES

Gross: The specimen is received in formalin in one container labeled "ovaries uterus" and con-sists of an 8.3 x 4.8 x 3.9 cm, 86 gm uterus with contiguous uterine cervix, as well as separate right and left ovaries, each with its corresponding fallopian tube.

Apart from the marks of surgical instrumentation, the uterine serosa and ectocervical mucosa are pink-tan, smooth and reflective. The uterus is dissected into anterior and posterior halves revealing a patent endocervical canal and an endometrial cavity lined by a thin, pink-tan mu-cosa. The cut surfaces of the cervix are unremarkable. The cut surfaces of the uterus show a myometrial thickness of 1.7 cm. No tumors are seen.

One ovary is 2.1 x 1.1 x 1.1 cm and the other, 2.2 x 1.1 x 1.0 cm. Each has a firm, convo-luted, pink-tan cortical surface. The fallopian tube corresponding to the former ovary is 4.0 cm long and 0.4–0.5 cm in diameter. The fallopian tube corresponding to the latter ovary is 3.9 cm long and 0.4–0.6 cm in diameter. Each has a pink-red, mostly smooth and reflective serosa. The fimbria are intact. The cut surfaces of both ovaries and fallopian tubes are unre-markable. Representative sections are submitted. Summary of sections: A = anterior uterus, B = posterior uterus, C = anterior cervix, D = posterior cervix, E-F = ovaries and fallopian tubes.

MICROSCOPIC: Microscopic examination is performed.

DIAGNOSIS: Myometrium with adenomyosis.
            Non secretory endometrium.
            Mild cervicitis and nonatypical squamous metaplasia.
            Uterus, cervix, bilateral fallopian tubes and ovaries removed during procedure.

ICD-9-CM/ICD-10-CM diagnosis code(s): _____

ICD-9-CM procedure and ICD-10-PCS procedure code(s): _____

MS-DRG: _____

Case 8-15

Health Record Face Sheet

Western Regional
Medical Center

Record Number:	28-12-11
Age:	39
Gender:	Female
Length of Stay:	3 days
Service Type:	Inpatient
Discharge Status:	Direct Admit
Diagnosis/Procedure:	Pelvic Relaxation Enterocele TAH Abdominoplasty

---

DISCHARGE SUMMARY

DATE OF ADMISSION: 6/29/xx
DATE OF DISCHARGE: 7/1/xx

DISCHARGE DIAGNOSIS:

Symptomatic pelvic relaxation, intertrigo with abdominal panniculus.

LABORATORY DATA:

WBC 7200, hemoglobin 11.1, hematocrit 32.2. SMAC essentially normal. UA within normal limits.

HOSPITAL COURSE:

The patient underwent an abdominal hysterectomy oophorectomy, and salpingectomy with preservation of the right ovary and salpinx. She also underwent a resection of a large abdominal panniculus and repair of a lax abdominal wall.

Postoperatively she had an uneventful course. Had fever which responded to IPPB. She ambulated early. Drains were removed. On 7/1/xx the wound showed, no compromise at the flaps and she was discharged on Velosef, Ferrous gluconate for a hemoglobin of 10. Benadryl. Phenergan suppositories. To wear an abdominal binder continuously and stay bent over.

She was discharged afebrile to contact both Dr. Lassiter's and Dr. Hugos' office on Monday for an appointment later in the week.

continued

Case 8-15, *continued*

ADMISSION HISTORY & PHYSICAL

ADMISSION DATE: 6/29/xx

PRESENT ILLNESS: This 39-year-old Gravida 0 female presents with a history of pelvic relaxation and the awareness of something causing increased pressure in the upper rectosigmaid causing actual obstruction to the passage of bowel movements. She is able to correct this somewhat with manually removing the stool by pressure in the posterior vagina. After a thorough discussion of the various options and concerns and with the realization on the patient's part that she is not at all interested in childbirth and with the further realization on examination that this represents prolapse of the cervix posteriorly and inferiorly into the rectovaginal septum, that certainly hysterectomy arid correction of what may very well be an enterocele would be in her best interests.

The patient has had significant difficulty with ovarian function and has been doing very well on oral contraceptives recently that the possibility of bilateral salpingo-oophorectomy and the need far subsequent Estrogen replacement therapy were all discussed and well understood by the patient. Her questions and her husband's questions were answered at length and I feel that she does have a good understanding of the risks of the procedure, the typical recovery, the concerns for the ovaries, and I feel does give an informed consent. In addition, since her gastric bypass procedure she has lost weight well and at this time has discussed with Dr. Lassiter the possibility of an abdominoplasty. This has been discussed with him and she does likewise give an informed consent for abdominoplasty and panniculectomy.

PAST HISTORY: She has had episodes of relative hypertension and there is certainly a history of hypertension in her mother and both grandmothers. However, she is on no current medication. She has had gallbladder disease and had a cholecystectomy with her gastric bypass 10 years ago. She has also had intermittent right lower quadrant pain which has been evaluated in the past with colonoscopy and found to probably indicate some functional bowel disorder.

She is allergic to no known medications, neither smokes nor drinks, and has never used drugs.

FAMILY HISTORY: Reveals diabetes in her grandmother and adult-onset diabetes in her father. Her grandfather died of carcinoma of the throat and both of her grandmothers suffered from heart disease.

PHYSICAL EXAMINATION: Reveals a well-developed, well-nourished female in no acute distress.

HEENT EXAM: Clear.
THYROID: Normal.
CHEST: Clear to auscultation.
HEART: Reveals regular rate and rhythm with no murmurs.
ABDOMEN: Soft and benign.
EXTERNAL GENITALIA: Normal. Cervix is central and clear. The uterus is anteflexed and normal size but pushes readily to beyond the spines with valsalva maneuver. The anterior vaginal wall is well supported with no urethral detachment and no evidence of cystocele. There is no rectocele, however, the upper one-third of the posterior vaginal wall does prolapse with voluntary straining and represents an enterocele. The uterus is anteflexed and normal size. The adnexa are clear to palpation.

EXTREMITIES: Clear.

IMPRESSION: Pelvic relaxation with large enterocele as well as large redundant panniculus following weight loss.

PLAN: Total abdominal hysterectomy, possible bilateral salpingo-oophorectomy and abdominoplasty.

Case 8-15, *continued*

OPERATIVE NOTE

DATE OF PROCEDURE: 6/29/xx

PREOPERATIVE DIAGNOSIS: Abdominal panniculus with intertriginous changes.

POSTOPERATIVE DIAGNOSIS: Same.

OPERATIVE PROCEDURE: Abdominoplasty.

SURGEON: Dr. Lassiter

ASSISTANT: Dr. Hugos

INDICATIONS: This 39-year-old female has a significant abdominal panniculus with problems of intertrigo and difficulty with hygiene in this regard. She presents for an abdominal panniculectomy, abdominoplasty in conjunction with a hysterectomy.

OPERATIVE PROCEDURE: After satisfactory induction under general endotracheal anesthesia, mid thigh to mid chest area were prepped and draped in the usual sterile manner. The area of resection was outlined just above the pubic hairline, carried out laterally. The midline was marked, the incision was then made and carried down to the underlying fascia. At this level with the use of the cutting and coagulating current on the Bovie, the abdominal panniculus as a flap was elevated to the level of the umbilicus. At this, level the umbilicus was circumscribed and separately dissected free. At this time after hemostasis was established. Dr. Smith performed the abdominal hysterectomy which will be separately dictated.

After the peritoneum and fascia were closed by Dr. Lassiter further dissection was carried up almost to the level of the xiphoid, carefully dissecting over a previous upper midline incision. Occasional stick-ties of 3-0 Vicryl suture were used in conjunction with coagulation. Due to a laxity of the abdominal wall, a plication of the fascia was performed with #1 Ethibond suture in a figure-of-eight manner. This gave considerable support to the abdominal wall. The patient was then brought into flexion at the hips and the amount of pannus to be removed was determined. Also the positioning of the umbilicus was decided upon.

An incision in a transverse manner over the previous scar was used to replace the umbilicus which was then brought through and sutured with interrupted 4 and 5-0 Prolene suture. After amputation of the pannus which removed 1015 grams from the left side, 1059 grams from the right side, hemostasis again was established and then closure performed with #1, 0 and 2-0 Vicryl suture in the dermal layer and a subcuticular 3-0 Prolene suture for the skin.

Two large Hemovac drains were placed laterally and secured into place with a suture. Steri-Strips were applied. The viability of the flap was good at the termination of the procedure.

Adaptic, dry dressing followed by an Elastoplast support dressing was applied. The patient tolerated the procedure well and was sent to the recovery area in satisfactory condition.

continued

Case 8-15, *continued*

OPERATIVE NOTE

DATE OF PROCEDURE: 6/29/xx

PREOPERATIVE DIAGNOSIS: Pelvic relaxation with large enterocele and large panniculus

POSTOPERATIVE DIAGNOSIS: Pelvic relaxation with large enterocele and large panniculus

PROCEDURE: Hysterectomy with left salpingo-oophorectomy performed by Dr. Smith with Dr. Machado assisting. Panniculectomy performed by Dr. Lassiter with Dr. Hugos assisting.

INSTRUMENT & SPONGE COUNT: Were correct.
ESTIMATED BLOOD LOSS: 600 cc's.

PROCEDURE & FINDINGS: After satisfactory level of general anesthesia was obtained, the patient was prepped and draped supine in the usual manner for abdominal surgery. The panniculectomy incisions were laid out by Dr. Lassiter and per his dictation, the skin incision and skin dissections proceeded.

When the umbilicus had been isolated, the skin was reflected laterally and the abdomen was entered through a midline incision. A self-retaining retractor was placed and the bowel was packed cephalad. The pelvic tissues were evaluated. The ovaries were bilaterally normal. The uterus was anteflexed and a normal size and indeed there was a very deep cul-de-sac. The round ligaments were clamped, divided and suture ligated and the peritoneum incised over the anterior cervix to develop a bladder flap. This bladder flap was dissected sharply. Inferiorly there was much adhesion of the bladder flap to the cervix. The peritoneum was then split exposing the peri-rectal spaces bilaterally. The ureters were palpated and on the left the infundibulopelvic ligament was isolated, clamped and divided. The utero-ovarian ligaments on the right together with the tube were then clamped, divided and suture ligated. The broad ligament tissues were clamped at the level of the internal os, divided and suture ligated.

With intrafascial technique, the cardinal ligaments and uterosacral ligaments were clamped divided and suture ligated and the lateral vaginal angles clamped. The uterus, its attached left adnexa was then removed by transacting the vaginal mucosa and the cervix was removed intact. The vaginal cuff was closed with interrupted figure-of-eights of 0 Vicryl with good hemostasis. Again, the ureters were palpated and found to be quite lateral and inferior to the previous sutures. The uterosacral ligaments were then developed and plicated in the midline posteriorly in its more anatomic position and to close the deep cul-de-sac to prevent further enterocele formation. This was accomplished with good tissue and a very adequate repair was felt to be accomplished.

The peritoneum was then closed over all pedicles, averting them in the retroperitoneal space and hemostasis was again adequate. There was approximately 250 cc's of blood loss to this point. The packs were removed and the upper abdomen was examined as the patient had concerns for a ventral hernia particularly in her left upper abdomen. Careful palpation of the incision as well as the abdominal wall revealed no evidence of fascial defect and no evidence of hernia. The instruments were removed and the peritoneum was closed with continuous 0 Vicryl. Fascia was approximated with continuous 0 Vicryl. The procedure was then returned to Dr. Lassiter to proceed with the panniculectomy as per his dictation.

ICD-9-CM/ICD-10-CM diagnosis code(s): _____

ICD-9-CM procedure and ICD-10-PCS procedure code(s): _____

MS-DRG: _____

Case 8-16

Health Record Face Sheet

Western Regional
Medical Center

Record Number: 55-09-10

Age: 33

Gender: Male

Length of Stay: 2 Days

Diagnosis/Procedure: Urethral Stricture
                             Pulmonary Edema
                             Operative Complication

                             Internal Urethrotomy

Service Type: Inpatient

Discharge Status: To Home

DISCHARGE SUMMARY

ADMISSION DATE: 1/18/xx

DISCHARGE DATE: 1/20/xx

Mr. Quekel was admitted with a diagnosis of gross hematuria. He was taken to the operating room and cystoscoped on 1/18/xx. There he was discovered to have a bulbous urethral stricture. Using the visual urethrotome I opened the stricture. He tolerated the procedure well and was returned to the recovery room. He had some coughing and by the time I saw him in the afternoon he had a lot of coughing.

LABORATORY DATA: Was normal except for an Iron high at 151 and Cholesterol of 245. He continued to cough and I called Dr. Hilum to see him, and he made a diagnosis of trauma to the lungs secondary to pressure at the time of arousal following surgery. His Hematocrit was 48.8 preoperative, 44.5 postoperatively. ACT time 1 minute 45 seconds. Blood gases showed an oxygen saturation of 68. Chest X-ray showed fluffy infiltrates. Chest films gradually showed improvement.

The patient was admitted on 1/18/xx and seen in consultation by Dr. Hilum, who made the diagnosis of noncardiogenic pulmonary edema related to Mueller maneuvers during emergence from anesthesia. Patient responded well to the oxygen and treatments, improved, and was discharged home, to be followed in my office and by Dr. Hilum, as needed.

continued

Case 8-16, *continued*

HISTORY & PHYSICAL

ADMISSION DATE: 1/18/xx

This is a 33-year-old who has a brother who is a physician. He came to see me originally on Monday. In July he had blood in his urine. Last week again he noted blood. No symptoms. General health is good. Medications none. Allergies none. We did a culture which was negative. IVP was obtained which was totally normal. His Urinalysis when I saw him on Monday was totally normal. There was no evidence of any blood whatsoever. We thus discussed gross hematuria and decided to just observe him for a period of time with the normal tests. He called me today. He bled again this morning. He had clots and bright red blood and so it's time to proceed. I will cystoscope him on Monday.

PAST MEDICAL HISTORY, SOCIAL HISTORY, PSYCHIATRIC HISTORY: Otherwise unremarkable.

REVIEW OF SYSTEMS: Otherwise normal.

PHYSICAL EXAMINATION: Well-developed, well-nourished young 33-year-old man with bleeding and no other significant symptomatology.

SKIN & LYMPHATICS: Normal.
HEAD: Normocephalic.
EARS: TM's normal. Hears well in left and right.
EYES: Pupils equal, round and reactive to light and accommodation. Extraocular movement normal.
NOSE, MOUTH & THROAT: Normal.
NECK: Supple.
CHEST: Clear to auscultation.
HEART: Regular sinus rhythm, no murmurs.
ABDOMEN: Soft without masses, organomegaly, tenderness or bruits.
BACK & EXTREMITIES: Normal.
NEUROLOGICAL: Normal.

FINAL IMPRESSION: Gross hematuria. For cysto, possible TUR bladder tumor.

CONSULTATION NOTE

DATE OF CONSULTATION: 1/18/xx

REQUESTING PHYSICIAN: Dr. Eels

HISTORY OF PRESENT ILLNESS: This 33-year-old white male underwent general anesthesia for repair of a urethral stricture earlier today. Patient was noted to have laryngospasm upon emergence from anesthesia. This resolved in a relatively short period of time but patient states that to his recollection within about 15 minutes of waking up he had the onset of cough productive of bloody sputum. During the afternoon the cough has persisted associated with the sensation of a need to hyperventilate. He has also had a sensation of gurgling in his chest. Coughing was made worse by talking. Since sitting up tonight, the sensation of shortness of breath and gurgling in the chest has markedly improved. He has not had any chest discomfort during the day. There is no prior history of pneumonias, chest injuries or hemoptysis.

MEDICATIONS PRIOR TO ADMISSION: None.

DRUG ALLERGIES: None known.

PAST MEDICAL HISTORY: He had tonsillectomy at age 18 and remembers that he was slow to come out of anesthesia at that time, but no other complications.

SOCIAL HISTORY: Patient quit smoking 10 years ago after about two years of an irregular habit. He quit chewing tobacco 3–4 years ago after about 15 years of regular use. He drinks ethanol rarely. He is employed as a wildlife biologist.

FAMILY HISTORY: Father died of emphysema. He had peptic ulcer disease requiring gastrectomy. Mother has low blood pressure. Grandmother has Alzheimer's disease.

REVIEW OF SYSTEMS: Negative for kidney disorders, heart disease, peptic ulcer disease, hepatitis, liver disease, deep venous thrombosis, thyroid disorder, dysphagia or heartburn.

PHYSICAL EXAM:

BP: 124/72. TEMP: 99.6 degrees. PULSE: 96. RESP: 28.
HEENT: Remarkable for thin, bloody fluid in the mouth after coughing.
NECK: Is without adenopathy or thyromegaly.
CHEST: Remarkable for bilateral inspiratory crackles which are more prominent anteriorly than posteriorly.
CARDIOVASCULAR: Regular rate and rhythm without murmur or gallop.
ABDOMEN: Soft without tenderness, masses or hepatosplenomegaly.
EXTREMITIES: Without clubbing, cyanosis or edema.
NEUROLOGIC EXAM: Intact grossly.

Room air arterial blood gases tonight show a pH 7.40, PCO2 37 and PO2 35. Chest X-ray PA and lateral shows diffuse alveolar and interstitial infiltrates with sparing of the lung bases. Serum Chemistries earlier today were within normal limits. CBC today showed a Hematocrit of 49, white count 5.8 and Platelets 231,000.

IMPRESSION: Noncardiogenic pulmonary edema related to Mueller maneuvers performed during emergence from anesthesia.

RECOMMENDATIONS: Supportive care, primarily with oxygen. As he has had intravenous fluids running during the day today, will give him one dose of Lasix to eliminate any volume overload which will accelerate the noncardiogenic capillary leak.

PROGNOSIS: Is felt to be good with most cases getting significant improvement within 48 hours and near complete resolution within about 1 week.

Thank you for allowing me to participate in this gentleman's care.

continued

Case 8-16, *continued*

DATE OF PROCEDURE: 1/18/xx

PREOPERATIVE DIAGNOSIS: Gross hematuria.

POSTOPERATIVE DIAGNOSIS: Bulbous urethral stricture.

PROCEDURE: The patient was placed supine on the operating table and attempt was made to pass the panendoscope. The urethral meatus was a little tight. I opened it and then passed the panendoscope.

Upon entering the bulbous area, there were two areas of stricture which were relatively hard to get through. I then passed a 5 French ureteral catheter through these areas and on into the bladder. Once it was in place I could then insert the visual urethrotome over the 5 French catheter to the area of the strictures and then cut the strictures at 1 o'clock thus opening up the strictured area. From there I passed large verumontanum on into the bladder. The prostate looked okay. The ureteral orifices were identified. The ureteral orifices were widely dilated, patulous and it wouldn't surprise me if they weren't refluxing because they were so large, probably because of the pressure. The bladder was large, the bladder was spacious, the bladder walls were not heavily trabeculated. They were slightly trabeculated. The bladder was examined carefully using the foroblique and right angle lenses without finding any bladder tumors or other abnormalities. The ureteral orifices were observed and no bleeding was found coming from the orifices. At that point in time there was not much bleeding from the urethra. As soon as I removed the cystoscope, he started bleeding profusely so I inserted a #20 French Foley catheter and placed a 4x4 around the tip of the penis and then pulled the balloon inflated to 10 cc's against the prostatic fossa to control the bleeding in the urethra.

FINAL DIAGNOSIS: Bulbous urethra stricture.

PROCEDURE CARRIED OUT: Internal urethrotomy using visual urethrotome.

RADIOLOGY REPORT

EXAM: Chest

DATE: 1/20/xx

HISTORY: Follow-up pulmonary infiltrates.

PA CHEST:

There has been partial clearing of the bilateral fluffy pulmonary infiltrates since the film taken yesterday. Again, this appearance is consistent with pulmonary hemorrhage. No other change is seen.

IMPRESSION:

Some improvement.

EXAM: PA Chest

DATE: 1/19/xx

HISTORY: Hemoptysis following surgery.

CHEST:

There are quite extensive bilateral fluffy infiltrates. The heart and other mediastinal structures are normal. Bony structures are unremarkable.

IMPRESSION:

Bilateral fluffy infiltrates. This combined with the history of hemoptysis would indicate this probably represents pulmonary hemorrhage.

Case 8-16, *continued*

ICD-9-CM/ICD-10-CM diagnosis code(s): _____

ICD-9-CM procedure and ICD-10-PCS procedure code(s): _____

MS-DRG: _____

Case 8-17

Health Record Face Sheet

Western Regional
Medical Center

Record Number:	04-99-06
Age:	46
Gender:	Female
Length of Stay:	1 Day
Diagnosis/Procedure:	Retained Foreign Body— Toothpick
	Removal FB
Service Type:	Inpatient
Discharge Status:	To Home

continued

DISCHARGE SUMMARY

DATE OF ADMISSION: 5/04/xx
DATE OF DISCHARGE: 5/05/xx

DIAGNOSIS:

1. Retained wooden toothpick foreign body with secondary foreign body reaction and low grade infection, right great toe.
2. Otherwise healthy female in no acute distress.

OPERATIONS & DIAGNOSTIC PROCEDURES PERFORMED:

1. Removal of wooden foreign body and exploration of toe through two incisions and removal of granulation tissue and culture and sensitivity of wound.

SURGEON: Dr. Marx
ANESTHESIA: General by mask anesthesia.

LABORATORY DATA: Admission WBC 7100, Hemoglobin 12.9, Hematocrit 38.4, Platelet count 279,000, Segs. 69, Bands. 1, Lymphs. 35, Monos. 3, Eosins. 1.

Admission EKG, normal EKG, mean QRS axis +10 degrees, QRS interval 0.08, QT interval 0.38.

HOSPITAL COURSE: 46-year-old female undergoing the above elective procedure without difficulty or incident. Postoperative course unremarkable. She did require admission overnight to the hospital on a short stay admission because of nausea preventing her from eating or mobilizing immediately postoperatively.

By morning this resolved and she was discharged in stable condition to return to the emergency room for dressing change in 48 hours.

DISCHARGE MEDICATIONS: Darvocet N–100 #40, Tylox tabs. #20, Velosef .5gr po qid #12. Cultures and sensitivities are pending at this time for aerobic and anaerobic and although bacteria may be present not responsive to the Velosef we will give this prophylactically anyway.

Case 8-17, *continued*

HISTORY & PHYSICAL

DATE OF ADMISSION: 5/04/xx

PRESENT ILLNESS: 46-year-female who stepped on a toothpick at home about three months ago. The notes are attached on the record and should be reviewed. Dr. Bernstein has tried on two previous occasions to remove what appears to be a retained wooden toothpick from the right great toe over the last 2 1/2 weeks. She remains with a painful draining sinus area over the plantar lateral aspect of the great toe in addition to a dorsal pointing abscess just distal to the web space involving the great toe itself. It does not appear that the MP joint itself is infected about the great toe. She is otherwise in good health. Attached are records. These are detailed and otherwise self-explanatory.

ALLERGIES: None.
PRESENT MEDICATIONS: Duricef.

PHYSICAL EXAMINATION:
BP: 129/78. RESP: 18. PULSE: 84. She is afebrile.
HEENT: PERLA, EFROM.
NECK: Supple, full range of nonpainful motion. No neck masses.
CHEST: Clear to P&A.
CARDIAC: Unremarkable.
ORTHOPEDIC: As noted.

IMPRESSION:

1. Retained foreign body, suspected broken toothpick, wooden, right great toe with dorsal point abscess.

2. No signs of osteomyelitis at this time or MP joint infection of right great toe.

DISPOSITION: She comes in for incision and drainage under anesthesia and removal of what we suspect to be a retained foreign body although it cannot be visualized directly by X-ray.

She consents to surgery understanding the options and care. She wishes to proceed at this time understanding I cannot guarantee the foreign body will be found. This may represent a low grade infection secondary to the inoculum itself and there is no way of knowing specifically if foreign body is actually retained in the great toe.

continued

OPERATIVE NOTE

DATE OF PROCEDURE: 5/04/xx

PREOPERATIVE DIAGNOSIS: Retained foreign body, wooden toothpick, right great toe since February with chronic running sinus. No signs of osteomyelitis or MP joint infection of right great toe.

POSTOPERATIVE DIAGNOSIS: Same.

OPERATION PERFORMED: Incision and drainage and removal of large 1.5-cm wooden toothpick retained foreign body, right great toe.

SURGEON: Dr. Marx
ANESTHESIA: General mask anesthesia.

PROCEDURE: Supine position, Betadine prep, alcohol rinse, with the tourniquet inflated after foot elevation. No exsanguination was utilized and under 4.5 power loupe magnification and fiberoptic illumination, the plantar aspect sinus drainage tract was opened, the sinus tract explored. Initially we could feel something firm inside the toe but we could not visualize it despite loupe magnification. A second dorsal incision was made in the dorsal pointing abscess. This dorsal pointing area was actually the wooden toothpick that had protruded almost through the skin dorsally.

The toothpick was removed thereafter. It measured 1.4 to 1.5 cm. overall length. Wound was irrigated thoroughly, debrided of its granulation tissue, and packed open with a Betadine saturated Iodoform gauze 1/4".

A sterile bulky compression dressing was applied and the patient awakened and returned to recovery in stable condition after diffuse and copious irrigation without difficulty.

She tolerated the procedure well and no untoward complications appreciated.

Case 8-17, *continued*

PHYSICIAN'S ORDERS & PROGRESS RECORD

DATE	ORDERS	✓	DATE	PROGRESS
5/4/xx	D/C IV oral meds prn Arrange for pt to come into ER at 5 p.m. Monday for dressing change. Elevate foot above chest.		5/4/xx	P.T. Pt. up amb. without crutches. No need for physical therapy. Stable - up with crutches
5/5/xx	D/C home tonight. for am 10 mg IM q 6 h prn N&V		5/5/xx	N&V - unable to go home until clears

continued

Case 8-17, *continued*

PATHOLOGY REPORT

OPERATION:

INCISION AND DRAINAGE
REMOVAL FOREIGN BODY, RIGHT GREAT TOE

GROSS: The specimen is the pointed end of a small stick consistent with a toothpick. The outer surface is discolored blue. The specimen measures 1.7 cm. long and 0.3 cm. in diameter at the broken end.

FINDINGS: Foreign body, right great toe, consistent with portion of toothpick.

ICD-9-CM/ICD-10-CM diagnosis code(s): _____

ICD-9-CM procedure and ICD-10-PCS procedure code(s): _____

MS-DRG: _____

Case 8-18

Health Record Face Sheet

Western Regional
Medical Center

Record Number:	67-08-99
Age:	78
Gender:	Male
Length of Stay:	1 Day
Service Type:	INPT Medical
Discharge Status:	Expired
Diagnosis/Procedure:	Anoxic ischemic encephalopathy Respiratory failure Pneumonia Exacerbation of COPD

Case 8-18, *continued*

DEATH SUMMARY

DATE OF ADMISSION: 9/02/xx

DATE OF DEATH: 9/03/xx

HISTORY OF PRESENT ILLNESS: This 78-year-old Native-American male was received in transfer from County Medical Center and Dr. Joseph for respiratory failure. Patient had been hospitalized there for increasing shortness of breath associated with infiltrates and leukocytosis. He subsequently had what appeared to be a respiratory arrest and upon immediate resuscitation regained spontaneous respirations but was noted to be in severe bronchospasm. He was transferred for further management of same.

PAST MEDICAL HISTORY: Patient was hospitalized in February for congestive heart failure. He's been on chronic home oxygen for COPD but continued to smoke. He had a history of chronic dyspepsia for which he had been on chronic Tagamet. He also had chronic atrial fibrillation. Only prior surgeries were cataract removal. He has a history of peripheral vascular disease for which he had been on Trental for a time and has a history of a chronic right inguinal hernia.

For social history and review of systems and family history, please see History & Physical.

PHYSICAL EXAM: Temperature was 100 degrees rectally. Blood pressure varied from 80 to 120 systolic with a pulse in the 110–120 range. Respirations were 28 before starting the ventilator. Respirations were quite labored and associated with abdominal paradox. HEENT, the pupils were constricted with the right pupil being sluggishly reactive and the left pupil not reactive. The neck was without adenopathy but there was prominent JVD during expiration. The abdomen was soft without tenderness, masses, or hepatosplenomegaly. Bowel sounds were initially not heard but were heard within the next few hours. The extremities had 1+/4+ edema and were cool and mottled. Neuro exam: The patient was completely unresponsive. In response to any stimulus he had diffuse myoclonic jerking in all extremities. The gaze was conjugate. Doll's eye reflexes were absent. All limbs moved with the myoclonic episodes. Deep tendon reflexes were 1+ to 2 bilaterally.

LABORATORY DATA: Blood gases upon patient's arrival with 6 liters running into his endotracheal tube showed a pH of 7.18, P02 76 and PC02 90. Chest X-ray showed patchy infiltrates in the upper and lower lobes with prominent emphysematous changes. Magnesium was 1.9, BUN 26, Creatinine 1.8, Glucose 189, Uric Acid 9.2, GOT was elevated at 92, LDH elevated at 403, Phosphorus elevated at 5.8, Sodium and Chloride mildly depressed at 133 and 90 respectively.

Urinalysis showed 5–10 white cells and greater than 100 red cells. CBC showed a white count of 36.8K with 73 segs., 19 bands. Hematocrit was 41, Platelet count 562,000. PT was 12.4, PTT 36.7.

HOSPITAL COURSE: The patient's wife related to me that the patient had made no express wishes regarding heroic support but that she felt we should go on with ventilatory support and not repeat the cardiac resuscitation if it became necessary. Accordingly he was started on infrequent bronchodilators, intravenous steroids, and continued on his Rocephin after repeat blood cultures, sputum and urine cultures were obtained. He was paralyzed in order to facilitate mechanical ventilation in the presence of severe bronchospasm and started on ventilator therapy. He had one episode of supraventricular tachycardia with a rate approximately 160. Systolic remained 120–140 at that time and attempt at cardioversion with Adenocard up to 12 mg IV was not successful. Dig. Level came back at 1.0 and patient was subsequently given a total of .5 mg intravenous Digoxin as well as a 3 gram Magnesium infusion since his Magnesium was 1.9. The SVT resolved shortly after initiating these maneuvers.

Neurology consultation was obtained and patient was felt to have anoxic/ischemic encephalopathy without evidence of focal or lateralizing lesions, subarachnoid hemorrhage or meningitis. Supportive care was recommended and this was undertaken. The patient continued to have severe bronchospasm despite inhaled bronchodilators and steroids. Sputum cultures did not grow any pathogens as did urine and blood cultures.

Patient was re-evaluated after 72 hours of support as per neurology recommendations and was found to have no significant improvement in his neurologic exam. Dr. Chontel felt that there was a zero chance of meaningful survival. When the family was informed of this assessment, which they had expected, the wife and son instructed me to discontinue ventilator support. This was accomplished after an adequate time period for Norcuron to have worn off. Patient was given 4 mg Morphine IV for comfort and died shortly after cessation of mechanical ventilation at 11 minutes after 10 a.m. on the 24th. No autopsy was requested.

FINAL DIAGNOSES:

1. Anoxic/ischemic encephalopathy.
2. Respiratory failure.
3. Bilateral pneumonia.
4. Exacerbation of chronic obstructive pulmonary disease.
5. History of congestive heart failure.
6. History of peripheral vascular disease.
7. Chronic atrial fibrillation.

continued

HISTORY & PHYSICAL

DATE OF ADMISSION: 9/02/xx

HISTORY OF PRESENT ILLNESS:

This 78-year-old Native-American male comes as a transfer from the County Medical Center in Adams for further therapy of respiratory failure. The patient had been on PO Keflex for productive sputum over the week but was hospitalized yesterday with increasing dyspnea with white count of 21,000. Chest x-ray showed bibasilar infiltrates and the patient was started on Rocephin 1 gram hours. At 1:30 this morning the patient had what appeared to be a respiratory arrest and after suctioning large amounts of purulent sputum upon intubation the patient resumed spontaneous ventilation. However, his ventilation was labored, there was severe bronchospasm and arterial blood gases showed pH 7.36, PO2 56, and PCO2 of 65 on 4 liters through the endotracheal tube. An EKG was obtained and showed no new changes. There have been no prior episodes of respiratory failure but he was hospitalized in April of this year for congestive heart failure. He has a long history of chronic obstructive pulmonary disease and continued to smoke up until the time of admission.

PAST MEDICAL HISTORY:

Congestive heart failure and COPD as in present illness. The patient has been on Tagamet intermittently for many years for dyspepsia. The wife knows of no bleeding from peptic ulcer disease. He has chronic atrial fibrillation for which he has been on Digoxin. He was using home oxygen for his COPD. His functional status was limited to walking level ground and very short distances. However, he was able to drive and maintain a functional existence. Prior surgeries have been cataract surgeries. He is blind in the left eye; wife does not know why. There is a history of peripheral vascular disease.

SOCIAL HISTORY:

The patient has been employed most of his life as a Long-haul truck driver. He has also done welding and rotated as a mechanic. He used Ethanol heavily until his hospitalization for congestive heart failure in April. See History and Physical.

REVIEW OF SYSTEMS:

There is no history of lower tract obstructive symptoms. There is no known history of myocardial infarction or rheumatic fever. There is no history of hepatitis, liver disease, or deep venous thrombosis. He chronically complains of being depressed and irritable.

FAMILY HISTORY:

Father died of prostate carcinoma. Mother died of an accidental shooting at age 81. One brother died of asthma. One sister died of meningitis. Brother has nephrolithiasis.

PHYSICAL EXAM:

Temperature is pending, BP is 120/84, pulse is 110–120, respirations were 28 before starting on the ventilator.

HEENT: The pupils are constricted. The right pupil is sluggishly reactive. The left pupil is not reactive (probably chronic secondary to blindness).

NECK: Without adenopathy. There is prominent JVD during exploration.

CHEST: Basilar rales bilaterally with loud wheezing and prolonged expiration.

ABDOMEN: Soft without masses or hepatosplenomegaly. Bowel sounds are not heard.

EXTREMITIES: 1+/4+ edema and are cool and mottled.

NEUROLOGICAL: Mental status: The patient is not responsive except to exhibited diffuse mild myoclonic jerking in response to nonspecific stimuli. This response is elicited with every stimulus such as performing physical exam. The gaze is conjugate and all limbs move with the myoclonic episodes.

Case 8-18, *continued*

RECTAL: Deferred.

LABORATORY DATA:

Blood Gases upon patient's arrival with 6 liters running into the endotracheal tube showed a pH of 7.18, PO2 76, and PCO2 90. Chest x-ray reveals patchy infiltrates in the upper lobes and lower lobes with prominent emphysematous changes. Labs are pending at this time.

IMPRESSION:

1. Respiratory failure with prominent bronchospasm.
2. Probable anoxic injury secondary to respiratory arrest.
3. Probable bibasilar pneumonia.
4. History of COPD.
5. History of congestive heart failure.
6. History of chronic atrial fibrillation.

PLAN:

Begin ventilator therapy. Will need to paralyze patient and maintain ventilation with his severe bronchospasm and prolonged expiration. Plan to give inhaled bronchodilators frequently as well as steroids to interrupt the bronchospasm. Sputum cultures are reported to be growing the Staph species. We will continue Rocephin at this time and diurese as necessary.

continued

Case 8-18, *continued*

NEUROLOGY CONSULTATION

DATE OF CONSULTATION: 9/2/xx

Inpatient of Dr. Williams in the intensive care unit. Mr. Ramos is a 78-year-old Native-American male of uncertain prognosis who I have been asked to see in neuroloagical consultation in the intensive care unit by Dr. Williams for evaluation of decreased level of consciousness. History is obtained from the patient's charts as well as from Dr. Williams. The patient has a history of congestive heart failure, chronic atrial fib and COPD treated chronically as an outpatient by Dr. Joseph records indicate the patient was not compliant with his treatment including not stopping smoking and not taking his medications as prescribed. She saw him on 8/28/xx for increasing shortness of breath and predicted cough. She felt that he had acute bronchitis. When he did not improve and had progressive symptoms he was admitted to the County Medical Facility yesterday to begin evaluation. At the time of admission his arterial blood gases on 2 liters per minute showed a pH of 7.31, PCO2 67, PO2 69 with temperature of 99.1. Chest x-ray showed bibasilar infiltrates. Therapy was begun with Rocephin, Alupent, Lasix, Lanoxin, Vasotec, and Oxygen. At about 1:30 this morning the nurse heard the patient fall. He was found on the floor without respiration or palpable pulse. He was immediately resuscitated. Suctioning revealed a large amount of purulent material. He returned a pulse with chronic atrial fib and a blood pressure of 120/60. Developed spontaneous respirations and was transferred to the service of Dr. Williams here. He has been on a respirator and has not regained consciousness. He assists the respirator but does not do it in an effective manner. His past medical history is as above. In addition, he has a right inguinal hernia, bilateral hearing loss, history of right tympanic membrane perforation, and history of peripheral vascular disease. Family medical history is said to be unremarkable. The patient is said to be a married and retired mechanic, welder, and truck driver. His medications are noted above. He is said to have an ALLERGY TO PENICILLIN. He is a chronic cigarette user. He also is a chronic heavy alcohol user.

PHYSICAL EXAM:

The patient is an elderly Native-American male lying in the respirator without spontaneous movement. His cervical spine is supple and without evidence of meningismus. Carotid pulses are 1/4 bilaterally and without bruits. There are no cranial bruits. HEAD: Normocephalic. BP 130/74. Monitor shows atrial fib with ventricular rate of 90 to 100. Temp is 100° rectally. He has abrasions over the right knee.

NEUROLOGIC EXAM:

MENTAL STATUS: The patient does not respond to verbal or painful stimulation. There is no spontaneous movement or attempt to verbalize. He does not open his eyes.

CRANIAL NERVES: The patient does not respond to visual stimuli including threatening stimuli or light. The right pupil is eccentric and appears as perhaps it has been operated on. Both pupils are approximately 4mm. Neither react to light. Funduscopic exam shows sharp disc margins with good optic cupping. No spontaneous extraocular motions are present. Doll's eyes maneuvers (occulocephalics) are absent, i.e., abnormal. No corneal reflexes are present. The face is symmetrical. He does not respond to painful stimuli over the face. The gag reflex is absent.

REFLEXES: Deep tendon reflexes are 1 to 2/4 throughout and are symmetrical. Plantar reflexes are plantar extensor (Babinski) bilaterally. There are no abnormal superficial reflexes present.

MOTOR: No spontaneous movement is present. There is no withdrawal, posturing, or movement to painful stimuli. The toe in the upper extremities is flaccid to tone in both lower extremities is slightly spastic.

SENSORY: No response to painful stimuli.

Case 8-18, *continued*

CONSULTATION REPORT CONTINUED

LABORATORY DATA:

Chest x-ray shows infiltrates in both upper lobes and both lower lobes in a patchy manner. Has an emphysematous appearance on the chest x-ray. Admitting arterial blood gases showed a pH of 7.18, PCO2 of 90, PO2 of 76, bicarb of 33, and total CO2 of 36. Most recent arterial blood gases showed a pH of 7.28, PCO2 of 74, PO2 83, bicarb of 35. Magnesium is normal at 1.9. Admitting chem screen shows a nonfasting blood sugar with glucose running in the IV of 189, BUN 26, creatinine 1.8, uric acid 9.2, SGOT 92, LDH 403, albumin of 2.7, phosphorus 5.8, sodium 133. Cholesterol is low at 122. Admitting hemoglobin is 13.6 with slightly macrocytic indices. White blood cell count on admission was 36,800 with 0.6% lymphocytes, 0.3% monocytes, 98.4% neutrophils, 0.7% eosinophils. Platelet count on admission was 562,000. Admitting protime was 12.4 with an APTT of 36.7. Digoxin level was 1.0 and he has subsequently received additional digoxin. Admitting EKG showed multiple atrial tachycardia, unifocal PVC's, and low voltage.

IMPRESSION:

Acute encephalopathy due to anoxic-ischemic encephalopathy. This is probably more anoxic than ischemic in etiology though there is most likely an ischemic component. There is no present evidence of focal or lateralizing lesions, subarachnoid hemorrhage, or meningitis. His prognosis is uncertain at the present time and it is risky to venture a prognosis in anoxic ischemic encephalopathy before 72 hours have passed.

RECOMMENDATIONS:

1. Supportive care as you are doing.
2. Re-evaluate at 72 hours unless the patient develops focal findings or marked change in neurologic status.
3. If there is no improvement after 72 hours, or if he develops new neurological features I would recommend obtaining a noncontrast CT head scan.

Thank you for the opportunity of consulting with you. I would be happy to re-evaluate the patient in the future if you so desire.

continued

Case 8-18, *continued*

ICD-9-CM/ICD-10-CM diagnosis code(s): _____

ICD-9-CM procedure and ICD-10-PCS procedure code(s): _____

MS-DRG: _____

Case 8-19

Health Record Face Sheet

Western Regional
Medical Center

Record Number: 87-09-98

Age: 7 months

Gender: Male

Length of Stay: 6 days

Diagnosis/Procedure: Ventricular Shunt Malfunction
with Repair

Service Type: Inpatient Surgical

Discharge Status: To Home

Case 8-19, *continued*

DISCHARGE SUMMARY

HISTORY: This seven-month-old boy was well known to the Neuro Surgery Service with a history of post hemorrhagic hydrocephalus. The patient was diagnosed with this following premature birth. He was status post placement of ventriculoperitoneal shunt on separate occasions. He had had multiple shunt revisions secondary to malfunction and/or infection in the past. The patient was discharged recently from the hospital following fourth ventricular cyst fenestration and communication with other ventricles and discharged in stable condition. On the morning of admission, the parents noted progressive irritability, lethargy as well as decrease in his p.o. intake. The patient also had nausea and vomiting. Subsequently, they noted worsening of his disconjugate gaze and subsequently brought the patient for further evaluation.

Past medical history was as per history of present illness. The patient also had a history of seizures. Medications included Phenobarbital 30 mg b.i.d. Allergies were none.

PHYSICAL EXAMINATION: Temperature was 36.8; pulse 140; respiration 24; blood pressure 125/81; weight approximately 5 kg. On general evaluation, the patient appeared somewhat irritable but easily consoled. His neurological examination revealed a disconjugate gaze with anisocoria. The left pupil was 6, right three and both briskly reactive to light. He seemed to have difficulty elevating his right eye. His fontanel was soft. Multiple scalp - incisions which were well healed were noted. A suture was in place over the occipital incision. A right frontal ventricular shunt was palpable without the fluid tracking. The patient otherwise was at baseline neurologically. His HEENT examination was as above. Oropharynx and nasopharynx were normal. A nasogastric tube was in place. Neck examination showed indwelling internal jugular catheter. Neck was supple otherwise. Chest appeared clear to auscultation. The cardiovascular examination showed a regular rate and rhythm. Abdomen was benign. Extremities showed no edema or cyanosis. Pulses were intact. A computerized tomogram scan upon admission revealed marked anterior interval change and size. There was evidence of small amount of residual intraventricular air. Lateral ventricular size was without change. Shunt series showed no evidence of disconnection.

HOSPITAL COURSE: Upon admission, it was clear that the patient's fourth ventricle pad had become loculated and trapped once again despite recent fenestration. Because of his symptomatic status, he was taken to the operating room for placement of a fourth ventriculoperitoneal shunt. The procedure was uneventful and the patient tolerated it well. Please refer to his records for details. Postoperatively, he did well. On the first postoperative day, a computerized tomogram scan and shunt series were satisfactory.

Despite this the patient was noted to continue to have intermittent nausea and vomiting. A pediatric evaluation was requested. It was thought maybe the patient had an underlying gastroenteritis. He was treated with active medical management with a minimal response. Subsequently, his scan was repeated on the second postoperative day. This revealed enlargement of the fourth ventricle. As a result, the decision was made to reinvestigate the etiology for this. Intraoperatively, it was found that his fourth ventricular catheter was nonfunctional and plugged with intraventricular tissue residue. Because of this, a decision was made to place an external ventricular drain in the patient until his cerebrospinal fluid cleared. Subsequently, he underwent a procedure for removal of shunt and replacement with the external ventricular drain. He did well from this procedure. Postoperatively, he was managed conservatively. He continued to have no difficulty with his nausea and vomiting after this procedure. Subsequently after two days of monitoring, he was taken back to the operating room for removal of this external ventricular drain with placement of the shunt. The procedure went well and the patient tolerated it well. A postoperative scan on the first day showed decompression of the fourth ventricle and apparent functioning shunt. Because the patient had returned to his baseline status regarding activities and diet, the decision was made to discharge him to home to be followed on an outpatient basis.

DISPOSITION: The patient's condition at discharge showed that the patient was afebrile and his vital signs were stable. He was tolerating his diet well. His activities were back to baseline. Neurologically, he remained unchanged with a slight improvement in his disconjugate gaze. He persisted to have a third nerve palsy with anisocoria. The surgical wound at the time of discharge was healing well. The stitches were intact. The parents received detailed instructions regarding wound care. The stitches were due to come on the tenth postoperative day. Discharge medications were that on admission except for an increase in the Phenobarbital level to 37.5 mg b.i.d. because of the patient's subtherapeutic levels and one episode of seizure while under our care. Follow-up care was scheduled with Dr. Parmosa in the clinic in approximately three weeks. The parents were instructed to call in the interim if there are any problems regarding the patient's condition.

DISCHARGE DIAGNOSES:
1. Fourth ventricular shunt malfunction.
2. Hydrocephalus with ventricular loculation.

PROCEDURES PERFORMED:
1. Placement of fourth ventricular shunt on
2. Removal of fourth ventricular shunt and placement of external ventricular drain.
3. Removal of external ventricular drain and replacement/revision of fourth ventricular shunt.

continued

HISTORY AND PHYSICAL

HISTORY OF PRESENT ILLNESS: This 7-month-old boy, is well known to the neurosurgery service with a history of hydro-cephalus secondary to intraventricular remunerate and prematurity, has undergone multiple shunt revisions since birth who most recently was discharged on 8/13/xx after undergoing a laser fenestration of the fourth ventricle to communicate it with the remainder of the ventricular system. He was left with one right frontal ventroperitoneal shunt. Over the preceding several hours the parents noted the patient has become increasingly lethargic, has not tolerated feeds and vomited after eating this morning. In addition, they noted dysconjugate gaze and incoordination. They deny any fevers, diarrhea, rashes or cough.

PAST MEDICAL HISTORY: No known drug allergies.

CURRENT MEDICATIONS: Phenobarbital 3.5cc's q 12 hours.

REVIEW OF SYSTEMS: Remarkable for nasal congestion.

PHYSICAL EXAM: Tm 36.8, pulse 140, resp 24, bp 125/81, wght 5kg's. The child appears irritable but is consolable, somewhat hypotonic.

NEUROLOGIC EXAM: Patient demonstrates dysconjugate gaze with anisocoria. Left pupil is 6mm's, right pupil is 3mm's, both are briskly reactive. He seems to have some difficulty elevating his right eye. His fontanelle is soft. Multiple scalp incisions are noted with sutures in place and steristrips. A new right frontal ventricular shunt is palpable. He moves all extremities purposefully. Toes are upgoing bilaterally.

HEENT: Tympanic membranes are clear. Oro and nasopharynx are clear. Nasogastric tube is in place. Neck reveals a left IJ indwelling catheter in place. Chest clear to auscultation. COR regular rate and rhythm without murmur. Abdomen is soft, non-tender bowel sounds positive. Extremities without edema. Pulses are intact X4.

CT SCAN OF HEAD: Marked Interval increase in fourth ventricular size. When compared with scan of right frontal ventricular shunt is in place. There is evidence of a small amount of residual intraventricular air. The lateral ventricular size and third ventricular size do not appear different from that of the first.

SHUNT SERIES: Shows no evidence of obvious catheter breakage or disconnection.

IMPRESSION: 7MO WITH COMPLICATED HISTORY OF HYDROCEPHALUS AND NON-COMMUNICATING VENTRICLES SECONDARY TO INTRAVENTRICULAR HEMORRHAGE STATUS POST MULTIPLE SHUNT REVISIONS AND ATTEMPTED LATERAL TO FOURTH VENTRICULAR LASER FENESTRATION PRESENTS WITH OBVIOUS FAILURE OF FOURTH VENTRICULAR FENESTRATION AND FOURTH VENTRICULAR HYDROCEPHALUS.

PLAN: Will admit this child for placement of fourth-ventricular shunt with prospect of repeat fourth ventricular fenestration in the near future. At this point shunt placement will be taken on an emergency basis and will be arranged for later today.

Case 8-19, *continued*

PROGRESS NOTES

DATE / TIME	NOTES
8/20/xx 0900	Neurosurgery note:
	Full dictated H&P to follow
	Briefly:
	7 mo knows to NSR with H @ 2° to IVH. Has noncommunicating ventricular system and NMS D/C home 1 wk ago following fenestration of 4th vent to communicate s- 3rd & lat. Ventr. Pt p/w v & lethargy, as well as dysconjugate gaze since early a.m. PMHX- NDSA meds ∅ barb
	Exam: mult scalp incisions c̄ sutures & SS in place. R frontal VPS pupils R 3mm L 5mm & R dysconjugate, fontanelle S.H. MAE consolable toes (↑ ↑).
	CT head: markedly enlarged 4th vent. R frontal VPS c̄ intra vent air
	A/P – failure of 4th ventricular fenestration & 4th ventricular hydrocephalus. Admit for revision & placement of 4th vent. shunt.

BRIEF OPERATIVE REPORT

8/20/xx 1300

Diagnosis: Hydrocephalus.

Procedure: Left suboccipital incision for creation of shunt: ventriculo-peritoneal

Indication: 4th ventricular enlargement

Anesthesia: GETA:

Pathology: None

Drains: None

Implants: PS Medical shunt with low-low pressure / flow valve, and 4 cm proximal catheter.

Notes: Patient tolerated procedure well. All counts correct. Transferred to PACU in stable condition. Dictation completed.

Fluids: In		Out		Balance
Crystaloid	100cc	EBL	25cc	75cc
	100cc		25cc	

continued

Case 8-19, *continued*

PROGRESS NOTES

DATE/TIME	NOTES
08/21/xx 0900	Neurosurgery POD #1
	Pt stable overnight. Had sz post op resolved spont LOC 0 B. labored. Looked & increased maintenance.
	O: Temp 37 5 VSS I/O IBO/370cc
	Neur: sleeping, easily aroused, baseline neurologically
	Head – font soft and CAD
	Lungs – CTA
	CV – RRR
	Abd – Wound CTD
	Head CT – a 4th Vent. Shunt cath with good placement
	I/P Doing well
	1 – spont seizure post op
	2 – check phen Barb level & adjust
	3 – decrease soon if cont to do well

Case 8-19, *continued*

DATE OF REQUEST 8/20/xx	TIME: 1100	REQUESTING PHYSICIAN: Dr. Neuralt	CONSULTING PHYSICIAN: Dr. Renaldi

REQUEST CONSULTATION:

OPINION ONLY ☑   CONCURRENT CARE ☐   REFERRAL FOR ASSUMPTION OF CARE ☐

REASON FOR CONSULTATION: *Continual vomiting*

FINDING AND RECOMMENDATIONS: DATE OF CONSULTATION: 8/20/xx

Consulation: continual vomiting

Dx/ vomiting

HPI: 7 m/o male c̄ hx of hydrocephalus 2° IVH c̄ ventricular shunt revision who presented Tuesday with 4th ventricular hydrocephalus p- o/c – R/R s/p 4th ventricular fenestration. Presented c̄ lethargy, decreased PO & Vomiting x 1. Also noted dysconjugate gaze. 4th ventricular shungt (VR) placed on Tuesday. Continued to have emesis post operatively. Increased with feedings but during feedings or immedialely afterwards vomiting. No bile or blood no diarrhea. Family stating frequency has decreased. Mother does not think shunt functioning. Baseline – child attentive and playful. No family members are ill. No complications but small amt congestion. Afebrile

Meds: phenobarbital IVF ds ½ NS c̄ 20 MG KCL /2 at Nel1

Orders: same Ass: CT scan – decrease 4th ven mal size

PE: Gen, alter resting in mother's lap, 0 crying, limited movement

HEENT: alert and playing, NC, vitals: T-36.9, HR-144, RR-50, BP 144/50, wt- 5 kg

Multiple suture wounds. Mother states pt vomiting.

Neuro: supple, chest/ lungs clear, no M, RR, 0 retraction.

abd/ tb x 2, gast, slightly distended. Gen: NL 0 toes (↓)

Exam p- 16, units

Imp/Plan: a-ā r/o gastroenteritis/enteritis at initial inspec & evaluation. Vent shunt malf 4th with shunt complications & an odd finding consistent c̄ obstruction. so switch IVF to 20 mg/kcl IVT to 20 mg/kcl, NPO, breastfeeding am c̄ pedialyte (supplement c̄ 15 cc)

PROGRESS NOTES

continued

OPERATION REPORT

SURGEON: Dr. Neuralt

ASSISTANT: Dr. Yettie

Date: 8/20/xx

PREOPERATIVE DIAGNOSIS:	Fourth ventricular hydrocephalus.
POSTOPERATIVE DIAGNOSIS:	Fourth ventricular hydrocephalus.
OPERATION PERFORMED:	Placement of fourth ventricular ventriculoperitoneal shunt
Estimated blood loss:	Minimal.
Fluids:	100 cc Crystalloid.
Specimens:	3 cc of cerebral spinal fluid for standard studies.
Drains:	None.
Complications:	None.

INDICATIONS: The patient is a 7-month-old male with a complicated history of hydrocephalus secondary to intraventricular hemorrhage and prematurity. He has had multiple shunts in the past and has had numerous revision. Most recently, he was discharged from the hospital on 8/13/xx after laser fenestration of the septum into the fourth ventricle. He was left with one frontal ventriculoperitoneal shunt.

Over the day preceding arrival at the hospital, the patient demonstrated increasing lethargy with vomiting, back arching, and dysconjugate gaze which are symptoms that have heralded shunt malfunctions in the past. A CT scan was obtained through the emergency room which showed evidence of a markedly dilated fourth ventricle indicating that the fenestration between this ventricle and the lateral ventricular system had closed. For this reason, plans to place a ventricular shunt in the fourth ventricle were undertaken and discussed with parents.

PROCEDURE: After preoperative informed consent was obtained from the patient's father, he was brought to the operating room and placed under general endotracheal anesthesia. A preoperative dose of 250 mg nafcillin was administered IV. The patient was positioned in the left lateral decubitus position for placement of a right suboccipital bur hole.

Perspective incisions were marked in the paramedian region in the right subocciput and in addition, in the right abdominal region lateral to an existing scar approximately 2 cm from the midline at the level of the umbilicus. These areas were prepped in standard fashion and infiltrated with 0.5% lidocaine and 1:200,000 epinephrine.

OPERATIVE REPORT

SURGEON: Dr. Neuralt

ASSISTANT: Dr. Yettie

DATE: 8/22/xx

PREOPERATIVE DIAGNOSIS:	Fourth ventricular shunt malfunction.
POSTOPERATIVE DIAGNOSIS:	Fourth ventricular shunt malfunction.
OPERATION PERFORMED:	1. Removal of complete shunt system without replacement.
	2. Insertion of fourth ventricular external drainage system.

PROCEDURE: Under suitable general endotracheal anesthesia and with the patient in the prone position, a sterile prep and drape of the posterior portion of his head was accomplished. An incision overlying the shunt was opened and the shunt system was easily identified. After disconnecting the shunt system at the level of the ventricular reservoir, there was found to be no flow. A new shunt catheter was passed but there was still no flow.

A-Becker drain was passed and there was evidence of multiloculated small cystic areas but the fourth ventricles appeared to be filled with clot and debris from previous surgeries. A different Becker was then passed into a larger cystic area and left as an external ventricular drain. The entire shunt system was removed and not replaced.

The wound was then irrigated with saline containing bacitracin and then closure was accomplished with 4-0 Vicryl in the muscle and fascial layers as well as the subcutaneous layer and 4-0 nylon was used for the skin.

The patient tolerated the procedure well and left operating room in satisfactory condition.

continued

Case 8-19, *continued*

OPERATIVE REPORT

SURGEON: Dr. Neuralt

ASSISTANT: Dr. Yettie

DATE: 8/25/xx

PREOPERATIVE DIAGNOSIS: Shunt malfunction.

POSTOPERATIVE DIAGNOSIS: Shunt malfunction.

OPERATION PERFORMED: Removal of external ventricular drain and placement of fourth ventriculoperitoneal shunt.

Anesthesia: General.
Estimated blood loss: 5 cc.
Drains: None.
Complications: None.

INDICATIONS: The patient is a 7-month-old male infant who came in with a shunt malfunction. His shunt was changed several days ago, and this did not work right, and an external ventricular drain was placed. This drained well. We did inject Iohexol and everything was communicating in the fourth ventricular region.

We, therefore, bring him to the operating room now, to remove his drain and place a shunt.

PROCEDURE: After satisfactory induction of general endotracheal anesthesia, the patient was placed in the supine position with the head turned to the left. The hair was shaved. The skin was prepped with Betadine, and the child was draped in the usual sterile fashion.

The previous suboccipital incision, where the drain entered, was opened with sharp dissection, and a retractor was placed. A second stab wound was made in the abdomen. A shunt passer was used to connect the suboccipital wound with the stab wound in the abdomen, and a low-pressure valve and distal catheter were passed through the shunt-passer sheath.

The ventricular drain was cut and removed, and a ventricular catheter, 8 cm in length, was passed into the fourth ventricle, with good return of CSF. This was collected for routine studies.

The valve was pulled into place, and the reservoir cap was attached to the ventricular catheter. There was good flow of CSF from the distal end; 2 mg of intrathecal vancomycin were injected into the reservoir. A trocar was used to enter the peritoneal cavity, and the distal catheter was passed easily into the peritoneal cavity.

OPERATION REPORT

The wounds were irrigated. The subcutaneous tissue at both sites was closed with 4-0 Vicryl in a simple, interrupted fashion. The skin on the head was closed with 4-0 nylon in a running, interlocking fashion, and the skin on the belly was approximated with Mastisol and Steri-Strips.

The child was undraped. The exit site of the drain was prepped, and the drain was removed. The exit site was closed with 4–0 nylon.

The child tolerated this procedure well, and was taken to the recovery room in stable condition.

RADIOLOGY REPORT

SHUNT SERIES
= SHUNT INSERTION

Admit Diagnosis: RULE OUT SHUNT MALFUNCTION

EXAM

AP and lateral views of the skull-neck and AP filming of the chest-abdomen were done separately, but are reported in combination to facilitate clinical review.

The skull films show multiple bur holes in the right parietal area as well as craniotomy changes in the posterior fossa. A posterior fossa catheter extends on up through the tentorial incisura into the region of the third ventricle and a right ventriculoperitoneal shunt is in place. The shunts appear intact and extend into the peritoneal cavity. An NG tube is in the stomach. A central catheter terminates in the innominate vein and changes related to a prior left thoracotomy, probably for PDA ligation, are evident. Comparison with a prior exam shows that the posterior fossa shunt has been revised since that time.

IMPRESSION: SHUNT SERIES SHOWING INTACT VENTRICULOPERITONEAL SHUNT SYSTEMS AS DESCRIBED.

*** End of Finalized Text ***

Signing Physician: Marcus Hoyt, M.D.

Date: 8/25/xx

CT Brain w/o Cnt
F/U SHUNT REVISION

Admit Diagnosis: RULE OUT SHUNT MALFUNCTION

EXAM

Scout digital radiograph shows two shunts in place, one entering from the coronal suture area and the other from the posterior fossa. Axial scans were then performed from the base of the skull to the vertex. The posterior fossa catheter has decompressed the fourth ventricle representing a significant change compared with the prior study of yesterday. In the supratentorial region, there is continued moderate dilatation of the left lateral ventricle and moderate to marked dilatation of the right lateral ventricle. Dystrophic or possibly post infectious periventricular calcifications are evident bilaterally. The size of the lateral ventricles is stable when compared with yesterday's exam.

IMPRESSION: FOLLOW-UP NONENHANCED CRANIAL CT SCAN SHOWING INTERIM EVACUATION OF THE DILATED FOURTH VENTRICLE BY THE POSTERIOR FOSSA CATHETER. CONTINUED MODERATE DILATATION OF THE LATERAL VENTRICLES STABLE COMPARED WITH YESTERDAY'S STUDY. CONTINUED PERIVENTRICULAR PARENCHYMAL CALCIFICATIONS.

*** End of Finalized Text ***

Date: 8/24/xx

continued

Case 8-19, *continued*

SHUNT SERIES
Cerebral Shunt, Valve or

Admit Diagnosis: RULE OUT SHUNT MALFUNCTION

EXAM

AP and lateral views of the skull-neck and AP filming of the chest-abdomen were done separately, but are reported in combination to facilitate clinical review. Shunt series films on 8/24/xx have been returned for interpretation and are compared with the study of 8/25/xx. The ventricular shunt has its tip in the body of the right lateral ventricle. The abdominal end is in the left lateral abdomen. The shunt tubing is intact with no kinking or discontinuity seen. The NG tube and left innominate central line are in satisfactory position.

IMPRESSION: VENTRICULOPERITONEAL SHUNT AS NOTED WITH NO KINKING OR DISCONTINUITY SEEN.

** End of Finalized Text **

ICD-9-CM/ICD-10-CM diagnosis code(s): _____

ICD-9-CM procedure and ICD-10-PCS procedure code(s): _____

MS-DRG: _____

Case 8-20

Health Record Face Sheet

Western Regional
Medical Center

Record Number: 51-09-11

Age: 81

Gender: Male

Length of Stay: 6 Days

Service Type: Inpatient

Discharge Status: Transitional Care Unit

Diagnosis/Procedure: Urinary Retention
Benign Prostate Enlargement

Prostate Resection

Case 8-20, *continued*

DISCHARGE SUMMARY

DISCHARGE DIAGNOSES:

1.   URINARY RETENTION WITH ASSOCIATED OBSTRUCTIVE UROPATHY CLEARED WITH CATHETER DRAINAGE AND PROSTATE RESECTION.
    A.   BENIGN PROSTATE ENLARGEMENT.
    B.   ASSOCIATED HISTORY OF URINARY INFECTION.
2   BOLUS PENPHIGOID WITH ASSOCIATED ERYTHRODERMA AND CELLULITIS.
3.   HISTORY OF DECREASED ONCOTIC PRESSURE WITH DECREASED ALBUMIN AND GENERALIZED EDEMA.
4.   HISTORY OF ATRIAL FIBRILLATION.
5.   HISTORY OF BLINDNESS.
6.   HISTORY OF HYPOTHYROIDISM.
7.   HISTORY OF HYPERTENSION.
8.   HISTORY OF DEGENERATIVE JOINT DISEASE.

PROCEDURE PERFORMED: Prostate resection with cystoscopy.

HOSPITAL COURSE: The patient is an 81-year-old gentleman who has had a history of blindness and was admitted to the hospital with generalized rash. He was also found to have edema and low oncotic pressure. He was on steroids. He did have a biopsy that revealed that he had bolus penphigoid. In addition, in the early part of his hospitalization, he had an elevated creatinine and BUN. Those reports I am not able to review, but as I recall the creatinine was around 5 or 6. In the process of x-rays studies being complete, it was noted that he had marked enlargement of his bladder, with what appeared to be obstruction of the bladder outlets. A catheter was placed. He had a marked diuresis and improvement in his renal function.

The patient eventually did undergo a prostate resection. Benign prostate tissue was noted. There was some question regarding where the patient would be cared for. Initially, he was applying for a bed in the East Valley Nursing home, however, that did not work out and he was discharged on Monday the 16th of February to the Birch Street Senior Living Center. He will be followed there by his physician. During this hospitalization, he was cared for primarily by Dr. Walcott.

At the time of discharge, his steroids were being tapered. He also for a time was in the Transitional Care Unit aid then was transferred back down to the third floor. This was for his recovery following his prostate resection.

continued

OPERATIVE REPORT

PREOPERATIVE DIAGNOSIS: URINARY RETENTION, PROSTATE ENLARGEMENT.

POSTOPERATIVE DIAGNOSIS: URINARY RETENTION, PROSTATE ENLARGEMENT.

OPERATION PERFORMED: CYSTOSCOPY, TRANSURETHRAL RESECTION OF THE PROSTATE.

SURGEON: DR. RANDOLPH

DESCRIPTION OF THE PROCEDURE: The patient was given a spinal anesthetic and was placed carefully in the lithotomy position. He had also been premedicated with Solu-Cortef. He has been on Prednisone for some time and also was given a gram of Ancef. He was carefully placed in the lithotomy position. The external genitalia were prepared and then draped. The O'Connor drape was also in place. A #21 panendoscope was inserted. The urethra was normal. The prostate appeared enlarged and was obstructive. He had 3+ trabeculation of the bladder. There was also moderate edema of the bladder. The orifices appeared normal. I did not see any bladder tumors.

The urethra was dilated to 32 French. A #28 resectoscope sheath was inserted over a Timberlake obturator. A prostate resection was completed. The O'Connor drape was in place and was used in helping define posterior limits of the resection. The resection was carried out in a 360-degree area working from the bladder outlet through the distal prostatic urethra. The orifices were not resected. Also, the verumontanum was preserved. The resection appeared complete. Around 25 grams of tissue was resected. All bleeding points were cauterized. Chips were irrigated from the bladder. A #24 three-way catheter was inserted. 60 cc of fluid were placed in the balloon. The return through the catheter was relatively clear. About 400 cc of blood loss was estimated. No transfusion was required. He was transferred to the recovery area in stable condition.

Abnormality of his skin was noted and a biopsy was taken of the lesions and sent to Pathology in specimen dish.

He was transferred to the recovery area in stable condition.

Case 8-20, *continued*

TISSUE REPORT

HISTORY: R/O BULLOUS PEMPHIGOID

Gross: Labeled with the patient's name and designated right arm, received in formalin are three 0.6 cm circular tan skin punches excised to depths ranging from 0.2 to 0.4 cm. The specimens are inked, yellow, blue, and black, bisected and entirely submitted in a single cassette.

MICROSCOPIC: H&E sections show a very dense perivascular infiltrate composed predominantly of lymphocytes, plasma cells, and numerous eosinophils. There is a large subepidermal blister. There is no necrosis of the overlying epidermis. In areas, the blister space contains eosinophils.

DIAGNOSIS: SKIN, RIGHT ARM, BIOPSIES

CONSISTENT WITH BULLOUS PEMPHIGOID

TISSUE REPORT

HISTORY: BPH, URINARY RETENTION

Gross: Labeled with the patient's name and prostate tissue received in formalin is a 30-gram 5 × 5 × 4.5 cm aggregate of rubbery tan-pink focally cauterized soft tissue fragments. Representative sections are submitted in cassettes A-F.

MICROSCOPIC: DONE

DIAGNOSIS: PROSTATE TISSUE, TURP
- GLANDULAR AND STROMAL HYPERPLASIA
- FOCAL ACUTE AND CHRONIC PROSTATITIS
- SEMINAL VESICLE
- BASAL CELL HYPERPLASIA
- NO EVIDENCE OF MALIGNANCY

continued

Case 8-20, *continued*

RADIOLOGY REPORT

EXAMS:

CT PELVIS W/CONTRAST,
CT CHEST COMP W/CONT,
CT ABDOMEN W&W/O CONTRAST

ABDOMEN/PELVIS:
PROCEDURE:

Standard axial CT images were obtained through the abdomen and pelvis following intravenous and oral contrast media administration using spiral technique with 7 mm collimation and 1.4:1 pitch. No comparison scans.

FINDINGS:

The liver, gallbladder, spleen, pancreas, and adrenals all show normal morphology and parenchymal attenuation/enhancement. No intra or extrahepatic biliary ductal dilatation is identified.

The kidneys contain several small low-density lesions (mostly at the upper pole of the left kidney and lateral mid portion of the right kidney), all of which measure less than 10 mm in diameter and most likely represent cysts. No hydronephrosis or hydroureter is identified. The urinary bladder contains a prominent filling defect, at its base where there is a contour abnormality as a result of an enlarged irregular prostate.

There is an apparent low anterior abdominal wall defect with herniated small bowel loops anterior to the urinary bladder. (Please see Images 82 and 83.) A portion of the hepatic flexure of the colon is interposed between the anterior abdominal wall and the liver, but there is no evidence for obstruction. No other abnormalities of bowel are identified.

There is no intra- or extraperitoneal lymphadenopathy or free fluid identified. No inguinal or pelvic lymphadenopathy is identified.

There are moderate degenerative changes throughout the lumbar spine, most advanced at the lumbosacral junction. Dense intimal calcification involves the arterial vasculature of the abdomen and pelvis.

Case 8-20, *continued*

ICD-9-CM/ICD-10-CM diagnosis code(s): _____

ICD-9-CM procedure and ICD-10-PCS procedure code(s): _____

MS-DRG: _____

Case 8-21

Health Record Face Sheet

Western Regional
Medical Center

Record Number:	64-21-09
Age:	47
Gender:	Female
Length of Stay:	2 Days
Service Type:	Inpatient
Discharge Status:	To Home
Diagnosis/Procedure:	Right Knee Loose Body
	Right Knee Arthroscopy Chondroplasty

continued

HISTORY AND PHYSICAL

PATIENT: Sylvia Swenilli

RECORD NUMBER: 64-21-09

ROOM: 512

ADMIT DATE: 12/15/xx

PHYSICIAN: Dr. Redi

PROBLEM:
> She twisted her knee in September. Despite conservative treatment she continues to have significant knee pain.

HISTORY OF PRESENT ILLNESS:
> She has had a MRI that showed a moderate knee joint effusion. The ligaments appeared to be intact as did the menisci. Because of her continued symptoms she has elected to have knee arthroscopy. We suspect there may be a loose body in the knee accounting for the effusion. The risks, benefits, and alternatives have been explained to her.

PAST MEDICAL HISTORY:
CURRENT MEDS:	Flexeril and Vicodin.
ALLERGIES:	**PENICILLIN.**
SURGERIES:	Bladder surgery. Hysterectomy. Left foot and left hand surgery.
MEDICAL ILLNESS:	No diabetes or heart disease.

PSYCHOSOCIAL HISTORY:
> Ten pack year smoking history. Occasional alcohol. Single.

FAMILY HISTORY:
> Her mother had diabetes and her mother, father, and brother had early heart attacks.

REVIEW OF SYSTEMS:

PHYSICAL EXAM:
GENERAL:	She is alert and oriented x 3.
HEENT:	Appears to be normal.
NECK:	Benign.
CHEST:	She is breathing easily without wheezes.
HEART:	Regular rate.
ABDOMEN:	Benign.
EXTREM:	Right Knee: Medial joint line tenderness, moderate effusion, no ligamentous laxity. Skin is in good condition.
GU:	Benign.
NEURO:	Benign.

ASSESSMENT: Right knee pain.

PLAN: 1. Right knee arthroscopy, looking for the source of her continued knee effusions and pain.
2. The knee pain correlated to the twisting injury and we do not suspect an inflammatory arthropathy.

Case 8-21, *continued*

OPERATIVE REPORT

PATIENT: Sylvia Swenilli

RECORD NUMBER: 64-21-09

ROOM: 512

ADMIT DATE: 12/15/xx

SURGERY DATE: 12/15/xx

SURGEON: Dr. Redi

ASSIST: Dr. Mayer

NOTE: An assistant was very valuable in allowing proper exposure to the knee compartments during the arthroscopic procedure.

PREOPERATIVE DIAGNOSIS:	Right knee loose body.
POSTOPERATIVE DIAGNOSIS:	Right knee loose body and chondromalacia of the medial femoral condyle.
OPERATIVE PROCEDURE:	Right knee arthroscopy, loose body removal, and limited chondroplasty medial femoral condyle.
ANESTHESIA:	General.
ESTIMATED BLOOD LOSS:	Less than 5 cc.
TOURNIQUET TIME:	21 minutes.

ARTHROSCOPIC PHOTOS:

The first page shows the posterior horn of the medial meniscus with the probe, Grade II and III chondromalacia of the medial femoral condyle, the 4.0 shaver before chondroplasty, medial femoral condyle after chondroplasty, ACL, PCL, and lateral meniscus with the probe. The next page showed normal lateral femoral condyle, loose body in the intercondylar notch region, the undersurface of the patella, the shaver freeing up the loose body for removal, the patellofemoral articulation, and the popliteal hiatus. The last page shows posteromedial aspect of the knee free of loose bodies.

DESCRIPTION OF OPERATIVE PROCEDURE:

After anesthesia, the patient's right knee was prepped and draped in the usual sterile fashion. The lower extremities were placed in well-padded holders. 5 cc. of fluid was withdrawn from the right knee and sent for analysis to the lab. Following this, the right lower extremity was exsanguinated with an Esmarch and the tourniquet inflated to 300 mm. of mercury. Standard anterior, lateral, and medial portals were made using needle guidance for the medial. Blunt obturators were used to enter the joint. The knee was explored in a systematic fashion with the above findings. The medial and lateral menisci were completely intact without any unstable tears. There was significant chondromalacia of the medial femoral condyle involving essentially its entire surface. Loose-cartilage edges were debrided with a 4.0 shaver. There was mild chondromalacia of the tibial plateau medially. The ACL and PCL were normal. The lateral compartment was normal. The trochlea had mild to moderate chondromalacia in its interior aspect. The undersurface of the patella had very mild chondromalacia. The patellar tracking was normal. There was what appeared to be a loose body that had attached at the inferior pole of the patellar region. This was delineated and then loosed from the surrounding soft tissue with the 4.0 shaver and then removed with the arthroscopic grasper. This possibly was contributing the chondromalacia in the trochlear region. The trochlea had mostly Grade I chondromalacia and the patellar undersurface was essentially normal for age. The popliteal hiatus did not have any loose bodies. All debris was removed from the knee. The knee was flexed to 90 degrees. The blunt obturator was used to gently enter the posteromedial aspect of the knee and this region appeared to be normal. Fluid was suctioned out in this region and no loose bodies were visible. The blunt obturator with scope cannula was then placed up into the suprapatellar pouch and the knee irrigated and suctioned to remove any remaining debris. The tourniquet was deflated. Hemostasis appeared to be good. 30 cc. of 1/2% Marcaine with epinephrine was injected about the portal sites and into the knee joint. The portals were closed with subcutaneous 4-0 Vicryl suture and a Xeroform gauze dressing and Ace from foot to thigh were placed.

continued

Case 8-21, *continued*

PATIENT PROGRESS NOTES

From beginning of stay: 12/15/xx   **TO: 12/16/xx**   **Page 1 of 2**

PHYSICAL ASSESSMENT

INTRAOPERATIVE RECORD 1
    OR-Patient Identification: Verbal, Chart, Armband.
    Allergies Yes: _PENICILLIN_____
    OR-Verification: NPO Status, H&P, Procedure location, Consent form.
    OR-Mental Status: Alert, Oriented.
    OR-Limitations: Visual.
    OR-Personal Items:
      Glasses, Personal items left in room. Denture Uppers, Denture Lowers, NOT REMOVED.
    Body Piercings: None.
    Nsg DX: Potential For Anxiety R/T Concerns About Surgery &
      Goal/Outcome. Patient exhibits: Minimal to moderate signs of anxiety.
    OR-Comfort Measures Implemented:
      Orient to environment. Limit unnecessary exposure. Reduce environmental expo-
      sure, Give emotional support and reassurance. Give clear concise explanations, warm
      blanket.
    Evaluation: Patient Demonstrated: Minimal Anxiety.
    Knowledge Deficit R/T Upcoming Procedure
      Goal/Outcome: Patient/Parent verbalizes: Understanding of education.
    OR-Pre-Op Education:
      Pain Control, Environment, Equipment, Operating times, Pain Scale 0-10 explained,
      Patient verbalizes understanding of educ.
    Evaluation: Patient/Parent Demonstrated:
      Good Understanding of Education.
    Pre-Op Assessment Complete?   Yes.
    OR-Operating Room: Room 1.
    OR-Time In/Surgery start:
      Patient in
      adm. Consent reviewed by _RC_____RN, Scheduled.
    OR-Anesthesia: General, RN Available during Induction.
    OR-Pre-OP Diagnosis: RT KNEE INTERNAL DERANGEMENT.
    OR-Procedure: Knee Arthroscopy _RT_____.
    OR-Surgeon:
    OR-First Assistant:
    OR-Staff:
      1st Scrub:_
      Other:_
    OR-Anesthesiologist/CRNA:
    OR-Skin Appearance {Plan/Implementation}: Warm, Dry, Pink.
    Nsg Dx:Pot. for Inj. R/T Sensory/Motor deficits 2nd to Sedation/
      Goal/Outcome: Pt will remain injury free.
    OR-Patient Positon{Plan/Implementation}:
      Supine, Arms extended on armboard < 90%, Safety strap on.
    OR-Positioning Aids {Plan/Implementation}: pillow under-head.
      LT LEG IN LOW STIRRUP, RT LEG IN BLUE LEG HOLDER, PT POSITIONED BY DR.
    OR-Patient Warming Devices {Plan/Implementation}:
      Warm Solution, Warm Blankets.

PATIENT PROGRESS NOTES

From beginning of stay: 12/15/xx   TO: 12/16/xx   **Page 2 of 2**

PHYSICAL ASSESSMENT

OR-Electrosurgery (Plan/Implementation}:
  Grounding Pad, Site _LT_THIGH_____, Skin intact: Yes, CAUTERY NOT USED.
OR-Pneumatic Stockings {Plan/Implementation} :   **N/A.**
INTRAOPERATIVE RECORD 2
  OR-X-Ray {Plan/Implementation}:   N/A.
  OR-Additional Equipment{Plan/Implementation}:
  Video Cart, Dyonics Shaver.
  OR-Tourniqiuet Unit/Other {Plan/Implementation}:
  Applied   _____, LOCATION _RT_THIGH_____
  OR-Sharp & Sponge Count {Plan/Implementation}   N/A.
  Evaluation: Patient tolerated procedure with no apparent injury R/T:
  patient positioning, positioning aids, tourniquet, equipment used. Goal met.
  Nsg Dx: Potential for infection   Pt will be protected from pot infection.
  OR-Urinary catheter {Plan/Implementation}:   NA.
  OR-Skin Prep {Plan/Implementation}:   Prevail, Betadine scrub.
  OR-Medications {Plan/Implementation} :
  0.5% Marcaine C EPI 1:200,000 _30_cc.
  OR-Operative Implants {Plan/Implementation}:   None.
  OR-Specimens {Plan/Implementation}:   SYNOVIAL FLUID OF RT KNEE, TO LAB.
  OR-Wound {Plan/Implementation}:   Class 1.
  OR-Dressing {Plan/Implementation}:   Xeroform, 4X4, Gauze roll, Ace wrap.
  OR-Dressing cont. {Plan/Implementation}:   N/A.
  OR-Irrigation {Plan/Implementation} :   Saline.
  OR-Drains {Plan/Implementation} :   N/A.
  OR-Packing {Plan/Implementation}:   N/A.
  Evaluation: Standards of Asepsis Utilized Regarding:
  Skin prep, Wound class, Irrigation, Dressings, Lab specimens, Yes.
  OR-Nurses Notes:
  THE WORD "NO" WAS NOTED ON PT'S LT KNEE. PT'S INTRA-OP TEMP 97. PT
  TRANSFERRED TO PACU IN STABLE CONDITION.
  OR-Transferred To:
  PACU, Post op Dx_RT_KNEE_INTERNAL_DERANGEMENT. Surgery end time:_0830_.
  Leave OR time: _0840__.
  OR-Transferred Via:
  Stretcher, Side rails UP, Report given to.
  OR-I&O End of Case Totals {Outcome Evaluation} :
  Est.Blood Loss _<_5_CC_____.

continued

Case 8-21, *continued*

PHYSICIAN PROGRESS NOTES

Date		Date	
12/15/xx	Dx: R knee with internal derangement		
	Proc: R knee arthroscopy c̄ loose body		
	removal		
	TT: 21 min		
	EBL - < 5 CC		
	Comp: ∅		
	Plan: 1-F/U 10 days sooner if increased		
	pain or swelling.		
	2 —remove dressing in 3 days. Keep		
	wounds covered.		
12/16/xx	D/C home to follow up in office in		
	10 days.		
			Patient stamp

ICD-9-CM/ICD-10-CM diagnosis code(s): ____ _____

ICD-9-CM procedure and ICD-10-PCS procedure code(s): _____

MS-DRG: _____ _____

Case 8-22

Health Record Face Sheet

Western Regional
Medical Center

Record Number:	13-19-41
Age:	70
Gender:	Male
Length of Stay:	5 Days
Service Type:	Inpatient
Discharge Status:	To Home
Diagnosis/Procedure:	Urosepsis

DISCHARGE SUMMARY

ADMISSION DATE: 3/03/xx
DISCHARGE DATE: 3/07/xx

REASON FOR ADMISSION: Patient was admitted for evaluation of weakness, shaking chills, and urinary frequency.

HISTORY OF THE PRESENT ILLNESS: The patient has been in fairly good health except for history of TURP. There was no evidence of malignancy at that time and he's had no history or renal stones or significant urinary tract infections. The patient became increasingly weak at home with some mild disorientation and was admitted for evaluation due to his very progressive obviously severe symptoms.

Initial evaluation revealed an elderly man in obvious distress. Vital signs: Refer to chart.
HEENT: Unremarkable. Full extraocular movements. Neck supple. Chest clear. Cardiac exam, regular rhythm. Abdomen without tenderness or masses. Extremities unremarkable. Petechia noted. Initial urine showed obvious pyuria.

HOSPITAL COURSE: The patient was cultured and one dose of Gentamicin was given due to difficulty starting IV and Fortaz was started. Patient made initial clinical progress, however, did have some headache and left jaw pain that seemed to be localized to the left temporomandibular joint. His mental status rapidly returned to normal. Abdominal ultrasound was done which suggested a mass on the kidney. This was felt to be pyelo by a CT scan. Due to his daily progress and return to baseline, he was discharged to home on oral antibiotics with 3 weeks of therapy.

DISCHARGE PLANS: The patient is to continue home treatment, continue analgesics as needed for left TMJ pain. Also to continue Duricef 500mg bid for 2 more weeks with follow-up at the office at that time.

DISCHARGE DIAGNOSIS:
1. Urosepsis.
2. Headache secondary to temporomandibular joint dysfunction.
3. Mild disorientation secondary to infection resolved.

continued

Case 8-22, *continued*

HISTORY & PHYSICAL

REASON FOR ADMISSION: Patient was admitted for evaluation of weakness, shaking chills and urinary frequency.

HISTORY OF PRESENT ILLNESS: The patient had been noted on the phone to have an acute febrile illness. The illness persisted and advanced to where the patient was having very marked urinary frequency and weakness. The patient has no history of urinary tract infection, however has had TURP of the prostate.

PAST MEDICAL HISTORY: Consists of history of pneumonia, pulmonary embolus, hypothyroidism on replacement therapy. Patient was not on any medications other than Synthroid prior to admission.

FAMILY HISTORY: Non-contributory.
SOCIAL HISTORY: The patient's wife is apparently demented in a home. He lives alone. Doesn't drink or smoke.

REVIEW OF SYSTEMS: The patient denies any significant eye, ear, nose, or throat complaints except for mild headache. Pulmonary/cardiovascular: - Negative. GI Negative. No diarrhea, abdominal pain, weight loss, constipation. GU: See present illness. Neuropsych: No motor or sensory deficits.

INITIAL EVALUATION: Revealed an acutely ill man. Febrile. No acute distress
VITAL SIGNS: Refer to Chart.
HEENT: Unremarkable.
NECK: Supple. No lymphadenopathy, bruits, masses.
PHARYNX: Unremarkable.
CHEST: Clear.
CARDIAC EXAM: Regular rhythm, no murmurs.
ABDOMEN: Nontender without masses. No flank tenderness.
GU: Unremarkable.
EXTREMITIES: Unremarkable. 1+ pulses.
NEURO: Cranial nerves, motor and sensory evaluation normal.

INITIAL IMPRESSION:
1. Acute Urosepsis.
2. History of TURP
3. History of pneumonia.
4. History of pulmonary embolus after prolonged bed rest.

Case 8-22, *continued*

CONSULTATION:

DATE OF CONSULTATION:

Requesting Physician: Dr. Mickel
Consulting Physician: Dr. Urey

The patient is a 70-year-old gentleman admitted with an acute urinary tract infection characterized by high, fever and possible sepsis. He has had a transurethral resection of the prostate gland approximately 7 years ago, for benign disease. He was cystoscoped in the office approximately a year ago showing a mild bladder neck contracture but otherwise the prostatic fossa was open. He denies any real difficulty in voiding recently.

On admission his UA showed 50–100 red cells per high power field, 3+ bacteria, and greater than 100 white cells per high power field. Urinary culture grew out 100,000 colonies of E coli. Ultrasound of both kidneys shows some irregularity in the contour and configuration of the left kidney. For that reason in the recovery period CT scan was performed. This shows some cortical scarring in the mid portion of the left kidney, probably the result of old infection. There is nothing acute on the scan and no evidence of tumor. The patient has been treated appropriately with antibiotics. It is our recommendation he should be treated for another 10 days following discharge.

FINAL DIAGNOSIS:

Acute urinary tract infection.

Thank you for allowing us to help in his care.

continued

Case 8-22, *continued*

RADIOLOGY REPORT

EXAM: Bi-manual Ultrasound and Bladder US

HISTORY: Acute UTI with fever, dysuria and weakness.

RENAL AND BLADDER ULTRASOUND:

Multiple real-times were obtained of both kidneys. There is no evidence of hydronephrosis or perinephric fluid collections. Overall, the echo texture of the kidneys appeared within normal limits. There appeared to be a duplication of the left kidney, but when referring to prior IVP's there was no evidence of any duplication. Therefore, this raises the possibility of significant parenchymal scarring in the mid portion or perhaps a mass. The renal outlines are slightly irregular on the left, which would be consistent with prior infection, scarring or with mass. Multiple real-time-images of the bladder showed a moderate amount of fluid present. The patient was asked to go to the bathroom, but was unable to urinate, and stated he had no urge. Patient had urinated 30 to 45 minutes prior to coming down for the ultrasound.

IMPRESSION:
Irregular contour and configuration of the left kidney.
Further evaluation is recommended with CT following resolution of the current UTI.

Moderate post void residual.

EXAM:

HISTORY: Urinary infection. Irregular contour of the left kidney on recent ultrasound – further evaluation.

CT KIDNEY SCAN:

With intravenous contrast, 10 mm axial slices were obtained through the kidneys and compared to the ultrasound of

There is considerable atrophy and residual parenchymal irregularity of the lateral margin of the upper pole of the left kidney. There is minimal dilatation of the adjacent calyx. The parenchymal abnormality is sharply marginated by adjacent fat and terminates in a small notch inferolaterally in the mid-portion of the kidney. Findings are most compatible with atrophy and scarring from infection.

There is no evidence of heterogeneity of the parenchyma of the kidneys to suggest acute pyelonephritis - the changes seen are more compatible with chronic atrophy.

The collecting structures are otherwise normal. No evidence of hydronephrosis. No other abnormality is seen.

IMPRESSION:

Sharply marginated parenchymal loss at the lateral margin of the upper pole of the left kidney most compatible with chronic scarring from previous infection. No evidence of heterogeneity of functioning parenchyma to suggest focal bacterial nephritis, abscess or mass.

ICD-9-CM/ICD-10-CM diagnosis code(s): _____

ICD-9-CM procedure and ICD-10-PCS procedure code(s): _____

MS-DRG: _____

Instructions for Accessing the ICD 10 CM and ICD 10 PCS Official Guidelines for Coding and Reporting

General Question for this page—Do we need the step by step instructions versus supplying the web URL. The internal pages or step by step will probably change over time and I really do not see the need to provide the "click on" instructions.

I propose to simply list the Resource and the associated URL.

Center for Disease Control and Prevention ICD
http://www.cdc.gov/nchs/icd/icd10cm.htm

1. ICD 10 CM Official Guidelines for Coding and Reporting. URL: http://www.cdc.gov/nchs/data/icd/ICD10cmguidelines_2015%209_26_2014.pdf

2. ICD 10 PCS Official Guidelines for Coding and Reporting. URL: https://www.cms.gov/Medicare/Coding/ICD10/Downloads/PCS-2014-guidelines.pdf

3. ICD 10 CM Official Guidelines for Coding and Reporting in the Outpatient Services. URL http://www.cdc.gov/nchs/data/icd/icd10cm_guidelines_2014.pdf

– See Section IV

4. ICD 10 CM Official Guidelines for Coding and Reporting for Inpatient Services. URL: http://www.cdc.gov/nchs/data/icd/ICD10cmguidelines_2015%209_26_2014.pdf

– See Section II

Appendix B

Instructions for Accessing the *Uniform Hospital Discharge Data Set Guidelines*

To access the Uniform Hospital Discharge Data Set Guidelines:

1. Go to www.cdc.gov.
2. In the *Search* box at the top right side of the page, type in UHDDS.

3. Click on the link for *The National Committee on Vital and Health Statistics, 1992*.

4. Principal diagnosis, secondary diagnosis, and other coding guidelines are in *Appendix V*, pages 81–85.

Instructions for Accessing the *1995* and *1997 Documentation Guidelines for Evaluation and Management Services*

To access the 1995 and 1997 Documentation Guidelines for Evaluation and Management Services:

1. Go to http://cms.gov.
2. In the *Search* box at the top right of the page, type *1995 1997 guidelines*.

3. You will then see search results that include a link to the *Evaluation and Management Services Guide*. Click on the link to view the guidelines.
4. In the guide, you will find both *1995* and *1997 Documentation Guidelines for Evaluation and Management Services*.

Glossary

administrative documentation–information documented in the healthcare record regarding patient name, address, date of birth, age, next of kin, religion, physician, and insurance coverage information. Administrative information also describes why the patient is seeking services, consent for treatment, and use of private healthcare information.

Ambulatory Payment Classification (APC) system–the outpatient prospective payment system (OPPS) used by Medicare to reimburse hospitals for outpatient services and procedures

AAPC–formerly the American Academy of Professional Coders, the AAPC is the national organization that provides education and professional certification to medical coders in the specialized areas of physician's office, hospital outpatient, interventional radiology, and cardiology

American Health Information Management Association (AHIMA)–national organization that focuses on the management of personal health information required in healthcare settings; offers resources for education, accreditation, and a variety of certification options

ancillary services–outpatient services in the hospital such as lab, x-ray, and therapy services

case-mix index–the average relative weight of all cases treated at a given healthcare facility, which reflects the intensity of the resources utilized or clinical severity of a specific group of patients in relation to other groups of patients in a classification system associated with the CMS prospective payment system(s)

Centers for Medicare and Medicaid Services (CMS)–the division of the Department of Health and Human Services that is responsible for developing healthcare policy in the United States and for administering the Medicare program and the federal portion of the Medicaid program

charge description master (CDM) or chargemaster–a comprehensive list of eligible charges for an individual provider or healthcare facility

chief complaint (CC)–patient-provided subjective description of the events or reason why the patient sought medical treatment

chronic condition–a condition that persists for a long period of time

classification system–a system that takes identified nomenclatures and arranges related entries. In coding, the nomenclature assigns code numbers to diagnoses and procedures.

clinical documentation–information documented in the healthcare record that records the patient's current condition, course of treatment, and relevant current or past medical diagnoses or procedures along with anything "medical" such as laboratory, radiology, pathology, and cytology reports

clinical terminology–a set of standardized terminology used for a nomenclature

Commission on Accreditation for Health Informatics and Information Management Education (CAHIIM)–accrediting organization for educational programs in health informatics and information management

comorbidity–condition that existed at admission and is thought to increase the length of stay by at least 1 day for approximately 75% of patients

completeness–the degree to which a professional coder captures all of the diagnoses and procedures documented by the physician in the health record

compliance plan–provides the mechanism by which a facility or provider ensures that it is providing and billing for services according to the laws, regulations, and guidelines that govern billing and coding practices to prevent fraud and abuse

complication–secondary condition that arises during hospitalization and is thought to increase the length of stay by at least 1 day in approximately 75% of patients

critical access hospital (CAH)–a hospital that provides 24-hour emergency services in a rural area and that is located more than 35 miles from another hospital

decision support system–utilized for administrative and business activities in a healthcare organization or physician practice to produce information regarding the actual cost, charges, and reimbursement for hospital services provided to one or multiple patients with the same diagnosis(es) and procedure(s) performed

Department of Health and Human Services (DHHS)–cabinet-level federal agency that oversees all of the health and human services activities of the federal government and administers federal regulations

discharge summary–the physician's documentation of an inpatient hospital stay

emergency room (ER)–the emergency room in a hospital

facility EM–a hospital's evaluation and management (EM) level used to capture resources utilized by the facility under the APC reimbursement system

family medical history–subjective description of immediate family members' illnesses and/or diseases

fiscal intermediary (FI)–third-party payer that has the Medicare contract for a specific state and administers the state's Medicare program, including processing the state's Medicare claims

hard coding–coding that is not done by a coder, but is instead done by a facility's chargemaster system

Health Insurance Portability and Accountability Act of 1996 (HIPAA)–federal legislation enacted to provide continuity of health coverage, control fraud and abuse in healthcare, reduce healthcare costs, and guarantee the security and privacy of health information

health record–a document created to record a patient's health and the services received during healthcare visits

history and physical (H&P)–the physician's documentation of a patient's history of illness and physical examination upon admission

ICD-9-CM *Official Guidelines for Coding and Reporting*–official coding guidelines provided by CMS and NCHS that are to be followed when assigning ICD-9-CM codes until the October 1, 2014 implementation date of ICD-10-CM and ICD-10-PCS

inpatient–a patient who is formally admitted to a facility for treatment

medical necessity–formal process to ensure that an appropriate level of service is performed in an efficient and cost-effective manner in an appropriate setting based on the patient's physical needs and quality of life

Medicare Code Edits (MCE) software–software that finds and reports errors in the coding of claims data. The MCE editor will identify and indicate the nature of the error but will not correct the error

National Correct Coding Initiative (NCCI)–a series of code edits on Medicare Part B claims that identifies incorrect CPT-4® code combinations being reported; incorrect code combinations result in improper payment to a provider

nomenclature–a set of terms used in a particular discipline

objective documentation–the physician's assessment of the patient's current health status

observation (OBSV)–occurs when a patient is not formally admitted as an inpatient but whose condition warrants a hospital observation and stay to investigate further

operative report (OP)–the physician's documentation of a procedure that was performed

outpatient–a patient who is not formally admitted to a facility

past medical history–subjective description of a patient's childhood and adult illnesses and medical conditions

patient record–the health record for a patient in a hospital setting

postoperative–the period of time after surgery

present illness–patient-stated subjective information regarding the current illness

present on admission (POA)–indicator on inpatient claims. The POA indicates whether a diagnosis code was present or not present at the time an order for an inpatient admission occurred.

principal diagnosis–as defined by the Uniform Hospital Discharge Data Set, the condition established after study to be chiefly responsible for occasioning the admission of the patient to the hospital for care

principal procedure–procedure that was performed for the definitive treatment (rather than diagnosis) of the main condition or complication of the condition

progress note–a chronological record of the patient's condition during an episode of care and/or while receiving treatment from a provider

prospective payment system (PPS)–a reimbursement methodology that uses a predetermined payment rate based on the treatment for a specific illness; first utilized by Medicare but now used by many payers to reimburse for healthcare services

reliability–the degree to which the same codes are consistently assigned to the same health record by different coding professionals

resident record–the health record for a patient in a long-term care setting

resource-based relative value scale (RBRVS)–Medicare payment system that reimburses physicians treating Medicare patients. Work performed by the physician, practice expenses, overhead, equipment, supplies, and medical malpractice insurance are all taken into account. This system is utilized to ensure that fair and accurate reimbursement is provided to physicians in all services and specialties

review of systems–subjective description of symptoms or illnesses pertaining to individual body systems.

same-day surgery (SDS)–surgery in which a patient presents for an outpatient procedure and goes home on the same day

secondary diagnosis–as defined by the Uniform Hospital Discharge Data Set, all conditions that coexist at the time of admission, or develop subsequently, which affect the treatment received and/or the length of stay in the hospital/facility

social and personal history–subjective description of personal health habits and social status

standing orders–established orders that direct procedures to follow for a particular diagnosis or procedure

subjective information–information collected from the patient or other patient representative

timeliness–the amount of time it takes for the health record to be coded

Uniform Hospital Discharge Data Set (UHDDS)–developed by the U.S. Department of Health, Education and Welfare in 1974 to ensure that all hospitals report a minimum set of data for all patient admissions and use uniform definitions when reporting that data

utilization management–the process of ensuring medical necessity is met for patients receiving care in the appropriate healthcare setting

validity–the degree to which the codes assigned accurately reflect the physician documentation for diagnoses and procedures in an episode of care

World Health Organization (WHO)–the United Nations' coordinating authority on international public health

Index